2.00

The Essential Medication Guidebook to Healthy Aging

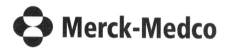 Merck-Medco

Merck-Medco Managed Care, L.L.C., a subsidiary of Merck & Co., Inc.

D1432469

BALLANTINE BOOKS   NEW YORK

A Ballantine Book
Published by The Ballantine Publishing Group

Copyright © 1998, 2001 by Merck-Medco Managed Care, L.L.C.
All rights reserved.

No part of this book may be reproduced or used in any form or by any means, electronic
or mechanical, including photography, or by any information storage and retrieval system,
without permission in writing from the publisher.

Merck-Medco Managed Care, L.L.C.
100 Parsons Pond Road
Franklin Lakes, NJ 07417

All rights reserved under International and Pan-American Copyright Conventions.
Published in the United States by The Ballantine Publishing Group, a division of Random
House, Inc., New York, and simultaneously in Canada by Random House of Canada
Limited, Toronto.

Ballantine is a registered trademark and the Ballantine colophon is a trademark of Random
House, Inc.

www.ballantinebooks.com

Library of Congress Cataloging-in-Publication Data: 2001119556

ISBN 0-345-45137-6

For more information about your health, safely using prescription drugs, and more, please visit us
online at www.merckmedco.com.

Manufactured in the United States of America

First Ballantine Books Edition: February 2002

10 9 8 7 6 5 4 3 2 1

Editors

Les Paul, MD, MS   Becky Nagle, PharmD, BCPS

Editorial Board

Richard M. Dupee, MD, FACP
Robert Epstein, MD, MS
Terry Fulmer, PhD, RN, FAAN
Mark Monane, MD, MS, FACP, AGSF
Mark Rubino, RPh
Todd Semla, PharmD

Contributors/Reviewers

Jean Barilla, MS
Keith Bradbury, RPh, MS
Kevin Cleary, PharmD, MBA
Amita Dasmahapatra, MD
Richard Feifer, MD
Daniel Ford, MD
George Fulop, MD
Leslie Gise, MD
Shelly Gray, PharmD
Paul Greenberg, MD
Marvin Konstam, MD
Alan Lotvin, MD

Randy A. McCoy, PharmD
Steve Montamat, MD
Heather-Ann Periconi, RPh
Walter Peterson, MD
Brent Pfeiffenberger
Michael Rich, MD
Myra Skluth, MD
Susan Squillace, MD
Jeffrey Susman, MD
Rhonda Wroble, PharmD
Sandra Yang, PharmD
Chun Wan Yin, PharmD

Editorial and Production Staff

Senior Staff Editor:	Gail Anne Chirico
Staff Editor:	Raquel Nael-Marrero, RN
Copy Editor:	Laurie Sammeth Campbell, MA
Marketing Communications:	Kim Brenner, Jill Scheer
Product Development:	Jeff Blankenship, Mark Davis

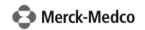 **Merck-Medco**

Editors

Les Paul, MD, MS
Vice President, Medical Policy
& Programs, Merck-Medco

Becky Nagle, PharmD, BCPS
Director, Clinical Practice & Education,
Merck-Medco

Editorial Board

Richard M. Dupee, MD, FACP
Chief, Geriatric Division, New England Medical Center, Boston, Massachusetts

Robert S. Epstein, MD, MS
Chief Medical Officer & Senior Vice President, Department of Medical Affairs,
Merck-Medco

Terry Fulmer, PhD, RN, FAAN
Professor & Director of The Muriel & Virginia Pless Center for Nursing Research,
Co-Director, Hartford Institute for Geriatric Nursing, New York University,
New York, New York

Mark Monane, MD, MS, FACP, AGSF
(Formerly) Senior Director, Medical Policy & Programs, Merck-Medco

Mark Rubino, RPh
Vice President, Clinical Services, Merck-Medco

Todd Semla, PharmD
Associate Director, Psychopharmacology Clinical Research Center,
Department of Psychiatry and Behavioral Science, Evanston Northwestern
Healthcare, Evanston, Illinois

Contributors/Reviewers

Jean Barilla, MS
Senior Manager
Medical Policy & Programs
Merck-Medco

Keith Bradbury, RPh, MS
Senior Director
Drug Information
Merck-Medco

Amita Dasmahapatra, MD
Senior Director
Medical Policy & Programs
Merck-Medco

Richard Feifer, MD
Associate Director
Medical Policy & Programs
Merck-Medco

Daniel Ford, MD
Associate Professor
Internal Medicine
Welch Center for Prevention,
Epidemiology, and Clinical
Research
Johns Hopkins Medical Institute
Baltimore, Maryland

George Fulop, MD
Senior Director
Medical Policy & Programs
Merck-Medco

Leslie Gise, MD
Clinical Professor
Department of Psychiatry
John A. Burns School of
Medicine
University of Hawaii
Honolulu, Hawaii

Shelly Gray, PharmD
Associate Professor
School of Pharmacy
University of Washington
Seattle, Washington

Paul Greenberg, MD
Director
Medical Policy & Programs
Merck-Medco

Marvin Konstam, MD
Chief of Cardiology
New England Medical
Center
Boston, Massachusetts

Alan Lotvin, MD
Chief Medical Officer
Health Plan Services
Merck-Medco

Randy A. McCoy, PharmD
Lead Pharmacist
Central Plains Clinic
Sioux Falls, South Dakota

Steve Montamat, MD
Internal Medicine Specialist
St. Luke's Internal Medicine
Boise, Idaho

Heather-Ann Periconi, RPh
Senior Manager
Clinical Product
Management
Merck-Medco

Walter Peterson, MD
Professor of Medicine
Director, Training Program
in Digestive Diseases
Dallas VA Medical Center
Dallas, Texas

Brent Pfeiffenberger
(Formerly) Pharmacy Intern
Clinical Practice &
Education
Merck-Medco

Michael Rich, MD
Director, Coronary Care
Unit & Geriatric Cardiology
Program
Barnes Jewish Hospital
St. Louis, Missouri

Myra Skluth, MD
Chief, General Internal
Medicine
Norwalk Hospital
Norwalk, Connecticut

Susan Squillace, MD
Associate Professor of Family
Medicine
University of Virginia Health
Sciences Center
Charlottesville, Virginia

Jeffrey Susman, MD
Director, Family Medicine
University of Cincinnati
Cincinnati, Ohio

Rhonda Wroble, PharmD
(Formerly) Pharmacy Resident
Merck-Medco

Sandra Yang, PharmD
Manager
Clinical Practice &
Education
Merck-Medco

Chun Wan Yin, PharmD
Manager
Clinical Practices &
Therapeutics
Merck-Medco

Special Note to Readers

Although efforts have been made to assure the accuracy of the information contained in the *Guidebook*, the information is presented without guarantees or warrantees regarding the information or the use of any product described in the *Guidebook*. The reader is advised to discuss information obtained in this book with a doctor, pharmacist, nurse, or other healthcare professional.

Inclusion of products listed in this book does not constitute endorsement, nor has every medication on the market been included.

Certain uses of medications discussed herein may not have been approved by the Food and Drug Administration (FDA) but, nonetheless, have been reported in the medical literature or represent accepted clinical practices.

The *Medication Guidebook to Healthy Aging* is not intended to take the place of your doctor or other healthcare professional. It is a resource designed to help you make the best decisions and get the most from medical services available to you as well as a reminder to discuss any health or medication problems with your doctor or other healthcare professional.

Contents

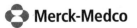

Contents

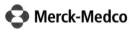

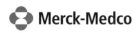

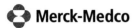

Dear Reader,

Americans are living longer and healthier lives than ever before. Advances in medical care and medications have helped make this possible. While medications are beneficial for many medical problems, their use comes with some risks. To receive the most benefit from your medications with the lowest risk of side effects, you should use them as directed by your doctor or other healthcare professional.

Older adults may have a greater chance of developing side effects from medications because aging causes our bodies to react differently to medications than when we were younger. As we age, we are more likely to have medical problems that require us to take more than one medication. The more medications we take, the more likely we are to have medication interactions and side effects. Understanding how changes that occur when you get older increase the risk of side effects from medications is very important. It can help you improve your medication safety and promote healthier living.

Several years ago Merck-Medco, in recognition of the health problems that may occur from unsafe medication use in older adults, developed the **Partners for Healthy Aging**® program. This award-winning program helps educate doctors and other healthcare professionals about the safe use of prescription medications in older adults. A study published in the *Journal of the American Medical Association* in October of 1998 showed that Merck-Medco's **Partners for Healthy Aging** program helped reduce the number of possibly unsafe medications used in older Americans.*

*Monane M, Matthias D, Nagle B, Kelly M. Improving prescribing patterns for the elderly through an online drug utilization review intervention: a system linking the computer, pharmacist, and physician. *JAMA* 1998;280:1249–52.

✪ Merck-Medco

The Medication Guidebook to Healthy Aging was designed to be an easy-to-use reference book to inform older adults, and those who care for them, about safe medication use. The *Guidebook* describes common medical problems and the medications that are often prescribed to treat those problems. Information in the *Guidebook* may help you work with your doctor or other healthcare professional to better understand your medications and to help you get the most benefit from them.

We hope you find the *Guidebook* a useful reference tool that helps you improve your health and quality of life.

Sincerely yours,

Les Paul, MD, MS
Editors

Becky Nagle, PharmD, BCPS

General Information

Special Medication Warnings for Older Adults

A triangle symbol ▲ appears next to the names of some medications throughout the *Guidebook*. It indicates medications that are more likely to cause unpleasant or dangerous side effects. These medications are generally not recommended for people over 65 years of age. The side effects caused by these medications in older adults may not be very obvious and may be mistaken for "just a part of getting older" but may be serious. If you are taking one of these medications, you might want to talk to your doctor or other healthcare professional to see if this medication is right for you. Safer medications may be available, and lower dosages may be required. You should not stop taking these medications without first talking to your doctor or other healthcare professional. The Warning! section in each chapter that has a medication marked with a ▲ will provide information about the specific risks and warnings for this medication.

A Warning about Grapefruit and Grapefruit Juice

Eating grapefruit or drinking grapefruit juice may change how your body handles some medications and may increase the side effects of these medications. Each time you take a medication, some of the medication is absorbed into the body, and the rest passes out of the body through the digestive tract (stomach and intestines). Research has shown that a substance in grapefruit and grapefruit juice blocks an intestinal enzyme that controls how much medication is absorbed by the body. When the enzyme is blocked, more medication is absorbed into the body. As a result, grapefruit or grapefruit juice may dramatically increase the amount of some medications in the body and then increase the side effects of the medication. There are many medications that may be affected by grapefruit or grapefruit juice. Some of the medications are listed in the table on the next page.

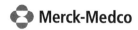

Talk to your doctor or other healthcare professional if you want to include grapefruit or grapefruit juice in your diet. You should try to eat or drink the same amount of grapefruit and/or grapefruit juice each day. For example, you should not drink a couple of glasses of grapefruit juice on one day and then not have any for a couple of days. If you have been taking any of the medications listed in the table on the next page, do not increase or decrease the amount of grapefruit in your diet without first talking to your doctor or other healthcare professional. He or she may want to change the dose of your medication(s) if you change your grapefruit or grapefruit juice intake.

Grapefruit May Interact with the Following Medications*

Brand Name	Generic Name	Brand Name	Generic Name
Adalat®	nifedipine	Neoral®	cyclosporine
Anafranil®	clomipramine	Norvasc®	amlodipine
Baycol®	cerivastatin	Plendil®	felodipine
BuSpar®	buspirone	Procardia®	nifedipine
Calan®	verapamil	Prograf®	tacrolimus
Cardene®	nicardipine	Propulsid®	cisapride
Halcion®	triazolam	Quinaglute®	quinidine
Hismanal®	astemizole	Quinidex®	quinidine
Invirase®	saquinavir	Sandimmune®	cyclosporine
Isoptin®	verapamil	Sporonox®	itraconazole
Lexxel®	felodipine/enalapril	Sular®	nisoldipine
Lipitor®	atorvastatin	Tarka®	verapamil/trandolapril
Lotrel®	amlodipine/benazepril	Tegretol®	carbamazepine
Mevacor®	lovastatin	Zocor®	simvastatin

*Other medications as well as other brands that may interact with grapefruit or grapefruit juice may not be listed above. Talk to your pharmacist or other healthcare professional about the interaction with food containing grapefruit or grapefruit juice with the medications you are currently taking.

Warning about Taking Another Person's Medications

You should not take another person's medications or give yours to anyone else, even if you appear to have symptoms similar to those of someone else. A medication that is right for one person may be dangerous for another.

How to Use *The Medication Guidebook to Healthy Aging*

The *Guidebook* is divided into three sections:

1. **General Information** (pages i to xxiv)
   This section provides information that is common to all medications, including how medications act differently in older adults and how to take medications as safely as possible. It will be helpful for you to read this general information first before you read the more specific information in the rest of the book.

2. **Medical Problem and Medication Chapters** (pages 1 to 691)
   This section is made up of 21 chapters. Each of the chapters contains information about a *specific* medical problem and the medications that are often used to treat it.

3. **Reference Guides and Index** (pages 693 to 833)
   This section offers medication listings, definitions of medical terms, and other useful references. The Medication and Chapter Table allows you to easily locate information on medications, categories of medication, and medical problems in the *Guidebook*.

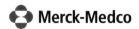

How to Find Information about Your Medications

There are several ways to find information about your medications in the *Guidebook*.

1. Contents

If you know for what medical problem the medication you are taking was prescribed, turn to the Contents in the front of the book. The Contents lists the chapters on all the medical problems and the medications or groups of medications that are discussed in the *Guidebook* with the page numbers where they can be found.

2. Medication and Chapter Table

To find out where information about your medication is located in the *Guidebook* (even if you do not know for what medical problem your medication has been prescribed), turn to the Medication and Chapter Table on page 693. The Medication and Chapter Table lists the medications that are discussed as treatment for the medical problems discussed in the *Guidebook*.

These medications are listed in alphabetic order by both generic (nonbrand) name and brand name (the name given by the manufacturer). If you do not see your medication listed in the Medication and Chapter Table, that means it is not discussed as a treatment for one of the medical problems in the *Guidebook*. It may, however, be listed as a medication that interacts with another medication. These medications, along with those that are discussed as treatment in the *Guidebook*, can be found in the Index on page 811.

3. Index

The Index, which starts on page 811, lists every medication and medical problem that is discussed in the *Guidebook*, along with the page number(s) on which it is discussed.

What Is Discussed in the Medical Problem and Medication Chapters?

The chapters in this section of the *Guidebook* discuss common medical problems and symptoms in older adults. Each of these chapters contains:

What is the medical problem? A description of the medical problem(s) appears in the beginning of each chapter. It may also include symptoms that may be present with that medical problem, causes of the medical problem, steps you may take to improve your condition, and special instructions.

A table of medications and/or categories of similar medications that may be used to treat the medical problem appears after the introduction to the medical problem. The medications are listed individually by brand name (name given by the manufacturer) in *italic type* and/or generic (nonbrand) name in plain type or as a category or group of medications.

The medication and/or category of medications sections: Each section starts with a description of how the medication or group of medications works. The following sections are included in many of the chapters:

How Will I Take This Medication?

This section has information on when and how often to take your medication and what to do if you miss a dose. It may also include information on how to store your medication, whether to take it with or without food, how long it takes to work, and other special instructions.

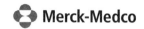

What Side Effects Can This Medication Cause?

This section lists some of the possible side effects that may occur when taking this medication or category of medications. Side effects that are listed in the *Guidebook* do not occur in everyone who takes this medication. Since some side effects occur more often than others, they are divided into groups by how often they usually occur: More Common, Less Common, and Rare. These lists may not be complete, and the frequency with which side effects occur may vary. Talk to your doctor or other healthcare professional if you have side effects that bother you, do not go away, make you worried about taking your medication, or make you want to stop taking your medication. It is important to remember that new side effects are sometimes identified after a medication becomes available, and these lists may not be complete.

Do Other Medications Interact with This Medication?

Sometimes when medications are taken together, they may cause each other to act differently. This is often called an interaction, and this section lists some common medication interactions. While not all interactions are serious, and many potentially interacting medications may be taken together safely under the supervision of your doctor or other healthcare professional, some may be very dangerous. Talk to your doctor or other healthcare professional if you are taking medications that may interact with each other. He or she may wish to change your medication or the dose of your medication to help prevent a problem from an interaction. It is important to remember that new interactions are sometimes identified after a medication becomes available, and these lists may not be complete.

Why Else Do People Take This Medication?

Some medications may be used for more than one medical condition. This section lists some of the other possible uses. Talk to your doctor or other healthcare professional before using any medication for something other than what it was originally prescribed for. (Not all medications have this section in the *Guidebook.*)

What Else Should I Know about This Medication?

This section contains useful information that is not covered in the other sections. (Not all medications have this section in the *Guidebook*.)

 # Warning!

This section contains warnings and important information about medical problems and medications. It includes warnings about some medical conditions that may worsen if you take this medication. It also provides information about blood tests and other special tests that may be needed, information about food or activities you should avoid, and signs of potential problems to watch out for. Tell your doctor or other healthcare professional about all your current and past medical problems to help make sure your medications can be used safely and effectively.

How Growing Older May Affect the Way Medications Work

As a person grows older, many changes in the body occur. These changes usually occur gradually and may happen so slowly that you may not even notice them. Some changes like poor eyesight, hearing trouble, or decreased endurance (strength) may be noticeable; others may not be. Changes that you cannot see or may not notice include how well your kidneys, liver, and other organs work. These changes may cause problems for you when you take medications because these organs control how your body handles medication.

It is important to know what happens when you take a medication. After the pill (tablet or capsule) is swallowed, it goes into the stomach where it mixes with fluids and breaks down into small particles. Then the medication passes through the stomach and intestines and goes into the bloodstream. The blood carries the medication to the part of the body where it is intended to act. Later, the medication is removed from the body. The kidneys and liver are the organs that remove most medications from the body.

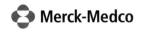

With aging, changes occur in the kidneys and the liver, and they do not remove medications as well as they did at a younger age. Before the kidneys may remove some medications from the body, the liver must break them down so they can be filtered or removed by the kidneys. If the liver does not break down medications as well as it should, they may build up in the bloodstream and cause side effects.

When kidneys slow down, the removal of some medications slows down. If you continue to take the same dose of the medication, medication blood levels may become higher because the medication is not removed as fast as it should be. High levels of medications in the blood may cause side effects.

Certain diseases may affect the kidney or liver and, thus, the way medications are handled in the body. For example, high blood pressure and diabetes may damage the kidneys. Some medications may reduce the ability of the kidneys or liver to remove medications from the body. Also, some medications simply cause a stronger effect in older adults than in younger people. Because medications often work differently in older adults than in younger adults, the recommended doses of many medications are lower for older adults. To help prevent side effects, your doctor or other healthcare professional may start by giving you a low dose of medication, increasing the amount slowly until it works well for you. You should not change the dose of your medication without talking to your doctor or other healthcare professional.

Changes in the body caused by aging and some medical problems may also affect your ability to take your medications properly. For example, because close-up vision worsens with age, it may be hard to read the directions on your medication bottle or the small print on the medication information booklets your pharmacist gives you. Be sure to tell your pharmacist if you have vision problems, and use your reading glasses when taking your medications to help prevent errors. If you have trouble seeing to read, talk to your doctor or other healthcare professional about scheduling an eye appointment.

Some medical problems may cause older adults to have trouble swallowing pills. Some medications may be very large or bitter tasting and may not be pleasant to take. Sometimes the medication may stick in your throat. To help prevent this, you should drink at least 8 ounces of fluid with your medications and avoid lying down right after taking your medications. Talk to your doctor or other healthcare professional if you have trouble swallowing because he or she may be able to change your medication to a liquid or to a smaller size pill to make it easier to swallow.

Arthritis (stiff, painful joints) is a common problem among older adults. If your hands are stiff, sore, or weak, you might have trouble removing the caps from medication bottles, using medication inhalers, or using syringes that are needed to give medication by injection. If you are having problems opening your medication bottles, let your pharmacist know. He or she can give you caps that are easier to open. If you have trouble using your inhaler, talk to your doctor or other healthcare professional about getting a device called a spacer, which can help you use the medication more easily. If you have trouble with syringes, talk to your doctor or pharmacist about getting medications already in the syringe or getting other devices that can help you use syringes more easily.

Many people experience changes in their memory as they grow older. Just as it may be hard to remember the name of a person you just met, it may be hard to remember if you took your morning doses of medication. This is often a normal part of aging and is not a cause for worry in most cases. Some medication schedules are harder to remember than others. For example, the instructions for some medications are to take them 3 times a day. It is often easier for people to take a medication once or twice a day instead of 3 or 4 times a day. If you are having problems remembering to take your medications, let your pharmacist, doctor, or other healthcare professional know. It may be possible to change to a medication that does not need to be taken so often. It is a good idea to develop a system to help you to remember to take your medications. See the section Other Tips for Taking Medication and Healthy Living on page xix.

Side Effects of Medications in Older Adults

Generally, the benefits of medication exceed their risks. However, sometimes medication may cause side effects or unwanted problems, and these may occur more often in older adults. There are many reasons for this. First, many older adults have several medical problems for which they take medications. Medications for one medical problem may worsen the symptoms of another medical problem. Side effects may occur when medications affect or interact with each other. The more medications a person takes, the more likely he or she is to have side effects. Another important reason why older adults have more side effects is that medications often act differently in the body as we age (see How Growing Older May Affect the Way Medications Work on page vii).

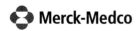

It may be hard to tell the difference between side effects, the symptoms of common illnesses, or changes that occur with aging. For this reason it may be difficult to know when you are having side effects from medications. For example, becoming confused or forgetful or having constipation, dizziness, or dry mouth may be caused by a certain medication, illness, or changes that occur with aging. If you notice any changes in your health or daily functioning, tell your doctor or other healthcare professional. He or she may be able to change your medication, lower the dose, or give you tips to help reduce side effects.

Using Over-the-Counter (OTC) Medications

Many older adults take over-the-counter (OTC) medications that may be bought without a prescription at a drugstore or grocery store. All medications described in the *Guidebook* are available by prescription only unless otherwise noted in the descriptions in the beginning of each medication section.

Although OTC medications may be very helpful in treating mild symptoms, it is important to remember that OTC medications may also cause side effects just like prescription medications may. The chance of developing serious side effects from OTC medications increases when they are not used properly. Read the label carefully and follow the directions or ask your doctor, pharmacist, or other healthcare professional for advice before taking any OTC medications.

Many OTC pain medications, antacids, cough and cold medications, laxatives, diarrhea medications, and sleep medications should only be used for short-term treatment. If your symptoms do not improve or get worse, it may be a sign of a more serious problem that needs to be evaluated by your doctor or other healthcare professional.

OTC medications may cause serious side effects. For example, some OTC pain medications such as *Advil®* or *Motrin®* (ibuprofen), *Orudis KT®* (ketoprofen), or *Aleve®* (naproxen), may cause bleeding stomach ulcers. However, used correctly, these pain medications may be safer than prescription medications because they contain a lower dose of medication, which may help avoid side effects that may occur with higher doses in prescription medications. Read the label to see what side effects may occur before you take OTC medications, and talk to your doctor or other healthcare professional if side effects occur.

OTC medications may interact with prescription medications. One medication may slow the removal of another medication from the body or prevent the proper absorption of another. For example, *Tagamet®* (cimetidine) may slow the removal of a breathing medication like theophylline and increase the amount of theophylline in the blood, which can cause side effects. Some antacids taken to relieve heartburn may block the absorption of other medications in the stomach. In this case, the other medication will not get into the bloodstream and be able to do what it is supposed to do. Be sure to read the label of the OTC medication to see what medications might interact with it. Talk to your doctor, pharmacist, or other healthcare professional if you have questions about taking an OTC medication with your other medications.

OTC medications may worsen some medical problems just like prescription medications may. For example, OTC sleep medications contain antihistamines and may cause trouble with urinating in men who have an enlarged prostate (benign prostatic hypertrophy). Be sure to read the label to find out which medical conditions may be worsened by an OTC medication before you take it. Talk to your doctor, pharmacist, or other healthcare professional if you have questions about taking an OTC medication.

Remember to tell your doctor, pharmacist, and other healthcare professionals about all of the OTC medications you take. They need to have this information so they can better understand your medical problems and help prevent interactions and side effects. Remember to include your use of vitamins and herbal or alternative medications because they may have side effects and interactions too.

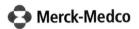

What Should I Know about My Medications?

- **What Am I Taking This Medication for, and How Will It Help Me?**
  Knowing the reason you are taking a medication will help you to
  understand why it is important to take it. For answers to this question
  and the questions below, read the medication information sheet that
  comes with your medication and the information about the medication
  in the *Guidebook*. Both provide information on how to take
  medications, what to do if you miss a dose, what side effects may occur,
  what medications might interact with each other, and other important
  facts about your medications. If you have questions about the
  medication information provided in the *Guidebook* or the medication
  information sheets that come with your medication, consult your doctor,
  pharmacist, or other healthcare professional.

- **When Should I Take This Medication, and How Much Should I
  Take?** Read the label of every prescription medication carefully. Follow
  the directions and pay attention to any warnings (such as not to drive
  while taking the medication). If you do not take a medication as
  prescribed, it may not work as well as it should or it may produce side
  effects. Some medications work best in the morning while others work
  best in the evening or at bedtime. Some medications may be given in
  the morning because side effects may keep you up at night if taken later
  in the day. Some medications are best taken in the evening or at
  bedtime to help reduce side effects during the day. Do not change the
  amount of medication you are taking unless directed to do so by your
  doctor or other healthcare professional. Taking more medication will
  not help you get better faster. It may actually cause side effects that may
  be dangerous. Not taking as much as prescribed may decrease how well
  the medication works for you. Taking the right dose of your medication
  at the right time will help you get the most from your medications and
  help you avoid side effects.

- **How Long Will It Take for This Medication to Work?** Not all
  medications work right away. They may take a few days or weeks—and
  sometimes even months—to work. Knowing when to expect a benefit
  from a medication will help you know how long to wait before
  contacting your doctor or other healthcare professional about the
  medication not working for you.

- **How Long Should I Take This Medication For?** Some medications are for short-term use, and some are for long-term use. Some medications will have to be taken even after your symptoms improve. Sometimes when medications are stopped too soon, the symptoms from the medical problem come back. Taking medications as long as prescribed may help you prevent a return of your symptoms.

  Some medications should not be stopped suddenly. If you have taken some medications for more than a couple of weeks and your doctor or other healthcare professional wants you to stop taking the medication, he or she may ask you to decrease it gradually, lowering the dose over a few weeks or months. Stopping suddenly may cause unpleasant withdrawal symptoms or may even worsen your medical problems. Pay careful attention to the instructions your doctor or other healthcare professional gives you about how much less to take and for how long. When starting a new medication, always ask your doctor or other healthcare professional how long you will need to take the medication.

- **How Should I Store This Medication?** Medication may lose potency (strength to do what it is supposed to do) if it is not stored properly. Medication will not work as well as it should if it loses potency. Keep all medications in their original containers, and follow the storage instructions listed in the medication information sheet that comes with your medication.

  All medications should have an expiration date. After this date, the medication may lose potency or may even be harmful. Throw away any medications when the expiration date has passed. Ask your pharmacist or other healthcare professional about how you should store your medications, and read the medication-storage information section in Other Tips for Taking Medication and Healthy Living on page xix.

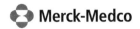

- **Can I Take This Medication with Food?** Some medications should be taken on an empty stomach to be absorbed properly while other medications should be taken with food to be absorbed properly. Sometimes taking medication with food will help prevent side effects like an upset stomach while other times certain foods must be avoided to help prevent side effects. To help your medication work best and help prevent side effects, find out if your medication should be taken with or without food.

- **Can I Drink Alcoholic Beverages (Such As Beer, Wine, Whiskey, and Others) While I Am Taking This Medication?** It is important to avoid drinking alcoholic beverages while taking many medications because drinking alcohol may increase the side effects of medications. Many medications cause drowsiness. You should avoid drinking alcohol while taking medications that cause drowsiness. Avoiding drinking alcoholic beverages while taking some medications may be important because drinking alcohol may worsen the medical condition for which you are taking the medication. In addition, when mixed with the medication, alcohol may cause nausea, vomiting, or other side effects. Always find out what effects alcoholic beverages will have on your medications.

- **What Should I Do If I Forget to Take a Dose?** From time to time, you may forget to take your medication. In some instances you should take the dose as soon as you remember. In other instances, you should skip the forgotten dose and take your regular dose of medication at the next scheduled time. In most cases taking two doses at the same time is not recommended. Check the specific information on your medications in the *Guidebook* and the medication information sheets that come with your prescription medications for information about missed doses. If you have questions about missed doses, talk to your doctor, pharmacist, or other healthcare professional. For more information about remembering to take your medications, see Other Tips for Taking Medication and Healthy Living on page xix.

- **What Side Effects Can This Medication Cause?** Medications may cause side effects. Many side effects occur when you first start taking a medication but stop in a few days or weeks. Other side effects may continue for as long as you take the medication. Tell your doctor or other healthcare professional if you have side effects that bother you, do not go away, make you worried about taking your medication, or make you want to stop taking your medication. If you develop side effects from your medication, your doctor or other healthcare professional may be able to prescribe a different medication, change the dose, or give you tips to help reduce your side effects.

- **What Medications Can Interact with This Medication?** Many medications interact with other medications. Some interactions may be minor, and some may cause serious problems. Tell all of your doctors, pharmacists, and other healthcare professionals about all of the prescription and nonprescription or over-the-counter (OTC) medications you take. OTC medications may have side effects and interactions just like prescription medications may. To keep track of your medications, fill out the Personal Medication Record in the back of the *Guidebook* and keep it up-to-date. Take your Personal Medication Record or a photocopy of it with you when you visit any healthcare professional and when you travel.

- **Will This Medication Make My Other Medical Problems Worse?** Sometimes medications for one medical problem may cause side effects that may worsen another medical problem. To help prevent side effects that may worsen your other medical problems, be sure to tell all of your doctors, pharmacists, and other healthcare professionals about all of the medical problems you have now and the problems you have had in the past.

- **Does This Medication Cause Drowsiness—Will I Be Able to Drive or Do Other Things I Need to Be Alert For?** Many medications cause drowsiness. Check with your doctor or other healthcare professional before driving when starting a new medication. It is important to avoid driving a car and other activities that require mental alertness, like using a knife or operating machinery, when taking medications that cause drowsiness.

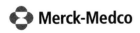

- **I Have Allergies to Some Medications. Will I Be Allergic to This Medication?** Many medications have more than one name, so it may be difficult for you to know if you have taken a particular medication before. Many medications belong to medication groups (categories) that cause similar side effects or allergic reactions. If you had a reaction to one medication, you may have a reaction to another medication in the same category. Sometimes, unrelated medications and categories of medications may cause allergies. Tell your doctor or other healthcare professional about any allergies or previous reactions you have had to medications to help prevent them in the future. Be sure to tell your doctor or other healthcare professional about serious medication reactions such as rash (skin redness, bumps, itching, or irritation), swelling of the face and throat, trouble breathing, or any other problems you have had with medications in the past.

- **Do I Have to Do Anything Special When I Take This Medication?** Sometimes you will have to avoid going out in the sun while taking certain medications. You may have to stop taking some medications before you have surgery or other medical procedures. Ask your doctor or other healthcare professional if you will have to limit any of your usual activities or stop taking your medications for medical or surgical procedures.

- **Will I Need to Have Any Blood Tests or Other Special Tests While I Am Taking This Medication?** Sometimes your doctor or other healthcare professional will order blood tests or other special tests to see if your medications are working as they should. Sometimes he or she may order blood tests to see if you are getting the right amount of medication, since many medications may cause side effects if you get too much and may not work well if you do not get enough. Some medications may affect the liver, kidneys, or other organs. Your doctor or other healthcare professional may order blood tests or other special tests to check to see if these problems occur. It is important to have these tests done as ordered.

Questions and Answers about Generic Medications

What Is the Difference between Brand-Name Medications and Generic Medications?

The Food and Drug Administration (FDA) is the government agency responsible for ensuring that medications in the United States are safe and effective. When the FDA approves a medication for use, the medication is given a generic name. The brand name is the name used by the company that discovered the medication. Generic names are usually more complicated and harder to remember than brand names. Many generic names are shorthand for the medication's chemical name, structure, or formula. Brand names are often used when a doctor or other healthcare professional writes a prescription. Not all brand-name medications have a generic form available. When the patent on a brand-name medication expires, other companies can make a generic form of that medication. The FDA must approve all generic forms of a brand-name medication. The FDA approval of a generic medication is based on scientific evidence that the generic medication produces an effect that is essentially the same as the brand-name medication. In the *Guidebook* medication brand names are listed in *italic type,* and the generic names are listed in plain type. If generic names are listed with the brand names, the generic name is in parentheses. For example, for the medication *Motrin*® (ibuprofen), *Motrin*® is the brand name, and ibuprofen is the generic name.

Why Are Generic Medications Less Expensive than Brand-Name Medications?

In the United States a company that develops a new medication can be granted a patent for the medication. Patents give the company exclusive rights to produce a medication for 20 years from the time the patent is applied for. However, usually many years go by between the time a medication is discovered and the time it is approved for use, usually leaving the manufacturer often less than half that time to exclusively sell a new medication. This gives the

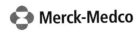

company a chance to make up some of the costs for developing, manufacturing, and advertising its medication. After a patent expires, other companies may sell a generic form of the medication. The price of a generic medication is usually much lower than that of the original brand-name medication, in part because there are no research and advertising costs as there were for the original brand-name medication. This creates competition between manufacturers of brand and generic medications, which, in turn, keeps prices lower when generic medications enter the market.

Who Decides If a Generic Medication Is OK or Not?

Approval of a generic medication is based on evidence that it produces an effect essentially identical (equivalent) to the brand-name medication. The FDA reviews the bioequivalency studies (studies done to assure a generic version of a medication releases its active ingredients into the bloodstream in the same way as the brand-name medication) to make sure they are equivalent. Although it contains the same active ingredient, a generic medication will usually differ from the brand-name medication in size, color, and shape. The FDA gives generic medications that are considered therapeutically equivalent to the brand-name medication an "A" rating. This means the generic medication contains the same active ingredient in the same strength and dosage form as the brand-name medication, and it is expected to produce the same effect.

Do I Always Receive a Generic Form of Medication for a Prescription?

No. First, not all brand-name medications have generic forms available. Second, if a generic medication is available, the FDA must approve it for substitution. The FDA publishes a book that lists all the generic medications that have been reviewed and considered safe and equivalent. If the generic medication is listed in the book, it may be substituted for the brand-name medication unless your doctor or other healthcare professional who writes the prescription specifically writes that no substitution may be made. Some state laws require that generic medications must be substituted for the brand-name medication when generics are available and equivalent. If your doctor or other healthcare professional believes that there are special reasons why you should not receive a generic medication, he or she can specify that you must receive the brand-name medication.

Why Should I Take Generic Medications?

Studies are reviewed by the FDA to make sure a generic medication releases its active ingredients into the bloodstream in the same manner as the brand-name medication does and that this medication should work in the same way as the brand-name medication. Because the generic medications cost significantly less than brand-name medications, you will get the same benefits at a lower cost. Therefore, if you use generics whenever possible, you may reduce prescription medication costs to you and your group health plan or insurance and, in turn, receive the most value.

Other Tips for Taking Medication and Healthy Living

Medication Containers and Storage

Unless otherwise directed, it is best to keep medications in their original containers. You should store most medications at room temperature (59ºF–86ºF) in an area where they will be protected from light and moisture. Do not keep your medications in the medicine cabinet in the bathroom because they may lose potency (strength) from moisture and humidity. Avoid keeping your medications near the stove where heat may cause them to lose potency. Avoid keeping them on a windowsill where the sunlight may cause them to lose potency.

Medication bottles come in childproof containers to prevent accidental poisoning. Do not keep the caps off the bottles or rest the caps on top of the bottles. Your medications could lose potency if stored like this, and they might not work as well as they should. If you have trouble opening these bottles, you may ask your pharmacist for easy-open containers. Be sure to keep your

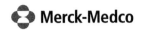

medication out of reach of children and pets. Ask your pharmacist if it is all right before putting medications in a pillbox. Pillboxes are not airtight containers, and some medications may lose potency if stored in these types of containers.

Remembering to Take Your Medications

It is important to take medications as prescribed. Try to set up your schedule to work them into your daily activities. If you have to take a medication twice a day, you might try taking it before you brush your teeth in the morning and at night. If you have trouble remembering to take your medication during the day, try setting a timer or alarm to remind you when to take it (ask your pharmacist about timer devices). Ask your friends and relatives to help remind you to take your medications. Also, talk to your doctor or other healthcare professional about any trouble you may be having remembering to take your medications. He or she may be able to find ways to simplify your medication schedule.

Tell your doctor or other healthcare professional about your preferences or habits related to taking your medications. Tell him or her if you are at home most of the day or out most of the day, what side effects have bothered you in the past, and any cost concerns you have about your medications.

Some people keep their medication bottles on the dining-room table, and this reminds them to take their medications whenever they sit down for a meal. Be sure to keep all medication out of the reach of children and pets, however. Some people find it helpful to use a pillbox in which you can keep all your doses of medications for a whole week at one time. This way, you may look in the box and see if you have taken your medication. Do not use a pillbox before talking with your pharmacist as some medications may lose potency if kept in a pillbox.

Advice about the Flu and Pneumonia

If you get the flu (influenza) or pneumonia when you are 65 years old or older, your chance of becoming seriously ill or even dying is higher than it would be if you were younger. It is recommended that anyone who is 50 years old or older and anyone who is in poor health with medical problems, such as congestive heart failure, diabetes, emphysema, or other conditions, get a flu shot every year.

Most people who get flu shots do not get the flu, and if they do get the flu, they will probably have a milder case than they would have had without the shot. The best time to get the shot is in October and early November. It is still effective and worth getting later in the flu season. Ask your doctor or other healthcare professional whether you should get a flu shot and when would be the best time for you to get it.

Your doctor or other healthcare professional may suggest that you get a vaccination called *Pneumovax®* to help prevent pneumonia. This shot helps prevent a common type of pneumonia caused by bacteria. One shot of the pneumonia vaccine usually lasts for many years. Most people 65 years old or older should get this shot because older adults are more likely to become very ill when they get pneumonia. Ask your doctor or other healthcare professional whether you should get a pneumonia vaccination.

Flu and pneumonia vaccines may be given safely to most people. You do not get the flu or pneumonia from getting the flu or the pneumonia shot. The most common side effect is a sore arm (pain where the shot was given). This usually lasts only a day or two. Allergic reactions from flu shots are rare. However, people who have allergies to eggs should not receive flu shots, because they contain some egg protein from chickens. Talk to your doctor or other healthcare professional if you have an egg allergy or any other allergy or previous reaction to a flu shot or a vaccination before getting a flu shot or a pneumonia vaccination.

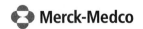

What to Remember when Traveling

Taking your medications correctly while traveling may be a challenge. But a little preparation may make it an easier, safer, and healthier trip.

Some medications cause side effects or have risks of medication interactions that may make it necessary for you to wear a medical identification bracelet in case you need emergency medical help. These bracelets will let emergency healthcare professionals know important information about your medical history so that they will not give you medications that could harm you. Ask your doctor or other healthcare professional whether you should wear a medical identification bracelet.

Important Information to Take with You while Traveling:

1. The names, telephone numbers (with area codes), addresses, and specialties of your doctors and other healthcare professionals

2. The names, telephone numbers (with area codes), and addresses of every pharmacy where you buy your medications

3. A list of your illnesses and medical conditions

4. A list of all your medications, their dosages (amount you take each time and how often), the conditions you are taking them for, and the length of time you have been taking them. Include nonprescription medications, vitamins, and herbal medications. This will be easy if you fill out and make a photocopy of the Personal Medication Record in the back of this book and carry it with you.

Consider Packing:

- A nonprescription medication to help relieve diarrhea (if you are traveling out of the country) because many people develop diarrhea when traveling out of the country

- A nonprescription pain reliever and fever reducer such as *Tylenol®* (acetaminophen)

- Sunblock or sunscreen to protect you against harmful ultraviolet rays of the sun that may lead to painful sunburn and skin cancer and because some medication may cause you to become more sensitive to the sun

- *Band-Aids®* for blisters from walking or minor cuts

- A nonprescription antibiotic ointment to help prevent infections from cuts or wounds

Store your medications properly when you travel. Most medications should be kept at room temperature. Check the directions that come on the medication information sheets with your medications for storage information. Ask your pharmacist any questions you have about proper storage. Follow these general tips:

Traveling by Air

When you travel by airplane, carry all your medications with you. Do not pack them in a suitcase that will be checked and stored on the plane where you will not be able to get to them. Some flights are delayed for hours or canceled. Luggage may be lost, usually just for a day or two, but long enough to cause a problem for you. The cargo areas of airplanes may become very cold or very hot, and such extreme temperatures may weaken or destroy some medications.

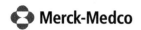

Traveling by Car

When you travel by car, do not store your medications in the trunk or glove compartment, where temperatures may become very hot or very cold. Do not place medications on the shelf in front of the back window of a car, where they may be exposed to direct sunlight and heat. Do not leave your medications in the car for any long periods.

Protecting Children

If you visit a place where children will be present, keep all medications out of their reach or in a locked suitcase. Store your medications in labeled, child-resistant containers. Do not underestimate how common it is for small children to climb to high places or how easily they may open drawers and cabinets. Tell the children's parent or guardian what medications you have and where you are putting them.

An Ample Supply

Bring along more medication than you expect to need for your entire trip. If anything happens to your medication or if you end up staying longer than planned, you may not be able to get a refill quickly. Do not wait until your medication has run out before you ask your doctor or other healthcare professional for a refill.

Chapter 1

Alzheimer's Disease

What Is Alzheimer's Disease?

Many older people have problems with their memory. They may forget what someone's name is or where they have put personal items like keys. A little forgetfulness is a normal part of aging.

However, some people forget so much that they have trouble taking care of themselves. They may forget to pay bills, shop for food, or even eat. They may get lost in familiar places, even in their own neighborhoods. Alzheimer's disease is the most common cause of this type of memory problem. Forgetting where you put the car keys is normal. Forgetting what the keys are used for could be a sign of Alzheimer's disease.

In Alzheimer's disease, memory problems get worse as the years go by. Often, people with Alzheimer's disease have more than just memory problems. They may feel depressed or nervous (anxious).

A number of medical conditions besides Alzheimer's disease can cause forgetfulness. For example, memory problems can come from depression, Parkinson's disease, or a series of mini-strokes.

The brain's chemistry changes in people who develop Alzheimer's disease. One change that seems to be important is that the brain has too little acetylcholine, a chemical that nerve cells use to communicate and store memories.

No cure has been found for Alzheimer's disease. However, taking certain medications may temporarily help to improve the memory of people with Alzheimer's disease or at least slow the progression (worsening) of the disease. Medications can also help to relieve some of the other symptoms of Alzheimer's disease—such as sadness, depression, or nervousness (anxiety).

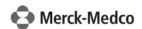

Medications for Alzheimer's Disease

Two types of medications may be used to treat Alzheimer's disease. This chapter discusses these categories of medications:

MEDICATIONS	See Page
Cholinesterase Inhibitors	2
Neuroleptic Medications	6

If you do not see the exact name of the medication that you take for Alzheimer's disease listed above, check the Medication and Chapter Table to find out which category your medication falls under or check the Index.

Cholinesterase Inhibitors

Acetylcholine is a chemical in the brain that nerve cells use to communicate and store memories. Cholinesterase inhibitors are medications that help keep the amount of acetylcholine in the brain at higher levels than it would be without the medications. They may temporarily help to improve memory or to keep it from getting worse.

Brand Name	Generic Name
Aricept®	donepezil
Cognex®	tacrine
Exelon®	rivastigmine

 ### How Will I Take Cholinesterase Inhibitors?

Cognex® (tacrine) is usually taken 4 times a day. *Cognex*® (tacrine) works best if it is taken on an empty stomach, 1 hour before meals. However, if it upsets your stomach, ask your doctor or other healthcare professional about taking it with food. *Aricept®* (donepezil) is usually taken once a day at bedtime. *Exelon®* (rivastigmine) is usually taken twice a day with breakfast and dinner.

To help prevent side effects, your doctor or other healthcare professional may start by giving you a low dose of this medication, increasing the amount slowly until it works well for you.

Cholinesterase inhibitors usually need to be taken for 4 to 12 weeks to work best. Do not stop taking these medications unless your doctor or other healthcare professional has directed you to do so.

If you miss a dose of this medication, take the dose you missed as soon as possible. However, if it is almost time for your next dose, skip the missed dose and just take the next one. Do not double your dose. Take your medication exactly as directed by your doctor or other healthcare professional. Do not stop taking a prescription medication unless directed by your doctor or other healthcare professional.

What Side Effects Can Cholinesterase Inhibitors Cause?

More Common

- Diarrhea
- Headache
- Muscle cramps
- Nausea
- Poor appetite
- Tiredness or sluggishness (fatigue)
- Trouble falling asleep or staying asleep (insomnia)
- Vomiting

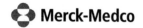

Less Common

- Abnormal dreams
- Dizziness when standing up from a bed or a chair
- Passing out or fainting
- Sadness, feeling blue or down, depressed mood (depression)
- Sweating
- Weight loss

Rare

- Liver problems that may cause yellowing of the skin or eyes (jaundice) with *Cognex®* (tacrine)
- Rash (skin redness, bumps, itching, or irritation)
- Seizures
- Ulcers in the stomach that may cause black, tarry-looking bowel movements

Tell your doctor or other healthcare professional if you have side effects that bother you, do not go away, make you worried about taking your medication, or make you want to stop taking your medication.

 ## Do Other Medications Interact with Cholinesterase Inhibitors?

Luvox® (fluvoxamine) **may increase** the side effects of *Cognex®* (tacrine).

Cognex® (tacrine) **may increase** the side effects of theophylline such as *Theo-Dur®*, *Uniphyl®*, and others—see Glossary.

Tell your doctor or other healthcare professional about all medications (both prescription and nonprescription [over-the-counter] medications) that you are taking.

What Else Should I Know about Cholinesterase Inhibitors?

Cholinesterase inhibitors may help prevent memory loss from getting worse or may slightly improve memory and the ability to get along independently. However, these medications are unlikely to make your memory as good as it was before you developed Alzheimer's disease.

Warning!

To give you the best care, your doctor or other healthcare professional needs to know about the diseases and medical conditions you have had—your full medical history. Tell your doctor or other healthcare professional if you have or have ever had any of the following:

- Allergy or previous reaction to cholinesterase inhibitors
- Breathing problems (asthma and COPD, including emphysema and chronic bronchitis)
- Heart rhythm problems (arrhythmia)
- Liver problems
- Passing out or fainting
- Seizures (epilepsy)
- Stomach problems (ulcers)

Cholinesterase inhibitors may make you unsteady on your feet, causing you to fall and possibly break a bone. If you have fallen recently, tell your doctor or other healthcare professional about it. Taking a different medication or a lower dose may make you less likely to fall. You should not stop taking this medication without first talking to your doctor or other healthcare professional.

If you have had seizures in the past, tell your doctor or other healthcare professional because cholinesterase inhibitors may cause seizures. Stopping this medication suddenly may also cause seizures. If your doctor or other healthcare professional decides that you should stop taking cholinesterase inhibitors, pay careful attention to the instructions he or she gives you about how much less to take and for how long.

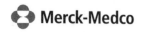

Since *Cognex®* (tacrine) may cause damage to your liver, your doctor or other healthcare professional may order blood tests to find out early on if the medication is causing liver problems, before they become serious.

Cholinesterase inhibitors may cause stomach pain, which may be a sign of an ulcer. However, you may have an ulcer without feeling any pain at all. If ulcers are not treated, they may cause serious stomach or intestinal bleeding. Tell your doctor or other healthcare professional if you have severe stomach pain or stomach pain that keeps returning or if you have ever had peptic ulcer disease. Call your doctor or other healthcare professional right away if you have black, tarry-looking bowel movements (stools), if you vomit dark material that looks like coffee grounds, or if you notice any blood in your bowel movements. Any of these symptoms may be a sign of a bleeding ulcer.

Under certain circumstances, your doctor or other healthcare professional may decide that you should stop taking this medication. If you have taken it for more than a couple of weeks, he or she may want you to decrease it gradually, lowering the dose over a few weeks or months. Stopping suddenly may cause unpleasant withdrawal symptoms or may worsen your medical problems. Pay careful attention to the instructions your doctor or other healthcare professional gives you about how much less to take and for how long.

Neuroleptic Medications

People with Alzheimer's disease may behave differently from the way they behaved before they had Alzheimer's disease. They may have delusions (a false belief that a person incorrectly believes to be true), feel upset (agitated), or act aggressively (irritably). The medications that are used to help prevent these problems are called neuroleptic medications.

Brand Name	Generic Name
Haldol®	haloperidol
Loxitane®	loxapine
Mellaril™	thioridazine
Moban®	molindone
Navane®	thiothixene
Prolixin®	fluphenazine
Risperdal®	risperidone
Serentil®	mesoridazine
Seroquel®	quetiapine
Stelazine®	trifluoperazine
Thorazine®	chlorpromazine
Trilafon®	perphenazine
Zyprexa®	olanzapine

How Will I Take Neuroleptic Medications?

These medications are usually taken once or twice a day. If taken once a day, they are usually taken at bedtime. Your doctor or other healthcare professional will tell you how many times a day to take your medication.

This medication is often used "as needed," so missing a dose should not be a problem. If you miss a dose and it is almost time for the next dose, you should skip the forgotten dose. Do not double the dose. Take your medication as directed by your doctor or other healthcare professional.

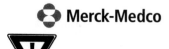

What Side Effects Can Neuroleptic Medications Cause?

More Common

- Constipation
- Dizziness when standing up from a bed or a chair
- Drowsiness
- Dry mouth
- Erection or ejaculation problems (erectile dysfunction)
- Nausea
- Nervousness (anxiety)*
- Shakiness or tremors
- Stiffness

Less Common

- Blurred vision
- Dry eyes
- Fast heartbeat (palpitations)
- Increased sensitivity to the sun (bad sunburn)
- Jerking motions, uncontrollable, repetitive movements of the face, neck, and arms (tics)
- Loss of interest in sex (decreased libido)
- Muscle aches and spasms
- Rash (skin redness, bumps, itching, or irritation)
- Trouble urinating or emptying the bladder
- Weight gain
- Worsening of behavior problems*
- Worsening of glaucoma (an eye disease)

*Sometimes medications may actually cause or worsen the same symptoms they are being used to help relieve. Talk to your doctor or other healthcare professional if your symptoms get worse instead of better while taking this medication.

Rare

- Heart rhythm problems (arrhythmia)
- Seizures

Tell your doctor or other healthcare professional if you have side effects that bother you, do not go away, make you worried about taking your medication, or make you want to stop taking your medication.

 Do Other Medications Interact with Neuroleptic Medications?

These medications *may increase* the side effects of *Seroquel*® (quetiapine):

- *Biaxin*® (clarithromycin)
- *Diflucan*® (fluconazole)
- Erythromycin such as *Ery-Tab*®, *Erythrocin*®, and others—see Glossary
- *Nizoral*® (ketoconazole)
- *Sporanox*® (itraconazole)

Lithium such as *Eskalith*®, *Lithobid*®, and others (see Glossary) *may increase* the side effects of neuroleptic medications.

Neuroleptic medications are generally not prescribed for anyone who is taking *Propulsid*® (cisapride [withdrawn from general distribution; available only by special arrangement with the manufacturer]), *Seldane*® (terfenadine [no longer commercially available]), or *Hismanal*® (astemizole [no longer commercially available]), because together they *may cause* serious, sometimes fatal, heart problems.

Neuroleptic medications *may increase* the side effects of other medications that cause drowsiness, including anticholinergic medications, antidepressants, antihistamines (allergy medications), antispasmodics, benzodiazepines (a type of tranquilizer), anxiety medications, narcotics (pain relievers), muscle relaxants,

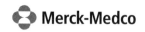

other neuroleptic medications, seizure medications, or sleep medications. Avoid driving a car and other activities that need mental alertness, like using a knife or operating machinery, while taking these medications together.

Drinking alcoholic beverages (such as beer, wine, whiskey, and others) *may increase* the side effects of neuroleptic medications.

Tegretol® (carbamazepine) and *Dilantin*® (phenytoin) *may decrease* how well some neuroleptic medications work.

Neuroleptic medications *may increase* the side effects of some high blood pressure (hypertension) medications—see Glossary.

Neuroleptic medications *may decrease* how well some Parkinson's disease medications work.

Smoking *may decrease* how well *Zyprexa*® (olanzapine) works.

Tell your doctor or other healthcare professional about all medications (both prescription and nonprescription [over-the-counter] medications) that you are taking.

Why Else Do People Take Neuroleptic Medications?

Neuroleptic medications are also taken for schizophrenia (a mental illness that causes delusions and hallucinations), behavior problems caused by head injuries, and some cases of severe depression.

What Else Should I Know about Neuroleptic Medications?

People whose behavior has been affected by Alzheimer's disease may not need to take neuroleptic medications for long periods of time. As the disease changes, the person may become less irritable, reducing the need for neuroleptic medications.

Warning!

To give you the best care, your doctor or other healthcare professional needs to know about the diseases and medical conditions you have had—your full medical history. Tell your doctor or other healthcare professional if you have or have ever had any of the following:

- Allergy or previous reaction to a neuroleptic medication
- Enlarged prostate (benign prostatic hypertrophy)
- Eye problems
- Glaucoma (an eye disease)
- Heart problems
- Kidney problems
- Liver problems
- Parkinson's disease
- Seizures (epilepsy)
- Trouble urinating or emptying the bladder

Neuroleptic medications may make you unsteady on your feet, causing you to fall and possibly break a bone. If you have fallen recently, tell your doctor or other healthcare professional about it. Taking a different medication or a lower dose may make you less likely to fall. You should not stop taking this medication without first talking to your doctor or other healthcare professional.

Neuroleptic medications may cause drowsiness. Avoid driving a car and other activities that need mental alertness, like using a knife or operating machinery, while taking this medication. Drinking alcoholic beverages (such as beer, wine, whiskey, and others) may increase the side effects.

People with Parkinson's disease may have worse symptoms (shakiness or tremors, stiffness in muscles) after starting to take neuroleptic medications. Tell your doctor or other healthcare professional if this happens to you.

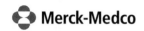

Neuroleptic medications may cause sudden (involuntary) muscle spasms of the face, neck, arms, and legs, which may not completely stop even after the person has stopped taking the medication. These medications should be taken for the shortest possible time. Tell your doctor or other healthcare professional if you have any of these side effects while taking the medication.

If you have had seizures in the past, tell your doctor or other healthcare professional because neuroleptic medications may cause seizures. Stopping these medications suddenly may also cause seizures. If your doctor or other healthcare professional decides that you should stop taking your neuroleptic medication, pay careful attention to the instructions he or she gives you about how much less to take and for how long.

Sometimes anticholinergic medications such as *Artane*® (trihexyphenidyl), *Cogentin*® (benztropine), and others (see Glossary) may be used with neuroleptic medications to help prevent side effects. In some people with Alzheimer's disease these medications may cause worsening of behavior or memory problems. Talk to your doctor or other healthcare professional if you are taking these medications.

If you are taking a neuroleptic medication, stay out of the sun as much as you can to avoid a serious sunburn. When you do go out in the sun, use sunblock or sunscreen, and wear protective clothing, such as a wide-brimmed hat and a long-sleeved shirt.

Under certain circumstances, your doctor or other healthcare professional may decide that you should stop taking this medication. If you have taken it for more than a couple of weeks, he or she may want you to decrease it gradually, lowering the dose over a few weeks or months. Stopping suddenly may cause unpleasant withdrawal symptoms or may worsen your medical problems. Pay careful attention to the instructions your doctor or other healthcare professional gives you about how much less to take and for how long.

Anxiety

What Is Anxiety (Nervousness)?

Everyone feels anxious (nervous) at one time or another. Anxiety is a feeling of fear, tension, or stress, and it is a natural response to danger and to dealing with difficult problems. At certain moments, such as when an actor has stage fright before a show or a student is about to take a test, a little anxiety may actually improve performance. But having a lot of anxiety when no real danger exists may get in the way of daily life. People who are anxious may have a fast heartbeat, rapid breathing, dizziness, headaches, muscle aches and pains, tiredness, shakiness, chest pain, or stomach pain. These symptoms may come and go.

They may shake, feel unsteady on their feet, or have a great deal of fear, and/or have trouble sleeping and thinking clearly. Some people who suffer from anxiety are also depressed (sadness, feeling blue or down, depressed mood) a lot of times.

Anxiety problems may also be caused by medications such as:

- Beta-adrenergic bronchodilators such as *Proventil*® (albuterol), *Serevent*® (salmeterol), and others—see Glossary

- Caffeine contained in some over-the-counter medications

- Cough, cold, and allergy medications

- *Eldepryl*® (selegiline)

- *Prozac*® (fluoxetine)

- *Ritalin*® (methylphenidate)

- *Symmetrel*® (amantadine)

- Theophylline such as *Theo-Dur*®, *Uniphyl*®, and others—see Glossary

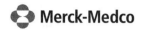

Talk to your doctor or other healthcare professional if you have anxiety (nervousness) and are taking any of these medications. He or she may be able to try a different medication or lower your dose to help reduce your anxiety. Do not stop taking the medications unless directed by your doctor or other healthcare professional.

Anxiety may be relieved in many ways. These include getting emotional support from family and friends, talking with a psychologist or other therapist, and taking medication.

Medications for Anxiety (Nervousness)

Several kinds of medications may be taken to help treat anxiety (nervousness). This chapter discusses these medications and/or categories of medications:

MEDICATIONS	See Page
Benzodiazepines	15
Antihistamines	21
BuSpar® (buspirone)	25
Effexor® (venlafaxine)	28
Meprobamate	32

If you do not see the exact name of the medication that you take for anxiety (nervousness) listed above, check the Medication and Chapter Table to find out which category your medication falls under or check the Index.

Benzodiazepines

Benzodiazepines may help relieve the symptoms of anxiety.

▲ Indicates medications that are more likely to cause unpleasant or dangerous side effects. These medications are generally not recommended for people over 65. The side effects may not be very obvious and may be mistaken for "just a part of getting older" but may be serious. If you are taking one of these medications, you might want to talk to your doctor or other healthcare professional to see if this medication is best for you. Safer medications may be available and lower dosages may be required. You should not stop taking these medications without first talking to your doctor or other healthcare professional.

See the WARNING section on page 19 for the specific safety problems associated with these medications ▲.

Brand Name	Generic Name
Ativan®	lorazepam
▲Klonopin®	clonazepam
▲Librax®	chlordiazepoxide/clidinium
▲Libritabs®	chlordiazepoxide
▲Librium®	chlordiazepoxide
▲Paxipam®	halazepam
Serax®	oxazepam
▲Tranxene®	clorazepate
▲Valium®	diazepam
Xanax®	alprazolam

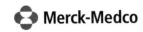

? How Will I Take Benzodiazepines?

Benzodiazepines are usually taken 1 to 4 times a day as needed for anxiety. Your doctor or other healthcare professional will tell you how many times a day to take your medication.

To help prevent side effects, your doctor or other healthcare professional may start by giving you a low dose of this medication, increasing the amount slowly until it works well for you.

This medication is often used "as needed," so missing a dose should not be a problem. If you miss a dose and it is almost time for the next dose, you should skip the forgotten dose. Do not double the dose. Take your medication as directed by your doctor or other healthcare professional.

What Side Effects Can Benzodiazepines Cause?

More Common

- Confusion
- Dizziness when standing up from a bed or a chair
- Drowsiness
- Falling
- Increased sensitivity to the sun (bad sunburn)
- Poor coordination or balance when walking
- Tiredness or sluggishness (fatigue)

Less Common

- Anxiety (nervousness)*
- Bitter taste

*Sometimes medications may actually cause or worsen the same symptoms they are being used to help relieve. Talk to your doctor or other healthcare professional if your symptoms get worse instead of better while taking this medication.

- Blurred or double vision
- Constipation
- Fast heartbeat (palpitations)
- Headache
- Increased chance of breaking a hip
- Long-term memory problems (amnesia)
- Low blood pressure (hypotension)
- Nausea
- Rash (skin redness, bumps, itching, or irritation)
- Sadness, feeling blue or down, depressed mood (depression)
- Seeing or hearing things that are not there (hallucinations)
- Shakiness or tremors
- Slurred speech
- Trouble breathing or shortness of breath
- Trouble urinating or emptying the bladder

Rare

- Frequent fever, sore throat, or flu-like symptoms that may be a sign of low white blood cells
- Increased breast size in men
- Liver problems that may cause yellowing of the skin or eyes (jaundice)
- Ringing in the ears (tinnitus)

Tell your doctor or other healthcare professional if you have side effects that bother you, do not go away, make you worried about taking your medication, or make you want to stop taking your medication.

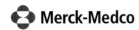

Do Other Medications Interact with Benzodiazepines?

Benzodiazepines *may increase* the side effects of other medications that cause drowsiness, including anticholinergic medications, antidepressants, antihistamines (allergy medications), antispasmodics, other benzodiazepines (a type of tranquilizer), other anxiety medications, narcotics (pain relievers), muscle relaxants, neuroleptic medications (a type of tranquilizer), seizure medications, or sleep medications. Avoid driving a car and other activities that need mental alertness, like using a knife or operating machinery, while taking these medications together.

Drinking alcoholic beverages (such as beer, wine, whiskey, and others) *may increase* the side effects of benzodiazepines.

These medications *may increase* the side effects of benzodiazepines:

- *Antabuse*® (disulfiram)
- *Biaxin*® (clarithromycin)
- *Crixivan*® (indinavir)
- Erythromycin such as *Ery-Tab*®, *Erythrocin*®, and others—see Glossary
- *Norvir*® (ritonavir)
- *Prilosec*® (omeprazole)
- *Sporanox*® (itraconazole)
- *Tagamet*® (cimetidine)
- *Zantac*® (ranitidine)

These medications *may decrease* how well benzodiazepines work:

- *Cerebyx*® (fosphenytoin)
- *Dilantin*® (phenytoin)
- *Rifadin*® (rifampin)
- *Tegretol*® (carbamazepine)

Grapefruit and grapefruit juice *may increase* the side effects of benzodiazepines. This interaction can happen whether you eat the grapefruit or drink the grapefruit juice at the same time as you take your medication or if you take the medication separately from the grapefruit or grapefruit juice. Talk to your doctor or other healthcare professional before eating grapefruit and drinking grapefruit juice if you are taking this medication. Please also read the discussion on A Warning about Grapefruit and Grapefruit Juice on pages i-ii.

Tell your doctor or other healthcare professional about all medications (both prescription and nonprescription [over-the-counter] medications) that you are taking.

Why Else Do People Take Benzodiazepines?

Some benzodiazepines may also be used to help reduce seizures, muscle spasms, and restless leg syndrome. Benzodiazepines are also used to treat insomnia.

 # Warning!

To give you the best care, your doctor or other healthcare professional needs to know about the diseases and medical conditions you have had—your full medical history. Tell your doctor or other healthcare professional if you have or have ever had any of the following:

- Allergy or previous reaction to benzodiazepines
- Breathing problems (asthma and COPD, including emphysema or chronic bronchitis)
- Glaucoma (an eye disease)
- High alcohol intake (drinking 3 or more alcoholic beverages, such as beer, wine, whiskey, and others, every day)
- Kidney problems
- Liver problems
- Sadness, feeling blue or down, depressed mood (depression)

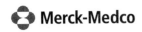

Klonopin® (clonazepam), *Libritabs*® (chlordiazepoxide), *Librium*® (chlordiazepoxide), *Paxipam*® (halazepam), *Tranxene*® (clorazepate), and *Valium*® (diazepam) are generally not recommended for use in people over the age of 65 because they are long-acting, and long-acting benzodiazepines have been associated with a higher risk of broken hips and car accidents than other, short-acting benzodiazepines. If you are taking any of these medications, ask your doctor or other healthcare professional if this medication is right for you. Do not stop taking this medication without talking to your doctor or other healthcare professional.

Benzodiazepines cause more side effects in older adults than in younger adults. Whenever possible, their use should be avoided. If a benzodiazepine is necessary, *Ativan*® (lorazepam), *Serax*® (oxazepam), and *Xanax*® (alprazolam) are generally recommended for anxiety.

If you are taking a benzodiazepine, stay out of the sun as much as you can to avoid a serious sunburn. When you do go out in the sun, use sunblock or sunscreen, and wear protective clothing, such as a wide-brimmed hat and a long-sleeved shirt.

After taking a benzodiazepine regularly, people may develop a strong need (dependence) for it. To help prevent this from happening, do not take benzodiazepines more often than prescribed by your doctor or other healthcare professional.

Benzodiazepines may cause drowsiness. Avoid driving a car and other activities that need mental alertness, like using a knife or operating machinery, while taking this medication. Drinking alcoholic beverages (such as beer, wine, whiskey, and others) may increase the side effects.

Benzodiazepines may make you unsteady on your feet, causing you to fall and possibly break a bone. If you have fallen recently, tell your doctor or other healthcare professional about it. Taking a different medication or a lower dose may make you less likely to fall. You should not stop taking this medication without first talking to your doctor or other healthcare professional.

Klonopin® (clonazepam) is sometimes confused with clonidine, which is taken for high blood pressure (hypertension). The names of the medications sound similar, but the medications themselves are very different. Talk to your doctor or other healthcare professional to make sure you are taking the right medications.

Under certain circumstances your doctor or other healthcare professional may decide that you should stop taking this medication. If you have taken it for more than a couple of weeks, he or she may want you to decrease it gradually, lowering the dose over a few weeks or months. Stopping suddenly may cause unpleasant withdrawal symptoms or may worsen your medical problems. Pay careful attention to the instructions your doctor or other healthcare professional gives you about how much less to take and for how long.

Antihistamines

Antihistamines that cause drowsiness may help relieve the symptoms of anxiety.

▲ Indicates medications that are more likely to cause unpleasant or dangerous side effects. These medications are generally not recommended for people over 65. The side effects may not be very obvious and may be mistaken for "just a part of getting older" but may be serious. If you are taking one of these medications, you might want to talk to your doctor or other healthcare professional to see if this medication is best for you. Safer medications may be available and lower dosages may be required. You should not stop taking these medications without first talking to your doctor or other healthcare professional.

See the WARNING section on page 24 for the specific safety problems associated with these medications ▲.

Brand Name	Generic Name
▲Atarax®	hydroxyzine
▲Vistaril®	hydroxyzine

How Will I Take Antihistamines?

Antihistamines are usually taken 1 to 4 times a day as needed for anxiety. Your doctor or other healthcare professional will tell you how many times a day to take your medication.

This medication is often used "as needed," so missing a dose should not be a problem. If you miss a dose and it is almost time for the next dose, you should skip the forgotten dose. Do not double the dose. Take your medication as directed by your doctor or other healthcare professional.

What Side Effects Can Antihistamines Cause?

More Common

- Blurred vision

- Constipation

- Diarrhea

- Dizziness when standing up from a bed or a chair

- Double vision

- Drowsiness

- Dry mouth, eyes, and nose

- Poor coordination and trouble walking

- Trouble urinating or emptying the bladder

Less Common

- Anxiety (nervousness)*

- Confusion

*Sometimes medications may actually cause or worsen the same symptoms they are being used to help relieve. Talk to your doctor or other healthcare professional if your symptoms get worse instead of better while taking this medication.

- Fainting

- Fast heartbeat (palpitations)

- Memory problems

- Nausea

- Poor appetite

- Reddening of the face (flushing)

- Shakiness or tremors

- Trouble breathing in asthma and COPD, including emphysema or chronic bronchitis

- Trouble falling asleep or staying asleep (insomnia)

- Vomiting

Tell your doctor or other healthcare professional if you have side effects that bother you, do not go away, make you worried about taking your medication, or make you want to stop taking your medication.

Do Other Medications Interact with Antihistamines?

Antihistamines *may increase* the side effects of other medications that cause drowsiness, including anticholinergic medications, antidepressants, other antihistamines (allergy medications), antispasmodics, benzodiazepines (a type of tranquilizer), other anxiety medications, narcotics (pain relievers), muscle relaxants, neuroleptic medications (a type of tranquilizer), seizure medications, or sleep medications. Avoid driving a car and other activities that need mental alertness, like using a knife or operating machinery, while taking these medications together.

Drinking alcoholic beverages (such as beer, wine, whiskey, and others) *may increase* the side effects of antihistamines.

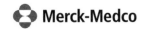

Many nonprescription (over-the-counter [OTC]) medications such as pain, cough, cold, allergy, and sleep medications contain antihistamines. If you are taking antihistamines regularly, you should talk to your doctor or other healthcare professional before taking any new OTC medications.

Tell your doctor or other healthcare professional about all medications (both prescription and nonprescription [over-the-counter] medications) that you are taking.

Why Else Do People Take Antihistamines?

Antihistamines may be taken for skin allergies, cold, flu, hay fever, and other allergic conditions. They may also be taken to help relieve insomnia.

 # Warning!

To give you the best care, your doctor or other healthcare professional needs to know about the diseases and medical conditions you have had—your full medical history. Tell your doctor or other healthcare professional if you have or have ever had any of the following:

- Allergy or previous reaction to antihistamines

- Breathing problems (asthma and COPD, including emphysema or chronic bronchitis)

- Enlarged prostate (benign prostatic hypertrophy)

- Glaucoma (an eye disease)

Antihistamines that cause drowsiness are generally not recommended for people over the age of 65 for anxiety because they may cause serious side effects, including dizziness, blurred vision, constipation, trouble urinating or emptying the bladder, confusion, and a fast heartbeat. If you are taking one of these medications, talk to your doctor or other healthcare professional to see if it is right for you. Do not stop taking this medication without first talking to your doctor or other healthcare professional.

Antihistamines may cause drowsiness. Avoid driving a car and other activities that need mental alertness, like using a knife or operating machinery, while taking this medication. Drinking alcoholic beverages (such as beer, wine, whiskey, and others) may increase the side effects.

Antihistamines may make you unsteady on your feet, causing you to fall and possibly break a bone. If you have fallen recently, tell your doctor or other healthcare professional about it. Taking a different medication or a lower dose may make you less likely to fall. You should not stop taking this medication without first talking to your doctor or other healthcare professional.

BuSpar® (buspirone)

BuSpar® (buspirone) may help relieve the symptoms of anxiety.

How Will I Take BuSpar® (buspirone)?

BuSpar® (buspirone) is usually taken 3 times a day. *BuSpar®* (buspirone) usually takes at least 2 weeks to work. Your doctor or other healthcare professional will tell you how many times a day to take your medication.

If you miss a dose of this medication, take the dose you missed as soon as possible. However, if it is almost time for your next dose, skip the missed dose and just take the next one. Do not double your dose. Take your medication exactly as directed by your doctor or other healthcare professional. Do not stop taking a prescription medication unless directed by your doctor or other healthcare professional.

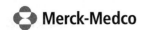

What Side Effects Can *BuSpar*® (buspirone) Cause?

More Common

- Anxiety (nervousness)*

- Dizziness

- Drowsiness

- Headache

- Nausea

Less Common

- Excitement*

- Sadness, feeling blue or down, depressed mood (depression)

- Weakness

*Sometimes medications may actually cause or worsen the same symptoms they are being used to help relieve. Talk to your doctor or other healthcare professional if your symptoms get worse instead of better while taking this medication.

Tell your doctor or other healthcare professional if you have side effects that bother you, do not go away, make you worried about taking your medication, or make you want to stop taking your medication.

Do Other Medications Interact with *BuSpar*® (buspirone)?

These medications *may increase* the side effects of *BuSpar*® (buspirone):

- *Biaxin*® (clarithromycin)

- *Diflucan*® (fluconazole)

- Diltiazem such as *Cardizem*®, *Cartia*®, *Tiazac*®, and others—see Glossary

- Erythromycin such as *Ery-Tab*®, *Erythrocin*®, and others—see Glossary

- *Nizoral*® (ketoconazole)

- *Sporanox*® (itraconazole)
- Verapamil such as *Calan*®, *Covera*®, *Verelan*®, and others—see Glossary

Rifadin® (rifampin) ***may decrease*** how well *BuSpar*® (buspirone) works.

BuSpar® (buspirone) is generally not prescribed for anyone who is taking MAO inhibitors, such as *Marplan*® (isocarboxazid), *Nardil*® (phenelzine), or *Parnate*® (tranylcypromine), because together they ***may cause*** serious or even fatal reactions. If your doctor or other healthcare professional wants you to stop taking one medication and start taking the other, you should wait at least 2 weeks between stopping one and starting the other.

BuSpar® (buspirone) ***may increase*** the side effects of other medications that cause drowsiness, including anticholinergic medications, antidepressants, antihistamines (allergy medications), antispasmodics, benzodiazepines (a type of tranquilizer), other anxiety medications, narcotics (pain relievers), muscle relaxants, neuroleptic medications (a type of tranquilizer), seizure medications, or sleep medications. Avoid driving a car and other activities that need mental alertness, like using a knife or operating machinery, while taking these medications together.

Grapefruit and grapefruit juice ***may increase*** the side effects of *BuSpar*® (buspirone). This interaction can happen whether you eat the grapefruit or drink the grapefruit juice at the same time as you take your medication or if you take the medication separately from the grapefruit or grapefruit juice. Talk to your doctor or other healthcare professional before eating grapefruit or drinking grapefruit juice if you are taking this medication. Please also read the discussion on A Warning about Grapefruit and Grapefruit Juice on pages i-ii.

Drinking alcoholic beverages (such as beer, wine, whiskey, and others) ***may increase*** the side effects of *BuSpar*® (buspirone).

Tell your doctor or other healthcare professional about all medications (both prescription and nonprescription [over-the-counter] medications) that you are taking.

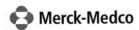

 # Warning!

To give you the best care, your doctor or other healthcare professional needs to know about the diseases and medical conditions you have had—your full medical history. Tell your doctor or other healthcare professional if you have or have ever had, or presently take, any of the following:

- Allergy or previous reaction to *BuSpar®* (buspirone)

- Liver problems

- MAO inhibitors such as *Marplan®* (isocarboxazid), *Nardil®* (phenelzine), or *Parnate®* (tranylcypromine)—see Glossary

BuSpar® (buspirone) may cause drowsiness. Avoid driving a car and other activities that need mental alertness, like using a knife or operating machinery, while taking this medication. Drinking alcoholic beverages (such as beer, wine, whiskey, and others) may increase the side effects.

Effexor® (venlafaxine)

Effexor® (venlafaxine) may help relieve the symptoms of anxiety.

How Will I Take *Effexor®* (venlafaxine)?

Effexor® (venlafaxine) is usually taken once a day with food. Your doctor or other healthcare professional will tell you how often to take this medication.

When a medication has initials after its name, such as XL, XR, SR, BID, DUR, and others, it usually means that the body absorbs the medication slowly over time, so you usually have to take it only once or twice a day. The body will absorb some medications of this type too fast if you crush or break them or dissolve them in liquid, and their effects will not last as long as they should. Check with your doctor or other healthcare professional before crushing or breaking your pills or dissolving your pills in liquid.

If you miss a dose of this medication, take the dose you missed as soon as possible. However, if it is almost time for your next dose, skip the missed dose and just take the next one. Do not double your dose. Take your medication exactly as directed by your doctor or other healthcare professional. Do not stop taking a prescription medication unless directed by your doctor or other healthcare professional.

What Side Effects Can *Effexor*® (venlafaxine) Cause?

More Common

- Anxiety (nervousness)*
- Blurred vision
- Constipation
- Dizziness when standing up from a bed or a chair
- Drowsiness
- Dry mouth
- Ejaculation problems (erectile dysfunction)
- Headache
- Increased or excessive sweating (perspiration)
- Nausea
- Trouble falling asleep or staying asleep (insomnia)

Less Common

- Fast heartbeat (palpitations)
- High blood pressure (hypertension)
- Rash (skin redness, bumps, itching, or irritation)

*Sometimes medications may actually cause or worsen the same symptoms they are being used to help relieve. Talk to your doctor or other healthcare professional if your symptoms get worse instead of better while taking this medication.

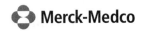
- Ringing in the ears (tinnitus)

- Trouble urinating or emptying the bladder

Rare

- Seizures

Tell your doctor or other healthcare professional if you have side effects that bother you, do not go away, make you worried about taking your medication, or make you want to stop taking your medication.

 ## Do Other Medications Interact with *Effexor®* (venlafaxine)?

Effexor® (venlafaxine) is generally not prescribed for anyone who is taking MAO inhibitors, such as *Marplan®* (isocarboxazid), *Nardil®* (phenelzine), or *Parnate®* (tranylcypromine), because together they ***may cause*** serious or even fatal reactions. If your doctor or other healthcare professional wants you to stop taking one medication and start taking the other, you should wait at least 2 weeks between stopping one and starting the other.

Effexor® (venlafaxine) is generally not prescribed for anyone who is taking triptans (migraine medications) such as *Imitrex®* (sumatriptan) and *Zomig®* (zolmitriptan) or for anyone who is taking *Meridia®* (sibutramine) or other appetite suppressants because together they ***may cause*** serious or even fatal reactions. Taken together, they may cause anxiety (nervousness), muscle weakness, confusion, and seizures.

Effexor® (venlafaxine) ***may increase*** the side effects of other medications that cause drowsiness, including anticholinergic medications, antidepressants, antihistamines (allergy medications), antispasmodics, benzodiazepines (a type of tranquilizer), other anxiety medications, narcotics (pain relievers), muscle relaxants, neuroleptic medications (a type of tranquilizer), seizure medications, or sleep medications. Avoid driving a car and other activities that need mental alertness, like using a knife or operating machinery, while taking these medications together.

Drinking alcoholic beverages (such as beer, wine, whiskey, and others) ***may increase*** the side effects of *Effexor®* (venlafaxine).

Tell your doctor or other healthcare professional about all medications (both prescription and nonprescription [over-the-counter] medications) that you are taking.

Why Else Do People Take *Effexor®* (venlafaxine)?

Effexor® (venlafaxine) is also taken for depression.

 # Warning!

To give you the best care, your doctor or other healthcare professional needs to know about the diseases and medical conditions you have had—your full medical history. Tell your doctor or other healthcare professional if you have or have ever had, or presently take, any of the following:

- Allergy or previous reaction to *Effexor®* (venlafaxine)

- Heart problems

- High blood pressure (hypertension)

- Kidney problems

- Liver problems

- Manic depression

- MAO inhibitors such as *Marplan®* (isocarboxazid), *Nardil®* (phenelzine), or *Parnate®* (tranylcypromine)—see Glossary

- Seizures (epilepsy)

- Trouble falling asleep or staying asleep (insomnia)

Effexor® (venlafaxine) may make you unsteady on your feet, causing you to fall and possibly break a bone. If you have fallen recently, tell your doctor or other

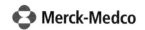
healthcare professional about it. Taking a different medication or a lower dose may make you less likely to fall. You should not stop taking this medication without first talking to your doctor or other healthcare professional.

Effexor® (venlafaxine) may cause drowsiness. Avoid driving a car and other activities that need mental alertness, like using a knife or operating machinery, while taking this medication. Drinking alcoholic beverages (such as beer, wine, whiskey, and others) may increase the side effects.

Under certain circumstances, your doctor or other healthcare professional may decide that you should stop taking this medication. If you have taken it for more than a couple of weeks, he or she may want you to decrease it gradually, lowering the dose over a few weeks or months. Stopping suddenly may cause unpleasant withdrawal symptoms or may worsen your medical problems. Pay careful attention to the instructions your doctor or other healthcare professional gives you about how much less to take and for how long.

Meprobamate

Meprobamate may help relieve the symptoms of anxiety.

▲ Indicates medications that are more likely to cause unpleasant or dangerous side effects. These medications are generally not recommended for people over 65. The side effects may not be very obvious and may be mistaken for "just a part of getting older" but may be serious. If you are taking one of these medications, you might want to talk to your doctor or other healthcare professional to see if this medication is best for you. Safer medications may be available and lower dosages may be required. You should not stop taking these medications without first talking to your doctor or other healthcare professional.

See the WARNING section on page 35 for the specific safety problems associated with these medications ▲.

Brand Name	Generic Name
▲Equanil®	meprobamate
▲Miltown®	meprobamate

How Will I Take Meprobamate?

Meprobamate is usually taken 2 to 4 times a day as needed for anxiety. Your doctor or other healthcare professional will tell you how to take this medication.

This medication is often used "as needed," so missing a dose should not be a problem. If you miss a dose and it is almost time for the next dose, you should skip the forgotten dose. Do not double the dose. Take your medication as directed by your doctor or other healthcare professional.

What Side Effects Can Meprobamate Cause?

More Common

- Diarrhea
- Dizziness
- Drowsiness
- Nausea
- Vomiting

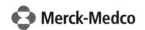
Less Common

- Excitement*

- Headache

- Weakness

Rare

- Allergic reaction such as rash (skin redness, bumps, itching, or irritation), swelling of the face and throat, or trouble breathing

- Bleeding that does not stop easily (nose bleeds, bleeding while brushing your teeth, and cuts)

- Blurred vision

- Easy bruising ("black-and-blue" marks on the skin)

- Frequent fever, sore throat, or flu-like symptoms that may be a sign of low white blood cells

- Irregular heartbeat (palpitations)

- Seizures

- Slurred speech

*Sometimes medications may actually cause or worsen the same symptoms they are being used to help relieve. Talk to your doctor or other healthcare professional if your symptoms get worse instead of better while taking this medication.

Tell your doctor or other healthcare professional if you have side effects that bother you, do not go away, make you worried about taking your medication, or make you want to stop taking your medication.

 Do Other Medications Interact with Meprobamate?

Meprobamate *may increase* the side effects of other medications that cause drowsiness, including anticholinergic medications, antidepressants, antihistamines (allergy medications), antispasmodics, benzodiazepines (a type of tranquilizer), other anxiety medications, narcotics (pain relievers), muscle relaxants, neuroleptic medications (a type of tranquilizer), seizure medications, or sleep medications. Avoid driving a car and other activities that need mental alertness, like using a knife or operating machinery, while taking these medications together.

Drinking alcoholic beverages (such as beer, wine, whiskey, and others) *may increase* the side effects of meprobamate.

Tell your doctor or other healthcare professional about all medications (both prescription and nonprescription [over-the-counter] medications) that you are taking.

Why Else Do People Take Meprobamate?

Meprobamate may also be used to treat trouble falling asleep or staying asleep (insomnia).

 # Warning!

To give you the best care, your doctor or other healthcare professional needs to know about the diseases and medical conditions you have had—your full medical history. Tell your doctor or other healthcare professional if you have or have ever had any of the following:

- Allergy or previous reaction to meprobamate
- Kidney problems
- Liver problems
- Seizures (epilepsy)

Meprobamate is generally not recommended for people over the age of 65 for anxiety because it may cause a strong need for the medication (dependence) and serious side effects, including dizziness and blurred vision. If you are taking this

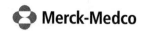

medication, talk to your doctor or other healthcare professional to see if it is right for you. Do not stop taking this medication without first talking to your doctor or other healthcare professional.

Meprobamate may cause drowsiness. Avoid driving a car and other activities that need mental alertness, like using a knife or operating machinery, while taking this medication. Drinking alcoholic beverages (such as beer, wine, whiskey, and others) may increase the side effects.

If you have had seizures in the past, tell your doctor or other healthcare professional because meprobamate may cause seizures. Stopping this medication suddenly may also cause seizures. If your doctor or other healthcare professional decides that you should stop taking meprobamate, pay careful attention to the instructions he or she gives you about how much less to take and for how long.

Meprobamate may make you unsteady on your feet, causing you to fall and possibly break a bone. If you have fallen recently, tell your doctor or other healthcare professional about it. Taking a different medication or a lower dose may make you less likely to fall. You should not stop taking this medication without first talking to your doctor or other healthcare professional.

After taking meprobamate regularly, people may develop a strong need (dependence) for it. To help prevent this from happening, do not take meprobamate more often than prescribed by your doctor or other healthcare professional.

Under certain circumstances your doctor or other healthcare professional may decide that you should stop taking this medication. If you have taken it for more than a couple of weeks, he or she may want you to decrease it gradually, lowering the dose over a few weeks or months. Stopping suddenly may cause unpleasant withdrawal symptoms or may worsen your medical problems. Pay careful attention to the instructions your doctor or other healthcare professional gives you about how much less to take and for how long.

Arthritis and Pain

What Is Arthritis?

Arthritis is a general term that includes several different conditions. Arthritis is usually caused by wear and tear on the joints or by inflammation (swelling, pain, and redness) from an overactive immune system. Osteoarthritis is the most common type of arthritis in people over 65 and is caused by wear and tear on the joints. In fact, osteoarthritis is one of the most common medical problems in older adults. Rheumatoid arthritis is caused by inflammation. Rheumatoid arthritis is less common in older adults than osteoarthritis.

Treatment of osteoarthritis may include weight reduction, exercise, physical therapy, pain medication, and sometimes surgery. Treatment of rheumatoid arthritis may include exercise, physical therapy, pain medication, and medications that help prevent the immune system from damaging the joints. Talk to your doctor or other healthcare professional before starting an exercise program to find out what types of exercise can help your arthritis symptoms without causing wear and tear on your joints.

This chapter focuses on pain medications used for osteoarthritis. Many of the pain medications discussed in the chapter may also be used to help relieve the pain of rheumatoid arthritis and other types of arthritis. Many medications used for rheumatoid arthritis that work by preventing the immune system from causing joint damage are not discussed in this chapter.

What Is Pain?

Pain is usually a sign that the body has been damaged or injured. Depending on the situation, the cause may be inflammation (pain, swelling, and redness), an infection, or a pressure on the tissues somewhere in the body.

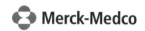
Pain that starts suddenly and lasts only a short while is called acute pain. Long-lasting pain is called chronic pain. Pain impulses usually start in nerve endings in the skin or in joints, muscles, or organs. The pain signals travel along nerves to areas in the brain that can receive those signals (pain receptors). The brain senses the pain and sends uncomfortable messages to different parts of the body.

Feeling pain is not "normal" for anyone. If you have pain for more than a week, tell your doctor or other healthcare professional. He or she can help you find out what is causing the pain and try to find ways to help you feel better.

Medications for Arthritis and Pain

Several kinds of medications may be taken for arthritis and pain. This chapter discusses these medications and/or categories of medications that can be taken for pain of both osteoarthritis and rheumatoid arthritis.

MEDICATIONS	See Page
Acetaminophen	39
Nonsteroidal Anti-inflammatory Drugs (NSAIDs)	42
COX-2 Inhibitors (Coxibs)	50
Aspirin and Aspirin-like Medications (Salicylates)	55
Narcotics and Narcotic-like Medications	60
Ultram® (tramadol)	68
Corticosteroids	72
Tricyclic Antidepressants	77
Tegretol® (carbamazepine) and Trileptal® (oxcarbazepine)	83
Neurontin® (gabapentin)	90
Capsaicin	93

If you do not see the exact name of the medication that you take for arthritis or pain listed above, check the Medication and Chapter Table to find out which category your medication falls under or check the Index.

Other medications (such as hydroxychloroquine and gold medications) help prevent damage to the joints caused by rheumatoid arthritis but are not used for osteoarthritis. These medications are not discussed in this chapter.

Acetaminophen

Acetaminophen works well for mild-to-moderate aches and pains. Unlike some other pain medications, acetaminophen does not irritate the stomach. Your doctor or other healthcare professional may suggest trying acetaminophen first for your osteoarthritis pain. Acetaminophen does not reduce swelling, but it can relieve the pain caused by inflammation (pain, swelling, and redness). Acetaminophen is available over-the-counter (OTC) without a prescription.

Brand Name	Generic Name
Anacin® Aspirin Free	acetaminophen
Genapap™	acetaminophen
Panadol®	acetaminophen
Tylenol®	acetaminophen

How Will I Take Acetaminophen?

Acetaminophen comes in a pill or liquid form and also as a suppository to be inserted into the rectum. It is usually taken as needed every 4 to 6 hours, either with or without food. The most acetaminophen that anyone should take in 1 day is 4000 mg (8 extra-strength 500-mg tablets or 12 regular-strength 325-mg tablets). Follow the instructions on the package or ask your doctor or other healthcare professional how much to take and how many times a day to take your medication.

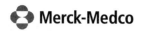

This medication is often used "as needed," so missing a dose should not be a problem. If you miss a dose and it is almost time for the next dose, you should skip the forgotten dose. Do not double the dose. Take your medication as directed by your doctor or other healthcare professional.

What Side Effects Can Acetaminophen Cause?

Rare

- Allergic reactions such as rash (skin redness, bumps, itching, or irritation), swelling of the face and throat, or trouble breathing

- Liver problems that may cause yellowing of the skin or eyes (jaundice)

Tell your doctor or other healthcare professional if you have side effects that bother you, do not go away, make you worried about taking your medication, or make you want to stop taking your medication.

Do Other Medications Interact with Acetaminophen?

Tylenol® (acetaminophen) taken regularly with the following medications *may increase* the side effects of these medications:

- *Anturane*® (sulfinpyrazone)

- *Coumadin*® (warfarin)

- *Dilantin*® (phenytoin)

Drinking alcoholic beverages (such as beer, wine, whiskey, and others) *may increase* the side effects of *Tylenol*® (acetaminophen).

Many nonprescription (over-the-counter [OTC]) medications such as pain, cough, cold, allergy, and sleep medications contain acetaminophen. If you are taking acetaminophen regularly, you should talk to your doctor or other healthcare professional before taking any new OTC medications.

Tell your doctor or other healthcare professional about all medications (both prescription and nonprescription [over-the-counter] medications) that you are taking.

Why Else Do People Take Acetaminophen?

Acetaminophen is also used for lowering a fever.

 # Warning!

To give you the best care, your doctor or other healthcare professional needs to know about the diseases and medical conditions you have had—your full medical history. Tell your doctor or other healthcare professional if you have or have ever had any of the following:

- Allergy or previous reaction to acetaminophen
- High alcohol intake (drinking 3 or more alcoholic beverages, such as beer, wine, whiskey, and others, every day)
- Liver problems

If you accidentally take too much acetaminophen (or any other medication), call your doctor or other healthcare professional immediately.

If you drink 3 or more alcoholic beverages, such as beer, wine, whiskey, and others, every day, you should not take more than 2000 mg of acetaminophen in a day (4 extra-strength 500-mg tablets or 6 regular-strength 325-mg tablets). Taking more than 2000 mg may cause or worsen liver problems.

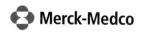

Nonsteroidal Anti-inflammatory Drugs (NSAIDs)

NSAIDs help to relieve pain and reduce swelling and redness. There are many different NSAIDs (see the list that follows). Most work in about the same way and cause similar side effects. Some, such as *Daypro®* (oxaprozin), have longer-lasting effects and may be taken once a day. Other NSAIDs, such as *Motrin®* (ibuprofen) and *Advil®* (ibuprofen), may work faster but do not last as long, so they must be taken more often. Most NSAIDs are available by prescription. Ibuprofen, naproxen, and ketoprofen are available without a prescription.

▲ Indicates medications that are more likely to cause unpleasant or dangerous side effects. These medications are generally not recommended for people over 65. The side effects may not be very obvious and may be mistaken for "just a part of getting older" but may be serious. If you are taking one of these medications, you might want to talk to your doctor or other healthcare professional to see if this medication is best for you. Safer medications may be available and lower dosages may be required. You should not stop taking these medications without first talking to your doctor or other healthcare professional.

See the WARNING section on page 48 for the specific safety problems associated with this medication ▲.

Brand Name	Generic Name
Advil®*	ibuprofen*
Aleve®*	naproxen*
Anaprox®	naproxen
Ansaid®	flurbiprofen
Arthrotec®	diclofenac/misoprostol
Cataflam®	diclofenac
Clinoril®	sulindac
Daypro®	oxaprozin
Feldene®	piroxicam
▲Indocin®	indomethacin
Lodine®	etodolac
Mobic®	meloxicam
Motrin®*	ibuprofen*
Nalfon®	fenoprofen
Naprelan®	naproxen
Naprosyn®	naproxen
Orudis®*	ketoprofen*
Oruvail®	ketoprofen
Relafen®	nabumetone
Tolectin®	tolmetin
Toradol®	ketorolac
Voltaren®	diclofenac
Various	meclofenamate

*These medications are available by prescription or can be purchased over-the-counter without a prescription.

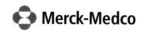

There is a newer kind of NSAID called a COX-2 inhibitor or coxib. These are also used for pain and arthritis, but they have different side effects. They are discussed in the next section of this chapter. Please see the next section if you are taking *Celebrex®* (celecoxib) or *Vioxx®* (rofecoxib).

 ## How Will I Take NSAIDs?

NSAIDs come in the form of pills, syrups, suppositories to be inserted into the rectum, and injections. NSAIDs are usually taken 1 to 4 times a day. Your doctor or other healthcare professional will tell you how many times a day to take your medication. NSAIDs are often taken with food to help prevent stomach upset. Take the medication with a full 8-ounce glass of water to keep the pills from sticking in your throat, which can cause irritation.

It may take a week or more before you feel the full effects of the medication. Your doctor or other healthcare professional may prescribe several different NSAIDs before finding the one that works best for you.

When a medication has initials such as XL, XR, SR, BID, or DUR after its name, it usually means that the body absorbs the medication slowly over time, so you usually have to take it only once or twice a day. The body will absorb some medications of this type too fast if you crush or break them or dissolve them in liquid, and their effects will not last as long as they should. Check with your doctor or other healthcare professional before crushing or breaking your pills or dissolving your pills in liquid.

This medication is often used "as needed," so missing a dose should not be a problem. If you miss a dose and it is almost time for the next dose, you should skip the forgotten dose. Do not double the dose. Take your medication as directed by your doctor or other healthcare professional.

What Side Effects Can NSAIDs Cause?

More Common

- Constipation
- Heartburn
- Nausea
- Stomach pain
- Vomiting

Less Common

- Allergic reactions such as rash (skin redness, bumps, itching, or irritation), swelling of the face and throat, or trouble breathing
- Diarrhea
- Dizziness
- Headache
- Hearing loss
- Increased sensitivity to the sun (bad sunburn)
- Kidney problems
- Ringing in the ears (tinnitus)
- Swelling or puffiness of the feet, ankles, or lower legs (edema)
- Ulcers in the stomach that may cause black, tarry-looking bowel movements

Rare

- Bleeding that does not stop easily (nose bleeds, bleeding while brushing your teeth, and cuts)
- Blurred vision
- Confusion, especially with *Indocin*® (indomethacin)
- Fast heartbeat (palpitations)
- Liver problems that may cause yellowing of the skin or eyes (jaundice)

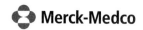

- Loss of taste or changes in the way things taste
- Sadness, feeling blue or down, depressed mood (depression)

Tell your doctor or other healthcare professional if you have side effects that bother you, do not go away, make you worried about taking your medication, or make you want to stop taking your medication.

 ## Do Other Medications Interact with NSAIDs?

Many nonprescription (over-the-counter [OTC]) medications such as pain, cough, cold, allergy, and sleep medications contain aspirin or NSAIDs. If you are taking NSAIDs regularly, you should talk to your doctor or other healthcare professional before taking any new OTC medications.

NSAIDs *may decrease* how well these medications work:

- Diuretics (water pills) such as *HydroDIURIL*® (hydrochlorothiazide or HCTZ), *Lasix*® (furosemide), and others—see Glossary
- High blood pressure (hypertension) medications—see Glossary

NSAIDs *may increase* the side effects of these medications:

- *Aggrenox*® (dipyridamole and aspirin)
- Aspirin, aspirin-containing medications, or aspirin-like medications (salicylates)—see Glossary
- Corticosteroids such as prednisone and others—see Glossary
- *Coumadin*® (warfarin)
- Heparin
- Lithium such as *Eskalith*®, *Lithobid*®, and others—see Glossary
- *Lovenox*® (enoxaparin)
- *Neoral*® (cyclosporine)

- *Persantine*® (dipyridamole)

- *Rheumatrex*® (methotrexate)

- *Sandimmune*® (cyclosporine)

Bile acid binders such as *Questran*® (cholestyramine) or *Colestid*® (colestipol) or bulk-forming laxatives like *Metamucil*® (psyllium) **may decrease** the effects of NSAIDs by preventing them from being absorbed completely. To help make sure they are absorbed so they can work properly, take NSAIDs 1 hour before or 4 to 6 hours after taking a bile acid binder or a bulk-forming laxative.

Drinking alcoholic beverages (such as beer, wine, whiskey, and others) **may increase** the side effects of NSAIDs.

Tell your doctor or other healthcare professional about all medications (both prescription and nonprescription [over-the-counter] medications) that you are taking.

Why Else Do People Take NSAIDs?

NSAIDs can also help to lower a fever. Some NSAIDs come as eyedrops for eye irritation and pain.

What Else Should I Know about NSAIDs?

Many NSAIDs are available without a prescription. These medications may cause the same unpleasant side effects as medications that do require a prescription.

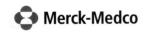

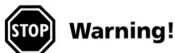 # Warning!

To give you the best care, your doctor or other healthcare professional needs to know about the diseases and medical conditions you have had—your full medical history. Tell your doctor or other healthcare professional if you have or have ever had, any of the following:

- Allergy or previous reaction to aspirin or NSAIDs

- Asthma or nasal polyps (overgrowth of tissue in the nose)

- Bleeding problems

- Congestive heart failure

- High alcohol intake (drinking 3 or more alcoholic beverages, such as beer, wine, whiskey, and others, every day)

- High blood pressure (hypertension)

- Kidney problems

- Liver problems

- Stomach problems (ulcer)

Indocin® (indomethacin) may cause confusion, nervousness (anxiety), and seeing or hearing things that are not there (hallucinations). It may also cause the stomach problems described below. This medication is not generally recommended for use in people over 65. If you are taking *Indocin*® (indomethacin), ask your doctor or other healthcare professional if it is the right medication for you. Do not stop taking the medication without talking to your doctor or other healthcare professional.

NSAIDs may cause stomach pain, which may be a sign of an ulcer. However, you may have an ulcer without feeling any pain at all. If ulcers are not treated, they may cause serious stomach or intestinal bleeding. Tell your doctor or other healthcare professional if you have severe stomach pain or stomach pain that keeps returning or if you have ever had peptic ulcer disease. Call your doctor or other healthcare professional right away if you have black, tarry-looking bowel movements (stools), if you vomit dark material that looks like coffee grounds, or if you notice any blood in your bowel movements. Any of these symptoms may be a sign of a bleeding ulcer.

Arthrotec® (diclofenac/misoprostol) can cause cramping stomach pain and diarrhea that usually start in the first few weeks of treatment and stop 1 to 2 weeks later. Tell your doctor or other healthcare professional if you have or have ever had inflammatory bowel disease (ulcerative colitis or Crohn's disease). Taking your pills with meals and at bedtime may decrease the diarrhea and cramping. Avoid antacids that contain magnesium such as *Maalox®* and *Mylanta®* (magnesium/aluminum), which may cause diarrhea. Talk to your doctor or other healthcare professional if the diarrhea and pain continue.

Taking NSAIDs may sometimes cause allergic reactions such as a rash, wheezing, and trouble breathing. People who have a bad reaction when they take aspirin are the ones most likely to get this kind of allergic reaction. If you have had a previous reaction to aspirin or any other NSAID, talk to your doctor or other healthcare professional before starting to take NSAIDs.

Toradol® (ketorolac) is usually taken for up to 5 days. Taking it for longer than that could cause bleeding in the stomach (an ulcer). If you are taking *Toradol®* (ketorolac) for more than 5 days, ask your doctor or other healthcare professional how long you should continue taking this medication.

Taking an NSAID if you have kidney problems, liver problems, high blood pressure, or congestive heart failure may make any of these conditions worse. If you have any of these conditions, talk with your doctor or other healthcare professional about it, especially before taking any nonprescription (over-the-counter) medications. Many over-the-counter medications contain NSAIDs and could be harmful.

NSAIDs may prevent blood from clotting as well as usual. If you are going to have surgery, you should talk to your doctor or other healthcare professional about whether you should stop taking NSAIDs before surgery. Depending on the kind of NSAID you are taking, you may need to stop your NSAID for a few days or a week before surgery. This problem does not occur with the kind of NSAIDs that are called COX-2 inhibitors, such as *Celebrex®* (celecoxib) or *Vioxx®* (rofecoxib).

If you are taking NSAIDs, stay out of the sun as much as you can to avoid a serious sunburn. When you do go out in the sun, use sunblock or sunscreen, and wear protective clothing, such as a wide-brimmed hat and a long-sleeved shirt.

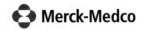

COX-2 Inhibitors (Coxibs)

COX is an abbreviation for cyclooxygenase, an enzyme in the body. Medications that block cyclooxygenase in the body help to relieve pain and reduce the swelling and redness of inflammation. There are 2 kinds of COX enzymes—COX-1 and COX-2. NSAIDs like *Motrin®* (ibuprofen), *Aleve®* (naproxen), and others (see Glossary), block both COX-1 and COX-2, and may cause the unwanted side effects of stomach irritation, ulcers, and bleeding. These side effects are mostly caused by blocking COX-1. COX-2 medications also reduce the swelling and redness of inflammation, but they do that by mainly blocking COX-2 (and not COX-1). While there are recent studies showing a reduced frequency of some stomach side effects when COX-2 inhibitors are used in people with osteoarthritis and rheumatoid arthritis, these drugs are, in general, associated with the same side effects as other NSAIDs and their risks compared to other NSAIDs are still being defined.

Brand Name	Generic Name
Celebrex®	celecoxib
Vioxx®	rofecoxib

 ## How Will I Take COX-2 Inhibitors?

COX-2 inhibitors are usually taken 1 to 2 times daily. They may be taken with or without food. If the medication upsets your stomach, it may be taken with food. Take the medication with a full 8-ounce glass of water to keep the pills from sticking in your throat, which can cause irritation. Your doctor or other healthcare professional will tell you how many times a day to take your medication.

This medication is often used "as needed," so missing a dose should not be a problem. If you miss a dose and it is almost time for the next dose, you should skip the forgotten dose. Do not double the dose. Take your medication as directed by your doctor or other healthcare professional.

What Side Effects Do COX-2 Inhibitors Cause?

More Common

- Constipation
- Diarrhea
- Heartburn
- Nausea
- Stomach pain
- Vomiting

Less Common

- Allergic reactions such as rash (skin redness, bumps, itching, or irritation), swelling of the face and throat, or trouble breathing
- Dizziness
- Headache
- Hearing loss
- Itching
- Kidney problems
- Swelling or puffiness of the feet, ankles, or lower legs (edema)

Rare

- Blurred vision
- Fast heartbeat (palpitations)
- Liver problems that may cause yellowing of the skin or eyes (jaundice)
- Ringing in the ears (tinnitus)
- Ulcers in the stomach that may cause black, tarry-looking bowel movements

---

Tell your doctor or other healthcare professional if you have side effects that bother you, do not go away, make you worried about taking your medication, or make you want to stop taking your medication.

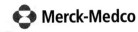

Do Other Medications Interact with COX-2 Inhibitors?

Many nonprescription (over-the-counter [OTC]) medications such as pain, cough, cold, allergy, and sleep medications contain aspirin or other NSAIDs, which *may increase* the side effects of COX-2 inhibitors. If you are taking COX-2 inhibitors regularly, you should talk to your doctor or other healthcare professional before taking any new OTC medications.

COX-2 inhibitors *may decrease* how well these medications work:

- Diuretics (water pills) such as *HydroDIURIL*® (hydrochlorothiazide or HCTZ), *Lasix*® (furosemide), and others—see Glossary

- High blood pressure (hypertension) medications—see Glossary

These medications *may increase* the side effects of *Celebrex*® (celecoxib):

- *Diflucan*® (fluconazole)

- *Nizoral*® (ketoconazole)

- *Sporanox*® (itraconazole)

COX-2 inhibitors *may increase* the side effects of these medications:

- *Aggrenox*® (dipyridamole and aspirin)

- Aspirin, aspirin-containing medications, and aspirin-like medications (salicylates)—see Glossary

- Corticosteroids such as prednisone and others—see Glossary

- *Coumadin*® (warfarin)

- Heparin

- Lithium such as *Eskalith*®, *Lithobid*®, and others—see Glossary

- *Lovenox*® (enoxaparin)

- *Rheumatrex*® (methotrexate)

Rifadin® (rifampin) *may decrease* how well *Vioxx*® (rofecoxib) works.

Drinking alcoholic beverages (such as beer, wine, whiskey, and others) *may increase* the side effects of COX-2 inhibitors.

Tell your doctor or other healthcare professional about all medications (both prescription and nonprescription [over-the-counter] medications) that you are taking.

What Else Should I Know about COX-2 Inhibitors?

The name of the COX-2 inhibitor, *Celebrex*® (celecoxib), is similar to the names of medications for very different problems. For example, *Celexa*™ (citalopram) is a medication for depression, and *Cerebyx*® (fosphenytoin) is a medication for seizures (epilepsy). Always read the label on the prescription bottle carefully to be sure you are taking the medication that was prescribed for you.

Warning!

To give you the best care, your doctor or other healthcare professional needs to know about the diseases and medical conditions you have had—your full medical history. Tell your doctor or other healthcare professional if you have or have ever had any of the following:

- Allergy or previous reaction to any of the following:

    ◆ Aspirin and aspirin-containing medications

    ◆ Carbonic anhydrase inhibitors such as *Azopt*® (brinzolamide), *Diamox*® (acetazolamide), *Trusopt*® (dorzolamide), and others—see Glossary

    ◆ Diabetes medications such as *Glucotrol*® (glipizide), *DiaBeta*® (glyburide), and others—see Glossary

    ◆ Diuretics (water pills) such as *HydroDIURIL*® (hydrochlorothiazide or HCTZ), *Lasix*® (furosemide), and others—see Glossary

    ◆ Nonsteroidal anti-inflammatory drugs (NSAIDs) such as *Motrin*® (ibuprofen), *Aleve*® (naproxen), *Vioxx*® (rofecoxib), *Celebrex*® (celecoxib), and others—see Glossary

    ◆ Sulfa medications such as *Bactrim*™, *Septra*®, and others—see Glossary

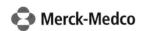

- Asthma or nasal polyps (overgrowth of tissue in the nose)
- Congestive heart failure
- High blood pressure (hypertension)
- Kidney problems
- Liver problems
- Stomach problems (ulcer)

Taking COX-2 inhibitors can sometimes cause allergic reactions such as a rash, wheezing, and trouble breathing. People who have a bad reaction when they take aspirin are the ones most likely to get this kind of allergic reaction. If you have had a previous unpleasant reaction to aspirin or any other NSAIDs, talk to your doctor or other healthcare professional before taking COX-2 inhibitors.

If you are allergic to sulfas, you may be allergic to *Celebrex*® (celecoxib). If you have had an allergic reaction to sulfa, which may be found in antibiotics such as *Septra*® (cotrimoxazole) and *Bactrim*™ (cotrimoxazole), diuretics such as *HydroDIURIL*® (hydrochlorothiazide or HCTZ), and diabetes medication such as *Diabinese*® (chlorpropamide), you may have an allergic reaction to *Celebrex*® (celecoxib). Tell your doctor or other healthcare professional about your allergies before taking *Celebrex*® (celecoxib).

COX-2 inhibitors may cause stomach pain, which may be a sign of an ulcer. However, you may have an ulcer without feeling any pain at all. If ulcers are not treated, they may cause serious stomach or intestinal bleeding. Tell your doctor or other healthcare professional if you have severe stomach pain or stomach pain that keeps returning or if you have ever had peptic ulcer disease. Call your doctor or other healthcare professional right away if you have black, tarry-looking bowel movements (stools), if you vomit dark material that looks like coffee grounds, or if you notice any blood in your bowel movements. Any of these symptoms may be a sign of a bleeding ulcer.

Aspirin and Aspirin-like Medications (Salicylates)

Aspirin and the other salicylates are often used for arthritis and pain. Like other NSAIDs, aspirin and other salicylates may help to relieve pain, reduce swelling, and control fever. To lessen inflammation (pain, swelling, and redness), salicylates must be taken in larger doses than you would need to relieve pain or control fever. Higher doses may be needed for rheumatoid arthritis than for osteoarthritis. Aspirin and some salicylates are available over-the-counter without a prescription, and some salicylates are available only with a prescription. Follow the directions on the package or ask your doctor or other healthcare professional how much and how often to take your medication.

Brand Name	Generic Name
Arthritis Pain Formula™*	aspirin*
Ascriptin®*	aspirin*
Bufferin®*	aspirin*
Disalcid®	salsalate
Doan's®*	magnesium salicylate*
Dolobid®	diflunisal
Ecotrin®*	aspirin*
Empirin®*	aspirin*
Magan®	magnesium salicylate
Mobidin®	magnesium salicylate
Trilisate®	choline magnesium trisalicylate
ZORprin®	aspirin

*Can be purchased over-the-counter without a prescription

How Will I Take Aspirin and Aspirin-like Medications (Salicylates)?

Salicylates come in the form of pills to be taken by mouth or suppositories to be inserted into the rectum. Keep suppositories in the refrigerator. Do not freeze. Salicylates are usually taken 1 to 2 times a day or as needed every 4 hours, depending on the kind you are taking. Follow the instructions on the package or ask your doctor or other healthcare professional how many times a day to take your medication.

They may be taken with food to help prevent stomach upset. Some salicylates are coated or combined with buffers (chemicals that help control the acidity) to make them less upsetting to the stomach. Coating and buffers can help make side effects less likely but do not prevent them all. Take the medication with a full 8-ounce glass of water to keep the pills from sticking in your throat, which can cause irritation. Do not crush or chew these pills unless directed by your doctor or other healthcare professional. The most aspirin that anyone should usually take in 1 day is 4000 mg (8 extra-strength 500-mg tablets or 12 regular-strength 325-mg tablets). Do not take more unless directed by your doctor or other healthcare professional.

This medication is often used "as needed," so missing a dose should not be a problem. If you miss a dose and it is almost time for the next dose, you should skip the forgotten dose. Do not double the dose. Take your medication as directed by your doctor or other healthcare professional.

What Side Effects Can Aspirin and Aspirin-like Medications (Salicylates) Cause?

More Common

- Heartburn

- Nausea

- Vomiting

Less Common

- Bleeding that does not stop easily (nose bleeds, bleeding while brushing your teeth, and cuts)
- Easy bruising ("black-and-blue" marks on the skin)
- Hearing loss
- Low red blood cells (anemia)
- Ringing in the ears (tinnitus)
- Ulcers in the stomach that may cause black, tarry-looking bowel movements

Rare

- A combination of dizziness, diarrhea, confusion, headache, sweating, and fast, troubled breathing (hyperventilation) called salicylism
- Allergic reactions such as rash (skin redness, bumps, itching, or irritation), swelling of the face and throat, or trouble breathing
- Kidney problems
- Liver problems
- Severe bleeding

Tell your doctor or other healthcare professional if you have side effects that bother you, do not go away, make you worried about taking your medication, or make you want to stop taking your medication.

 ## Do Other Medications Interact with Aspirin or Aspirin-like Medications (Salicylates)?

Many nonprescription (over-the-counter [OTC]) medications such as pain, cough, cold, allergy, and sleep medications contain aspirin or NSAIDs. If you are taking aspirin or other aspirin-like medications regularly, you should talk to your doctor or other healthcare professional before taking any new OTC medications.

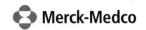

Aspirin and aspirin-like medications *may increase* the side effects of these medications:

- *Aggrenox®* (dipyridamole and aspirin)
- Corticosteroids such as prednisone—see Glossary
- *Coumadin®* (warfarin)
- *Depakene®* (valproate)
- *Depakote®* (divalproex)
- Diabetes medications such as *DiaBeta®* (glyburide), *Glucophage®* (metformin), *Glucotrol®* (glipizide), and others—see Glossary
- Heparin
- Insulin
- *Lovenox®* (enoxaparin)
- Nonsteroidal anti-inflammatory drugs (NSAIDs) such as *Motrin®* (ibuprofen), *Aleve®* (naproxen), *Vioxx®* (rofecoxib), *Celebrex®* (celecoxib), and others—see Glossary
- *Pepto-Bismol®* (bismuth subsalicylate)
- *Persantine®* (dipyridamole)
- *Plavix®* (clopidogrel)
- *Rheumatrex®* (methotrexate)
- *Ticlid®* (ticlopidine)

Aspirin *may decrease* how well these medications work:

- *Anturane®* (sulfinpyrazone)
- *Benemid®* (probenecid)

Drinking alcoholic beverages (such as beer, wine, whiskey, and others) *may increase* the side effects of aspirin and aspirin-like medications.

Tell your doctor or other healthcare professional about all medications (both prescription and nonprescription [over-the-counter] medications) that you are taking.

Why Else Do People Take Aspirin and Aspirin-like Medications (Salicylates)?

Aspirin and aspirin-like medications can also help to lower a fever. Aspirin can help to prevent stroke and heart attacks. Using aspirin to help prevent a heart attack or stroke is not recommended for everyone. Talk to your doctor or other healthcare professional before taking aspirin to help prevent heart attacks and strokes.

What Else Should I Know about Aspirin and Aspirin-like Medications (Salicylates)?

Many aspirin and aspirin-like medications are available without a prescription. However, they may have the same side effects as the prescription medications containing aspirin and aspirin-like medications. Always check with your doctor or other healthcare professional before using any new medication, including those that do not need a prescription.

 # Warning!

To give you the best care, your doctor or other healthcare professional needs to know about the diseases and medical conditions you have had—your full medical history. Tell your doctor or other healthcare professional if you have or have ever had any of the following:

- Allergy or previous reaction to aspirin, aspirin-like medications (salicylates) or nonsteroidal anti-inflammatory drugs (NSAIDs) such as *Motrin*® (ibuprofen), *Aleve*® (naproxen), *Vioxx*® (rofecoxib), *Celebrex*® (celecoxib), and others—see Glossary

- Asthma or nasal polyps (overgrowth of tissue in the nose)

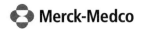

- Bleeding problems
- High alcohol intake (drinking 3 or more alcoholic beverages, such as beer, wine, whiskey, and others, every day)
- Liver problems
- Stomach problems (ulcer)

Aspirin and aspirin-like medications may cause stomach pain, which may be a sign of an ulcer. However, you may have an ulcer without feeling any pain at all. If ulcers are not treated, they may cause serious stomach or intestinal bleeding. Tell your doctor or other healthcare professional if you have severe stomach pain or stomach pain that keeps returning or if you have ever had peptic ulcer disease. Call your doctor or other healthcare professional right away if you have black, tarry-looking bowel movements (stools), if you vomit dark material that looks like coffee grounds, or if you notice any blood in your bowel movements. Any of these symptoms may be a sign of a bleeding ulcer.

If you have asthma or a history of polyps in the nose, ask your doctor or other healthcare professional whether you can take aspirin safely.

Aspirin or aspirin-like medications may prevent blood from clotting as well as usual. If you are going to have surgery, you should talk to your doctor or other healthcare professional about whether you should stop taking these medications before surgery. Depending on the kind of medication, you may need to stop for a few days or a week before surgery.

Aspirin may cause a serious, even fatal, illness called Reye's syndrome when given to children who have flu-like symptoms. Do not give aspirin to children without talking to a doctor or other healthcare professional.

Narcotics and Narcotic-like Medications

Narcotics are powerful pain relievers and usually used only for severe pain because they may cause unpleasant side effects and can be addictive. Narcotics are often used for cancer pain, pain after surgery, and other severe pain that is not relieved by other medications or when other pain medications cause side effects.

▲ Indicates medications that are more likely to cause unpleasant or dangerous side effects. These medications are generally not recommended for people over 65. The side effects may not be very obvious and may be mistaken for "just a part of getting older" but may be serious. If you are taking one of these medications, you might want to talk to your doctor or other healthcare professional to see if this medication is right for you. Safer medications may be available and lower dosages may be required. You should not stop taking these medications without first talking to your doctor or other healthcare professional.

See the WARNING section on page 65 for the specific safety problems associated with these medications ▲.

Brand Name	Generic Name
▲*Darvon*®	propoxyphene
▲*Demerol*®	meperidine
Dilaudid®	hydromorphone
Duragesic®	fentanyl
Hycodan®	hydrocodone
Kadian®	morphine
Levo-Dromoran®	levorphanol
MS Contin®	morphine
Oramorph®	morphine
OxyContin®	oxycodone
Stadol®	butorphanol
▲*Talwin*®	pentazocine
Various	codeine
Various	morphine

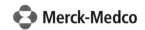

Narcotics may be combined with other pain relievers such as acetaminophen and aspirin to improve pain relief. If you are taking a combination, see the earlier sections in this chapter that discuss side effects, drug interactions, and warnings for acetaminophen on page 39 or aspirin on page 55.

Pain Medications Combined with Aspirin or Acetaminophen

Brand Name	Generic Name
▲*Darvocet-N®*	propoxyphene/acetaminophen
▲*Darvon® Compound-65*	propoxyphene/aspirin
Lorcet®	hydrocodone/acetaminophen
Lortab®	hydrocodone/acetaminophen
Percocet®	oxycodone/acetaminophen
Percodan®	oxycodone/aspirin
Phenaphen® with Codeine	codeine/acetaminophen
▲*Talacen®*	pentazocine/acetaminophen
▲*Talwin® Compound*	pentazocine/aspirin
Tylenol® with Codeine	codeine/acetaminophen
Tylox™	oxycodone/acetaminophen
Vicodin®	hydrocodone/acetaminophen
▲*Wygesic®*	propoxyphene/acetaminophen

How Will I Take Narcotics or Narcotic-like Medications?

Narcotics come in the form of pills, syrups, suppositories to be inserted into the rectum, patches that contain medication to be applied to the skin like a *Band-Aid®* bandage, lozenges, and injections (shots). Narcotics may be taken with or without food. Do not take more medication than your doctor or other healthcare professional has prescribed.

To help prevent side effects, your doctor or other healthcare professional may start by giving you a low dose of this medication, increasing the amount slowly until it works well for you.

When a medication has initials after its name, such as XL, XR, SR, BID, "contin," or others, it usually means that the body absorbs the medication slowly over time, so you usually have to take it only once or twice a day. The body will absorb some medications of this type too fast if you crush or break them or dissolve them in liquid, and their effects will not last as long as they should. Check with your doctor or other healthcare professional before crushing or breaking your pills or dissolving your pills in liquid.

This medication is often used "as needed," so missing a dose should not be a problem. If you miss a dose and it is almost time for the next dose, you should skip the forgotten dose. Do not double the dose. Take your medication as directed by your doctor or other healthcare professional.

What Side Effects Can Narcotics Cause?

More Common

- Constipation
- Decrease in the size of the pupils of the eyes (constriction)
- Drowsiness
- Nausea
- Poor appetite
- Trouble urinating or emptying the bladder

Less Common

- Blurred vision
- Confusion
- Dizziness
- Itching

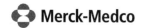
- Low blood pressure (hypotension)
- Reddening of the face (flushing)
- Vomiting

Rare

- Allergic reactions such as rash (skin redness, bumps, or irritation), swelling of the face and throat, or trouble breathing
- Seeing or hearing things that are not there (hallucinations)
- Seizures
- Shortness of breath
- Slow heartbeat (palpitations)

Tell your doctor or other healthcare professional if you have side effects that bother you, do not go away, make you worried about taking your medication, or make you want to stop taking your medication.

 ## Do Other Medications Interact with Narcotics?

Darvon® (propoxyphene/aspirin), *Darvocet®* (propoxyphene/acetaminophen), and *Wygesic®* (propoxyphene/acetaminophen) *may increase* the side effects of *Tegretol®* (carbamazepine).

Quinidine such as *Quinaglute®*, *Quinidex®*, and others (see Glossary) *may decrease* how well codeine works.

Drinking alcoholic beverages (such as beer, wine, whiskey, and others) *may increase* the side effects of narcotics.

Narcotics *may increase* the side effects of other medications that cause drowsiness, including anticholinergic medications, antidepressants, antihistamines (allergy medications), antispasmodics, benzodiazepines (a type of tranquilizer), anxiety medications, other narcotics (pain relievers), muscle relaxants, neuroleptic medications (a type of tranquilizer) seizure medications, or sleep medications. Avoid driving a car and other activities that need mental alertness, like using a knife or operating machinery, while taking these medications together.

Many nonprescription (over-the-counter [OTC]) medications such as pain, cough, cold, allergy, and sleep medications contain aspirin, NSAIDs, or *Tylenol*® (acetaminophen). If you are taking a pain reliever that has a narcotic plus aspirin or acetaminophen (combination narcotics) regularly, you should talk to your doctor or other healthcare professional before taking any new OTC medications.

Morphine ***may increase*** the side effects of *Glucophage*® (metformin).

Narcotics are generally not prescribed for anyone who is taking MAO inhibitors, such as *Marplan*® (isocarboxazid), *Nardil*® (phenelzine), or *Parnate*® (tranylcypromine), because together they ***may cause*** serious or even fatal reactions. If your doctor or other healthcare professional wants you to stop taking one medication and start taking the other, you should wait at least 2 weeks between stopping one and starting the other.

Tell your doctor or other healthcare professional about all medications (both prescription and nonprescription [over-the-counter] medications) that you are taking.

What Else Can Narcotics Be Used For?

Morphine, a narcotic, is sometimes used for severe congestive heart failure or pain of a heart attack. Narcotics may also be used to quiet coughing (cough suppressant).

 # Warning!

To give you the best care, your doctor or other healthcare professional needs to know about the diseases and medical conditions you have had—your full

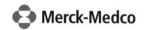

medical history. Tell your doctor or other healthcare professional if you have
or have ever had, or presently take, any of the following:

- Allergy or previous reaction to narcotics

- Breathing problems (asthma and COPD, including emphysema or
  chronic bronchitis)

- Constipation or blockage

- Enlarged prostate (benign prostatic hypertrophy)

- Gallbladder problems

- Kidney problems

- Liver problems

- MAO inhibitors such as *Marplan*® (isocarboxazid), *Nardil*® (phenelzine),
  or *Parnate*® (tranylcypromine)

- Seizures (epilepsy)

- Underactive thyroid (hypothyroidism)

Darvon®, *Darvon*® Compound, *Darvocet*®, and *Wygesic*® (medications that contain
propoxyphene) may not relieve pain any better than *Tylenol*® (acetaminophen)
but may cause the same side effects as other narcotics. These medications are
not generally recommended for use in people over 65. If you are taking one
of them, ask your doctor or other healthcare professional if it is the right
medication for you. Do not stop taking the medication without talking to
your doctor or other healthcare professional.

Talwin® (pentazocine) may cause confusion and seeing or hearing things that are
not there (hallucinations). This medication is not generally recommended for
use in people over 65. If you are taking *Talwin*® (pentazocine), ask your doctor
or other healthcare professional if it is the right medication for you. Do not
stop taking the medication without talking to your doctor or other healthcare
professional.

Demerol® (meperidine) may build up in the body and cause serious side effects
such as seizures. This medication is generally not recommended for use in
people over 65. If you are taking *Demerol*® (meperidine), ask your doctor or

other healthcare professional if it is the right medication for you. Do not stop taking the medication without talking to your doctor or other healthcare professional.

Narcotics may cause drowsiness. Avoid driving a car and other activities that need mental alertness, like using a knife or operating machinery, while taking this medication. Drinking alcoholic beverages (such as beer, wine, whiskey, and others) may increase the side effects.

Narcotics may make you unsteady on your feet, causing you to fall and possibly break a bone. If you have fallen recently, tell your doctor or other healthcare professional about it. Taking a different medication or a lower dose may make you less likely to fall. You should not stop taking this medication without first talking to your doctor or other healthcare professional.

After taking a narcotic regularly, people may develop a strong need (dependence) for it. To prevent this from happening, do not take a narcotic more often than prescribed by your doctor or other healthcare professional.

Constipation caused by taking narcotics is very common and may be very uncomfortable. If you are taking narcotics or are about to start, ask your doctor or other healthcare professional how to help prevent constipation.

Narcotics may be dangerous to children or pets if they take them accidentally. To throw away a used *Duragesic®* (fentanyl) patch, fold it in half (medication side in), and flush it down the toilet. If you are using *Duragesic®* (fentanyl) patches, you should not expose the narcotic patches to heat. Heat makes the narcotic come out of the patch faster.

Under certain circumstances, your doctor or other healthcare professional may decide that you should stop taking this medication. If you have taken it for more than a couple of weeks, he or she may want you to decrease it gradually, lowering the dose over a few weeks or months. Stopping suddenly may cause unpleasant withdrawal symptoms or may worsen your medical problems. Pay careful attention to the instructions your doctor or other healthcare professional gives you about how much less to take and for how long.

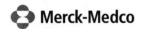
Ultram® (tramadol)

Ultram® (tramadol) is not a narcotic but works in a similar way and has similar side effects. It is used for moderate-to-severe pain.

How Will I Take *Ultram*® (tramadol)?

Ultram® (tramadol) comes as a pill that is usually taken as needed for pain every 4 to 6 hours. Your doctor or other healthcare professional will tell you how much of this medication to take and when.

To help prevent side effects, your doctor or other healthcare professional may start by giving you a low dose of this medication, increasing the amount slowly until it works well for you.

This medication is often used "as needed," so missing a dose should not be a problem. If you miss a dose and it is almost time for the next dose, you should skip the forgotten dose. Do not double the dose. Take your medication as directed by your doctor or other healthcare professional.

What Side Effects Can *Ultram*® (tramadol) Cause?

More Common

- Constipation
- Diarrhea
- Dizziness
- Drowsiness
- Dry mouth
- Headache
- Heartburn

- Increased or excessive sweating (perspiration)
- Itching
- Nausea
- Vomiting

Rare

- Seeing or hearing things that are not there (hallucinations)
- Seizures

Tell your doctor or other healthcare professional if you have side effects that bother you, do not go away, make you worried about taking your medication, or make you want to stop taking your medication.

Do Other Medications Interact with *Ultram®* (tramadol)?

Tegretol® (carbamazepine) ***may decrease*** how well *Ultram®* (tramadol) works.

Ultram® (tramadol) ***may increase*** the chances of seizures when taken with these medications:

- *Celexa™* (citalopram)
- *Compazine®* (prochlorperazine)
- *Flexeril®* (cyclobenzaprine)
- *Luvox®* (fluvoxamine)
- Neuroleptic medications such as *Risperdal®* (risperidone), *Thorazine®* (chlorpromazine), *Zyprexa®* (olanzapine), and others—see Glossary
- *Paxil®* (paroxetine)
- *Phenergan®* (promethazine)
- *Prozac®* (fluoxetine)
- *Tegretol®* (carbamazepine)

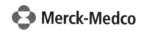
- Tricyclic antidepressants such as *Elavil*® (amitriptyline), *Pamelor*® (nortriptyline), *Sinequan*® (doxepin), and others—see Glossary

- *Wellbutrin*® (bupropion)

- *Zoloft*® (sertraline)

- *Zyban*® (bupropion)

Ultram® (tramadol) is generally not prescribed for anyone who is taking MAO inhibitors such as *Marplan*® (isocarboxazid), *Nardil*® (phenelzine), or *Parnate*® (tranylcypromine), because together they **may cause** serious or even fatal reactions. If your doctor or other healthcare professional wants you to stop taking one medication and start taking the other, you should wait at least 2 weeks between stopping one and starting the other.

Ultram® (tramadol) **may increase** the side effects of other medications that cause drowsiness, including anticholinergic medications, antidepressants, antihistamines (allergy medications), antispasmodics, benzodiazepines (a type of tranquilizer), anxiety medications, narcotics (pain relievers), muscle relaxants, neuroleptic medications (a type of tranquilizer), seizure medications, or sleep medications. Avoid driving a car and other activities that need mental alertness, like using a knife or operating machinery, while taking these medications together.

Drinking alcoholic beverages (such as beer, wine, whiskey, and others) **may increase** the side effects of *Ultram*® (tramadol).

Tell your doctor or other healthcare professional about all medications (both prescription and nonprescription [over-the-counter] medications) that you are taking.

 # Warning!

To give you the best care, your doctor or other healthcare professional needs to know about the diseases and medical conditions you have had—your full

medical history. Tell your doctor or other healthcare professional if you have or have ever had, or presently take, any of the following:

- Allergy or previous reaction to *Ultram®* (tramadol) or narcotics

- Kidney problems

- Liver problems

- MAO inhibitors such as *Marplan®* (isocarboxazid), *Nardil®* (phenelzine), or *Parnate®* (tranylcypromine)

- Seizures (epilepsy)

- Underactive thyroid (hypothyroidism)

If you have had seizures in the past, tell your doctor or other healthcare professional because *Ultram®* (tramadol) may cause seizures. Stopping this medication suddenly may also cause seizures. If your doctor or other healthcare professional decides that you should stop taking *Ultram®* (tramadol), pay careful attention to the instructions he or she gives you about how much less to take and for how long.

Ultram® (tramadol) may cause drowsiness. Avoid driving a car and other activities that need mental alertness, like using a knife or operating machinery, while taking this medication. Drinking alcoholic beverages (such as beer, wine, whiskey, and others) may increase the side effects.

Ultram® (tramadol) may make you unsteady on your feet, causing you to fall and possibly break a bone. If you have fallen recently, tell your doctor or other healthcare professional about it. Taking a different medication or a lower dose may make you less likely to fall. You should not stop taking this medication without first talking to your doctor or other healthcare professional.

Although *Ultram®* (tramadol) is not a narcotic, after taking it regularly, people may develop a strong need (dependence) for it. To prevent this from happening, do not take *Ultram®* (tramadol) more often than prescribed by your doctor or other healthcare professional.

Under certain circumstances, your doctor or other healthcare professional may decide that you should stop taking this medication. If you have taken it for more than a couple of weeks, he or she may want you to decrease it gradually,

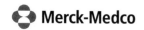

lowering the dose over a few weeks or months. Stopping suddenly may cause unpleasant withdrawal symptoms or may worsen your medical problems. Pay careful attention to the instructions your doctor or other healthcare professional gives you about how much less to take and for how long.

Corticosteroids

Corticosteroids are among the most powerful medications for reducing inflammation (pain, swelling, and redness). They are sometimes used to treat the inflammation caused by rheumatoid arthritis.

Brand Name	Generic Name
Aristocort®	triamcinolone
Celestone®	betamethasone
Medrol®	methylprednisolone
Various	cortisone
Various	dexamethasone
Various	hydrocortisone
Various	prednisolone
Various	prednisone

How Will I Take Corticosteroids?

Corticosteroids for arthritis are taken in pill form or by injection (shot). Injections may be helpful if only a few joints are painful and are usually given only a few times every 2 to 3 weeks. Corticosteroid pills are usually taken once daily. Taking oral corticosteroids with food will help prevent stomach upset. Your doctor or other healthcare professional will prescribe the lowest dose possible for the shortest time to relieve your pain and swelling. Your doctor or other healthcare professional will tell you how often to take your medication.

If you miss a dose of this medication, take the dose you missed as soon as possible. However, if it is almost time for your next dose, skip the missed dose and just take the next one. Do not double your dose. Take your medication exactly as directed by your doctor or other healthcare professional. Do not stop taking a prescription medication unless directed by your doctor or other healthcare professional.

What Side Effects Can Corticosteroids Cause?

In the first few weeks after you start taking them (short-term):

- High blood pressure (hypertension)
- Increased appetite
- Increased blood sugar (hyperglycemia)
- Increased chances for infection
- Mood swings
- Nausea
- Stomach pain
- Swelling or puffiness of the feet, ankles, or lower legs (edema)
- Trouble falling asleep or staying asleep (insomnia)
- Ulcers in the stomach that may cause black, tarry-looking bowel movements
- Vomiting
- Weakness or muscle cramps that may be a sign of low potassium in your blood (hypokalemia)

After months or years of taking them (long-term):

- Acne
- Cataracts
- Easy bruising ("black-and-blue" marks on the skin)

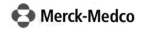
- Hair growth in unwanted places
- Muscle weakness
- Poor wound healing
- Redness of the face
- Thin skin
- Thinning bones from decreased bone density (osteoporosis)
- Weight gain
- Worsening of glaucoma (an eye disease)

Tell your doctor or other healthcare professional if you have side effects that bother you, do not go away, make you worried about taking your medication, or make you want to stop taking your medication.

 ## Do Other Medications Interact with Corticosteroids?

These medications *may decrease* how well corticosteroids work:

- Barbiturates such as *Butisol®* (butabarbital), *Luminal®* (phenobarbital), *Mebaral®* (mephobarbital), and others—see Glossary
- *Dilantin®* (phenytoin)
- *Rifadin®* (rifampin)

Corticosteroids *may decrease* how well these medications work:

- *Mestinon®* (pyridostigmine)
- *Prostigmin®* (neostigmine)

These medications *may increase* the side effects of corticosteroids:

- *Biaxin®* (clarithromycin)
- *Diflucan®* (fluconazole)

- Erythromycin such as *Ery-Tab®*, *Erythrocin®*, and others—see Glossary
- Estrogens such as *Estrace®*, *Premarin®*, *Prempro™*, and others—see Glossary
- *Nizoral®* (ketoconazole)
- *Sporanox®* (itraconazole)

Corticosteroids *may increase* the side effects of these medications:

- Aspirin, medications that contain aspirin, and aspirin-like medications (salicylates)—see Glossary
- *Coumadin®* (warfarin)
- Diuretics (water pills) such as *HydroDIURIL®* (hydrochlorothiazide or HCTZ), *Lasix®* (furosemide), and others—see Glossary
- *Lanoxin®* (digoxin)
- Nonsteroidal anti-inflammatory drugs (NSAIDs) such as *Motrin®* (ibuprofen), *Aleve®* (naproxen), *Vioxx®* (rofecoxib), *Celebrex®* (celecoxib), and others—see Glossary

Many nonprescription (over-the-counter [OTC]) medications such as pain, cough, cold, allergy, and sleep medications contain aspirin or nonsteroidal anti-inflammatory drugs (NSAIDs) that can increase the side effects of corticosteroids. If you are taking corticosteroids, you should talk to your doctor or other healthcare professional before taking any new OTC medications.

Drinking alcoholic beverages (such as beer, wine, whiskey, and others) *may increase* the side effects of corticosteroids.

Tell your doctor or other healthcare professional about all medications (both prescription and nonprescription [over-the-counter] medications) that you are taking.

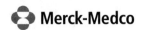

Why Else Do People Take Corticosteroids?

Corticosteroids have many uses. For example, they can also be used for breathing problems (asthma and COPD, including emphysema or chronic bronchitis), allergies, skin conditions, liver problems, blood problems, kidney problems, and gout.

 # Warning!

To give you the best care, your doctor or other healthcare professional needs to know about the diseases and medical conditions you have had—your full medical history. Tell your doctor or other healthcare professional if you have or have ever had any of the following:

- Allergy or previous reaction to corticosteroids
- Diabetes
- Fungal infections
- Glaucoma (an eye disease)
- High blood pressure (hypertension)
- Inflammatory bowel disease (ulcerative colitis or Crohn's disease).
- Kidney problems
- Stomach problems (ulcer)
- Thinning bones from decreased bone density (osteoporosis)
- Tuberculosis
- Underactive thyroid (hypothyroidism)

Because corticosteroids can cause low potassium blood levels (hypokalemia) and high blood sugar (hyperglycemia), your doctor or other healthcare professional may order blood tests to check your potassium levels and blood sugar (glucose).

Corticosteroids can hide symptoms of an infection and can weaken the body's defenses against infection. Call your doctor or other healthcare professional if you have a fever, sore throat, or flu-like symptoms that will not go away.

Corticosteroids may cause stomach pain, which may be a sign of an ulcer. However, you may have an ulcer without feeling any pain at all. If ulcers are not treated, they may cause serious stomach or intestinal bleeding. Tell your doctor or other healthcare professional if you have severe stomach pain or stomach pain that keeps returning or if you have ever had peptic ulcer disease. Call your doctor or other healthcare professional right away if you have black, tarry-looking bowel movements (stools), if you vomit dark material that looks like coffee grounds, or if you notice any blood in your bowel movements. Any of these symptoms may be a sign of a bleeding ulcer.

If you use corticosteroids for a long time, thinning of your bones (osteoporosis) can occur. Talk to your doctor or other healthcare professional about whether you are at increased risk for osteoporosis and about calcium, vitamin D, and other medications you may take to help keep your bones strong.

When taken for more than 6 months, corticosteroids may cause or worsen cataracts and glaucoma (an eye disease). Your doctor or other healthcare professional may check your eyes to see if the corticosteroids are causing or worsening cataracts or glaucoma.

Under certain circumstances, your doctor or other healthcare professional may decide that you should stop taking this medication. If you have taken it for more than a couple of weeks, he or she may want you to decrease it gradually, lowering the dose over a few weeks or months. Stopping suddenly may cause unpleasant withdrawal symptoms or may worsen your medical problems. Pay careful attention to the instructions your doctor or other healthcare professional gives you about how much less to take and for how long.

Tricyclic Antidepressants

Tricyclic antidepressants are often used for long-lasting (chronic) pain caused by nerve damage (neuropathy). They may be used for pain from diabetic neuropathy, trigeminal neuralgia, post-herpetic neuralgia, amputation, and other types of nerve pain.

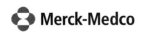

▲ Indicates medications that are more likely to cause unpleasant or dangerous side effects. These medications are generally not recommended for people over 65. The side effects may not be very obvious and may be mistaken for "just a part of getting older" but may be serious. If you are taking one of these medications, you might want to talk to your doctor or other healthcare professional to see if this medication is best for you. Safer medications may be available and lower dosages may be required. You should not stop taking these medications without first talking to your doctor or other healthcare professional.

See the WARNING section on page 82 for the specific safety problems associated with these medications ▲.

Brand Name	Generic Name
▲*Anafranil*®	clomipramine
▲*Asendin*®	amoxapine
▲*Elavil*®	amitriptyline
▲*Ludiomil*®*	maprotiline
Norpramin®	desipramine
Pamelor®	nortriptyline
▲*Sinequan*®	doxepin
▲*Surmontil*®	trimipramine
▲*Tofranil*®	imipramine

*Tetracyclic antidepressant—works in ways similar to a tricyclic antidepressant

How Will I Take Tricyclic Antidepressants for Chronic Pain?

Tricyclic antidepressants are pills that are usually taken 1 to 3 times a day. If taken only once a day, they are usually taken at bedtime to decrease the chance of side effects during the day. Your doctor or other healthcare professional will tell you how often to take your medication.

To help prevent side effects, your doctor or other healthcare professional may start by giving you a low dose of this medication, increasing the amount slowly until it works well for you.

If you miss a dose of this medication, take the dose you missed as soon as possible. However, if it is almost time for your next dose, skip the missed dose and just take the next one. Do not double your dose. Take your medication exactly as directed by your doctor or other healthcare professional. Do not stop taking a prescription medication unless directed by your doctor or other healthcare professional.

What Side Effects Can Tricyclic Antidepressants Cause?

More Common

- Constipation

- Dizziness when standing up from a bed or a chair

- Drowsiness

- Dry mouth, eyes, and nose

- Trouble urinating or emptying the bladder

Less Common

- Confusion

- Fast, slow, or irregular heartbeat (palpitations)

- Increased sensitivity to the sun (bad sunburn)

- Loss of interest in sex (decreased libido)

- Rash (skin redness, bumps, itching, or irritation)

- Worsening of glaucoma (an eye disease)

Rare

- Hair loss

- Increased breast size and tenderness (in both men and women)

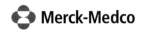

- Seizures

- Shakiness or tremors

Tell your doctor or other healthcare professional if you have side effects that bother you, do not go away, make you worried about taking your medication, or make you want to stop taking your medication.

 ## Do Other Medications Interact with Tricyclic Antidepressants?

These medications *may increase* the side effects of tricyclic antidepressants:

- Quinidine such as *Quinaglute®*, *Quinidex®*, and others—see Glossary

- *Ritalin®* (methylphenidate)

- *Rythmol®* (propafenone)

- *Tagamet®* (cimetidine)

Tricyclic antidepressants *may increase* the side effects of other medications that cause drowsiness, including anticholinergic medications, other antidepressants, antihistamines (allergy medications), antispasmodics, benzodiazepines (a type of tranquilizer), anxiety medications, narcotics (pain relievers), muscle relaxants, neuroleptic medications (a type of tranquilizer), seizure medications, or sleep medications. Avoid driving a car and other activities that need mental alertness, like using a knife or operating machinery, while taking this medication.

Drinking alcoholic beverages (such as beer, wine, whiskey, and others) *may increase* the side effects of tricyclic antidepressants.

These medications *may decrease* how well tricyclic antidepressants work:

- Barbiturates such as *Butisol®* (butabarbital), *Luminal®* (phenobarbital), *Mebaral®* (mephobarbital), and others—see Glossary

- *Rifadin®* (rifampin)

- *Tegretol®* (carbamazepine)

Taking a tricyclic antidepressant with *Catapres®* (clonidine) or *Ismelin®* (guanethidine) ***may raise*** your blood pressure to dangerously high levels.

Tricyclic antidepressants are not usually prescribed for anyone who is taking MAO inhibitors, such as *Marplan®* (isocarboxazid), *Nardil®* (phenelzine), or *Parnate®* (tranylcypromine), because together they ***may cause*** serious or even fatal reactions. If your doctor or other healthcare professional wants you to stop taking an MAO inhibitor and start taking a tricyclic antidepressant or to stop taking a tricyclic antidepressant and start taking an MAO inhibitor, you should stop one at least 2 weeks before you start the other.

Grapefruit and grapefruit juice ***may increase*** the side effects of *Anafranil®* (clomipramine). This interaction can happen whether you eat the grapefruit or drink the grapefruit juice at the same time as you take your medication or if you take the medication separately from the grapefruit or grapefruit juice. Talk to your doctor or other healthcare professional before eating grapefruit or drinking grapefruit juice if you are taking this medication. Please also read the discussion on A Warning about Grapefruit and Grapefruit Juice on pages i-ii.

Tricyclic antidepressants are generally not prescribed for anyone who is taking *Propulsid®* (cisapride [withdrawn from general distribution; available only by special arrangement with the manufacturer]), *Seldane®* (terfenadine [no longer commercially available]), or *Hismanal®* (astemizole [no longer commercially available]), because together they ***may cause*** serious, sometimes fatal, heart problems.

Tell your doctor or other healthcare professional about all medications (both prescription and nonprescription [over-the-counter] medications) that you are taking.

Why Else Do People Take Tricyclic Antidepressants?

Tricyclic antidepressants can be used to treat depression, abnormal fears (phobias), panic attacks, inability to hold urine in (urinary incontinence), obsessive-compulsive disorders, and eating disorders such as anorexia and

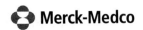

bulimia. Tricyclic antidepressants can also be used to help prevent migraine headaches.

 # Warning!

To give you the best care, your doctor or other healthcare professional needs to know about the diseases and medical conditions you have had—your full medical history. Tell your doctor or other healthcare professional if you have or have ever had, or presently take, any of the following:

- Allergy or previous reaction to tricyclic antidepressants, *Tegretol®* (carbamazepine), or *Trileptal®* (oxcarbazepine)

- Enlarged prostate (benign prostatic hypertrophy)

- Glaucoma (an eye disease)

- Liver problems

- Manic depression

- MAO inhibitors such as *Marplan®* (isocarboxazid), *Nardil®* (phenelzine), or *Parnate®* (tranylcypromine)

- Overactive thyroid (hyperthyroidism)

- Schizophrenia

- Seizures (epilepsy)

- Trouble urinating or emptying the bladder

Asendin® (amoxapine), *Elavil®* (amitriptyline), *Ludiomil®* (maprotiline), *Sinequan®* (doxepin), *Surmontil®* (trimipramine), and *Tofranil®* (imipramine) are generally not recommended for use in people over the age of 65 because these types of tricyclic antidepressants have been associated with a higher risk of broken hips than other tricyclic antidepressants. If you are taking any of these medications, ask your doctor or other healthcare professional if this medication is right for you. Do not stop taking this medication without talking to your doctor or other healthcare professional.

Tricyclic antidepressants may cause drowsiness. Avoid driving a car and other activities that need mental alertness, like using a knife or operating machinery, while taking this medication. Drinking alcoholic beverages (such as beer, wine, whiskey, and others) may increase the side effects.

If you have had seizures in the past, tell your doctor or other healthcare professional because tricyclic antidepressants may cause seizures. Stopping this medication suddenly may also cause seizures. If your doctor or other healthcare professional decides that you should stop taking tricyclic antidepressants, pay careful attention to the instructions he or she gives you about how much less to take and for how long.

If you are taking a tricyclic antidepressant, stay out of the sun as much as you can to avoid a serious sunburn. When you do go out in the sun, use sunblock or sunscreen, and wear protective clothing, such as a wide-brimmed hat and a long-sleeved shirt.

Under certain circumstances, your doctor or other healthcare professional may decide that you should stop taking this medication. If you have taken it for more than a couple of weeks, he or she may want you to decrease it gradually, lowering the dose over a few weeks or months. Stopping suddenly may cause unpleasant withdrawal symptoms or may worsen your medical problems. Pay careful attention to the instructions your doctor or other healthcare professional gives you about how much less to take and for how long.

Tegretol® (carbamazepine) and *Trileptal*® (oxcarbazepine)

Tegretol® (carbamazepine) and *Trileptal*® (oxcarbazepine) help to relieve pain that comes from nerve damage (neuropathy). They may be used for pain from diabetic neuropathy, trigeminal neuralgia, post-herpetic neuralgia, amputation, and other types of nerve pain.

How Will I Take *Tegretol*® (carbamazepine) and *Trileptal*® (oxcarbazepine)?

Tegretol® (carbamazepine) comes in pill or liquid form, and *Trileptal*® (oxcarbazepine) is available in a pill form. These medications are usually taken 1 to 4 times daily. To help prevent stomach upset, *Tegretol*® (carbamazepine) may be taken with food. Your doctor or other healthcare professional will tell you how often to take your medication.

When a medication has initials such as XL, XR, SR, BID, or DUR after its name, it usually means that the body absorbs the medication slowly over time, so you usually have to take it only once or twice a day. The body will absorb some medications of this type too fast if you crush or break them or dissolve them in liquid, and their effects will not last as long as they should. Check with your doctor or other healthcare professional before crushing or breaking your pills or dissolving your pills in liquid.

If you miss a dose of this medication, take the dose you missed as soon as possible. However, if it is almost time for your next dose, skip the missed dose and just take the next one. Do not double your dose. Take your medication exactly as directed by your doctor or other healthcare professional. Do not stop taking a prescription medication unless directed by your doctor or other healthcare professional.

What Side Effects Can *Tegretol*® (carbamazepine) and *Trileptal*® (oxcarbazepine) Cause?

More Common

- Blurred vision
- Dizziness when standing up from a bed or a chair
- Double vision
- Drowsiness

- Nausea

- Vomiting

Less common

- Confusion, nervousness, agitation, or hostility

- Constant, uncontrollable back-and-forth eye movements

- Diarrhea

- Headache

- Numbness or tingling in the hands, arms, legs, and feet

Rare

- Allergic reactions such as rash (skin redness, bumps, itching, or irritation) or swelling of the face and throat

- Bleeding that does not stop easily (nose bleeds, bleeding while brushing your teeth, and cuts)

- Easy bruising ("black-and-blue" marks on the skin)

- Frequent fever, sore throat, or flu-like symptoms that may be a sign of low white blood cells

- Liver problems that may cause yellowing of the skin or eyes (jaundice)

- Severe rash (skin redness, bumps, itching, or irritation) with peeling skin

- Shortness of breath

- Sores, ulcers, or white spots on lips or in mouth

- Tightness in chest

Tell your doctor or other healthcare professional if you have side effects that bother you, do not go away, make you worried about taking your medication, or make you want to stop taking your medication.

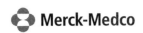

Do Other Medications Interact with *Tegretol*® (carbamazepine) and *Trileptal*® (oxcarbazepine)?

Tegretol® (carbamazepine) *may decrease* how well these medications work:

- Benzodiazepines such as *Ativan*® (lorazepam), *Klonopin*® (clonazepam), *Xanax*® (alprazolam), and others—see Glossary

- *Coumadin*® (warfarin)

- *Haldol*® (haloperidol)

- *Neoral*® (cyclosporine)

- *Plendil*® (felodipine)

- *Sandimmune*® (cyclosporine)

- Seizure medications such as *Dilantin*® (phenytoin), *Depakote*® (valproic acid), *Neurontin*® (gabapentin), and others—see Glossary

- Theophylline such as *Theo-Dur*®, *Uniphyl*®, and others—see Glossary

- Tricyclic antidepressants such as *Elavil*® (amitriptyline), *Pamelor*® (nortriptyline), *Sinequan*® (doxepin), and others—see Glossary

- *Vibramycin*® (doxycycline)

- *Wellbutrin*® (bupropion)

- *Zyban*® (bupropion)

Tegretol® (carbamazepine) *may increase* the side effects of lithium such as *Eskalith*®, *Lithobid*®, and others—see Glossary.

These medications *may increase* the side effects of *Tegretol*® (carbamazepine):

- *Biaxin*® (clarithromycin)

- *Danocrine*® (danazol)

- *Darvocet*® (propoxyphene)

- *Darvon*® (propoxyphene)

- *Diflucan*® (fluconazole)

- Diltiazem such as *Cardizem*®, *Cartia*®, *Tiazac*®, and others—see Glossary

- Erythromycin such as *Ery-Tab*®, *Erythrocin*®, and others—see Glossary

- Isoniazid

- *Nizoral*® (ketoconazole)

- *Prozac*® (fluoxetine)

- *Sporanox*® (itraconazole)

- *Tagamet*® (cimetidine)

- Tricyclic antidepressants such as *Elavil*® (amitriptyline), *Pamelor*® (nortriptyline), *Sinequan*® (doxepin), and others—see Glossary

- Verapamil such as *Calan*®, *Covera*®, *Verelan*®, and others—see Glossary

These medications *may decrease* how well *Tegretol*® (carbamazepine) works:

- Barbiturates such as *Butisol*® (butabarbital), *Luminal*® (phenobarbital), *Mebaral*® (mephobarbital), and others—see Glossary

- *Dilantin*® (phenytoin)

- *Felbatol*® (felbamate)

- *Rifadin*® (rifampin)

- *Ultram*® (tramadol)

Tegretol® (carbamazepine) and *Trileptal*® (oxcarbazepine) *may increase* the side effects of other medications that cause drowsiness, including anticholinergic medications, antidepressants, antihistamines (allergy medications), antispasmodics, benzodiazepines (a type of tranquilizer), anxiety medications, narcotics (pain relievers), muscle relaxants, neuroleptic medications (a type of tranquilizer), seizure medications, or sleep medications. Avoid driving a car and other activities that need mental alertness, like using a knife or operating machinery, while taking these medications together.

Drinking alcoholic beverages (such as beer, wine, whiskey, and others) *may increase* the side effects of *Tegretol*® (carbamazepine) or *Trileptal*® (oxcarbazepine).

If *Tegretol*® (carbamazepine) or *Trileptal*® (oxcarbazepine) is taken by someone who is also taking a medication to prevent seizures, neither type of medication may work the way it should.

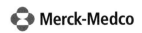

Tegretol® (carbamazepine) or *Trileptal*® (oxcarbazepine) are generally not prescribed for anyone who is taking MAO inhibitors, such as *Marplan*® (isocarboxazid), *Nardil*® (phenelzine), or *Parnate*® (tranylcypromine), because together they *may cause* serious or even fatal reactions. If your doctor or other healthcare professional wants you to stop taking one medication and start taking the other, you should wait at least 2 weeks between stopping one and starting the other.

Tegretol® (carbamazepine) or *Trileptal*® (oxcarbazepine) is generally not prescribed for anyone who is taking *Propulsid*® (cisapride [withdrawn from general distribution; available only by special arrangement with the manufacturer]), *Seldane*® (terfenadine [no longer commercially available]), or *Hismanal*® (astemizole [no longer commercially available]), because together they *may cause* serious, sometimes fatal, heart problems.

Tell your doctor or other healthcare professional about all medications (both prescription and nonprescription [over-the-counter] medications) that you are taking.

Why Else Do People Take *Tegretol*® (carbamazepine) and *Trileptal*® (oxcarbazepine)?

Tegretol® (carbamazepine) or *Trileptal*® (oxcarbazepine) may also be used for seizures. *Tegretol*® (carbamazepine) may be used for some mental conditions and behavioral problems.

What Else Should I Know about *Tegretol*® (carbamazepine) and *Trileptal*® (oxcarbazepine)?

If you find out that you need dental work or surgery on your teeth, tell your dentist that you are taking *Tegretol*® (carbamazepine) or *Trileptal*® (oxcarbazepine). It may interfere with some medications used in dental procedures and surgery.

Warning!

To give you the best care, your doctor or other healthcare professional needs to know about the diseases and medical conditions you have had—your full medical history. Tell your doctor or other healthcare professional if you have or have ever had, or presently take, any of the following:

- Allergy or previous reaction to *Tegretol*® (carbamazepine), *Trileptal*® (oxcarbazepine), or tricyclic antidepressants such as *Elavil*® (amitriptyline), *Pamelor*® (nortriptyline), *Sinequan*® (doxepin), and others—see Glossary

- Blood problems

- Kidney problems

- Liver problems

- MAO inhibitors such as *Marplan*® (isocarboxazid), *Nardil*® (phenelzine), or *Parnate*® (tranylcypromine)

- Mental illness such as schizophrenia

Tegretol® (carbamazepine) or *Trileptal*® (oxcarbazepine) may make you unsteady on your feet, causing you to fall and possibly break a bone. If you have fallen recently, tell your doctor or other healthcare professional about it. Taking a different medication or a lower dose may make you less likely to fall. You should not stop taking this medication without first talking to your doctor or other healthcare professional.

Tegretol® (carbamazepine) or *Trileptal*® (oxcarbazepine) may cause drowsiness. Avoid driving a car and other activities that need mental alertness, like using a knife or operating machinery, while taking this medication. Drinking alcoholic beverages (such as beer, wine, whiskey, and others) may increase the side effects.

Grapefruit and grapefruit juice ***may increase*** the side effects of *Tegretol*® (carbamazepine). This interaction can happen whether you eat the grapefruit or drink the grapefruit juice at the same time as you take your medication or if you take the medication separately from the grapefruit or grapefruit juice. Talk to your doctor or other healthcare professional before eating grapefruit or drinking grapefruit juice if you are taking this medication. Please also read the discussion on A Warning about Grapefruit and Grapefruit Juice on pages i-ii.

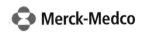

Under certain circumstances, your doctor or other healthcare professional may decide that you should stop taking this medication. If you have taken it for more than a couple of weeks, he or she may want you to decrease it gradually, lowering the dose over a few weeks or months. Stopping suddenly may cause unpleasant withdrawal symptoms or may worsen your medical problems. Pay careful attention to the instructions your doctor or other healthcare professional gives you about how much less to take and for how long.

Neurontin® (gabapentin)

Neurontin® (gabapentin) is a medication used to help relieve pain from neuropathy (nerve damage).

How Should I Take *Neurontin*® (gabapentin)?

Neurontin® (gabapentin) may be taken with or without food and is usually taken 1 to 3 times daily. Your doctor or other healthcare professional will tell you how often to take this medication.

If you miss a dose of this medication, take the dose you missed as soon as possible. However, if it is almost time for your next dose, skip the missed dose and just take the next one. Do not double your dose. Take your medication exactly as directed by your doctor or other healthcare professional. Do not stop taking a prescription medication unless directed by your doctor or other healthcare professional.

What Side Effects Can *Neurontin*® (gabapentin) Cause?

More Common
- Blurred vision
- Confusion

- Dizziness

- Drowsiness

Less Common

- Nausea

- Nervousness (anxiety)

- Poor appetite

- Shakiness or tremors

- Vomiting

- Weight gain

Rare

- Bleeding that does not stop easily (nose bleeds, bleeding while brushing your teeth, and cuts)

- Easy bruising ("black-and-blue" marks on the skin)

- Rash (skin redness, bumps, itching, or irritation)

Tell your doctor or other healthcare professional if you have side effects that bother you, do not go away, make you worried about taking your medication, or make you want to stop taking your medication.

 Do Other Medications Interact with *Neurontin*® (gabapentin)?

Antacids such as *Maalox*® or *Mylanta*® (aluminum hydroxide and magnesium hydroxide), *Rolaids*® or *Tums*® (calcium carbonate), or *Amphojel*® (aluminum hydroxide) ***may decrease*** the effects of *Neurontin*® (gabapentin) when taken at the same time. If you are using antacids, take *Neurontin*® (gabapentin) 1 hour before or 2 hours after taking your antacid.

Neurontin® (gabapentin) ***may increase*** the side effects of other medications that cause drowsiness, including anticholinergic medications, antidepressants,

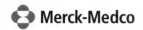

antihistamines (allergy medications), antispasmodics, benzodiazepines (a type of tranquilizer), anxiety medications, narcotics (pain relievers), muscle relaxants, neuroleptic medications (a type of tranquilizer), seizure medications, or sleep medications. Avoid driving a car and other activities that need mental alertness, like using a knife or operating machinery, while taking these medications together.

Drinking alcoholic beverages (such as beer, wine, whiskey, and others) *may increase* the side effects of *Neurontin*® (gabapentin).

Tell your doctor or other healthcare professional about all medications (both prescription and nonprescription [over-the-counter] medications) that you are taking.

Why Else Do People Take *Neurontin*® (gabapentin)?

Neurontin® (gabapentin) may also be used to help prevent seizures (epilepsy).

 # Warning!

To give you the best care, your doctor or other healthcare professional needs to know about the diseases and medical conditions you have had—your full medical history. Tell your doctor or other healthcare professional if you have or have ever had any of the following:

- Allergy or previous reaction to *Neurontin*® (gabapentin)
- Kidney problems
- Pancreas problems (pancreatitis)
- Seizures (epilepsy)

Neurontin® (gabapentin) may cause drowsiness. Avoid driving a car and other activities that need mental alertness, like using a knife or operating machinery, while taking this medication. Drinking alcoholic beverages (such as beer, wine, whiskey, and others) may increase the side effects.

Neurontin® (gabapentin) may make you unsteady on your feet, causing you to fall and possibly break a bone. If you have fallen recently, tell your doctor or other healthcare professional about it. Taking a different medication or a lower dose may make you less likely to fall. You should not stop taking this medication without first talking to your doctor or other healthcare professional.

Under certain circumstances, your doctor or other healthcare professional may decide that you should stop taking this medication. If you have taken it for more than a couple of weeks, he or she may want you to decrease it gradually, lowering the dose over a few weeks or months. Stopping suddenly may cause unpleasant withdrawal symptoms or may worsen your medical problems. Pay careful attention to the instructions your doctor or other healthcare professional gives you about how much less to take and for how long.

Capsaicin

Capsaicin is a medication used to help relieve pain from arthritis, neuropathy (nerve damage), shingles (post-herpetic neuralgia), and other painful conditions. Capsaicin is available over-the-counter (OTC) without a prescription.

Brand Name	Generic Name
Capsin®	capsaicin
Zostrix®	capsaicin

 ## How Should I Use Capsaicin?

Capsaicin comes as a cream or a lotion that is usually applied 3 to 4 times daily. It usually takes at least 2 weeks to work; it may take up to 1 month. It may cause stinging or burning when applied to the skin, but this usually improves

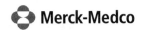
after continued use. Follow the instructions on the package or ask your doctor or other healthcare professional how often to use this medication.

If you miss a dose of this medication, use it as soon as possible. However, if it is almost time for your next dose, skip the missed dose and go back to your regular dosing schedule. Do not double your dose. Use your medication exactly as directed by your doctor or other healthcare professional. Do not stop using a prescription medication unless directed by your doctor or other healthcare professional.

 ## What Side Effects Can Capsaicin Cause?

More Common

- Burning
- Redness
- Stinging

Less Common

- Cough

Tell your doctor or other healthcare professional if you have side effects that bother you, do not go away, make you worried about taking your medication, or make you want to stop taking your medication.

 ## Do Other Medications Interact with Capsaicin?

Capsaicin does not have any known medication interactions.

Warning!

To give you the best care, your doctor or other healthcare professional needs to know about the diseases and medical conditions you have had—your full medical history. Tell your doctor or other healthcare professional if you have or have had an allergy or previous reaction to capsaicin.

Wash your hands thoroughly with soap and water after each use. If you are using capsaicin for arthritis in your hands, you should wait 30 minutes before washing your hands. During that time, be sure to keep your hands away from your eyes, nose, and mouth to avoid irritation. If you accidentally get capsaicin in your eyes, rinse them with large amounts of cool water. Call your doctor or other healthcare professional if you develop pain or redness that does not go away.

You may feel burning or stinging when you start to use capsaicin. This usually stops after a few days of use. Burning or stinging is more common when it is used less than 3 to 4 times daily. Talk to your doctor or other healthcare professional if burning or stinging continues.

Do not use capsaicin on an open wound or minor cuts and scrapes (abrasions).

Do not apply a heating pad to the area where you have applied capsaicin. Avoid tightly wrapping or bandaging the area where you applied the medication.

Asthma, Emphysema, and Chronic Bronchitis

Breathing problems may occur with asthma, emphysema, and chronic bronchitis. Asthma occurs when the breathing passages in the lungs are tightened (constricted), inflamed (swollen) or blocked by mucus (phlegm), limiting the amount of air that can get through. People with asthma often have allergies to dust, pollen, molds, and other substances in the air.

Emphysema and chronic bronchitis usually occur as a result of damage to the lungs from long-standing exposure to inhaled irritants, the most common of which is cigarette smoke. Emphysema and chronic bronchitis are also called chronic obstructive pulmonary disease or COPD. Symptoms of COPD include frequent coughing with mucus for months or years (chronic cough) and shortness of breath.

Treatment for asthma and COPD includes avoiding irritants (things that make your breathing more difficult), taking medications as prescribed by your doctor or other healthcare professional, quitting smoking, and staying away from other people who are smoking. If you still smoke, ask your doctor or other healthcare professional about ways to help you stop smoking.

Treatment for asthma is divided into two kinds of medications called "quick-relief medications" and "controller medications." Quick-relief medications help reduce or relieve shortness of breath and wheezing during an asthma attack. Quick-relief medications are fast-acting and are usually used as needed when asthma symptoms start. Controller medications are medications that help prevent or control asthma so that asthma attacks do not occur. Controller medications are slow-acting and are usually used daily to help prevent an asthma attack from occurring. Some of the same medications are used for

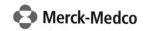
emphysema and chronic bronchitis and work similarly for each of these conditions.

Symptoms of asthma, emphysema, and chronic bronchitis may be worsened if you get the flu (influenza) or pneumonia. Ask your doctor or other healthcare professional about getting a flu shot every fall to help prevent the flu. Also, ask about a vaccination to help prevent pneumonia.

Medications for Asthma and COPD

Several kinds of medications may be taken for asthma and COPD. This chapter discusses these medications and/or categories of medications:

MEDICATIONS	See Page
Beta-adrenergic Bronchodilators	99
Theophylline	106
Atrovent® (ipratropium)	112
Corticosteroids	117
Intal® (cromolyn) and *Tilade*® (nedocromil)	125
Leukotriene Modifiers	129

If you do not see the exact name of the medication that you take for asthma or COPD listed above, check the Medication and Chapter Table to find out which category your medication falls under or check the Index.

Beta-adrenergic Bronchodilators

Beta-adrenergic bronchodilators help to relax constricted (narrowed) breathing passages that cause shortness of breath in people with asthma and COPD. This helps to open the breathing passages and allow air to pass in and out of the lungs more freely. Most inhaled beta-adrenergic bronchodilators are called "quick-relief medications" because they are used as needed to help relieve shortness of breath and wheezing during an asthma attack.

The long-acting beta-adrenergic bronchodilator inhaler *Serevent®* (salmeterol) is called a "controller medication" because it is used daily to help control asthma to help prevent asthma attacks from happening. It cannot be used for quick relief of wheezing and shortness of breath during an asthma attack because it takes too long to take effect.

Beta-adrenergic bronchodilator pills are called "controller medications" because they are used daily to help prevent and control asthma so that asthma attacks do not occur. They do not work quickly and cannot be taken for quick relief of wheezing and shortness of breath during an asthma attack. Talk to your doctor or other healthcare professional to see which beta-adrenergic bronchodilators are right for you.

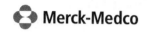

Brand Name	Generic Name	Types of Medications
Alupent®	metaproterenol	spray inhaler, oral liquid, oral tablets, nebulizer solution
AsthmaNefrin®	epinephrine	nebulizer solution
Brethine®	terbutaline	oral tablets
Bricanyl®	terbutaline	oral tablets
Combivent®†	albuterol/ipratropium	spray inhaler
Isuprel®	isoproterenol	oral tablets, spray inhaler
Maxair®	pirbuterol	spray inhaler
Medihaler ISO®	isoproterenol	spray inhaler
Metaprel®	metaproterenol	oral tablets, oral liquid, spray inhaler, nebulizer solution
Primatene® *Mist**	epinephrine	spray inhaler
Proventil®	albuterol	oral tablets, oral syrup, spray inhaler, nebulizer solution
Serevent®	salmeterol	spray inhaler, disk inhaler
Tornalate®	bitolterol	spray inhaler, nebulizer solution
Ventolin®	albuterol	oral tablets, oral syrup, spray inhaler, capsule inhaler, nebulizer solution
Xopenex™	levalbuterol	nebulizer solution

*Available over-the-counter without a prescription

†For convenience, albuterol is combined with ipratropium for people who need both medications. Please also read the section called *Atrovent*® (ipratropium) on page 112.

How Will I Take Beta-adrenergic Bronchodilators?

Beta-adrenergic bronchodilator "quick-relief medications" come in inhalers or liquid medications to put in a nebulizer (see below). Quick-relief medications are usually used every 4 to 6 hours as needed for wheezing and shortness of breath during asthma attacks. They usually work in 15 to 30 minutes when used in an inhaler or a nebulizer. Your doctor or other healthcare professional may instruct you to use your quick-relief inhaler 15 minutes before you exercise or go outside in cold weather to help prevent wheezing or shortness of breath.

Beta-adrenergic bronchodilators may also be used to help prevent asthma and COPD. When used to help prevent symptoms, inhaled beta-adrenergic bronchodilators are usually taken regularly 2 to 4 times daily.

Serevent® (salmeterol) is an inhaled "controller medication" that is usually used twice daily to help control asthma and help prevent attacks from occurring. Your doctor or other healthcare professional may also instruct you to take your *Serevent*® (salmeterol) 30 to 60 minutes before you exercise or go outside in cold weather to help prevent wheezing or shortness of breath.

Beta-adrenergic bronchodilator pills are "controller medications" and are usually taken 1 to 4 times daily. Your doctor or other healthcare professional will tell you how often to use your medication and when to take your medication.

If you miss a dose of this medication, take the dose you missed as soon as possible. However, if it is almost time for your next dose, skip the missed dose and just take the next one. Do not double your dose. Take your medication exactly as directed by your doctor or other healthcare professional. Do not stop taking a prescription medication unless directed by your doctor or other healthcare professional.

Beta-adrenergic Bronchodilator Inhalers

Inhalers are aerosol sprays or disk or capsule devices that help you breathe your medication directly into the lungs where it needs to work. This is more helpful during an asthma attack than oral tablets or liquids because many inhalers

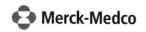

provide quicker relief when you are having shortness of breath or an asthma attack. Inhalers contain low doses of medications because the medication goes straight to the lungs, unlike a pill that has to be absorbed and then move through your bloodstream to get to the lungs. Consequently, they lower the chance of side effects that may occur when you take a higher dose of oral medication.

To get the most benefit from an inhaler, you must carefully follow all of the steps for its proper use. Inhaler use can sometimes be difficult because you have to coordinate your breathing with pressing down on the inhaler. Inhalers may also be hard to use if you have trouble with weakness or steadiness in your hands from arthritis, stroke, Parkinson's disease, and other medical problems. See directions for using aerosol spray inhalers at the end of this chapter on pages 132–133. Ask your doctor or other healthcare professional to watch you use your inhaler to make sure you are using it correctly. If you have trouble using the inhaler, you may be given a tube-like device called a spacer. A spacer helps to increase the amount of medication that gets into your lungs and also helps lower your chance of mouth and throat irritation from the inhaled medication.

Beta-adrenergic Bronchodilator Medications for Nebulizers

Beta-adrenergic bronchodilator liquid medication is put into a small machine called a nebulizer to create a mist of medication that you breathe in through a tube directly into the lungs. Like inhalers, this medication goes right into the lungs where it needs to work. Nebulizers are sometimes used when people have severe asthma and COPD or if they have trouble using inhalers. To get the most benefit from a nebulizer, you must follow the directions for use provided with your nebulizer. You should also clean the machine as directed to help prevent lung infections. Do not use your liquid medication in your nebulizer if it has specks or particles floating in the liquid or if the liquid becomes cloudy or discolored. Talk to your doctor or other healthcare professional if you have questions about using your nebulizer.

Beta-adrenergic Bronchodilator Pills and Liquids

Pills and liquids contain higher doses of beta-adrenergic bronchodilators than inhalants, so pills and liquids may cause more side effects than inhalants. Pills and liquids take longer to work than inhalants. People who have trouble using inhalers may have to take pills or liquids for their asthma and COPD.

What Side Effects Can Beta-adrenergic Bronchodilators Cause?

More Common

- Fast or irregular heartbeat (palpitations)
- Nervousness (anxiety)
- Shakiness or tremors
- Trouble falling asleep or staying asleep (insomnia)

Less Common

- Headache
- High blood pressure (hypertension)

Rare

- Trouble urinating or emptying the bladder

Tell your doctor or other healthcare professional if you have side effects that bother you, do not go away, make you worried about taking your medication, or make you want to stop taking your medication.

Do Other Medications Interact with Beta-adrenergic Bronchodilators?

Many nonprescription (over-the-counter [OTC]) medications, such as pain, cough, cold, and allergy medications contain medications that *may increase* the

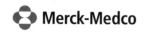

side effects of beta-adrenergic bronchodilators. If you are taking beta-adrenergic bronchodilators regularly, you should talk to your doctor or other healthcare professional before taking any new OTC medications.

Beta blockers, such as *Inderal®* (propranolol), *Tenormin®* (atenolol), *Toprol®* (metoprolol), and others (see Glossary), ***may increase*** the symptoms of asthma, emphysema, chronic bronchitis, and COPD, causing shortness of breath or trouble breathing.

Beta-adrenergic bronchodilators are generally not prescribed for anyone who is taking MAO inhibitors, such as *Marplan®* (isocarboxazid), *Nardil®* (phenelzine), or *Parnate®* (tranylcypromine), because together they ***may cause*** serious or even fatal reactions. If your doctor or other healthcare professional wants you to stop taking one medication and start taking the other, you should wait at least 2 weeks between stopping one and starting the other.

Comtan® (entacapone) ***may increase*** the side effects of beta-adrenergic bronchodilators.

Tell your doctor or other healthcare professional about all medications (both prescription and nonprescription [over-the-counter] medications) that you are taking.

What Else Should I Know about Beta-adrenergic Bronchodilators?

You cannot tell whether an inhaler is empty by shaking it. It contains a propellant (something that drives the medication out of the inhaler) as well as your medication. Some propellant may be left in the canister, even though the medicine is used up. Spraying into the air or trying to taste the medication will not help you tell if it is empty and wastes medication. Floating your canister in water to see whether it is empty will not work either. The best way to tell if an aerosol inhaler is empty is to count the number of doses you have taken. The number of doses in an aerosol inhaler is written on the canister. Ask your doctor or other healthcare professional to help you calculate the number of doses you have left by counting the number of puffs you take each day. Make sure you always have an extra inhaler so you will not run out.

 # Warning!

To give you the best care, your doctor or other healthcare professional needs to know about the diseases and medical conditions you have had—your full medical history. Tell your doctor or other healthcare professional if you have or have ever had, or presently take, any of the following:

- Allergy or previous reaction to beta-adrenergic bronchodilators
- Diabetes
- Heart problems (angina)
- Heart rhythm problems (arrhythmia)
- High blood pressure (hypertension)
- MAO inhibitors such as *Marplan*® (isocarboxazid), *Nardil*® (phenelzine), or *Parnate*® (tranylcypromine)
- Overactive thyroid (hyperthyroidism)

Do not use more medication than your doctor or other healthcare professional recommends. Needing more medication than prescribed may be a sign that you have worsening of your condition, which can be serious, even fatal, if not treated. Talk to your doctor or other healthcare professional if your medications are not helping to relieve your symptoms.

Some inhalers are called "quick-relief medications" because they help relieve wheezing and shortness of breath during an asthma attack. Other inhalers are called "controller medications" because they control asthma and help prevent asthma attacks from occurring. To get the most benefit from your inhalers, you need to know which to use when. If you are using more than one inhaler, ask your doctor or other healthcare professional to tell you what each inhaler is for and when it should be used. If you have a quick-relief inhaler for shortness of breath and asthma attacks, you should remember to take it with you when you leave the house.

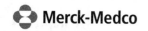

Serevent® (salmeterol), a long-acting beta-adrenergic bronchodilator, must not be used to relieve wheezing and shortness of breath during an asthma attack. It is used only as a "controller medication" to help prevent and control asthma so that asthma attacks do not occur.

Epinephrine such as *AsthmaNefrin®* and *Primatene® Mist* may cause problems with anesthesia used in surgery. Tell your doctor or other healthcare professional if you will be having surgery or major dental work in case he or she wants you to stop your medication for a few days.

Theophylline

Theophylline helps open the breathing passages and helps the diaphragm (muscle under the lungs) bring air into the lungs. Theophylline is called a "controller medication" because it is taken daily to help prevent and control asthma so that asthma attacks do not occur. Theophylline is used to help prevent symptoms of asthma and COPD from occurring. Theophylline pills and syrups cannot be used to help relieve wheezing or shortness of breath during an asthma attack.

Brand Name	Generic Name
Slo-bid™	theophylline
Slo-Phyllin®	theophylline
Theo-24®	theophylline
Theobid®	theophylline
Theo-Dur®	theophylline
Theolair™	theophylline
T-Phyl®	theophylline
Uni-Dur®	theophylline
Uniphyl®	theophylline

How Will I Take Theophylline?

Theophylline is usually taken as a pill 1 to 4 times a day. Theophylline may also be taken as a syrup, which may help people who have trouble swallowing pills. Your doctor or other healthcare professional will tell you how many times a day to take your medication.

When a medication has initials after its name, such as XL, XR, SR, BID, DUR, and others, it usually means that the body absorbs the medication slowly over time, so you usually have to take it only once or twice a day. The body will absorb some medications of this type too fast if you crush or break them or dissolve them in liquid, and their effects will not last as long as they should. Check with your doctor or other healthcare professional before crushing or breaking your pills or dissolving your pills in liquid.

If you miss a dose of this medication, take the dose you missed as soon as possible. However, if it is almost time for your next dose, skip the missed dose and just take the next one. Do not double your dose. Take your medication exactly as directed by your doctor or other healthcare professional. Do not stop taking a prescription medication unless directed by your doctor or other healthcare professional.

What Side Effects Can Theophylline Cause?

More Common

- Headache
- Heartburn
- Nausea
- Need to urinate more often
- Nervousness (anxiety)
- Shakiness or tremors
- Trouble falling asleep or staying asleep (insomnia)

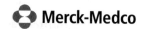

Less Common

- Dizziness

- Fast heartbeat (palpitations)

- Irritability

- Rash (skin redness, bumps, itching, or irritation)

- Seizures

- Ulcers in the stomach that may cause black, tarry-looking bowel movements

- Vomiting

Tell your doctor or other healthcare professional if you have side effects that bother you, do not go away, make you worried about taking your medication, or make you want to stop taking your medication.

 Do Other Medications Interact with Theophylline?

These medications *may increase* the side effects of theophylline:

- Amiodarone such as *Cordarone*® or *Pacerone*®

- *Antabuse*® (disulfiram)

- *Biaxin*® (clarithromycin)

- Calcium channel blockers such as *Cardizem*® (diltiazem), *Norvasc*® (amlodipine), *Procardia*® (nifedipine), and others—see Glossary

- *Cognex*® (tacrine)

- *Dynabac*® (dirithromycin)

- Erythromycin such as *Ery-Tab*®, *Erythrocin*®, and others—see Glossary

- *Ethmozine*® (moricizine)

- Interferon such as *Intron*® A (interferon alfa-2b), *Betaseron*® (interferon beta-1b), and others—see Glossary

- *Luvox®* (fluvoxamine)

- *Mexitil®* (mexiletine)

- *Mintezol®* (thiabendazole)

- *Prevacid®* (lansoprazole)

- *Prilosec®* (omeprazole)

- Propylthiouracil (PTU)

- Quinolone antibiotics such as *Cipro®* (ciprofloxacin), *Floxin®* (ofloxacin), and *Levaquin®* (levofloxacin)—see Glossary

- *Rythmol®* (propafenone)

- *Tagamet®* (cimetidine)

- *Tapazole®* (methimazole)

- *Ticlid®* (ticlopidine)

- *Zithromax®* (azithromycin)

- *Zovirax®* (acyclovir)

- *Zyflo®* (zileuton)

- *Zyloprim®* (allopurinol)

These medications ***may decrease*** how well theophylline works:

- *Anturane®* (sulfinpyrazone)

- Barbiturates such as *Butisol®* (butabarbital), *Luminal®* (phenobarbital), *Mebaral®* (mephobarbital), and others—see Glossary

- *Cytadren®* (aminoglutethimide)

- *Dilantin®* (phenytoin)

- Isoniazid

- *Rifadin®* (rifampin)

- *Tegretol®* (carbamazepine)

- Thyroid medications such as *Cytomel®* (liothyronine), *Levoxyl®* (levothyroxine), *Synthroid®* (levothyroxine), and others—see Glossary

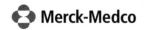

Theophylline *may decrease* how well these medications work:

- *Accolate*® (zafirlukast)

- *Dilantin*® (phenytoin)

Beta blockers, such as *Inderal*® (propranolol), *Tenormin*® (atenolol), *Toprol*® (metoprolol), and others (see Glossary), *may increase* the symptoms of asthma, emphysema, chronic bronchitis, and COPD, causing shortness of breath or trouble breathing.

Many nonprescription (over-the-counter [OTC]) medications such as pain, cough, cold, and allergy medications, contain medications that *may increase* the side effects of theophylline. If you are taking theophylline, you should talk to your doctor or other healthcare professional before taking any new OTC medications.

Tell your doctor or other healthcare professional about all medications (both prescription and nonprescription [over-the-counter] medications) that you are taking.

What Else Should I Know about Theophylline?

Caffeine may increase the side effects of theophylline. Do not eat or drink large amounts of food or beverages that contain caffeine, such as coffee, tea, chocolate, colas, and some other soft drinks.

 # Warning!

To give you the best care, your doctor or other healthcare professional needs to know about the diseases and medical conditions you have had—your full medical history. Tell your doctor or other healthcare professional if you have or have ever had any of the following:

- Allergy or previous reaction to theophylline

- Congestive heart failure

- Heart problems

- Heart rhythm problems (arrhythmia)

- Liver problems

- Seizures (epilepsy)

- Stomach problems (ulcers)

- Overactive thyroid (hyperthyroidism)

Since theophylline may cause side effects if you get too much medication and may not work well if you do not get enough, your doctor or other healthcare professional may order blood tests to see if you are getting the right amount of this medication. Nausea, vomiting, nervousness, or trouble sleeping may be early signs that you are getting too much medication. Talk to your doctor or other healthcare professional if you have any of these symptoms, and be sure to get your blood tests as ordered. Do not change your dose or stop taking this medication unless directed by your doctor or other healthcare professional.

Changes in diet can affect how quickly theophylline is removed from your body. High- or low-protein diets or eating char-broiled or grilled food can affect your theophylline blood levels. Talk to your doctor or other healthcare professional before making any major changes in your diet while you are taking theophylline.

In addition to worsening your asthma and COPD, smoking cigarettes can affect how quickly theophylline is removed from your body. Talk to your doctor or other healthcare professional about ways to quit smoking. Let your doctor or other healthcare professional know when you quit so he or she can test your theophylline blood level to see if your dose of theophylline needs to be changed.

Theophylline is a "controller medication" and is used to help prevent shortness of breath and other symptoms from asthma and COPD from happening. It is important to know that this medication will not help when you are having sudden shortness of breath or an asthma attack. Taking extra theophylline will not help and may cause more side effects. Talk to your doctor or other healthcare professional to make sure you know what medication to take and what to do when you have sudden shortness of breath or an asthma attack. If you have a quick-relief inhaler for shortness of breath and asthma attacks, you should remember to take it with you when you leave the house.

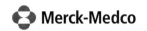
Theophylline may cause stomach pain, which may be a sign of an ulcer. However, you may have an ulcer without feeling any pain at all. If ulcers are not treated, they may cause serious stomach or intestinal bleeding. Tell your doctor or other healthcare professional if you have severe stomach pain or stomach pain that keeps returning or if you have ever had peptic ulcer disease. Call your doctor or other healthcare professional right away if you have black, tarry-looking bowel movements (stools), if you vomit dark material that looks like coffee grounds, or if you notice any blood in your bowel movements. Any of these symptoms may be a sign of a bleeding ulcer.

Atrovent® (ipratropium)

Atrovent® (ipratropium) helps to relax constricted (narrowed) breathing passages. This helps to open the breathing passages and allow air to pass in and out of the lungs more freely. *Atrovent*® (ipratropium) is usually used to help prevent and relieve shortness of breath from COPD, including emphysema and chronic bronchitis. It is sometimes used as a "quick-relief medication" in asthma because it can help relieve shortness of breath and wheezing.

Brand Name	Generic Name	Types of Medications
Atrovent®	ipratropium	spray inhaler, nebulizer solution
Combivent®†	ipratropium/albuterol†	spray inhaler

†For convenience, albuterol is combined with ipratropium for people who need both medications. Please also read the section called Beta-adrenergic Bronchodilators on page 99.

 How Will I Take *Atrovent*® (ipratropium)?

Atrovent® (ipratropium) comes in an inhaler or in a liquid medication to put in a nebulizer. When used to help prevent symptoms of emphysema or chronic bronchitis, it is usually used regularly 2 to 4 times daily.

For quick relief from wheezing and shortness of breath during asthma attacks, *Atrovent®* (ipratropium) inhalers and nebulizers are usually used as needed every 4 to 6 hours. They usually work in 15 to 30 minutes. Your doctor or other healthcare professional will tell you how much and how often to use this medication.

If you miss a dose of this medication, take the dose you missed as soon as possible. However, if it is almost time for your next dose, skip the missed dose and just take the next one. Do not double your dose. Take your medication exactly as directed by your doctor or other healthcare professional. Do not stop taking a prescription medication unless directed by your doctor or other healthcare professional.

Atrovent® (ipratropium) Inhalers

Atrovent® (ipratropium) inhalers are aerosol sprays that help you breathe your medication directly into the lungs where it needs to work. This is more helpful than oral tablets or liquids because it provides quicker relief when you are having shortness of breath or an asthma attack. Inhalers contain low doses of medications because the medication goes straight to the lungs, unlike a pill that has to be absorbed and then move through your bloodstream to get to the lungs. Consequently, inhalers may lower the chance of side effects that may occur when you take a higher dose of oral medication.

To get the most benefit from an inhaler, you must carefully follow all of the steps for its proper use. Inhaler use can sometimes be difficult because you have to coordinate your breathing with pressing down on the inhaler. Inhalers may also be hard to use if you have trouble with weakness or steadiness in your hands from arthritis, stroke, Parkinson's disease, and other medical problems. See directions for using aerosol spray inhalers at the end of this chapter on pages 132–133. Ask your doctor or other healthcare professional to watch you use your inhaler to make sure you are using it correctly. If you have trouble using the inhaler, you may be given a tube-like device called a spacer. A spacer helps to increase the amount of medication that gets into your lungs and also helps lower your chance of mouth and throat irritation from the inhaled medication.

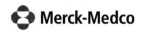

Atrovent® (ipratropium) Medications for Nebulizers

Atrovent® (ipratropium) liquid medication is put into a small machine called a nebulizer to create a mist of medication that you breathe in through a tube directly into the lungs. Like inhalers, this medication goes right into the lungs where it needs to work. Nebulizers are sometimes used when people have severe asthma and COPD or if they have trouble using inhalers. To get the most benefit from your nebulizer, you must follow the directions for use provided with your nebulizer. You should also clean the machine as directed to help prevent lung infections. Do not use your liquid medication in your nebulizer if it has specks or particles floating in the liquid or if the liquid becomes cloudy or discolored. Talk to your doctor or other healthcare professional if you have questions about using your nebulizer.

What Side Effects Can *Atrovent®* (ipratropium) Cause?

More Common

- Dry mouth

Less Common

- Blurred or double vision
- Cough
- Dizziness
- Headache
- Nervousness (anxiety)
- Trouble urinating or emptying the bladder

Tell your doctor or other healthcare professional if you have side effects that bother you, do not go away, make you worried about taking your medication, or make you want to stop taking your medication.

Do Other Medications Interact with *Atrovent*® (ipratropium)?

Beta blockers such as *Inderal*® (propranolol), *Tenormin*® (atenolol), *Toprol*® (metoprolol), and others (see Glossary) *may increase* the symptoms of asthma, and COPD, including emphysema and chronic bronchitis, causing shortness of breath or trouble breathing.

Combivent® (ipratropium/albuterol) is generally not prescribed for anyone who is taking MAO inhibitors, such as *Marplan*® (isocarboxazid), *Nardil*® (phenelzine), or *Parnate*® (tranylcypromine), because together they *may cause* serious or even fatal reactions. If your doctor or other healthcare professional wants you to stop taking one medication and start taking the other, you should wait at least 2 weeks between stopping one and starting the other.

Tell your doctor or other healthcare professional about all medications (both prescription and nonprescription [over-the-counter] medications) that you are taking.

What Else Should I Know about *Atrovent*® (ipratropium)?

You cannot tell whether an inhaler is empty by shaking it. It contains a propellant (something that drives the medication out of the inhaler) as well as your medication. Some propellant may be left in the canister, even though the medicine is used up. Spraying into the air or trying to taste the medication will not help you tell if it is empty and wastes medication. Floating your canister in water to see whether it is empty will not work either. The best way to tell if an aerosol inhaler is empty is to count the number of doses you have taken. The number of doses in an aerosol inhaler is written on the canister. Ask your doctor or other healthcare professional to help you calculate the number of doses you have left by counting the number of puffs you take each day. Make sure you always have an extra inhaler so you will not run out.

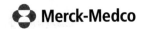

Warning!

To give you the best care, your doctor or other healthcare professional needs to know about the diseases and medical conditions you have had—your full medical history. Tell your doctor or other healthcare professional if you have or have ever had, or presently take, any of the following:

- Allergy or previous reaction to *Atrovent®* (ipratropium) or *Combivent®* (ipratropium/albuterol)

- Enlarged prostate (benign prostatic hypertrophy)

- Glaucoma (an eye disease)

- Heart problems

- Liver problems

- MAO inhibitors such as *Marplan®* (isocarboxazid), *Nardil®* (phenelzine), or *Parnate®* (tranylcypromine)

- Trouble urinating or emptying the bladder

Be careful not to spray the inhalant in your eyes, especially if you have the eye condition, glaucoma. Call your doctor or other healthcare professional if you experience sudden and severe pain in the eye.

Do not use more medication than your doctor or other healthcare professional recommends. Needing more medication than prescribed may be a sign that you have worsening of your condition, which can be serious, even fatal, if not treated. Talk to your doctor or other healthcare professional if your medications are not helping to relieve your symptoms.

Some inhalers are called "quick-relief medications" because they help relieve wheezing and shortness of breath during an asthma attack. Other inhalers are called "controller medications" because they control asthma and help prevent asthma attacks from occurring. To get the most benefit from your inhalers, you need to use them at the right time. If you are using more than one inhaler, ask your doctor or other healthcare professional to tell you what each inhaler is for and when it should be used. If you have a quick-relief inhaler for shortness of breath and asthma attacks, you should remember to take it with you when you leave the house.

Corticosteroids (Steroids)

Corticosteroid inhalers and pills help to reduce inflammation (swelling and irritation) of the breathing passages and help air pass in and out of the lungs more freely. Inhaled corticosteroids are called "controller medications" because they are used to control asthma and help prevent asthma attacks from occurring. Inhaled corticosteroids are not "quick-relief medications" and do not relieve wheezing or shortness of breath during an asthma attack. Corticosteroid pills or injections may be used with a "quick-relief inhaled medication" to provide relief during an asthma attack. Corticosteroid pills may also improve the breathing in people with COPD that has worsened. Your doctor or other healthcare professional will tell you when and how often to use corticosteroid inhalers and pills.

Brand Name	Generic Name
AeroBid® Inhaler	flunisolide
Aristocort®	triamcinolone
Azmacort® Inhaler	triamcinolone
Beclovent® Inhaler	beclomethasone
Celestone®	betamethasone
Decadron®	dexamethasone
Flovent® Inhaler	fluticasone
Hexadrol®	dexamethasone
Medrol®	methylprednisolone
Pulmicort® Inhaler	budesonide
Vanceril® Inhaler	beclomethasone
Various	prednisone
Various	hydrocortisone
Various	prednisolone

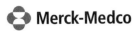

How Will I Take Corticosteroids?

Corticosteroid inhalers are usually used 2 to 4 times daily. Pills are usually taken once a day in the morning or once every other day. Taking corticosteroid pills with food or milk may help prevent stomach upset from the medication. Your doctor or other healthcare professional will tell you how often to take the medication.

If you miss a dose of this medication, take the dose you missed as soon as possible. However, if it is almost time for your next dose, skip the missed dose and just take the next one. Do not double your dose. Take your medication exactly as directed by your doctor or other healthcare professional. Do not stop taking a prescription medication unless directed by your doctor or other healthcare professional.

Corticosteroid Inhalers

Inhalers are aerosol sprays or disk devices that help you breathe your medication directly into the lungs where it needs to work. Inhalers contain low doses of medications because the medication goes straight to the lungs, unlike a pill that has to be absorbed and then move through your bloodstream to get to the lungs. Consequently, inhalers may lower the chance of side effects that may occur when you take a higher dose of oral medication.

To get the most benefit from an inhaler, you must carefully follow all of the steps for its proper use. Inhaler use can sometimes be difficult because you have to coordinate your breathing with pressing down on the inhaler. Inhalers may also be hard to use if you have trouble with weakness or steadiness in your hands from arthritis, stroke, Parkinson's disease, and other medical problems. See directions for using aerosol spray inhalers at the end of this chapter on pages 132–133. Ask your doctor or other healthcare professional to watch you use your inhaler to make sure you are using it correctly. If you have trouble using the inhaler, you may be given a tube-like device called a spacer. A spacer helps to increase the amount of medication that gets into your lungs and also helps lower your chance of mouth and throat irritation from the inhaled medication.

Corticosteroid Pills and Liquids

Pills and liquids contain higher doses of corticosteroids than inhalants, so pills and liquids may cause more side effects than inhalants. People with worsening or severe asthma or COPD may have to take corticosteroid pills or liquids to help control their symptoms.

What Side Effects Can Corticosteroids Cause?

In the first few weeks after you start taking corticosteroid pills (short-term)*:

- High blood pressure (hypertension)
- Increased appetite
- Increased blood sugar (hyperglycemia)
- Increased chance of infection
- Mood swings
- Nausea
- Stomach pain
- Swelling or puffiness of the feet, ankles, or lower legs (edema)
- Trouble falling asleep or staying asleep (insomnia)
- Ulcers in the stomach that may cause black, tarry-looking bowel movements
- Vomiting
- Weakness or muscle cramps that may be a sign of low potassium in your blood (hypokalemia)

After months or years of taking corticosteroids (long-term)*:

- Acne
- Cataracts

*The side effects of corticosteroid pills rarely occur with corticosteroid inhalers.

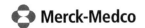

- Easy bruising ("black-and-blue" marks on the skin)
- Hair growth in unwanted places
- Muscle weakness
- Poor wound healing
- Reddening of the face (flushing)
- Thinning bones from decreased bone density (osteoporosis)
- Thin skin
- Weight gain
- Worsening of glaucoma (an eye disease)

Inhaled Corticosteroids Only

- Coughing and wheezing
- Dry mouth
- Hoarseness or voice changes
- Oral thrush (yeast infection of the mouth)
- Sore throat

Tell your doctor or other healthcare professional if you have side effects that bother you, do not go away, make you worried about taking your medication, or make you want to stop taking your medication.

 ## Do Other Medications Interact with Corticosteroids?

These medications **may decrease** how well corticosteroids work:

- Barbiturates such as *Butisol*® (butabarbital), *Luminal*® (phenobarbital), *Mebaral*® (mephobarbital), and others—see Glossary

- *Dilantin®* (phenytoin)
- *Rifadin®* (rifampin)

Corticosteroids ***may decrease*** how well these medications work:
- *Mestinon®* (pyridostigmine)
- *Prostigmin®* (neostigmine)

These medications ***may increase*** the side effects of corticosteroids:
- *Biaxin®* (clarithromycin)
- *Diflucan®* (fluconazole)
- Erythromycin such as *Ery-Tab®*, *Erythrocin®*, and others—see Glossary
- Estrogens such as *Estrace®*, *Premarin®*, *Prempro™*, and others—see Glossary
- *Nizoral®* (ketoconazole)
- *Sporanox®* (itraconazole)

Corticosteroids ***may increase*** the side effects of these medications:
- Aspirin and medications that contain aspirin
- *Coumadin®* (warfarin)
- Diuretics (water pills) such as *HydroDIURIL®* (hydrochlorothiazide or HCTZ), *Lasix®* (furosemide), and others—see Glossary
- *Lanoxin®* (digoxin)
- Nonsteroidal anti-inflammatory drugs (NSAIDs) such as *Motrin®* (ibuprofen), *Aleve®* (naproxen), *Celebrex®* (celecoxib), *Vioxx®* (rofecoxib), and others—see Glossary

Many nonprescription (over-the-counter [OTC]) medications such as pain, cough, cold, allergy, and sleep medications contain aspirin or nonsteroidal anti-inflammatory drugs (NSAIDs) that ***may increase*** the side effects of corticosteroids. If you are taking corticosteroids, you should talk to your doctor or other healthcare professional before taking any new OTC medications.

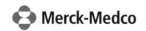

Beta blockers, such as *Inderal*® (propranolol), *Tenormin*® (atenolol), *Toprol*® (metoprolol), and others (see Glossary), ***may increase*** the symptoms of asthma and COPD, including emphysema and chronic bronchitis, causing shortness of breath or trouble breathing.

Tell your doctor or other healthcare professional about all medications (both prescription and nonprescription [over-the-counter] medications) that you are taking.

Why Else Do People Take Corticosteroids?

Corticosteroid pills are also sometimes used for arthritis and related diseases, allergies, some skin conditions, some chronic (long-term) liver problems, blood disorders, kidney problems, and conditions in which inflammation is a problem, including gout and bursitis.

What Else Should I Know about Corticosteroids?

After each time you use your inhaler, rinse your mouth well with water or mouthwash. Doing this may help prevent mouth and throat irritation and infection.

You cannot tell whether an inhaler is empty by shaking it. It contains a propellant (something that drives the medication out of the inhaler) as well as your medication. Some propellant may be left in the canister, even though the medication is used up. Spraying into the air or trying to taste the medication will not help you tell if it is empty and wastes medication. Floating your canister in water to see whether it is empty will not work either. The best way to tell if an aerosol inhaler is empty is to count the number of doses you have taken. The number of doses in an aerosol inhaler is written on the canister. Ask your doctor or other healthcare professional to help you calculate the number of doses you have left by counting the number of puffs you take each day. Make sure you always have an extra inhaler so you will not run out.

Warning!

To give you the best care, your doctor or other healthcare professional needs to know about the diseases and medical conditions you have had—your full medical history. Tell your doctor or other healthcare professional if you have or have ever had any of the following:

- Allergy or previous reaction to corticosteroids

- Diabetes

- Fungal infections

- Glaucoma (an eye disease)

- High blood pressure (hypertension)

- Inflammatory bowel disease (ulcerative colitis or Crohn's disease)

- Kidney problems

- Stomach problems (ulcer)

- Thinning bones from decreased bone density (osteoporosis)

- Tuberculosis

- Underactive thyroid (hypothyroidism)

Because corticosteroid pills may cause low potassium blood levels (hypokalemia) and high blood sugar (hyperglycemia), your doctor or other healthcare professional may order blood tests to check your blood sugar (glucose) and potassium levels.

Corticosteroid pills may hide symptoms of an infection and may weaken the body's defenses against infection. Call your doctor or other healthcare professional if you have a fever, sore throat, or flu-like symptoms that do not go away.

Corticosteroid pills may cause stomach pain, which may be a sign of an ulcer. However, you may have an ulcer without feeling any pain at all. If ulcers are not treated, they may cause serious stomach or intestinal bleeding. Tell your doctor or other healthcare professional if you have severe stomach pain or stomach pain that keeps returning or if you have ever had peptic ulcer disease.

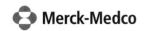

Call your doctor or other healthcare professional right away if you have black, tarry-looking bowel movements (stools), if you vomit dark material that looks like coffee grounds, or if you notice any blood in your bowel movements. Any of these symptoms may be a sign of a bleeding ulcer.

If you use corticosteroid pills for more than a couple of weeks, thinning of your bones (osteoporosis) may occur. Talk to your doctor or other healthcare professional about whether you are at increased risk for osteoporosis and about calcium, vitamin D, and other medications you can take to help keep your bones strong.

When taken for more than 6 months, corticosteroid pills may cause or worsen cataracts and glaucoma (an eye disease). Ask your doctor or other healthcare professional about scheduling an eye appointment to see whether the corticosteroids are causing or worsening cataracts or glaucoma.

Do not use more medication than your doctor or other healthcare professional recommends. Needing more medication than prescribed may be a sign that you have worsening of your condition, which can be serious, even fatal, if not treated. Talk to your doctor or other healthcare professional if your medications are not helping to relieve your symptoms.

Some inhalers are called "quick-relief medications" because they help relieve wheezing and shortness of breath during an asthma attack. Other inhalers are called "controller medications" because they control asthma and help prevent asthma attacks from occurring. To get the most benefit from your inhalers, you need to use them at the right time. If you are using more than one inhaler, ask your doctor or other healthcare professional to tell you what each inhaler is for and when it should be used. If you have a quick-relief inhaler for shortness of breath and asthma attacks, you should remember to take it with you when you leave the house.

Under certain circumstances, your doctor or other healthcare professional may decide that you should stop taking this medication. If you have taken it for more than a couple of weeks, he or she may want you to decrease it gradually, lowering the dose over a few weeks or months. Stopping suddenly may cause unpleasant withdrawal symptoms or may worsen your medical problems. Pay careful attention to the instructions your doctor or other healthcare professional gives you about how much less to take and for how long.

Intal® (cromolyn) and *Tilade*® (nedocromil)

Intal® (cromolyn) and *Tilade*® (nedocromil) help prevent the release of substances in the lungs that may cause inflammation (swelling and irritation) that produces asthma symptoms. *Intal*® (cromolyn) and *Tilade*® (nedocromil) are called "controller medications" because they help prevent and control asthma so that asthma attacks do not occur. These medications do not work quickly so they cannot be used to relieve wheezing or shortness of breath during an asthma attack.

How Will I Take *Intal*® (cromolyn) or *Tilade*® (nedocromil)?

Intal® (cromolyn) or *Tilade*® (nedocromil) is usually taken 4 times a day. These medications may not provide their full benefit for 2 to 3 weeks. Your doctor or other healthcare professional may instruct you to take 2 puffs at least 15 to 60 minutes before you exercise or go outside in cold weather to help prevent wheezing or shortness of breath. Your doctor or other healthcare professional will tell you how often and when to take your medication.

If you miss a dose of this medication, take the dose you missed as soon as possible. However, if it is almost time for your next dose, skip the missed dose and just take the next one. Do not double your dose. Take your medication exactly as directed by your doctor or other healthcare professional. Do not stop taking a prescription medication unless directed by your doctor or other healthcare professional.

Intal® (cromolyn) or *Tilade*® (nedocromil) Inhalers

Inhalers are aerosol sprays and powdered capsule devices that help you breathe your medication directly into the lungs where it needs to work. Inhalers contain low doses of medications because the medication goes straight to the lungs, unlike a pill that has to be absorbed and then move through your bloodstream to get to the lungs. Consequently, inhalers may lower the chance of side effects that may occur when you take a higher dose of oral medication.

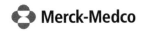
To get the most benefit from an inhaler, you must carefully follow all of the steps for its proper use. Inhaler use can sometimes be difficult because you have to coordinate your breathing with pressing down on the inhaler. Inhalers may also be hard to use if you have trouble with weakness or steadiness in your hands from arthritis, stroke, Parkinson's disease, and other medical problems. See directions for using aerosol spray inhalers at the end of this chapter on pages 132–133. Ask your doctor or other healthcare professional to watch you use your inhaler to make sure you are using it correctly. If you have trouble using the inhaler, you may be given a tube-like device called a spacer. A spacer helps to increase the amount of medication that gets into your lungs and also helps lower your chance of mouth and throat irritation from the inhaled medication.

Intal® (cromolyn) Medication for Nebulizers

Intal® (cromolyn) liquid medication is put into a small machine called a nebulizer to create a mist of medication that you breathe in through a tube directly into the lungs. As with inhalers, nebulizers send this medication right into the lungs where it needs to work. Nebulizers are sometimes used when people have severe asthma and COPD or if they have trouble using inhalers. To get the most benefit from your nebulizer, you must follow the directions for use provided with your nebulizer. You should also clean the machine as directed to help prevent lung infections. Do not use your liquid medication in your nebulizer if it has specks or particles floating in the liquid or if the liquid becomes cloudy or discolored. Talk to your doctor or other healthcare professional if you have questions about using your nebulizer.

 ## What Side Effects Can *Intal*® (cromolyn) or *Tilade*® (nedocromil) Cause?

More Common

- Bitter taste in mouth

- Cough

- Headache

Less Common

- Allergic reactions such as rash (skin redness, bumps, itching, or irritation), swelling of the face and throat, or trouble breathing

- Drowsiness

- Muscle aches and pains

- Nausea

- Throat irritation

Tell your doctor or other healthcare professional if you have side effects that bother you, do not go away, make you worried about taking your medication, or make you want to stop taking your medication

---

 ## Do Other Medications Interact with *Intal*® (cromolyn) or *Tilade*® (nedocromil)?

Beta blockers, such as *Inderal*® (propranolol), *Tenormin*® (atenolol), *Toprol*® (metoprolol), and others (see Glossary), **may increase** the symptoms of asthma and COPD, including emphysema and chronic bronchitis, causing shortness of breath or trouble breathing.

Why Else Do People Take *Intal*® (cromolyn) or *Tilade*® (nedocromil)?

Cromolyn and nedocromil are sometimes used in eyedrops for eye irritation (conjunctivitis) and in nasal sprays for allergy symptoms.

What Else Should I Know about *Intal*® (cromolyn) or *Tilade*® (nedocromil)?

You cannot tell whether an inhaler is empty by shaking it. It contains a propellant (something that drives the medication out of the inhaler) as well as

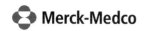
your medication. Some propellant may be left in the canister, even though the medicine is used up. Spraying into the air or trying to taste the medication will not help you tell if it is empty and wastes medication. Floating your canister in water to see whether it is empty will not work either. The best way to tell if an aerosol inhaler is empty is to count the number of doses you have taken. The number of doses in an aerosol inhaler is written on the canister. Ask your doctor or other healthcare professional to help you calculate the number of doses you have left by counting the number of puffs you take each day. Make sure you always have an extra inhaler so you will not run out.

 # Warning!

To give you the best care, your doctor or other healthcare professional needs to know about the diseases and medical conditions you have had—your full medical history. Tell your doctor or other healthcare professional if you have or have ever had any of the following:

- Allergy or previous reaction to *Intal*® (cromolyn) or *Tilade*® (nedocromil)
- Heart problems (angina)
- Irregular heartbeat (arrhythmia)
- Kidney problems
- Liver problems

Do not use more medication than your doctor or other healthcare professional recommends. Needing more medication than prescribed may be a sign that you have worsening of your condition, which can be serious, even fatal, if not treated. Talk to your doctor or other healthcare professional if your medications are not helping to relieve your symptoms.

Some inhalers are called "quick-relief medications" because they help relieve wheezing and shortness of breath during an asthma attack. Other inhalers are called "controller medications" because they control asthma and help prevent asthma attacks from occurring. To get the most benefit from your inhalers, you need to use them at the right time. If you are using more than one inhaler, ask your doctor or other healthcare professional to tell you what each inhaler is for and when it should be used. If you have a quick-relief inhaler for shortness of breath and asthma attacks, you should remember to take it with you when you leave the house.

Leukotriene Modifiers

Leukotriene modifiers help prevent inflammation (swelling and irritation) of the breathing passages. This helps allow air to pass in and out of the lungs more freely. These medications are called "controller medications" because they help prevent and control asthma symptoms so that asthma attacks do not occur. These medications do not work quickly so they cannot be used to relieve wheezing or shortness of breath during an asthma attack.

Brand Name	Generic Name
Accolate®	zafirlukast
Singulair®	montelukast
Zyflo®	zileuton

How Will I Take Leukotriene Modifiers?

Leukotriene modifiers are taken as pills, usually 1 to 4 times a day. *Accolate*® (zafirlukast) should be taken on an empty stomach 1 hour before meals or 2 hours after meals. *Singulair*® (montelukast) and *Zyflo*® (zileuton) can be taken with or without food. *Singulair*® (montelukast) is usually taken once a day in the evening. Your doctor or other healthcare professional will tell you how many times a day to take your medication.

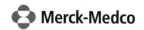

If you miss a dose of this medication, take the dose you missed as soon as possible. However, if it is almost time for your next dose, skip the missed dose and just take the next one. Do not double your dose. Take your medication exactly as directed by your doctor or other healthcare professional. Do not stop taking a prescription medication unless directed by your doctor or other healthcare professional.

What Side Effects Can Leukotriene Modifiers Cause?

More Common

- Headache

Less Common

- Diarrhea

- Dizziness

- Nausea

- Stomach pain

- Trouble falling asleep or staying asleep (insomnia)

Rare

- Liver problems that may cause yellowing of the skin or eyes (jaundice)

- Rash (skin redness, bumps, itching, or irritation)

Tell your doctor or other healthcare professional if you have side effects that bother you, do not go away, make you worried about taking your medication, or make you want to stop taking your medication.

Do Other Medications Interact with Leukotriene Modifiers?

Accolate® (zafirlukast) ***may increase*** the side effects of *Coumadin*® (warfarin).

Zyflo® (zileuton) ***may increase*** the side effects of these medications:

- *Coumadin*® (warfarin)
- *Inderal*® (propranolol)
- Theophylline such as *Theo-Dur*®, *Uniphyl*®, and others—see Glossary

Aspirin or aspirin-containing medications ***may increase*** the side effects of *Accolate*® (zafirlukast).

These medications ***may decrease*** how well *Accolate*® (zafirlukast) works:

- Erythromycin such as *Ery-Tab*®, *Erythrocin*®, and others—see Glossary
- Theophylline such as *Theo-Dur*®, *Uniphyl*®, and others—see Glossary

These medications ***may decrease*** how well *Singulair*® (montelukast) works:

- *Rifadin*® (rifampin)
- *Tegretol*® (carbamazepine)

Beta blockers, such as *Inderal*® (propranolol), *Tenormin*® (atenolol), *Toprol*® (metoprolol), and others (see Glossary), ***may increase*** the symptoms of asthma, and COPD, including emphysema and chronic bronchitis, causing shortness of breath or trouble breathing.

Tell your doctor or other healthcare professional about all medications (both prescription and nonprescription [over-the-counter] medications) that you are taking.

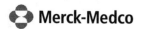

Warning!

To give you the best care, your doctor or other healthcare professional needs to know about the diseases and medical conditions you have had—your full medical history. Tell your doctor or other healthcare professional if you have or have ever had any of the following:

- Allergy or previous reaction to leukotriene modifiers

- High alcohol intake (drinking 3 or more alcoholic beverages such as beer, wine, whiskey, and others, every day)

- Liver problems

Leukotriene modifiers are "controller medications" used to help control asthma and help prevent asthma attacks from occurring. It is important to know that this medication will not help relieve wheezing or shortness of breath during an asthma attack. Taking extra leukotriene modifier medication will not help during the attack either and may cause more side effects. Talk to your doctor or other healthcare professional to make sure you know what to take and what to do if you have sudden shortness of breath or an asthma attack. If you have a quick-relief inhaler for shortness of breath and asthma attacks, you should remember to take it with you when you leave the house.

Since some leukotriene modifiers may cause damage to your liver, your doctor or other healthcare professional may order blood tests to find out early on if the medication is causing liver problems, before they become serious.

Steps for Using an Aerosol Spray Inhaler Correctly

1. Remove the cap, and shake the inhaler for at least 30 seconds to mix up the medication.

2. Breathe out slowly and deeply to empty the lungs as much as possible, so you have room in your lungs to breathe in the medication.

3. Place the inhaler in your mouth or 1 to 2 inches away from the front of your mouth, as instructed by your doctor or other healthcare professional. Keep your tongue from blocking the spray of medication.

4. As you begin to breathe in slowly and deeply, press the inhaler once and continue to breathe in as long as you can. Do not breathe in too quickly because it may increase the amount of medication that sticks in the back of your throat instead of going down into your lungs.

5. Hold your breath for 10 seconds or as close to that as you can. This will help keep the medication in your lungs. Then gently breathe out slowly and completely.

6. If you are using more than 1 puff or spray of the medication, repeat all of the previous steps, including shaking the inhaler. If you are using a quick-relief medication, wait 1 minute between puffs or sprays to give the medication a chance to open up your breathing passages, so the next spray will go deeper into your lungs.

7. If you are using a corticosteroid inhaler, rinse your mouth or gargle with water to help prevent mouth or throat irritation and infection.

8. At your next appointment, ask your doctor or other healthcare professional to watch you use your inhaler to make sure you are using it correctly.

Chapter 5

Congestive Heart Failure

What Is Congestive Heart Failure?

When the heart cannot pump enough blood to meet the body's needs, the condition is called congestive heart failure (CHF). Congestive heart failure may occur after a heart attack (myocardial infarction) or with high blood pressure (hypertension), heart valve problems, and some types of heart rhythm problems (arrhythmia).

In congestive heart failure the heart does not work as well as it should. Blood may back up in the veins, fluid may fill the lungs, and the legs and ankles may become swollen and puffy. You may feel weak, have trouble breathing, and gain weight from fluid retention. Your doctor or other healthcare professional may ask you to weigh yourself regularly to watch for fluid retention.

The treatment for congestive heart failure includes getting plenty of rest, eating a low-salt (sodium) diet, limiting the amount of fluids you drink, and taking medication. Medications used for congestive heart failure may either help strengthen the heart itself or help make the heart's work easier by decreasing the fluid in the body or by relaxing the blood vessels. No medications can cure congestive heart failure, but they may help to relieve the symptoms of congestive heart failure.

Medications for Congestive Heart Failure

Several kinds of medications may be taken for congestive heart failure. This chapter discusses these medications and/or categories of medications:

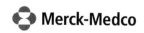

MEDICATIONS	See Page
Digoxin	136
Diuretics (Water Pills)	141
Angiotensin-Converting Enzyme (ACE) Inhibitors	146
Nitrates	150
Apresoline® (hydralazine)	155
Beta Blockers	159
Aldactone® (spironolactone)	164

If you do not see the exact name of the medication that you take for congestive heart failure listed above, check the Medication and Chapter Table to find out which category your medication falls under or check the Index.

Digoxin

Digoxin has been used for many years to treat congestive heart failure and some heart rhythm problems (arrhythmia), palpitations, and a type of rapid heartbeat (atrial fibrillation). Digoxin helps increase the strength of each beat of the heart and helps make the heart slow down when it starts to beat too quickly due to a rhythm abnormality.

Brand Name	Generic Name
Lanoxicaps®	digoxin
Lanoxin®	digoxin

How Will I Take Digoxin?

Digoxin is usually taken as a pill or liquid once a day or possibly once every other day. Some people take different doses on different days to get the right amount of medication into the blood. Your doctor or other healthcare professional will tell you how often to take your medication.

If you miss a dose of this medication, take the dose you missed as soon as possible. However, if it is almost time for your next dose, skip the missed dose and just take the next one. Do not double your dose. Take your medication exactly as directed by your doctor or other healthcare professional. Do not stop taking a prescription medication unless directed by your doctor or other healthcare professional.

What Side Effects Can Digoxin Cause?

More Common

- Diarrhea
- Headache
- Nausea
- Poor appetite
- Slow heartbeat (palpitations)
- Vomiting

Less Common

- Blurred vision
- Confusion
- Dizziness
- Heart rhythm problems (arrhythmia)
- Passing out or fainting

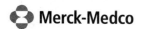
- Seeing "halos" around bright objects
- Tiredness or sluggishness (fatigue)

Rare

- Increased breast size in men

Tell your doctor or other healthcare professional if you have side effects that bother you, do not go away, make you worried about taking your medication, or make you want to stop taking your medication.

 Do Other Medications Interact with Digoxin?

These medications *may increase* the side effects of digoxin:

- Beta blockers such as *Inderal®* (propranolol), *Tenormin®* (atenolol), *Toprol®* (metoprolol), and others—see Glossary
- *Biaxin®* (clarithromycin)
- Calcium channel blockers such as *Cardizem®* (diltiazem), *Norvasc®* (amlodipine), *Procardia®* (nifedipine), and others—see Glossary
- Corticosteroids such as prednisone and others—see Glossary
- *Diflucan®* (fluconazole)
- Diuretics (water pills) such as *HydroDIURIL®* (hydrochlorothiazide or HCTZ), *Lasix®* (furosemide), and others—see Glossary
- Erythromycin such as *Ery-Tab®*, *Erythrocin®*, and others—see Glossary
- Heart rhythm problem (arrhythmia) medications—see Glossary
- *Micardis®* (telmisartan)
- *Neoral®* (cyclosporine)
- *Nizoral®* (ketoconazole)
- *Plaquenil®* (hydroxychloroquine)
- Propylthiouracil or PTU

- Quinidine such as *Quinaglute*®, *Quinidex*®, and others—see Glossary

- *Sandimmune*® (cyclosporine)

- *Serzone*® (nefazodone)

- *Sporanox*® (itraconazole)

- *Tapazole*® (methimazole)

- Tetracycline antibiotics such as *Dynacin*® (minocycline), *Sumycin*® (tetracycline), *Vibramycin*® (doxycycline), and others—see Glossary

These medications **may decrease** how well digoxin works:

- *Azulfidine*® (sulfasalazine)

- *Neo-Tabs*™ (neomycin)

- *Precose*® (acarbose)

- *Reglan*® (metoclopramide)

- *Rheumatrex*® (methotrexate)

- Thyroid medications such as *Cytomel*® (liothyronine), *Levoxyl*® (levothyroxine), *Synthroid*® (levothyroxine), and others—see Glossary

Nonsteroidal anti-inflammatory drugs (NSAIDs) such as *Motrin*® (ibuprofen), *Aleve*® (naproxen), *Vioxx*® (rofecoxib), *Celebrex*® (celecoxib), and others (see Glossary), **may increase** the symptoms of congestive heart failure. Check with your doctor or other healthcare professional before taking any of these medications.

Antacids such as *Maalox*® or *Mylanta*® (aluminum hydroxide/magnesium hydroxide), *Rolaids*® or *Tums*® (calcium carbonate), or *Amphojel*® (aluminum hydroxide) **may decrease** the effects of digoxin when taken at the same time. If you are taking antacids, take digoxin 1 hour before or 2 hours after taking your antacid.

Bile acid binders such as *Questran*® (cholestyramine) or *Colestid*® (colestipol) or bulk-forming laxatives like *Metamucil*® (psyllium) **may decrease** the effects of digoxin by preventing it from being absorbed completely. To help make sure it is absorbed so it can work properly, take digoxin 1 hour before or 4 to 6 hours after taking a bile acid binder or a bulk-forming laxative.

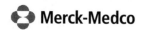

Many nonprescription (over-the-counter [OTC]) medications such as antacids, laxatives, pain, cough, cold, and allergy medications contain medications that *may increase* the symptoms of congestive heart failure. If you are taking any medications for congestive heart failure, you should talk to your doctor or other healthcare professional before taking any new OTC medications.

Tell your doctor or other healthcare professional about all medications (both prescription and nonprescription [over-the-counter] medications) that you are taking.

Why Else Do People Take Digoxin?

Digoxin is also taken for heart rhythm problems (arrhythmia).

 # Warning!

To give you the best care, your doctor or other healthcare professional needs to know about the diseases and medical conditions you have had—your full medical history. Tell your doctor or other healthcare professional if you have or have ever had any of the following:

- Allergy or previous reaction to digoxin
- Heart attack (myocardial infarction)
- Kidney problems
- Low potassium in your blood (hypokalemia)
- Overactive thyroid (hyperthyroidism)
- Underactive thyroid (hypothyroidism)

Not having enough potassium in the blood (hypokalemia) may lead to increased side effects from digoxin and make the heart beat abnormally. If you are taking any of the medications listed below, they may lower potassium levels in your blood. Follow your doctor or other healthcare professional's instructions about what to eat or whether to take potassium supplements (pills or powder) to keep your potassium at the right level, and have your blood tested as recommended. The following medications may lower potassium levels in your blood:

- Diuretics (water pills) such as *HydroDIURIL*® (hydrochlorothiazide or HCTZ), *Lasix*® (furosemide), and others—see Glossary

- Corticosteroids such as prednisone and others—see Glossary

Since digoxin may cause side effects if you get too much medication and may not work well if you do not get enough, your doctor or other healthcare professional may order blood tests to see if you are getting the right amount of this medication. Nausea, vomiting, diarrhea, and dizziness may be early signs that you are getting too much medication. Talk to your doctor or other healthcare professional if you have any of these symptoms, and be sure to get your blood tests as ordered. Do not change your dose or stop taking this medication unless directed by your doctor or other healthcare professional.

Digoxin may make you unsteady on your feet, causing you to fall and possibly break a bone. If you have fallen recently, tell your doctor or other healthcare professional about it. Taking a different medication or a lower dose may make you less likely to fall. You should not stop taking this medication without first talking to your doctor or other healthcare professional.

Diuretics

Diuretics (water pills) increase the amount of urine that your body makes. This helps your kidneys to remove salt (sodium) and water from the body. Diuretics are used to help reduce the symptoms of congestive heart failure.

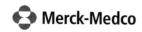
Brand Name	Generic Name
Bumex®	bumetanide
Demadex®	torsemide
Edecrin®	ethacrynic acid
Lasix®	furosemide
Lozol®	indapamide
Zaroxolyn®	metolazone

How Will I Take Diuretics?

Diuretics are usually taken 1 to 2 times daily. If taken only once a day, diuretics are usually taken in the morning. If you need to take diuretics twice a day, do not wait to take the second dose until the evening since it may keep you up at night with frequent urination. If it causes you to have to urinate frequently, you may want to take it after you get home from activities outside the house. Your doctor or other healthcare professional will tell you how many times a day to take your medication.

If you miss a dose of this medication, take the dose you missed as soon as possible. However, if it is almost time for your next dose, skip the missed dose and just take the next one. Do not double your dose. Take your medication exactly as directed by your doctor or other healthcare professional. Do not stop taking a prescription medication unless directed by your doctor or other healthcare professional.

What Side Effects Can Diuretics Cause?

More Common

- Gout (very painful, swollen joints)
- Headache

- Increased sensitivity to the sun (bad sunburn)
- Tiredness or sluggishness (fatigue)
- Weakness or muscle cramps that may be a sign of low potassium in your blood (hypokalemia)

Less Common

- Dizziness when standing up from a bed or a chair
- Erection problems (erectile dysfunction)
- Increased blood sugar (hyperglycemia)
- Increased thirst and dry mouth with dizziness when standing that may be a sign of excessive water loss (dehydration)

Rare

- Allergic reactions such as rash (skin redness, bumps, itching, or irritation), swelling of the face and throat, or trouble breathing
- Easy bruising ("black-and-blue" marks on the skin)
- Skin rash with fever and joint pain or swelling that may be a sign of lupus

---

Tell your doctor or other healthcare professional if you have side effects that bother you, do not go away, make you worried about taking your medication, or make you want to stop taking your medication.

 Do Other Medications Interact with Diuretics?

Diuretics may cause low potassium blood levels (hypokalemia) which *may increase* the side effects of *Lanoxin*® (digoxin).

Nonsteroidal anti-inflammatory drugs (NSAIDs) such as *Motrin*® (ibuprofen), *Aleve*® (naproxen), *Vioxx*® (rofecoxib), *Celebrex*® (celecoxib), and others (see Glossary) *may decrease* how well diuretics work.

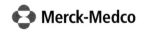

Many nonprescription (over-the-counter [OTC]) medications such as antacids, laxatives, pain, cough, cold, and allergy medications contain medications that *may increase* the symptoms of congestive heart failure. If you are taking any medications for congestive heart failure, you should talk to your doctor or other healthcare professional before taking any new OTC medications.

Diuretics *may increase* the side effects of lithium such as *Eskalith®*, *Lithobid®*, and others—see Glossary.

High blood pressure (hypertension) medications (see Glossary) *may increase* the effects of diuretics.

Bile acid binders such as *Questran®* (cholestyramine) or *Colestid®* (colestipol) or bulk-forming laxatives like *Metamucil®* (psyllium) *may decrease* the effects of diuretics by preventing them from being absorbed completely. To help make sure they are absorbed so they can work properly, take your diuretic 1 hour before or 4 to 6 hours after taking a bile acid binder or a bulk-forming laxative.

Diuretics *may decrease* how well diabetic medications such as *Glynase®* (glyburide), *Glucotrol®* (glipizide), and others work—see Glossary.

Diuretics must be used carefully if prescribed for anyone who is taking *Propulsid®* (cisapride [withdrawn from general distribution; available only by special arrangement with the manufacturer]), *Seldane®* (terfenadine [no longer commercially available]), or *Hismanal®* (astemizole [no longer commercially available]), because the low potassium blood levels that may be caused by diuretics *may cause* serious, sometimes fatal, heart problems when taken with these medications.

Tell your doctor or other healthcare professional about all medications (both prescription and nonprescription [over-the-counter] medications) that you are taking.

Why Else Do People Take Diuretics?

Diuretics are sometimes used to help reduce puffiness or swelling of the legs and ankles (edema) and to help treat kidney problems, high blood pressure (hypertension), and liver problems.

 # Warning!

To give you the best care, your doctor or other healthcare professional needs to know about the diseases and medical conditions you have had—your full medical history. Tell your doctor or other healthcare professional if you have or have ever had any of the following:

- Allergy or previous reaction to any of the following:
    - Diabetes medications such as *DiaBeta*® (glyburide), *Glucophage*® (metformin), *Glucotrol*® (glipizide), and others—see Glossary
    - Sulfa medications such as *Bactrim*™, *Septra*®, and others—see Glossary
    - Diuretics (water pills) such as *HydroDIURIL*® (hydrochlorothiazide or HCTZ), *Lasix*® (furosemide), and others—see Glossary
    - Carbonic anhydrase inhibitors such as *Azopt*® (brinzolamide), *Diamox*® (acetazolamide), *Trusopt*® (dorzolamide), and others—see Glossary
- Diabetes
- Gout
- Kidney problems
- Liver problems
- Lupus

Because diuretics may cause low potassium blood levels (hypokalemia) and high blood sugar (hyperglycemia), your doctor or other healthcare professional may order blood tests to check your potassium levels and blood sugar (glucose).

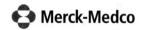

Dehydration (excessive water loss) may be a problem for older adults. Increased thirst, dry mouth, weakness or dizziness when standing up from a bed or a chair, and darkening or decreased urine may be signs of dehydration. Diuretics may cause dehydration by themselves, but it is more likely to occur during very hot weather, after vigorous exercise, or when you have severe diarrhea or vomiting. If not treated, this may be serious. Call your doctor or other healthcare professional if you develop these symptoms.

If you are taking diuretics, stay out of the sun as much as you can to avoid a serious sunburn. When you do go out in the sun, use sunblock or sunscreen, and wear protective clothing, such as a wide-brimmed hat and a long-sleeved shirt.

Angiotensin-Converting Enzyme (ACE) Inhibitors

Angiotensin-converting enzyme (ACE) inhibitors relax blood vessels and help relieve the symptoms of congestive heart failure.

Brand Name	Generic Name
Accupril®	quinapril
Aceon®	perindopril
Altace®	ramipril
Capoten®	captopril
Lotensin®	benazepril
Mavik®	trandolapril
Monopril®	fosinopril
Prinivil®	lisinopril
Univasc®	moexipril
Vasotec®	enalapril
Zestril®	lisinopril

How Will I Take ACE Inhibitors?

ACE inhibitors are usually taken 1 to 3 times a day. *Capoten*® (captopril) and *Univasc*® (moexipril) should be taken on an empty stomach 1 hour before or 2 hours after meals. Other ACE inhibitors may be taken with or without food. Your doctor or other healthcare professional will tell you how many times a day to take your medication.

If you miss a dose of this medication, take the dose you missed as soon as possible. However, if it is almost time for your next dose, skip the missed dose and just take the next one. Do not double your dose. Take your medication exactly as directed by your doctor or other healthcare professional. Do not stop taking a prescription medication unless directed by your doctor or other healthcare professional.

What Side Effects Can ACE Inhibitors Cause?

More Common

- Dizziness when standing up from a bed or a chair
- Dry cough that will not go away
- High potassium in your blood (hyperkalemia)
- Rash (skin redness, bumps, itching, or irritation)
- Tiredness or sluggishness (fatigue)

Less Common

- Changes in taste
- Diarrhea
- Kidney problems
- Nausea
- Swelling of the face, lips, tongue, arms, and legs (angioedema)

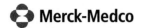

Rare

- Easy bruising ("black-and-blue" marks on the skin)

- Erection problems (erectile dysfunction)

- Frequent fever, sore throat, or flu-like symptoms that may be a sign of low white blood cells

---

Tell your doctor or other healthcare professional if you have side effects that bother you, do not go away, make you worried about taking your medication, or make you want to stop taking your medication.

 ## Do Other Medications Interact with ACE Inhibitors?

Many nonprescription (over-the-counter [OTC]) medications such as antacids, laxatives, pain, cough, cold, and allergy medications contain medications that **may increase** the symptoms of congestive heart failure. If you are taking any medications for congestive heart failure, you should talk to your doctor or other healthcare professional before taking any new OTC medications.

ACE inhibitors **may increase** the side effects of lithium such as *Eskalith®*, *Lithobid®*, and others—see Glossary.

Nonsteroidal anti-inflammatory drugs (NSAIDs) such as *Motrin®* (ibuprofen), *Aleve®* (naproxen), *Vioxx®* (rofecoxib), *Celebrex®* (celecoxib), and others (see Glossary) **may decrease** how well ACE inhibitors work.

ACE inhibitors **may increase** the side effects of high blood pressure (hypertension) medications—see Glossary.

The following **may increase** potassium blood levels and **may increase** the side effects of ACE inhibitors:

- Potassium-sparing diuretics such as *Aldactazide®* (spironolactone/ hydrochlorothiazide), *Dyazide®* (triamterene/hydrochlorothiazide), *Moduretic®* (amiloride/hydrochlorothiazide), and others—see Glossary

- Potassium supplements such as *K-Dur®*, *Klor-Con®*, *Slow K®*, and others—see Glossary

- Salt substitutes

Tell your doctor or other healthcare professional about all medications (both prescription and nonprescription [over-the-counter] medications) that you are taking.

Why Else Do People Take ACE Inhibitors?

ACE inhibitors may be used for high blood pressure (hypertension) and to help prevent kidney problems in people with diabetes.

Warning!

To give you the best care, your doctor or other healthcare professional needs to know about the diseases and medical conditions you have had—your full medical history. Tell your doctor or other healthcare professional if you have or have ever had, or presently take, any of the following:

- Allergy or previous reaction to ACE inhibitors

- Congestive heart failure

- Cough

- Diuretics (water pills) such as *HydroDIURIL®* (hydrochlorothiazide or HCTZ), *Lasix®* (furosemide), and others—see Glossary

- High potassium in your blood (hyperkalemia)

- Kidney problems

- Liver problems

- Low blood pressure (hypotension)

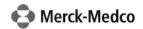

- Potassium supplements such as *K-Dur®*, *Klor-Con®*, *Slow K®*, and others—see Glossary

- Swelling of the face, lips, tongue, arms, and legs (angioedema)

Kidney problems or diabetes may increase the amount of potassium in the blood. Your doctor or other healthcare professional may order blood tests to make sure your potassium blood levels do not get too high while taking ACE inhibitors.

Ask your doctor or other healthcare professional before using salt substitutes because many contain an ingredient that could increase your potassium blood levels.

ACE inhibitors may make you unsteady on your feet, causing you to fall and possibly break a bone. If you have fallen recently, tell your doctor or other healthcare professional about it. Taking a different medication or a lower dose may make you less likely to fall. You should not stop taking this medication without first talking to your doctor or other healthcare professional.

Cough may be a common and annoying side effect of ACE inhibitors. Talk to your doctor or other healthcare professional if you develop a cough. This should be checked because it may be a sign of worsening congestive heart failure or another medical problem.

Nitrates

Nitrates open up (dilate) the blood vessels in the body. They are sometimes used with *Apresoline®* (hydralazine) to help reduce symptoms of congestive heart failure.

Brand Name	Generic Name
Deponit® Patches	nitroglycerin
Dilatrate® Tablets	isosorbide dinitrate
Imdur® Tablets	isosorbide mononitrate
Ismo® Tablets	isosorbide mononitrate
Isordil® Tablets	isosorbide dinitrate
Minitran® Patches	nitroglycerin
Monoket® Tablets	isosorbide mononitrate
Nitro-Bid® Capsules	nitroglycerin
Nitrodisc® Patches	nitroglycerin
Nitro-Dur® Patches	nitroglycerin
Sorbitrate® Tablets	isosorbide dinitrate
Transderm-Nitro® Patches	nitroglycerin

How Will I Take Nitrates?

For congestive heart failure, nitrates may be taken as a pill or a patch applied to the skin like a *Band-Aid*®. Nitrate pills are usually taken 1 to 3 times a day. Your doctor or other healthcare professional will tell you how often to take this medication.

When a medication has initials after its name, such as XL, XR, SR, BID, DUR, and others, it usually means that the body absorbs the medication slowly over time, so you usually have to take it only once or twice a day. The body will absorb some medications of this type too fast if you crush or break them or dissolve them in liquid, and their effects will not last as long as they should. Check with your doctor or other healthcare professional before crushing or breaking your pills or dissolving your pills in liquid.

Patches are usually used once a day for about 12 to 16 hours. Nitroglycerin patches are easy to apply. Put the patch on the skin of your chest, back (trunk),

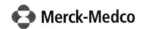

or upper arms. You can help to keep the patches from irritating your skin by putting each new one in a different place. Put on a new patch if the first one falls off.

Your skin absorbs the nitrate medication that is in the patch. There will usually be about 8 to 12 hours in a 24-hour time period that you will not have a patch on. This is to give your body the chance to let the medication work well. If you do not give your body time off the patch, you may notice that your patch does not work as well as it used to work. Your doctor or other healthcare professional will tell you how long to leave your patches on.

When taking off or disposing of an old patch, make sure you throw it away where children and pets cannot get it as it will still contain medication that may be harmful to them.

If you miss a dose of this medication, take the dose you missed as soon as possible. However, if it is almost time for your next dose, skip the missed dose and just take the next one. Do not double your dose. Take your medication exactly as directed by your doctor or other healthcare professional. Do not stop taking a prescription medication unless directed by your doctor or other healthcare professional.

 ## What Side Effects Can Nitrates Cause?

More Common

- Dizziness when standing up from a bed or a chair
- Fainting
- Fast heartbeat (palpitations)
- Headache
- Rash (skin redness, bumps, itching, or irritation), possible with patches
- Reddening of the face (flushing)

Tell your doctor or other healthcare professional if you have side effects that bother you, do not go away, make you worried about taking your medication, or make you want to stop taking your medication.

Do Other Medications Interact with Nitrates?

Many nonprescription (over-the-counter [OTC]) medications such as antacids, laxatives, pain, cough, cold, and allergy medications contain medications that *may increase* the symptoms of congestive heart failure. If you are taking any medications for congestive heart failure, you should talk to your doctor or other healthcare professional before taking any new OTC medications.

Nitrates *may increase* the side effects of high blood pressure (hypertension) medications—see Glossary.

If you are taking nitrates, do not take *Viagra*® (sildenafil). This combination of medications *may cause* serious side effects and even death.

DHE-45® (dihydroergotamine) *may decrease* how well nitrates work.

Drinking alcoholic beverages (such as beer, wine, whiskey, and others) *may increase* the side effects of nitrates.

Tell your doctor or other healthcare professional about all medications (both prescription and nonprescription [over-the-counter] medications) that you are taking.

Why Else Do People Take Nitrates?

Nitrates may be used for coronary artery disease and cardiac chest pain (angina).

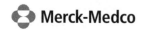

What Else Should I Know about Nitrates?

Headaches are common side effects of nitrates. In fact, getting a headache soon after taking a nitrate usually means the medication is working. These headaches usually go away in a couple of weeks. Talk to your doctor or other healthcare professional about taking over-the-counter (OTC) pain medications for headache relief if they become bothersome.

 # Warning!

To give you the best care, your doctor or other healthcare professional needs to know about the diseases and medical conditions you have had—your full medical history. Tell your doctor or other healthcare professional if you have or have ever had any of the following:

- Allergy or previous reaction to adhesives, skin (transdermal) patches
- Allergy or previous reaction to nitrates
- Dizziness when standing up from a bed or a chair
- Glaucoma (an eye disease)
- Heart attack (myocardial infarction)
- Kidney problems
- Liver problems
- Low red blood cells (anemia)

Nitrates may make you unsteady on your feet, causing you to fall and possibly break a bone. If you have fallen recently, tell your doctor or other healthcare professional about it. Taking a different medication or a lower dose may make you less likely to fall. You should not stop taking this medication without first talking to your doctor or other healthcare professional.

If you are taking nitrates, do not take *Viagra*® (sildenafil). This combination of medications ***may cause*** serious side effects and even death. Death after use of *Viagra*® (sildenafil) most often occurs in men with heart disease or risks for developing heart disease. *Viagra*® (sildenafil) has not been studied in men with congestive heart failure.

Under certain circumstances, your doctor or other healthcare professional may decide that you should stop taking this medication. If you have taken it for more than a couple of weeks, he or she may want you to decrease it gradually, lowering the dose over a few weeks or months. Stopping suddenly may cause unpleasant withdrawal symptoms or may worsen your medical problems. Pay careful attention to the instructions your doctor or other healthcare professional gives you about how much less to take and for how long.

Apresoline® (hydralazine)

Apresoline® (hydralazine) is a vasodilator that relaxes blood vessels to help reduce the symptoms of congestive heart failure.

How Will I Take *Apresoline*® (hydralazine)?

Apresoline® (hydralazine) is usually taken 2 to 4 times a day. It may be taken with or without food. However, the way you take it should be consistent. It should either always be taken with food or always be taken without food. Your doctor or other healthcare professional will tell you how many times a day to take your medication.

If you miss a dose of this medication, take the dose you missed as soon as possible. However, if it is almost time for your next dose, skip the missed dose and just take the next one. Do not double your dose. Take your medication exactly as directed by your doctor or other healthcare professional. Do not stop taking a prescription medication unless directed by your doctor or other healthcare professional.

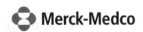

What Side Effects Can *Apresoline*® (hydralazine) Cause?

More Common

- Diarrhea
- Fast heartbeat (palpitations)
- Headache
- Increased sensitivity to the sun (bad sunburn)
- Nausea
- Poor appetite

Less Common

- Cardiac chest pain (angina)
- Constipation
- Dizziness
- Increased tearing (watery eyes)
- Liver problems that may cause yellowing of the skin or eyes (jaundice)
- Skin rash with fever and joint pain or swelling that may be a sign of lupus
- Tingling, pain, or weakness in hands and feet
- Reddening of the face (flushing)
- Stuffy, runny nose (rhinitis)
- Swelling or puffiness of the feet, ankles, or lower legs (edema)

Tell your doctor or other healthcare professional if you have side effects that bother you, do not go away, make you worried about taking your medication, or make you want to stop taking your medication.

Do Other Medications Interact with *Apresoline*® (hydralazine)?

Apresoline® (hydralazine) ***may increase*** the side effects of high blood pressure (hypertension) medications—see Glossary.

Apresoline® (hydralazine) ***may decrease*** how well diuretics (water pills) such as *HydroDIURIL*® (hydrochlorothiazide or HCTZ), *Lasix*® (furosemide), and others (see Glossary) work.

Many nonprescription (over-the-counter [OTC]) medications such as antacids, laxatives, pain, cough, cold, and allergy medications contain medications that ***may increase*** the symptoms of congestive heart failure. If you are taking any medications for congestive heart failure, you should talk to your doctor or other healthcare professional before taking any new OTC medications.

Nonsteroidal anti-inflammatory drugs (NSAIDs) such as *Motrin*® (ibuprofen), *Aleve*® (naproxen), *Vioxx*® (rofecoxib), *Celebrex*® (celecoxib), and others (see Glossary) ***may decrease*** how well *Apresoline*® (hydralazine) works.

Tell your doctor or other healthcare professional about all medications (both prescription and nonprescription [over-the-counter] medications) that you are taking.

Why Else Do People Take *Apresoline*® (hydralazine)?

Apresoline® (hydralazine) is sometimes used for high blood pressure (hypertension).

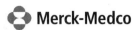

 # Warning!

To give you the best care, your doctor or other healthcare professional needs to know about the diseases and medical conditions you have had—your full medical history. Tell your doctor or other healthcare professional if you have or have ever had any of the following:

- Allergy or previous reaction to *Apresoline®* (hydralazine)

- Cardiac chest pain (angina)

- Coronary artery disease

- Kidney problems

- Liver problems

- Low blood pressure (hypotension)

- Lupus

- Stroke

If you get a skin rash with pain or swelling in your joints (elbows, knees, and others), especially while taking *Apresoline®* (hydralazine), call your doctor or other healthcare professional.

If you are taking *Apresoline®* (hydralazine), stay out of the sun as much as you can to avoid a serious sunburn. When you do go out in the sun, use sunblock or sunscreen, and wear protective clothing, such as a wide-brimmed hat and a long-sleeved shirt.

Apresoline® (hydralazine) may cause fluid retention and swelling or puffiness of the feet, ankles, or lower legs (edema). This medication is sometimes prescribed with a diuretic (water pill) to help prevent swelling. Ask your doctor or other healthcare professional about diuretics if you have edema.

Apresoline® (hydralazine) may make you unsteady on your feet, causing you to fall and possibly break a bone. If you have fallen recently, tell your doctor or other healthcare professional about it. Taking a different medication or a lower dose may make you less likely to fall. You should not stop taking this medication without first talking to your doctor or other healthcare professional.

Under certain circumstances, your doctor or other healthcare professional may decide that you should stop taking this medication. If you have taken it for more than a couple of weeks, he or she may want you to decrease it gradually, lowering the dose over a few weeks or months. Stopping suddenly may cause unpleasant withdrawal symptoms or may worsen your medical problems. Pay careful attention to the instructions your doctor or other healthcare professional gives you about how much less to take and for how long.

Beta Blockers

Beta blockers slow the heartbeat and help to lower blood pressure and reduce the symptoms of congestive heart failure.

Brand Name	Generic Name
Blocadren®	timolol
Coreg®	carvedilol
Corgard®	nadolol
Inderal®	propranolol
Kerlone®	betaxolol
Lopressor®	metoprolol
Normodyne®	labetalol
Tenormin®	atenolol
Toprol®	metoprolol
Zebeta®	bisoprolol

How Will I Take Beta Blockers?

Beta blockers are usually taken 1 to 3 times a day. They may be taken with or without food. However, the way you take most beta blockers should be consistent. They should either always be taken with food or always be taken

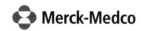

without food. Your doctor or other healthcare professional will tell you how often to take your medication.

When a medication has initials after its name, such as XL, XR, SR, BID, DUR, and others, it usually means that the body absorbs the medication slowly over time, so you usually have to take it only once or twice a day. The body will absorb some medications of this type too fast if you crush or break them or dissolve them in liquid, and their effects will not last as long as they should. Check with your doctor or other healthcare professional before crushing or breaking your pills or dissolving your pills in liquid.

If you miss a dose of this medication, take the dose you missed as soon as possible. However, if it is almost time for your next dose, skip the missed dose and just take the next one. Do not double your dose. Take your medication exactly as directed by your doctor or other healthcare professional. Do not stop taking a prescription medication unless directed by your doctor or other healthcare professional.

 ## What Side Effects Can Beta Blockers Cause?

More Common

- Dizziness when standing up from a bed or a chair
- Erection problems (erectile dysfunction)
- Loss of interest in sex (decreased libido)
- Tiredness or sluggishness (fatigue)
- Weakness

Less Common

- Change in blood sugar
- Congestive heart failure*

*Sometimes medications may actually cause or worsen the same symptoms they are being used to help relieve. Talk to your doctor or other healthcare professional if your symptoms get worse instead of better while taking this medication.

- Heartburn

- Leg pain when walking

- Rash (skin redness, bumps, itching, or irritation)

- Sadness, feeling blue or down, depressed mood (depression)

- Slow or irregular heartbeat (palpitations)

- Strange dreams and nightmares

- Trouble breathing or shortness of breath with asthma and COPD, including emphysema or chronic bronchitis

---

Tell your doctor or other healthcare professional if you have side effects that bother you, do not go away, make you worried about taking your medication, or make you want to stop taking your medication.

Do Other Medications Interact with Beta Blockers?

Many nonprescription (over-the-counter [OTC]) medications such as antacids, laxatives, pain, cough, cold, and allergy medications contain medications that **may increase** the symptoms of congestive heart failure. If you are taking any medications for congestive heart failure, you should talk to your doctor or other healthcare professional before taking any new OTC medications.

Beta blockers **may decrease** how well these medications work:

- Diabetes medications such as *DiaBeta*® (glyburide), *Glucophage*® (metformin), *Glucotrol*® (glipizide), and others—see Glossary

These medications **may increase** the side effects of beta blockers:

- Heart rhythm problem (arrhythmia) medications—see Glossary

- High blood pressure (hypertension) medications and diuretics (water pills)—see Glossary

- *Lanoxin*® (digoxin)

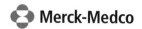

- Neuroleptic medications such as *Risperdal®* (risperidone), *Thorazine®* (chlorpromazine), *Zyprexa®* (olanzapine), and others—see Glossary

- Propylthiouracil or PTU

- *Tagamet®* (cimetidine)

- *Tapazole®* (methimazole)

Beta blockers *may increase* the side effects of these medications:

- *DHE-45®* (dihydroergotamine)

- *Ergomar®* (ergotamine)

- *Migranal®* (dihydroergotamine)

These medications *may decrease* how well beta blockers work:

- Barbiturates such as *Butisol®* (butabarbital), *Luminal®* (phenobarbital), *Mebaral®* (mephobarbital), and others—see Glossary

- NSAIDs such as *Motrin®* (ibuprofen), *Aleve®* (naproxen), *Vioxx®* (rofecoxib), *Celebrex®* (celecoxib), and others—see Glossary

- *Rifadin®* (rifampin)

- Theophylline such as *Theo-Dur®*, *Uniphyl®*, and others—see Glossary

- Thyroid medications such as *Cytomel®* (liothyronine), *Levoxyl®* (levothyroxine), *Synthroid®* (levothyroxine), and others—see Glossary

---

Tell your doctor or other healthcare professional about all medications (both prescription and nonprescription [over-the-counter] medications) that you are taking.

Why Else Do People Take Beta Blockers?

Beta blockers may also help prevent a heart attack (myocardial infarction), high blood pressure (hypertension), heart rhythm problems (arrhythmias), cardiac chest pain (angina), migraine headaches, and shakiness (tremors).

Warning!

To give you the best care, your doctor or other healthcare professional needs to know about the diseases and medical conditions you have had—your full medical history. Tell your doctor or other healthcare professional if you have or have ever had any of the following:

- Allergy or previous reaction to beta blockers

- Breathing problems (asthma and COPD, including emphysema or chronic bronchitis)

- Diabetes

- Overactive thyroid (hyperthyroidism)

- Poor circulation (peripheral vascular disease)

- Sadness, feeling blue or down, depressed mood (depression)

Beta blockers may worsen the symptoms of some lung problems, especially asthma and COPD, including emphysema or chronic bronchitis. Tell your doctor or other healthcare professional if you have trouble breathing or shortness of breath.

Taking beta blockers may hide the symptoms of low blood sugar (hypoglycemia). This may cause problems for people with diabetes. Ask your doctor or other healthcare professional whether you need to check your blood sugar to help prevent the dangers of hypoglycemia or other side effects.

Beta blockers may worsen the symptoms of poor circulation (peripheral vascular disease). Tell your doctor or other healthcare professional if you develop symptoms of poor circulation such as pain, numbness, or coldness of your legs, feet, and hands.

Beta blockers may make you unsteady on your feet, causing you to fall and possibly break a bone. If you have fallen recently, tell your doctor or other healthcare professional about it. Taking a different medication or a lower dose may make you less likely to fall. You should not stop taking this medication without first talking to your doctor or other healthcare professional.

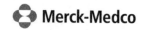

Under certain circumstances, your doctor or other healthcare professional may decide that you should stop taking this medication. If you have taken it for more than a couple of weeks, he or she may want you to decrease it gradually, lowering the dose over a few weeks or months. Stopping suddenly may cause unpleasant withdrawal symptoms or may worsen your medical problems. Pay careful attention to the instructions your doctor or other healthcare professional gives you about how much less to take and for how long.

Aldactone® (spironolactone)

Aldactone® (spironolactone) inhibits aldosterone (a hormone) to help reduce the symptoms of congestive heart failure.

How Will I Take *Aldactone*® (spironolactone)?

Aldactone® (spironolactone) is usually taken 1 to 4 times a day. Your doctor or other healthcare professional will tell you how many times a day to take your medication.

If you miss a dose of this medication, take the dose you missed as soon as possible. However, if it is almost time for your next dose, skip the missed dose and just take the next one. Do not double your dose. Take your medication exactly as directed by your doctor or other healthcare professional. Do not stop taking a prescription medication unless directed by your doctor or other healthcare professional.

What Side Effects Can *Aldactone®* (spironolactone) Cause?

More Common

- Nausea

- Poor appetite

- Too much potassium in the blood (hyperkalemia)

Less common

- Decreased interest in sex

- Diarrhea

- Dizziness

- Erection problems (erectile dysfunction)

- Increased breast size in men

- Vomiting

Rare

- Increased sensitivity to the sun (bad sunburn)

- Rash (skin redness, bumps, itching, or irritation)

Tell your doctor or other healthcare professional if you have side effects that bother you, do not go away, make you worried about taking your medication, or make you want to stop taking your medication.

Do Other Medications Interact with *Aldactone®* (spironolactone)?

Nonsteroidal anti-inflammatory drugs (NSAIDs) such as *Motrin®* (ibuprofen), *Aleve®* (naproxen), *Vioxx®* (rofecoxib), *Celebrex®* (celecoxib), and others (see Glossary) *may decrease* how well *Aldactone®* (spironolactone) works.

Many nonprescription (over-the-counter [OTC]) medications such as antacids, laxatives, pain, cough, cold, and allergy medications contain medications that

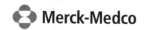

may increase the symptoms of congestive heart failure. If you are taking any medications for congestive heart failure, you should talk to your doctor or other healthcare professional before taking any new OTC medications.

The following *may increase* potassium blood levels and increase the side effects of *Aldactone®* (spironolactone):

- ACE inhibitors such as *Accupril®* (quinapril), *Vasotec®* (enalapril), *Zestril®* (lisinopril), and others—see Glossary

- Potassium supplements such as *K-Dur®*, *Klor-Con®*, *Slow K®*, and others—see Glossary

- Salt substitutes

Tell your doctor or other healthcare professional about all medications (both prescription and nonprescription [over-the-counter] medications) that you are taking.

Why Else Do People Take *Aldactone®* (spironolactone)?

Aldactone® (spironolactone) may sometimes be used for severe liver problems.

 # Warning!

To give you the best care, your doctor or other healthcare professional needs to know about the diseases and medical conditions you have had—your full medical history. Tell your doctor or other healthcare professional if you have or have ever had, or presently take, any of the following:

- ACE inhibitors such as *Accupril®* (quinapril), *Vasotec®* (enalapril), *Zestril®* (lisinopril), and others—see Glossary

- Allergy or previous reaction to *Aldactone®* (spironolactone)

- Diabetes

- High potassium in your blood (hyperkalemia)

- Kidney problems

- Low potassium in your blood (hypokalemia)

- Potassium supplements such as *K-Dur®*, *Klor-Con®*, *Slow K®*, and others—see Glossary

Kidney problems or diabetes may increase the amount of potassium in the blood. Your doctor or other healthcare professional may order blood tests to make sure your potassium blood levels do not get too high.

Ask your doctor or other healthcare professional before using salt substitutes because many contain potassium that could increase your potassium blood levels.

If you are taking *Aldactone®* (spironolactone), stay out of the sun as much as you can to avoid a serious sunburn. When you do go out in the sun, use sunblock or sunscreen, and wear protective clothing, such as a wide-brimmed hat and a long-sleeved shirt.

Chapter 6

Constipation

What Is Constipation?

Constipation is having bowel movements less often than usual, difficulty having bowel movements, or both. Constipation often causes a feeling of fullness and discomfort in the abdomen (stomach).

Older people are much more likely than younger people to be constipated. Sometimes older people worry too much about having a bowel movement every day. Some people have bowel movements twice a day and others only three times a week. Both are normal. If you are having regular bowel movements without pain or difficulty, you are probably not constipated.

You can help to keep your bowel movements regular by staying active, drinking a lot of water, and eating plenty of fresh fruits, vegetables, whole-grain cereals, and breads. The fiber in these kinds of food adds bulk to bowel movements and keeps the bowels moving.

Many of the following medications may cause or worsen constipation:

- Antacids containing aluminum hydroxide such as *AlternaGEL®*, *Amphojel®*, and others—see Glossary

- Antacids containing calcium such as *Rolaids®* (calcium carbonate), *Tums®* (calcium carbonate), and others—see Glossary

- Anticholinergic medications such as *Artane®* (trihexyphenidyl), *Cogentin®* (benztropine), and others—see Glossary

- Antihistamines such as *Allegra®* (fexofenadine), *Benadryl®* (diphenhydramine), *Zyrtec®* (cetirizine), and others—see Glossary

- Antispasmodics such as *Bentyl®* (dicyclomine), *Levsin®* (hyoscyamine), and others—see Glossary

- Calcium channel blockers such as *Cardizem®* (diltiazem), *Norvasc®* (amlodipine), *Procardia®* (nifedipine), and others—see Glossary

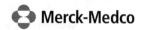

- Diuretics (water pills) such as *HydroDIURIL*® (hydrochlorothiazide or HCTZ), *Lasix*® (furosemide), and others—see Glossary

- Iron supplements (ferrous sulfate, ferrous gluconate, and ferrous fumarate)

- Muscle relaxants such as *Flexeril*® (cyclobenzaprine), *Soma*® (carisoprodol), and others—see Glossary

- Neuroleptic medications such as *Risperdal*® (risperidone), *Thorazine*® (chlorpromazine), *Zyprexa*® (olanzapine), and others—see Glossary

- Narcotics such as codeine, morphine, *Roxicet*™ (oxycodone), *Vicodin*® (hydrocodone), and others—see Glossary

- Tricyclic antidepressants such as *Elavil*® (amitriptyline), *Pamelor*® (nortriptyline), *Sinequan*® (doxepin), and others—see Glossary

---

Talk to your doctor or other healthcare professional if you have constipation and are taking one of these medications. Do not stop taking these medications unless directed by your doctor or other healthcare professional.

Medications to Help Prevent or Relieve Constipation

Several kinds of medications may be taken for constipation. This chapter discusses these medications and/or categories of medications:

MEDICATIONS	See Page
Fiber and Bulk-forming Laxatives	171
Stool Softeners	175
Enemas	177
Mineral Oil	180
Glycerin Suppositories	182
Saline Laxatives	184
Lactulose	187
Stimulant Laxatives	189

If you do not see the exact name of the medication that you take for constipation listed above, check the Medication and Chapter Table to find out which category your medication falls under or check the Index.

Fiber and Bulk-forming Laxatives

Taking bulk-forming laxatives may help people who do not eat enough fiber (fruits, vegetables, whole grains, and others) to have regular bowel movements. Fiber and bulk-forming laxatives increase the size (bulk) of bowel movements without making them watery. Bulk-forming laxatives keep bowel movements soft but well-formed and easy to pass through the rectum. Whole-grain cereals and vegetables are excellent natural sources of fiber. Wheat bran is the least expensive bulk-forming laxative and one that has been used successfully for many years. Bulk-forming laxatives are available without a prescription.

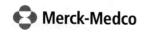

Brand Name	Generic Name
Citrucel®	methylcellulose
Fiberall®	psyllium
FiberCon®	polycarbophil
Konsyl®	psyllium
Maltsupex®	malt soup extract
Metamucil®	psyllium
Mitrolan®	polycarbophil
Perdiem® Fiber	psyllium
Unifiber®	cellulose

How Will I Take Bulk-forming Laxatives?

Bulk-forming laxatives must be taken with at least 8 ounces of water or juice to help prevent bowel movements from becoming hard. If you do not drink enough water or juice with your bulk-forming laxative, it may make your constipation worse.

Bulk-forming laxatives may be mixed in with food (such as cereal, applesauce, pudding, or mashed potatoes) or taken with water or juice soon after a meal. Taking a bulk-forming laxative with orange juice is also a popular choice, as this helps disguise the taste of the medication. Bulk-forming laxatives usually produce a soft, formed bowel movement in 1 to 3 days, although it may take longer. Follow the instructions given on the package, or ask your doctor or other healthcare professional how often to take this medication.

This medication is often used "as needed," so missing a dose should not be a problem. If you miss a dose and it is almost time for the next dose, you should skip the forgotten dose. Do not double the dose. Take your medication as directed by your doctor or other healthcare professional.

What Side Effects Can Bulk-forming Laxatives Cause?

More Common

- Diarrhea
- Gas or bloating

Less Common

- Allergic reactions such as rash (skin redness, bumps, itching, or irritation), swelling of the face and throat, or trouble breathing
- Severe constipation
- Stomach pain
- Trouble swallowing

Tell your doctor or other healthcare professional if you have side effects that bother you, do not go away, make you worried about taking your medication, or make you want to stop taking your medication.

Do Other Medications Interact with Bulk-forming Laxatives?

Bulk-forming laxatives *may decrease* the effects of other medications by preventing them from being absorbed completely. To help make sure they are absorbed so they may work properly, take your other medications 1 hour before or 4 to 6 hours after taking the bulk-forming laxative.

Tell your doctor or other healthcare professional about all medications (both prescription and nonprescription [over-the-counter] medications) that you are taking.

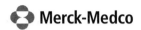

Why Else Do People Take Bulk-forming Laxatives?

Bulk-forming laxatives may improve the symptoms of irritable bowel syndrome, a long-lasting condition that causes abdominal pain, diarrhea, constipation, or bowel movements that switch from diarrhea to constipation.

What Else Should I Know about Bulk-forming Laxatives?

Drink at least one 8-ounce glass of water or juice with each dose of a bulk-forming laxative. If you do not drink enough fluid at the same time, the bulk-forming laxative may not work, or it may worsen constipation.

 # Warning!

To give you the best care, your doctor or other healthcare professional needs to know about the diseases and medical conditions you have had—your full medical history. Tell your doctor or other healthcare professional if you have or have ever had any of the following:

- Allergy or previous reaction to fiber and bulk-forming laxatives

- Bowel obstruction (blockage)

- Inflammatory bowel disease (ulcerative colitis or Crohn's disease)

- Rectal bleeding

- Severe abdominal (stomach) pain

Some bulk-forming laxatives contain dextrose (sugar) which may increase blood sugar if you have diabetes. Talk to your doctor or other healthcare professional before taking bulk-forming laxatives if you have diabetes.

Constipation may cause additional problems such as hemorrhoids or small tears around the opening of the rectum (fissures) or bleeding due to straining when moving your bowels. It is important to note, however, that if you see blood in your bowel movements, you should contact your doctor or other healthcare professional as this may be a sign of a more serious problem.

If you have constipation or diarrhea that persists for more than a week and does not get better, this may be a sign of a more serious condition. Talk to your doctor or other healthcare professional if this occurs.

Stool Softeners

Stool softeners hold water in the bowel and help soften the bowel movement. Taking a stool softener may help to relieve the strain or pain of having bowel movements if you are constipated. Stool softeners are mainly used to help prevent constipation. Stool softeners are available without a prescription.

Brand Name	Generic Name
Colace®	docusate sodium
Diocto-K®	docusate potassium
Surfak®	docusate calcium

How Will I Take Stool Softeners?

Most stool softeners are pills that are swallowed with at least 8 ounces of water or juice once or twice a day. Stool softeners work best when they are taken before bedtime. Stool softeners usually work in 1 to 3 days. Stool softeners are also available as liquids that may be stirred into milk or juice to improve their flavor. Follow the instructions given on the package, or ask your doctor or other healthcare professional how often to take this medication.

This medication is often used "as needed," so missing a dose should not be a problem. If you miss a dose and it is almost time for the next dose, you should skip the forgotten dose. Do not double the dose. Take your medication as directed by your doctor or other healthcare professional.

What Side Effects Can Stool Softeners Cause?

- Diarrhea

Tell your doctor or other healthcare professional if you have side effects that bother you, do not go away, make you worried about taking your medication, or make you want to stop taking your medication.

Do Other Medications Interact with Stool Softeners?

Stool softeners *may increase* the side effects of mineral oil.

Tell your doctor or other healthcare professional about all medications (both prescription and nonprescription [over-the-counter] medications) that you are taking.

What Else Should I Know about Stool Softeners?

Sometimes stool softeners cause bowel movements to become too soft and watery. If this happens, talk to your doctor or other healthcare professional about a lower dose of the stool softener.

Stool softeners may also be combined with stimulants such as *Peri-Colace*® (docusate/casanthranol), *Senokot S*® (docusate/senna), and others. See the section in this chapter on pages 189–192 for more information on stimulant laxatives.

Warning!

To give you the best care, your doctor or other healthcare professional needs to know about the diseases and medical conditions you have had—your full medical history. Tell your doctor or other healthcare professional if you have or have ever had any of the following:

- Allergy or previous reaction to stool softeners

- Bowel obstruction (blockage)

- Inflammatory bowel disease (ulcerative colitis or Crohn's disease)

- Rectal bleeding

- Severe abdominal (stomach) pain

Constipation may cause additional problems such as hemorrhoids or small tears around the opening of the rectum (fissures) or bleeding due to straining when moving your bowels. It is important to note, however, that if you see blood in your bowel movements, you should contact your doctor or other healthcare professional as this may be a sign of a more serious problem.

If you have constipation or diarrhea that persists for more than a week and does not get better, this may be a sign of a more serious condition. Talk to your doctor or other healthcare professional if this occurs.

Enemas

Enemas work quickly and powerfully. They increase the amount of fluid in the rectum and in the lower large intestine. With more water inside, the walls of the intestine become stretched. As a result, the person feels the urge to have a bowel movement.

Enemas may contain plain water or may be combined with mineral oil, stimulant medications, or softeners. Before you use an enema, ask your doctor or other healthcare professional if that would be a good idea.

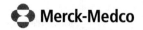
Brand Name	Generic Name
Fleet® Bisacodyl	bisacodyl
Therevac® Plus	docusate sodium/glycerin/ benzocaine
Therevac®-SB	docusate sodium/glycerin
Various	mineral oil
Various	sodium phosphate/sodium biphosphate

How Will I Use Enemas?

Enemas are inserted into the rectum as one single dose. Enemas usually work in 30 to 60 minutes. Follow the instructions given on the package, or ask your doctor or other healthcare professional how often to use this medication.

What Side Effects Can Enemas Cause?

More Common

- Rectal pain and irritation

Less Common

- Diarrhea

- Stomach pain or cramping

- Tiredness or sluggishness (fatigue)

- Weakness or muscle cramps that may be a sign of low potassium in your blood (hypokalemia)

Tell your doctor or other healthcare professional if you have side effects that bother you, do not go away, make you worried about taking your medication, or make you want to stop taking your medication.

Do Other Medications Interact with Enemas?

Enemas do not have any known medication interactions.

Why Else Do People Use Enemas?

Enemas are sometimes used to help clear the bowels before a rectal exam or medical procedure such as a colonoscopy.

Warning!

To give you the best care, your doctor or other healthcare professional needs to know about the diseases and medical conditions you have had—your full medical history. Tell your doctor or other healthcare professional if you have or have ever had any of the following:

- Allergy or previous reaction to an enema

- Bowel obstruction (blockage)

- Inflammatory bowel disease (ulcerative colitis or Crohn's disease)

- Kidney problems

- Rectal bleeding

- Severe abdominal (stomach) pain

Enemas should only be used on an "as needed" basis. Using enemas on a regular basis may make your constipation worse. With long-term use of enemas, your body begins to rely on the enema to produce bowel movements, and it forgets how to work on its own. If you now use or have used enemas on a regular basis, you may need to gradually stop using them. Your doctor or other healthcare professional can help you with reducing your use of enemas.

Constipation may cause additional problems such as hemorrhoids or small tears around the opening of the rectum (fissures) or bleeding due to straining when moving your bowels. It is important to note, however, that if you see blood in

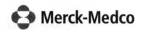

your bowel movements, you should contact your doctor or other healthcare professional, as this may be a sign of a more serious problem.

If you have constipation or diarrhea that persists for more than a week and does not get better, this may be a sign of a more serious condition. Talk to your doctor or other healthcare professional if this occurs.

Mineral Oil

Mineral oil may make it easier for the bowels to move by lubricating the intestines and by keeping water in bowel movements. Mineral oil is available without a prescription.

How Will I Take Mineral Oil?

Mineral oil is a thick liquid that is usually swallowed once or twice a day on an empty stomach, 1 hour before meals or 2 hours after meals. The oral liquid usually works in 6 to 8 hours. Follow the instructions given on the package, or ask your doctor or other healthcare professional how often to take this medication.

What Side Effects Can Mineral Oil Cause?

Less Common

- Diarrhea

- Rectal pain and irritation

- Stomach pain or cramping

- Tiredness or sluggishness (fatigue)

- Weakness or muscle cramps that may be a sign of low potassium in your blood (hypokalemia)

Rare

- Pneumonia

Tell your doctor or other healthcare professional if you have side effects that bother you, do not go away, make you worried about taking your medication, or make you want to stop taking your medication.

Do Other Medications Interact with Mineral Oil?

Mineral oil *may decrease* how well some vitamins work.

Stool softeners *may increase* the side effects of mineral oil.

Tell your doctor or other healthcare professional about all medications (both prescription and nonprescription [over-the-counter] medications) that you are taking.

Warning!

To give you the best care, your doctor or other healthcare professional needs to know about the diseases and medical conditions you have had—your full medical history. Tell your doctor or other healthcare professional if you now have or have ever had any of the following:

- Allergy or previous reaction to mineral oil
- Bowel obstruction (blockage)
- Difficulty swallowing
- Inflammatory bowel disease (ulcerative colitis or Crohn's disease)
- Rectal bleeding
- Severe abdominal (stomach) pain

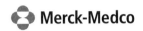

Do not lie down for at least 1 hour after taking mineral oil. This will help prevent the mineral oil from going into your lungs and help to decrease the chance of pneumonia.

Talk to your doctor or other healthcare professional before taking mineral oil daily. Regular use may decrease absorption of vitamins.

Constipation may cause additional problems such as hemorrhoids or small tears around the opening of the rectum (fissures) or bleeding due to straining when moving your bowels. It is important to note, however, that if you see blood in your bowel movements, you should contact your doctor or other healthcare professional as this may be a sign of a more serious problem.

If you have constipation or diarrhea that persists for more than a week and does not get better, this may be a sign of a more serious condition. Talk to your doctor or other healthcare professional if this occurs.

Glycerin Suppositories

Glycerin suppositories cause the rectum to contract and push out bowel movements. Glycerin suppositories help to soften bowel movements (stools) and lubricate the rectal area. Glycerin suppositories are available without a prescription.

 ## How Will I Use Glycerin Suppositories?

Suppositories are inserted into the rectum as needed. Glycerin suppositories usually work in about 15 to 60 minutes. Follow the instructions given on the package or ask your doctor or other healthcare professional how often to use this medication.

What Side Effects Can Glycerin Suppositories Cause?

- Diarrhea

- Rectal pain and irritation

Tell your doctor or other healthcare professional if you have side effects that bother you, do not go away, make you worried about taking your medication, or make you want to stop taking your medication.

Do Other Medications Interact with Glycerin Suppositories?

Glycerin suppositories do not have any known medication interactions.

Warning!

To give you the best care, your doctor or other healthcare professional needs to know about the diseases and medical conditions you have had—your full medical history. Tell your doctor or other healthcare professional if you have or have ever had any of the following:

- Allergy or previous reaction to glycerin suppositories

- Bowel obstruction (blockage)

- Inflammatory bowel disease (ulcerative colitis or Crohn's disease)

- Rectal bleeding

- Severe abdominal (stomach) pain

Glycerin suppositories should only be used on an "as needed" basis. Using them on a regular basis may make your constipation worse. With chronic use of glycerin suppositories, your body begins to rely on the suppositories to produce bowel movements, and it forgets how to work on its own. If you now use or have used glycerin suppositories on a regular basis, you may need to gradually stop using them. Your doctor or other healthcare professional can help you with this process.

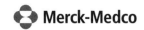 **Merck-Medco**

Constipation

Constipation may cause additional problems such as hemorrhoids or small tears around the opening of the rectum (fissures) or bleeding due to straining when moving your bowels. It is important to note, however, that if you see blood in your bowel movements, you should contact your doctor or other healthcare professional as this may be a sign of a more serious problem.

If you have constipation or diarrhea that persists for more than a week and does not get better, this may be a sign of a more serious condition. Talk to your doctor or other healthcare professional if this occurs.

Saline Laxatives

Saline laxatives draw water into the intestines and help to increase the squeezing motions (contractions) that move food through the intestines. Saline laxatives are available without a prescription.

Brand Name	Generic Name
Fleet® Phospho-soda	sodium diphosphate/ sodium phosphate
Phillips'® Milk of Magnesia	magnesium hydroxide
Various	magnesium citrate

 How Will I Take Saline Laxatives?

Saline laxatives are usually oral liquids taken only as needed. Most work in a few hours. Follow the instructions given on the package, or ask your doctor or other healthcare professional how often to take this medication.

What Side Effects Can Saline Laxatives Cause?

Less Common

- Diarrhea

- High magnesium in your blood from laxatives that contain magnesium

- Stomach pain or cramping

- Tiredness or sluggishness (fatigue)

- Weakness or muscle cramps that may be a sign of low potassium in your blood (hypokalemia)

Tell your doctor or other healthcare professional if you have side effects that bother you, do not go away, make you worried about taking your medication, or make you want to stop taking your medication.

Do Other Medications Interact with Saline Laxatives?

Saline laxatives *may decrease* the effects of other medications when taken at the same time. If you are using saline laxatives, take your other medications 1 hour before or 2 hours after taking your saline laxative.

Tell your doctor or other healthcare professional about all medications (both prescription and nonprescription [over-the-counter] medications) that you are taking.

Why Else Do People Take Saline Laxatives?

Saline laxatives may be used to help clear the bowel before a medical procedure such as a colonoscopy.

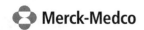

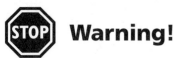 # Warning!

To give you the best care, your doctor or other healthcare professional needs to know about the diseases and medical conditions you have had—your full medical history. Tell your doctor or other healthcare professional if you have or have ever had any of the following:

- Allergy or previous reaction to saline laxatives
- Bowel obstruction (blockage)
- Congestive heart failure
- High blood pressure (hypertension)
- Inflammatory bowel disease (ulcerative colitis or Crohn's disease)
- Kidney problems
- Rectal bleeding
- Severe abdominal (stomach) pain

Some saline laxatives should only be used on an "as needed" basis. Using them on a regular basis may make your constipation worse. With chronic use of some saline laxatives, your body begins to rely on them to produce bowel movements, and it forgets how to work on its own. If you now use or have used saline laxatives on a regular basis, you may need to gradually stop using them. Your doctor or other healthcare professional can help you with this process.

Constipation may cause additional problems such as hemorrhoids or small tears around the opening of the rectum (fissures) or bleeding due to straining when moving your bowels. It is important to note, however, that if you see blood in your bowel movements, you should contact your doctor or other healthcare professional, as this may be a sign of a more serious problem.

If you have constipation or diarrhea that persists for more than a week and does not get better, this may be a sign of a more serious condition. Talk to your doctor or other healthcare professional if this occurs.

Many saline laxatives, like sodium phosphate, contain high amounts of salt (sodium). People who have high blood pressure, heart problems, or who are on a low-sodium diet should not take saline laxatives with high sodium content. If you have high blood pressure (hypertension) or congestive heart failure, or are on a low-sodium diet, talk to your doctor or other healthcare professional before taking any saline laxatives.

Many saline laxatives contain magnesium, which is removed from the body by the kidneys. If you have kidney problems, talk to your doctor or other healthcare professional before taking any saline laxatives.

Lactulose

Lactulose is not an over-the-counter laxative; it requires a prescription. Lactulose is a form of sugar that draws water into the colon to help make a soft, well-formed bowel movement (stool).

Brand Name	Generic Name
Cephulac®	lactulose
Chronulac®	lactulose
Dephulac®	lactulose

 ## How Will I Take Lactulose?

Lactulose is usually taken once or twice a day with water. It usually works in 1 to 2 days. You may mix lactulose with fruit juice or milk to improve its taste. Your doctor or other healthcare professional will tell you how often to take this medication.

This medication is often used "as needed," so missing a dose should not be a problem. If you miss a dose and it is almost time for the next dose, you should skip the forgotten dose. Do not double the dose. Take your medication as directed by your doctor or other healthcare professional.

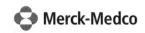

What Side Effects Can Lactulose Cause?

Less Common

- Diarrhea

- Gas or bloating

- Stomach pain or cramping

- Tiredness or sluggishness (fatigue)

- Weakness or muscle cramps that may be a sign of low potassium in your blood (hypokalemia)

Tell your doctor or other healthcare professional if you have side effects that bother you, do not go away, make you worried about taking your medication, or make you want to stop taking your medication.

Do Other Medications Interact with Lactulose?

Antacids such as *Maalox*® or *Mylanta*® (aluminum hydroxide/magnesium hydroxide) or *Amphojel*® (aluminum hydroxide) ***may decrease*** the effects of lactulose when taken at the same time. If you are using antacids, take lactulose 1 hour before or 2 hours after taking your antacid.

Tell your doctor or other healthcare professional about all medications (both prescription and nonprescription [over-the-counter] medications) that you are taking.

Why Else Do People Take Lactulose?

Lactulose may be used to help treat some of the symptoms from severe liver problems.

Warning!

To give you the best care, your doctor or other healthcare professional needs to know about the diseases and medical conditions you have had—your full medical history. Tell your doctor or other healthcare professional if you have or have ever had any of the following:

- Allergy or previous reaction to lactulose

- Bowel obstruction (blockage)

- Diabetes

- Inflammatory bowel disease (ulcerative colitis or Crohn's disease)

- Rectal bleeding

- Severe abdominal (stomach) pain

Constipation may cause additional problems such as hemorrhoids or small tears around the opening of the rectum (fissures) or bleeding due to straining when moving your bowels. It is important to note, however, that if you see blood in your bowel movements, you should contact your doctor or other healthcare professional, as this may be a sign of a more serious problem.

If you have constipation or diarrhea that persists for more than a week and does not get better, this may be a sign of a more serious condition. Talk to your doctor or other healthcare professional if this occurs.

Stimulant Laxatives

Stimulant laxatives stimulate muscles of the bowel to help cause bowel movements. They may be combined with stool softeners. Stimulant laxatives are available without a prescription.

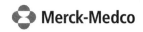
Brand Name	Generic Name
Agoral®	senna
Correctol®	bisacodyl
Doxidan™	casanthranol/docusate calcium
Dulcolax®	bisacodyl
Ex•Lax®	senna
Nature's Remedy®	cascara/aloe
Neoloid®	castor oil
Peri-Colace®	casanthranol/docusate sodium
Senokot®	senna
Senokot S®	senna/docusate sodium

How Will I Take Stimulant Laxatives?

Stimulant laxatives come as pills and liquids to be taken by mouth or as suppositories that are inserted in the rectum and are usually used as needed. The suppositories usually take 15 to 60 minutes to work. Pills or liquids usually take 6 to 8 hours to work. Stimulant laxatives that are hard-coated pills should be swallowed whole. Crushing, breaking, or chewing the tablets may cause painful stomach cramping. Follow the instructions given on the package, or ask your doctor or other healthcare professional how often to take this medication.

What Side Effects Can Stimulant Laxatives Cause?

Less Common

- Diarrhea

- Rectal pain or irritation

- Stomach pain or cramping

- Tiredness or sluggishness (fatigue)

- Weakness or muscle cramps that may be a sign of low potassium in your blood (hypokalemia)

Tell your doctor or other healthcare professional if you have side effects that bother you, do not go away, make you worried about taking your medication, or make you want to stop taking your medication.

Do Other Medications Interact with Stimulant Laxatives?

Antacids such as *Maalox®* or *Mylanta®* (aluminum hydroxide/magnesium hydroxide) or *Amphojel®* (aluminum hydroxide) ***may increase*** the side effects of some stimulant laxative pills when taken at the same time. If you are using antacids, take stimulant laxative pills 1 hour before or 2 hours after taking your antacid.

Tell your doctor or other healthcare professional about all medications (both prescription and nonprescription [over-the-counter] medications) that you are taking.

Why Else Do People Take Stimulant Laxatives?

Stimulant laxatives may be used to help clear the bowel before a rectal exam or a medical procedure such as a colonoscopy.

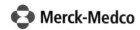

 # Warning!

To give you the best care, your doctor or other healthcare professional needs to know about the diseases and medical conditions you have had—your full medical history. Tell your doctor or other healthcare professional if you have or have ever had any of the following:

- Allergy or previous reaction to stimulant laxatives

- Bowel obstruction (blockage)

- Inflammatory bowel disease (ulcerative colitis or Crohn's disease)

- Rectal bleeding

- Severe abdominal (stomach) pain

Stimulant laxatives should only be used on an "as needed" basis. Using them on a regular basis may make your constipation worse. With chronic use of stimulant laxatives, your body begins to rely on them to produce bowel movements, and it forgets how to work on its own. If you now use or have used stimulant laxatives on a regular basis, you may need to gradually stop using them. Your doctor or other healthcare professional can help you with this process.

Constipation may cause additional problems such as hemorrhoids or small tears around the opening of the rectum (fissures) or bleeding due to straining when moving your bowels. It is important to note, however, that if you see blood in your bowel movements, you should contact your doctor or other healthcare professional, as this may be a sign of a more serious problem.

If you have constipation or diarrhea that persists for more than a week and does not get better, this may be a sign of a more serious condition. Talk to your doctor or other healthcare professional if this occurs.

Chapter 7

Coronary Artery Disease and Cardiac Chest Pain (Angina)

What Is Coronary Artery Disease?

For the heart to beat and pump blood through the body, the heart muscle needs oxygen, which it gets from the blood. But it cannot get the oxygen directly from the blood it is pumping. Instead, the heart has special arteries called coronary arteries that bring oxygen-rich blood directly to the heart muscle that needs it. In coronary artery disease, the arteries that bring blood to the heart muscle become clogged. Because the space inside the arteries gets narrower, too little blood can flow to the heart muscle. A sudden constriction (spasm) of the arteries can also block the flow of blood. The heart muscle may become damaged from lack of oxygen. A heart attack (myocardial infarction) can occur when the heart muscle does not get enough oxygen. If a doctor or other healthcare professional does not treat coronary artery disease, it can lead to a heart attack or death.

What Causes Coronary Artery Disease?

The usual cause of coronary artery disease is a buildup of deposits of fat (plaque) inside the walls of the arteries. You are at higher risk of developing coronary artery disease if you have high cholesterol or high blood pressure, if you smoke cigarettes, or if you have a family history of coronary artery disease. High cholesterol (hypercholesterolemia) can cause buildup of fat deposits (plaque) that clog the arteries. If you have high cholesterol, keeping it under control is important to try to prevent coronary artery disease. For more information about high cholesterol, please see the High Cholesterol chapter, which begins on page 431. High blood pressure (hypertension) makes the heart work too hard, and it can also injure the arteries that supply the heart muscle with blood. If you have high blood pressure, keeping it under control is important to try to prevent coronary artery disease. For more information about high blood pressure, please see the High Blood Pressure chapter, which begins on page 373. Cigarette smoking can increase the chance that you might develop coronary artery disease, particularly if combined with one of the other risk factors mentioned above. If you smoke, talk to your doctor or other healthcare professional about quitting smoking.

Many different factors increase your risk of coronary artery disease. Risk factors are habits or traits that make a person more likely to develop a disease. You can control many risk factors, but others you cannot. The more risk factors you have, the greater your chance of getting coronary artery disease. Become familiar with the risks of coronary artery disease and ask your doctor or other healthcare professional how to help reduce them.

Risk Factors for Coronary Artery Disease

Age

If you are a man over 45 years old

If you are a women over 55 years old

Women's Issues

If you are past menopause and are not taking estrogen

If you had your ovaries removed and are not taking estrogen

Family History

If your father or brother had a heart attack before age 55

If your mother or sister had a heart attack before age 65

Smoking

If you smoke

If you live or work with people who smoke every day

Cholesterol

If your total cholesterol blood level is 240 mg/dL or higher

If your HDL ("good") cholesterol blood level is less than 35 mg/dL

Blood Pressure

If your blood pressure is 140/90 mm Hg or higher

If you have been told that your blood pressure is too high

Physical Inactivity

If you get less than a total of 30 minutes of exercise or physical activity on most days

Body Weight

If you are 20 pounds or more overweight for your height and build

Diabetes

If you have diabetes

If you have a fasting blood sugar of 126 mg/dL or higher

If you need medicine to control your blood sugar

What Is Cardiac Chest Pain (Angina)?

Chest pain caused by coronary artery disease is called angina pectoris, often called angina. Cardiac chest pain can result when the arteries are narrowed or blocked, and the blood flow to the heart muscle cannot meet the heart's need for oxygen.

Not everyone with poor blood supply to the heart muscle feels pain or other symptoms. When there is pain, it usually starts under the breastbone (sternum). It can also hurt in the left shoulder, down the inside of the left arm, or in the throat, jaw, teeth, back (between the shoulder blades), or stomach area. Many people with angina pectoris do not feel a "pain sensation." Instead, they have sensations of fullness, pressure, heaviness, discomfort, numbness, or tightness in the chest.

People who have angina pectoris often get chest pain when they are physically active. That pain often lasts for several minutes and gets better when the person rests. People may get to know which kinds of physical activity will cause chest pain. For example, the pain may start when they exercise right after a meal, walk into the wind, or move from a warm room into cold air.

Types of treatment for angina and coronary artery disease include medications, angioplasty (a medical procedure that opens or unclogs the blood vessel with a flexible tube that has something like a balloon at the end), and heart bypass surgery. People can also make other changes in their life to help prevent coronary artery disease. Quitting smoking, eating a low-fat and low-cholesterol diet, losing weight, and exercising may help to prevent coronary artery disease. Talk to your doctor or other healthcare professional before starting a diet and exercise program.

Medications for Cardiac Chest Pain (Angina) and Coronary Artery Disease

Several kinds of medications may be taken for cardiac chest pain and coronary artery disease. This chapter discusses these categories of medications:

MEDICATIONS	See Page
Nitrates	197
Calcium Channel Blockers	206
Beta Blockers	212

If you do not see the exact name of the medication that you take for cardiac chest pain and coronary artery disease listed above, check the Medication and Chapter Table to find out which category your medication falls under or check the Index.

Nitrates

Nitrates are one of the oldest and most common types of medications for cardiac chest pain. These medications open up (dilate) the narrowed blood vessels in the body. When the blood can travel through wider blood vessels, the heart does not have to work as hard to pump the blood. By opening the coronary arteries, nitrates let more blood flow to the heart, and the pain that arises from the oxygen-starved heart muscle decreases.

Aerosol or Pump Sprays

Brand Name	Generic Name
Nitrolingual®	nitroglycerin

Chewable Tablets

Brand Name	Generic Name
Sorbitrate®	isosorbide dinitrate

Ointments

Brand Name	Generic Name
Nitro-Bid®	nitroglycerin
Nitrol®	nitroglycerin

Pills

Brand Name	Generic Name
Dilatrate®	isosorbide dinitrate
Imdur®	isosorbide mononitrate
Ismo®	isosorbide mononitrate
Isordil®	isosorbide dinitrate
Monoket®	isosorbide mononitrate
Nitro-Bid®	nitroglycerin
Nitrogard®	nitroglycerin
Nitroglyn®	nitroglycerin
Nitrong®	nitroglycerin
Sorbitrate®	isosorbide dinitrate

Under-the-Tongue (Sublingual) Tablets

Brand Name	Generic Name
Isordil®	isosorbide dinitrate
NitroQuick®	nitroglycerin
Nitrostat®	nitroglycerin
Sorbitrate®	isosorbide dinitrate

Skin (Transdermal) Patches

Brand Name	Generic Name
Deponit®	nitroglycerin
Minitran®	nitroglycerin
Nitrodisc®	nitroglycerin
Nitro-Dur®	nitroglycerin
Transderm-Nitro®	nitroglycerin

How Will I Take Nitrates?

Nitrate Pills that Dissolve under the Tongue (Sublingual)

Nitrate pills that dissolve under the tongue (sublingual) are usually used to help prevent angina or to help relieve cardiac chest pain once it starts. They work fast, providing relief from pain within minutes, and are easy to use. If you take nitrate pills that dissolve under your tongue, you may also take them before doing any exercise or hard physical activity. To use these pills, you should sit down first and then put them under your tongue until they disappear. Dissolving rapidly helps the medication to enter your bloodstream quickly. Do not swallow these pills. Be sure to carry these pills with you at all times.

You may repeat a dose once every 5 minutes until you feel better, but do not take more than 3 pills within 15 minutes unless directed to do so by your doctor or other healthcare professional. If the dose that has been prescribed for you does not relieve your symptoms, go to the emergency room of the nearest hospital right away where you will be evaluated and your doctor or other healthcare professional will be contacted.

Nitrate pills lose their effect over time. When that happens, they have to be thrown away. Keep all nitrate pills in their original containers with tight-fitting caps, and take the cotton out of the bottle when you get a new bottle. Keep them away from heat and sunlight. Do not keep them in a bathroom medicine cabinet. Heat and steam can make them "age" faster. It is also important that you do not keep your pills in your pants pocket because the body heat caused by walking can cause your pills to get too hot and lose potency (strength). Because nitrate pills lose potency over time, you should throw away any pills 6 months after the bottle has been opened. Always keep some nitrate pills with you.

Aerosol or Pump Sprays

Spray aerosol medications on your tongue or under your tongue. Do not breathe them in (inhale them) through your nose. Aerosol sprays are easy to use, work as well as under-the-tongue pills and may be taken for the same reasons. The people who tend to use them most are those who have difficulty taking pills. Be sure to carry your spray with you at all times.

You may repeat a dose once every 5 minutes until you feel better, but do not take more than 3 sprays within 15 minutes unless directed to do so by your doctor or other healthcare professional. If the dose that has been prescribed for you does not relieve your symptoms, go to the emergency room of the nearest hospital right away where you will be evaluated and your doctor or other healthcare professional will be contacted.

Chewable and Nonchewable Pills (Pills that Are Swallowed)

Chewable nitroglycerin may be chewed to help relieve cardiac chest pain. Chewable nitroglycerin pills may be taken before the cardiac chest pain starts and may help prevent cardiac chest pain.

Oral (nonchewable) nitrate pills are long-acting pills that are usually taken to help keep cardiac chest pain from happening. Because these pills are longer acting and do not start working right away, they are usually not used to relieve chest pain once you are having it. They are usually taken 1 to 3 times a day. Your doctor or other healthcare professional will tell you how often to take this medication.

When a medication has initials after its name, such as XL, XR, SR, BID, DUR, and others, it usually means that the body absorbs the medication slowly over time, so you usually have to take it only once or twice a day. The body will absorb some medications of this type too fast if you crush or break them or dissolve them in liquid, and their effects will not last as long as they should. Check with your doctor or other healthcare professional before crushing or breaking your pills or dissolving your pills in liquid.

If you miss a dose of this medication, take the dose you missed as soon as possible. However, if it is almost time for your next dose, skip the missed dose and just take the next one. Do not double your dose. Take your medication exactly as directed by your doctor or other healthcare professional. Do not stop taking a prescription medication unless directed by your doctor or other healthcare professional.

Ointments

Nitroglycerin ointments are used to help prevent cardiac chest pain (angina). Because ointments are longer acting and do not start working right away, they are usually not used to relieve cardiac chest pain once you are having it. Ointments can be messy, and some people find them hard to apply. The amount (dose) to spread on the skin is usually measured by a paper or applicator in inches of ointment squeezed out of the tube. You may spread your nitroglycerin ointment almost anywhere on the skin of your chest, back (trunk), or upper arms, usually 1 to 3 times a day. Do not rub or massage the nitrate ointment into your skin. Spread it in a thin, even layer, covering an area of the same size each time you use it, but not in the exact same place. Put the ointment on a different area every time you use it to avoid irritation of your skin. Wash your hands to remove any ointment you get on your hands. Your doctor or other healthcare professional will tell you how often to use your medication.

If you miss a dose of this medication, take the dose you missed as soon as possible. However, if it is almost time for your next dose, skip the missed dose and just take the next one. Do not double your dose. Take your medication exactly as directed by your doctor or other healthcare professional. Do not stop taking a prescription medication unless directed by your doctor or other healthcare professional.

Skin (Transdermal) Patches

Nitroglycerin patches are used to help prevent cardiac chest pain (angina). Because patches are longer acting and do not start working right away, they are not usually used to relieve cardiac chest pain once you are having it. Skin (transdermal) patches, which help to prevent angina, are easy to apply. Patches are usually used once a day for about 12 to 16 hours. Put the patch on the skin of your chest, back (trunk), or upper arms. You can help to keep the patches from irritating your skin by putting each new one in a different place. Put on a new patch if the first one falls off. When taking off or disposing of an old patch, make sure you throw it away where children and pets cannot get it because it will still contain some medication that may be harmful to them.

Your skin absorbs the nitrate medication that is in the patch. Usually, you will take the patch off for about 8 to 12 hours in a 24-hour time period. This is to give your body the chance to let the medication work well. If you do not give your body time off the patch, you may notice that your patch does not work as well as it used to work. Your doctor or other healthcare professional will tell you how long to leave your patches on.

If you miss a dose of this medication, take the dose you missed as soon as possible. However, if it is almost time for your next dose, skip the missed dose and just take the next one. Do not double your dose. Take your medication exactly as directed by your doctor or other healthcare professional. Do not stop taking a prescription medication unless directed by your doctor or other healthcare professional.

What Side Effects Can Nitrates Cause?

More Common

- Burning sensation under the tongue (under-the-tongue pill or spray only)

- Dizziness when standing up from a bed or a chair

- Fast heartbeat (palpitations)

- Headache

- Passing out or fainting

- Rash (skin redness, bumps, itching, or irritation), possible with ointments or patches

- Reddening of the face (flushing)

Tell your doctor or other healthcare professional if you have side effects that bother you, do not go away, make you worried about taking your medication, or make you want to stop taking your medication.

Do Other Medications Interact with Nitrates?

Nitrates *may increase* the side effects of high blood pressure (hypertension) medications and other medications for angina.

If you are taking nitrates, do not take *Viagra®* (sildenafil). This combination of medications *may cause* serious side effects and even death.

DHE-45® (dihydroergotamine) *may decrease* how well nitrates work.

Drinking alcoholic beverages (such as beer, wine, whiskey, and others) *may increase* the side effects of nitrates.

Tell your doctor or other healthcare professional about all medications (both prescription and nonprescription [over-the-counter] medications) that you are taking.

Why Else Do People Take Nitrates?

Nitrates may be used for heart failure. The nitroglycerin ointment is sometimes used for people who have poor blood flow to their hands (Raynaud's disease).

What Else Should I Know about Nitrates?

Headaches are common side effects of nitrates. In fact, getting a headache soon after taking a nitrate usually means the medication is working. These headaches usually go away in a couple of weeks if you are taking nitrates daily. Talk to your doctor or other healthcare professional about taking over-the-counter (OTC) pain medications for headache relief if they become bothersome.

 # Warning!

To give you the best care, your doctor or other healthcare professional needs to know about the diseases and medical conditions you have had—your full medical history. Tell your doctor or other healthcare professional if you have or have ever had any of the following:

- Allergy or previous reaction to adhesives, skin (transdermal) patches
- Allergy or previous reaction to nitrates
- Dizziness when standing up from a bed or a chair
- Glaucoma (an eye disease)
- Kidney problems
- Liver problems
- Low red blood cells (anemia)

Very soon after you take a nitrate medication for chest pain, your blood pressure may drop suddenly, which may make you feel dizzy and faint. To be sure you do not fall, sit or lie down whenever you take certain forms of nitrate such as the ones that dissolve under the tongue (sublingual medications), the ones you spray under your tongue (aerosol medications), and the ones that you chew.

Nitrates may make you unsteady on your feet, causing you to fall and possibly break a bone. If you have fallen recently, tell your doctor or other healthcare professional about it. Taking a different medication or a lower dose may make you less likely to fall. You should not stop taking this medication without first talking to your doctor or other healthcare professional.

Taking a nitrate medication may keep you from having cardiac chest pain while you exercise. Not having angina attacks or pain when exercising may tempt you to be more active than you really should be. Talk to your doctor or other healthcare professional to find out how much exercise you may do safely before you increase your activity.

If you are taking nitrates, do not take *Viagra*® (sildenafil). This combination of medications may cause serious side effects and even death. Death after use of *Viagra*® (sildenafil) most often occurs in men with heart disease or risks for developing heart disease.

If you are having chest pain, pain in the left shoulder, down the inside of the left arm, or pain in the throat, jaw, teeth, back (between the shoulder blades), or abdomen (stomach), you may be having a heart attack. Other symptoms of a heart attack might include fullness, pressure, heaviness, discomfort, numbness, or tightness on your chest. If you take nitroglycerin and the dose that has been prescribed for you does not relieve your symptoms, or you do not have nitroglycerin, go to the emergency room of the nearest hospital right away where you will be evaluated and your doctor or other healthcare professional will be contacted.

Under certain circumstances, your doctor or other healthcare professional may decide that you should stop taking this medication. If you have taken it for more than a couple of weeks, he or she may want you to decrease it gradually, lowering the dose over a few weeks or months. Stopping suddenly may cause unpleasant withdrawal symptoms or may worsen your medical problems. Pay careful attention to the instructions your doctor or other healthcare professional gives you about how much less to take and for how long.

Calcium Channel Blockers

Calcium channel blockers help relax blood vessels, so that more blood and oxygen flow to the heart, and the heart does not have to work so hard to pump blood through the blood vessels.

Brand Name	Generic Name
Adalat®	nifedipine
Calan®	verapamil
Cardene®	nicardipine
Cardizem®	diltiazem
Covera®	verapamil
Dilacor®	diltiazem
DynaCirc®	isradipine
Isoptin®	verapamil
Norvasc®	amlodipine
Plendil®	felodipine
Procardia®	nifedipine
Sular®	nisoldipine
Tiamate®	diltiazem
Tiazac®	diltiazem
Vascor®	bepridil
Verelan®	verapamil

How Will I Take Calcium Channel Blockers?

Calcium channel blockers are generally taken 1 to 3 times a day. *Plendil®* (felodipine), *Cardene®* (nicardipine), nifedipine, and diltiazem should be taken on an empty stomach 1 hour before or 2 hours after meals. Verapamil should be taken with food or meals. *DynaCirc®* (isradipine) should be taken with food to help prevent an upset stomach. *Sular®* (nisoldipine) should not be taken with high-fat meals. Your doctor or other healthcare professional will tell you how many times a day to take your medication.

When a medication has initials after its name, such as XL, XR, SR, BID, DUR, and others, it usually means that the body absorbs the medication slowly over time, so you usually have to take it only once or twice a day. The body will absorb some medications of this type too fast if you crush or break them or dissolve them in liquid, and their effects will not last as long as they should. Check with your doctor or other healthcare professional before crushing or breaking your pills or dissolving your pills in liquid.

If you miss a dose of this medication, take the dose you missed as soon as possible. However, if it is almost time for your next dose, skip the missed dose and just take the next one. Do not double your dose. Take your medication exactly as directed by your doctor or other healthcare professional. Do not stop taking a prescription medication unless directed by your doctor or other healthcare professional.

What Side Effects Can Calcium Channel Blockers Cause?

More Common

- Constipation
- Dizziness when standing up from a bed or a chair
- Headache
- Reddening of the face (flushing)
- Swelling or puffiness of feet, ankles, or lower legs (edema)

Less Common

- Congestive heart failure

- Diarrhea

- Nausea

- Rash (skin redness, bumps, itching, or irritation)

- Slow, fast, or irregular heartbeat (palpitations)

Tell your doctor or other healthcare professional if you have side effects that bother you, do not go away, make you worried about taking your medication, or make you want to stop taking your medication.

Do Other Medications Interact with Calcium Channel Blockers?

Calcium channel blockers **may increase** the side effects of these medications:

- *BuSpar*® (buspirone)

- Heart rhythm problem (arrhythmia) medications—see Glossary

- High blood pressure (hypertension) medications and diuretics (water pills)—see Glossary

- *Lanoxin*® (digoxin)

- Lithium such as *Eskalith*®, *Lithobid*®, and others—see Glossary

- *Neoral*® (cyclosporine)

- Quinidine such as *Quinaglute*®, *Quinidex*®, and others—see Glossary

- *Sandimmune*® (cyclosporine)

- Statins such as *Lipitor*® (atorvastatin), *Pravachol*® (pravastatin), *Zocor*® (simvastatin), and others—see Glossary

- *Tegretol*® (carbamazepine)

- Theophylline such as *Theo-Dur*®, *Uniphyl*®, and others—see Glossary

These medications *may increase* the side effects of calcium channel blockers:

- *Tagamet®* (cimetidine)
- *Zantac®* (ranitidine)

Ethmozine® (moricizine) *may decrease* how well diltiazem works, and diltiazem *may increase* the side effects of *Ethmozine®* (moricizine).

These medications *may decrease* how well calcium channel blockers work:

- Barbiturates such as *Butisol®* (butabarbital), *Luminal®* (phenobarbital), *Mebaral®* (mephobarbital), and others—see Glossary
- *Rifadin®* (rifampin)

These medications *may increase* the side effects of *Adalat®* (nifedipine), *Cardene®* (nicardipine), *DynaCirc®* (isradipine), *Plendil®* (felodipine), *Procardia®* (nifedipine), and *Sular®* (nisoldipine):

- *Diflucan®* (fluconazole)
- *Nizoral®* (ketoconazole)
- *Sporanox®* (itraconazole)

Erythromycin such as *Ery-Tab®*, *Erythrocin®*, and others (see Glossary) *may increase* the side effects of *Plendil®* (felodipine).

Norvir® (ritonavir) *may cause* serious or life-threatening side effects if taken by someone who is also taking *Vascor®* (bepridil).

Vascor® (bepridil) is generally not prescribed for anyone who is taking *Propulsid®* (cisapride [withdrawn from general distribution; available only by special arrangement with the manufacturer]), *Seldane®* (terfenadine [no longer commercially available]), or *Hismanal®* (astemizole [no longer commercially available]), because together they *may cause* serious, sometimes fatal, heart problems.

Grapefruit and grapefruit juice *may increase* the side effects of calcium channel blockers. This interaction can happen whether you eat the grapefruit or drink the grapefruit juice at the same time as you take your medication or if you take the medication separately from the grapefruit or grapefruit juice. Talk to your doctor or other healthcare professional before eating grapefruit or drinking grapefruit juice if you are taking this medication. Please also read the discussion on A Warning about Grapefruit and Grapefruit Juice on pages i-ii.

Tell your doctor or other healthcare professional about all medications (both prescription and nonprescription [over-the-counter] medications) that you are taking.

Why Else Do People Take Calcium Channel Blockers?

Calcium channel blockers are helpful for high blood pressure (hypertension), some heart rhythm problems (arrhythmia), and to help prevent migraine headaches. They are sometimes used for people who have poor blood flow to their hands (Raynaud's disease).

What Else Should I Know about Calcium Channel Blockers?

Take your medication every day as directed by your doctor or other healthcare professional, even if you feel fine. These medications have to be taken every day to work as well as possible and to help keep you from having cardiac chest pain (angina) and other symptoms.

 # Warning!

To give you the best care, your doctor or other healthcare professional needs to know about the diseases and medical conditions you have had—your full medical history. Tell your doctor or other healthcare professional if you have or have ever had any of the following:

- Allergy or previous reaction to calcium channel blockers
- Congestive heart failure

- Heart rhythm problems (arrhythmia)

- Kidney problems

- Liver problems

- Low blood pressure (hypotension)

Sustained-released or long-acting types of calcium channel blockers (released into the body slowly over 12 to 24 hours) are usually recommended for coronary artery disease because short-acting calcium channel blockers may cause more serious side effects than long-acting types. Long-acting medications usually have initials after their names such as CD, CR, CC, XL, XR, SR, HS, BID, or others. If you are not taking a medication with these initials after the name, talk to your doctor or other healthcare professional to see if this medication is right for you.

Calcium channel blockers may make you unsteady on your feet, causing you to fall and possibly break a bone. If you have fallen recently, tell your doctor or other healthcare professional about it. Taking a different medication or a lower dose may make you less likely to fall. You should not stop taking this medication without first talking to your doctor or other healthcare professional.

Taking a calcium channel blocker may keep you from having cardiac chest pain while you exercise. Not having angina attacks or pain when exercising may tempt you to be more active than you really should be. Talk to your doctor or other healthcare professional to find out how much exercise you may do safely before you increase your activity.

If you are having chest pain, pain in the left shoulder, down the inside of the left arm, or pain in the throat, jaw, teeth, back (between the shoulder blades), or abdomen (stomach), you may be having a heart attack. Other symptoms of a heart attack might include fullness, pressure, heaviness, discomfort, numbness, or tightness on your chest. If you take nitroglycerin and the dose that has been prescribed for you does not relieve your symptoms, or you do not have nitroglycerin, go to the emergency room of the nearest hospital right away where you will be evaluated and your doctor or other healthcare professional will be contacted.

Under certain circumstances, your doctor or other healthcare professional may decide that you should stop taking this medication. If you have taken it for more than a couple of weeks, he or she may want you to decrease it gradually, lowering the dose over a few weeks or months. Stopping suddenly may cause unpleasant withdrawal symptoms or may worsen your medical problems. Pay careful attention to the instructions your doctor or other healthcare professional gives you about how much less to take and for how long.

Beta Blockers

Some beta blockers are used to help prevent cardiac chest pain (angina). Taking a beta blocker helps to keep the heart from working too hard. The heart of someone who is taking a beta blocker does not beat as fast and uses less oxygen. The beta blocker also helps to lower blood pressure, which makes it easier for the heart to pump blood.

Brand Name	Generic Name
Blocadren®	timolol
Corgard®	nadolol
Inderal®	propranolol
Kerlone®	betaxolol
Lopressor®	metoprolol
Normodyne®	labetalol
Tenormin®	atenolol
Toprol®	metoprolol
Zebeta®	bisoprolol

How Will I Take Beta Blockers?

Beta blockers are usually taken 1 to 3 times daily. They may be taken with or without food. You should be consistent with most beta blockers: either always take them with food or always take them without food. Your doctor or other healthcare professional will tell you how often to take your medication.

When a medication has initials after its name, such as XL, XR, SR, BID, DUR, and others, it usually means that the body absorbs the medication slowly over time, so you usually have to take it only once or twice a day. The body will absorb some medications of this type too fast if you crush or break them or dissolve them in liquid, and their effects will not last as long as they should. Check with your doctor or other healthcare professional before crushing or breaking your pills or dissolving your pills in liquid.

If you miss a dose of this medication, take the dose you missed as soon as possible. However, if it is almost time for your next dose, skip the missed dose and just take the next one. Do not double your dose. Take your medication exactly as directed by your doctor or other healthcare professional. Do not stop taking a prescription medication unless directed by your doctor or other healthcare professional.

What Side Effects Can Beta Blockers Cause?

More Common

- Dizziness when standing up from a bed or a chair

- Erection problems (erectile dysfunction)

- Loss of interest in sex (decreased libido)

- Tiredness or sluggishness (fatigue)

- Weakness

Less Common

- Change in blood sugar

- Congestive heart failure

- Heartburn

- Leg pain when walking

- Rash (skin redness, bumps, itching, or irritation)

- Sadness, feeling blue or down, depressed mood (depression)

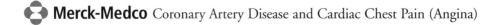

- Slow or irregular heartbeat (palpitations)

- Strange dreams and nightmares

- Trouble breathing or shortness of breath in asthma and COPD, including emphysema or chronic bronchitis

---

Tell your doctor or other healthcare professional if you have side effects that bother you, do not go away, make you worried about taking your medication, or make you want to stop taking your medication.

 ## Do Other Medications Interact with Beta Blockers?

Beta blockers *may decrease* how well diabetes medications such as *DiaBeta®* (glyburide), *Glucophage®* (metformin), *Glucotrol®* (glipizide), and others (see Glossary) work.

These medications *may increase* the side effects of beta blockers:

- Heart rhythm problem (arrhythmia) medications—see Glossary

- High blood pressure (hypertension) medications and diuretics (water pills)—see Glossary

- *Lanoxin®* (digoxin)

- Neuroleptic medications such as *Risperdal®* (risperidone), *Thorazine®* (chlorpromazine), *Zyprexa®* (olanzapine), and others—see Glossary

- Propylthiouracil (PTU)

- *Tagamet®* (cimetidine)

- *Tapazole®* (methimazole)

Beta blockers *may increase* the side effects of these medications:

- *DHE-45®* (dihydroergotamine)

- *Ergomar®* (ergotamine)

- *Migranal®* (dihydroergotamine)

These medications *may decrease* how well beta blockers work:

- Barbiturates such as *Butisol*® (butabarbital), *Luminal*® (phenobarbital), *Mebaral*® (mephobarbital), and others—see Glossary

- Nonsteroidal anti-inflammatory drugs (NSAIDs) such as *Motrin*® (ibuprofen), *Aleve*® (naproxen), *Vioxx*® (rofecoxib), *Celebrex*® (celecoxib), and others—see Glossary

- *Rifadin*® (rifampin)

- Theophylline such as *Theo-Dur*®, *Uniphyl*®, and others—see Glossary.

- Thyroid medications such as *Cytomel*® (liothyronine), *Levoxyl*® (levothyroxine), *Synthroid*® (levothyroxine), and others—see Glossary

---

Tell your doctor or other healthcare professional about all medications (both prescription and nonprescription [over-the-counter] medications) that you are taking.

Why Else Do People Take Beta Blockers?

Beta blockers can help prevent a heart attack (myocardial infarction), heart rhythm problems (arrhythmia), migraine headaches, and shakiness or tremors. Some people take beta blockers for high blood pressure or congestive heart failure.

 # Warning!

To give you the best care, your doctor or other healthcare professional needs to know about the diseases and medical conditions you have had—your full medical history. Tell your doctor or other healthcare professional if you have or have ever had any of the following:

- Allergy or previous reaction to beta blockers

- Breathing problems (asthma and COPD, including emphysema or chronic bronchitis)

- Congestive heart failure

- Diabetes

- Poor circulation (peripheral vascular disease)

- Sadness, feeling blue or down, depressed mood (depression)

Beta blockers may increase the symptoms of some lung problems, especially asthma and COPD, including emphysema or chronic bronchitis. Tell your doctor or other healthcare professional if you have trouble breathing or shortness of breath.

Beta blockers may hide the symptoms of low blood sugar (hypoglycemia). This can cause problems for people with diabetes. Ask your doctor or other healthcare professional how often you should check your blood sugar.

Beta blockers may increase the symptoms of poor circulation (peripheral vascular disease). Tell your doctor or other healthcare professional if you develop symptoms of poor circulation such as pain, numbness, or coldness of your legs, feet, and hands.

Beta blockers may make you unsteady on your feet, causing you to fall and possibly break a bone. If you have fallen recently, tell your doctor or other healthcare professional about it. Taking a different medication or a lower dose may make you less likely to fall. You should not stop taking this medication without first talking to your doctor or other healthcare professional.

Taking a beta blocker may keep you from having cardiac chest pain while you exercise. Not having angina attacks or pain when exercising may tempt you to be more active than you really should be. Talk to your doctor or other healthcare professional to find out how much exercise you may do safely before you increase your activity.

If you are having chest pain, pain in the left shoulder, down the inside of the left arm, or in the throat, jaw, teeth, back (between the shoulder blades), or abdomen (stomach), you may be having a heart attack. Other symptoms of a heart attack might include fullness, pressure, heaviness, discomfort, numbness, or tightness on your chest. If you take nitroglycerin and the dose that has been prescribed for you does not relieve your symptoms, or you do not have nitroglycerin, go to the emergency room of the nearest hospital right away where you will be evaluated and your doctor or other healthcare professional will be contacted.

Under certain circumstances, your doctor or other healthcare professional may decide that you should stop taking this medication. If you have taken it for more than a couple of weeks, he or she may want you to decrease it gradually, lowering the dose over a few weeks or months. Stopping suddenly may cause unpleasant withdrawal symptoms or may worsen your medical problems. Pay careful attention to the instructions your doctor or other healthcare professional gives you about how much less to take and for how long.

Chapter 8

Depression

What Is Depression?

Feeling sad from time to time is common. People who feel "blue" may say they are "depressed." But true depression (clinical depression) means more than having brief periods of sadness or feeling a little low. Clinical depression is a medical disorder that can affect the whole body, the way you think, and the way you feel. If you have a combination of these symptoms listed below for more than 2 weeks, talk with your doctor or other healthcare professional to find out whether you might have more than "the blues":

- Change in appetite (eating more or less than usual and gaining or losing weight)

- Excessive tiredness

- Extreme sadness

- Loss of interest in activities you usually enjoy

- Overwhelming hopelessness or guilt

- Restlessness, pacing, fidgeting, or the opposite—staying unusually still

- Sleep problems (either trouble falling asleep or staying asleep or constant drowsiness)

- Thoughts of death or suicide

- Trouble concentrating

In older people depression can be confused with many other conditions. It is not "normal" for older people to feel depressed. Older people do not always have the usual symptoms when they are depressed. Instead, they may have headaches, backaches, joint pain, or stomach problems—aches and pains that return again and again and are not helped by treatment.

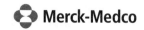

No one is sure what causes depression, but it probably involves changes in the chemical signals in the brain. Depression can be caused by other illnesses, such as cancer or stroke, certain medications, genetics, and painful life events, such as the loss of a loved one.

Fortunately, taking medication (antidepressants), talking with a trained therapist, or both can often help people with depression feel much better.

Medications for Depression

Several kinds of medications may be taken for depression. This chapter discusses these medications and/or categories of medications:

MEDICATIONS	See Page
Tricyclic Antidepressants	221
Selective Serotonin Reuptake Inhibitors (SSRIs)	227
Effexor® (venlafaxine)	232
Desyrel® (trazodone) and *Serzone*® (nefazodone)	236
Remeron® (mirtazapine)	240
Wellbutrin® (bupropion)	244
Ritalin® (methylphenidate)	247
Monoamine Oxidase (MAO) Inhibitors	250

If you do not see the exact name of the medication that you take for depression listed above, check the Medication and Chapter Table to find out which category your medication falls under or check the Index.

Tricyclic Antidepressants

▲ Indicates medications that are more likely to cause unpleasant or dangerous side effects. These medications are generally not recommended for people over 65. The side effects may not be very obvious and may be mistaken for "just a part of getting older" but may be serious. If you are taking one of these medications, you might want to talk to your doctor or other healthcare professional to see if this medication is best for you. Safer medications may be available and lower dosages may be required. You should not stop taking these medications without first talking to your doctor or other healthcare professional.

See the WARNING section on page 225 for the specific safety problems associated with these medications ▲.

Brand Name	Generic Name
▲*Anafranil*®	clomipramine
▲*Asendin*®	amoxapine
▲*Elavil*®	amitriptyline
Ludiomil®*	maprotiline*
Norpramin®	desipramine
Pamelor®	nortriptyline
▲*Sinequan*®	doxepin
▲*Surmontil*®	trimipramine
▲*Tofranil*®	imipramine
▲*Vivactil*®	protriptyline

*tetracyclic antidepressant (works in ways similar to tricyclic antidepressant).

Merck-Medco

How Will I Take Tricyclic Antidepressants?

Tricyclic antidepressants are pills that are usually taken 1 to 3 times a day. If taken only once a day, they are usually taken at bedtime to decrease the side effects during the day. If tricyclic antidepressants are prescribed for you, be patient; they may take 2 to 6 weeks to start working. Your doctor or other healthcare professional will tell you how often to take your medications.

To help prevent side effects, your doctor or other healthcare professional may start by giving you a low dose of this medication, increasing the amount slowly until it works well for you.

If you miss a dose of this medication, take the dose you missed as soon as possible. However, if it is almost time for your next dose, skip the missed dose and just take the next one. Do not double your dose. Take your medication exactly as directed by your doctor or other healthcare professional. Do not stop taking a prescription medication unless directed by your doctor or other healthcare professional.

What Side Effects Can Tricyclic Antidepressants Cause?

More Common

- Constipation

- Dizziness when standing up from a bed or a chair

- Drowsiness

- Dry mouth, eyes, and nose

- Trouble urinating or emptying the bladder

Less Common

- Confusion

- Fast or irregular heartbeat (palpitations)

- Loss of interest in sex (decreased libido)

- Rash (skin redness, bumps, itching, or irritation)
- Worsening of glaucoma (an eye disease)

Rare

- Breast enlargement and tenderness (in both men and women)
- Hair loss
- Seizures
- Shakiness or tremors

Tell your doctor or other healthcare professional if you have side effects that bother you, do not go away, make you worried about taking your medication, or make you want to stop taking your medication.

Do Other Medications Interact with Tricyclic Antidepressants?

These medications *may increase* the side effects of tricyclic antidepressants:

- Quinidine such as *Quinaglute*®, *Quinidex*®, and others—see Glossary
- *Ritalin*® (methylphenidate)
- *Rythmol*® (propafenone)
- *Tagamet*® (cimetidine)

Tricyclic antidepressants *may increase* the side effects of other medications that cause drowsiness, including anticholinergic medications, other antidepressants, antihistamines (allergy medications), antispasmodics, benzodiazepines (a type of tranquilizer), anxiety medications, narcotics (pain relievers), muscle relaxants, neuroleptic medications (a type of tranquilizer), seizure medications, or sleep medications. Avoid driving a car and other activities that need mental alertness, like using a knife or operating machinery, while taking these medications together.

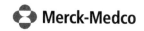

Drinking alcoholic beverages (such as beer, wine, whiskey, and others) *may increase* the side effects of tricyclic antidepressants.

These medications *may decrease* how well tricyclic antidepressants work:

- Barbiturates such as *Butisol®* (butabarbital), *Luminal®* (phenobarbital), *Mebaral®* (mephobarbital), and others—see Glossary

- *Rifadin®* (rifampin)

- *Tegretol®* (carbamazepine)

Taking a tricyclic antidepressant and *Catapres®* (clonidine) or *Ismelin®* (guanethidine) *may raise* a person's blood pressure to dangerously high levels.

Tricyclic antidepressants are generally not prescribed for anyone who is taking MAO inhibitors such as *Marplan®* (isocarboxazid), *Nardil®* (phenelzine), or *Parnate®* (tranylcypromine), because together they *may cause* serious or even fatal reactions. If your doctor or other healthcare professional wants you to stop taking one medication and start taking the other, you should wait at least 2 weeks between stopping one and starting the other.

Tricyclic antidepressants are generally not prescribed for anyone who is taking *Propulsid®* (cisapride [withdrawn from general distribution; available only by special arrangement with the manufacturer]), *Seldane®* (terfenadine [no longer commercially available]), or *Hismanal®* (astemizole [no longer commercially available]), because together they *may cause* serious, sometimes fatal, heart problems.

Grapefruit and grapefruit juice *may increase* the side effects of *Anafranil®* (clomipramine). This interaction can happen whether you eat the grapefruit or drink the grapefruit juice at the same time as you take your medication or if you take the medication separately from the grapefruit or grapefruit juice. Talk to your doctor or other healthcare professional before eating grapefruit or drinking grapefruit juice if you are taking this medication. Please also read the discussion on A Warning about Grapefruit and Grapefruit Juice on pages i-ii.

Tell your doctor or other healthcare professional about all medications (both prescription and nonprescription [over-the-counter] medications) that you are taking.

Why Else Do People Take Tricyclic Antidepressants?

Tricyclic antidepressants can help relieve long-term pain, abnormal fears (phobias), panic attacks, inability to hold urine in (urinary incontinence), obsessive-compulsive disorders, and eating disorders such as anorexia and bulimia. They are also used to help prevent migraine headaches.

 # Warning!

To give you the best care, your doctor or other healthcare professional needs to know about the diseases and medical conditions you have had—your full medical history. Tell your doctor or other healthcare professional if you have or have ever had, or presently take, any of the following:

- Allergy or previous reactions to tricyclic antidepressants, *Tegretol®* (carbamazepine), or *Trileptal®* (oxcarbazepine)

- Enlarged prostate (benign prostatic hypertrophy)

- Glaucoma (an eye disease)

- Liver problems

- Manic depression

- MAO inhibitors such as *Marplan®* (isocarboxazid), *Nardil®* (phenelzine), or *Parnate®* (tranylcypromine)

- Overactive thyroid (hyperthyroidism)

- Schizophrenia

- Seizures (epilepsy)

- Urinary retention

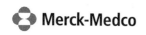

Anafranil® (clomipramine), *Asendin*® (amoxapine), *Elavil*® (amitriptyline), *Sinequan*® (doxepin), *Surmontil*® (trimipramine), *Tofranil*® (imipramine), and *Vivactil*® (protriptyline) are generally not recommended for use in people over the age of 65 because these types of tricyclic antidepressants have been associated with a higher risk of broken hips and car accidents than other tricyclic antidepressants. If you are taking any of these medications, ask your doctor or other healthcare professional if this medication is right for you. Do not stop taking this medication without talking to your doctor or other healthcare professional.

Tricyclic antidepressants may make you unsteady on your feet, causing you to fall and possibly break a bone. If you have fallen recently, tell your doctor or other healthcare professional about it. Taking a different medication or a lower dose may make you less likely to fall. You should not stop taking this medication without first talking to your doctor or other healthcare professional.

Tricyclic antidepressants may cause drowsiness. Avoid driving a car and other activities that need mental alertness, like using a knife or operating machinery, while taking this medication. Drinking alcoholic beverages (such as beer, wine, whiskey, and others) may increase the side effects.

If you have had seizures in the past, tell your doctor or other healthcare professional because tricyclic antidepressants may cause seizures. Stopping this medication suddenly may also cause seizures. If your doctor or other healthcare professional decides that you should stop taking your tricyclic antidepressant, pay careful attention to the instructions he or she gives you about how much less to take and for how long.

If you are taking tricyclic antidepressants, stay out of the sun as much as you can to avoid a serious sunburn. When you do go out in the sun, use sunblock or sunscreen and wear protective clothing, such as a wide-brimmed hat and a long-sleeved shirt.

Under certain circumstances, your doctor or other healthcare professional may decide that you should stop taking this medication. If you have taken it for more than a couple of weeks, he or she may want you to decrease it gradually, lowering the dose over a few weeks or months. Stopping suddenly may cause unpleasant withdrawal symptoms or may worsen your medical problems. Pay

careful attention to the instructions your doctor or other healthcare professional gives you about how much less to take and for how long.

Selective Serotonin Reuptake Inhibitors (SSRIs)

Brand Name	Generic Name
Celexa™	citalopram
Luvox®	fluvoxamine
Paxil®	paroxetine
Prozac®	fluoxetine
Zoloft®	sertraline

 ## How Will I Take SSRIs?

SSRIs are pills that are usually taken 1 to 2 times a day with or without meals. If taken once a day, they are usually taken in the morning. If they cause drowsiness, they can be taken at bedtime to decrease the side effects during the day. If SSRIs are prescribed for you, be patient; they may take 2 to 6 weeks to start working. Your doctor or other healthcare professional will tell you how often to take your medication.

To help prevent side effects, your doctor or other healthcare professional may start by giving you a low dose of this medication, increasing the amount slowly until it works well for you.

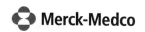
If you miss a dose of this medication, take the dose you missed as soon as possible. However, if it is almost time for your next dose, skip the missed dose and just take the next one. Do not double your dose. Take your medication exactly as directed by your doctor or other healthcare professional. Do not stop taking a prescription medication unless directed by your doctor or other healthcare professional.

What Side Effects Can SSRIs Cause?

More Common

- Diarrhea

- Dizziness when standing up from a bed or a chair

- Drowsiness

- Ejaculation problems (erectile dysfunction)

- Headache

- Nausea

- Nervousness (anxiety)

- Poor appetite

- Shakiness or tremors

- Trouble falling asleep or staying asleep (insomnia)

Less Common

- Constipation

- Rash (skin redness, bumps, itching, or irritation)

- Stomach pain

Rare

- Seizures

Tell your doctor or other healthcare professional if you have side effects that bother you, do not go away, make you worried about taking your medication, or make you want to stop taking your medication.

Do Other Medications Interact with SSRIs?

The medications listed below *may increase* the side effects of SSRIs:

- *Tagamet*® (cimetidine)
- Tricyclic antidepressants such as *Elavil*® (amitriptyline), *Pamelor*® (nortriptyline), *Sinequan*® (doxepin), and others—see Glossary

SSRIs *may increase* the side effects of these medications:

- *Cerebyx*® (fosphenytoin)
- *Coumadin*® (warfarin)
- *Dilantin*® (phenytoin)
- *Haldol*® (haloperidol)
- *Lanoxin*® (digoxin)
- Lithium such as *Eskalith*®, *Lithobid*®, and others—see Glossary
- *Neoral*® (cyclosporine)
- *Sandimmune*® (cyclosporine)
- Theophylline such as *Theo-Dur*®, *Uniphyl*®, and others—see Glossary

Taking SSRIs and *Ultram*® (tramadol) *may increase* your chance of seizures.

SSRIs *may decrease* how well *BuSpar*® (buspirone) works.

SSRIs are generally not prescribed for anyone who is taking MAO inhibitors, such as *Marplan*® (isocarboxazid), *Nardil*® (phenelzine), or *Parnate*® (tranylcypromine), because together they *may cause* serious or even fatal reactions. If your doctor or other healthcare professional wants you to stop taking one medication and start taking the other, you should wait at least 2

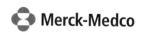

to 6 weeks between stopping one and starting the other, depending on which SSRI you are taking.

SSRIs are generally not prescribed for anyone who is taking triptans (migraine medications) such as *Imitrex*® (sumatriptan), *Zomig*® (zolmitriptan), and others (see Glossary) or *Meridia*® (sibutramine) and other appetite suppressants, because together they *may cause* serious or even fatal reactions. Taken together, they *may cause* nervousness (anxiety), muscle weakness, confusion, and seizures.

Luvox® (fluvoxamine) is generally not prescribed for anyone who is taking *Propulsid*® (cisapride [withdrawn from general distribution; available only by special arrangement with the manufacturer]), *Seldane*® (terfenadine [no longer commercially available]), or *Hismanal*® (astemizole [no longer commercially available]), because together they *may cause* serious, sometimes fatal, heart problems.

SSRIs *may increase* the side effects of other medications that cause drowsiness, including anticholinergic medications, other antidepressants, antihistamines (allergy medications), antispasmodics, benzodiazepines (a type of tranquilizer), anxiety medications, narcotics (pain relievers), muscle relaxants, neuroleptic medications (a type of tranquilizer), seizure medications, or sleep medications. Avoid driving a car and other activities that need mental alertness, like using a knife or operating machinery, while taking these medications together.

Drinking alcoholic beverages (such as beer, wine, whiskey, and others) *may increase* the side effects of SSRIs.

Tell your doctor or other healthcare professional about all medications (both prescription and nonprescription [over-the-counter] medications) that you are taking.

Why Else Do People Take SSRIs?

SSRIs can help relieve obsessive-compulsive disorder, bulimia (an eating disorder), panic disorder, and social phobia.

Warning!

To give you the best care, your doctor or other healthcare professional needs to know about the diseases and medical conditions you have had—your full medical history. Tell your doctor or other healthcare professional if you have or have ever had, or presently take, any of the following:

- Allergy or previous reaction to SSRIs

- Changes in appetite or weight

- Diabetes

- Liver problems

- Manic depression

- MAO inhibitors such as *Marplan*® (isocarboxazid), *Nardil*® (phenelzine), or *Parnate*® (tranylcypromine)

- Nervousness (anxiety)

- Seizures (epilepsy)

- Trouble falling asleep or staying asleep (insomnia)

Some SSRIs may cause drowsiness. Avoid driving a car and other activities that need mental alertness, like using a knife or operating machinery, while taking this medication. Drinking alcoholic beverages (such as beer, wine, whiskey, and others) may increase the side effects.

Some SSRIs may make you unsteady on your feet, causing you to fall and possibly break a bone. If you have fallen recently, tell your doctor or other healthcare professional about it. Taking a different medication or a lower dose may make you less likely to fall. You should not stop taking this medication without first talking to your doctor or other healthcare professional.

Under certain circumstances, your doctor or other healthcare professional may decide that you should stop taking this medication. If you have taken it for more than a couple of weeks, he or she may want you to decrease it gradually, lowering the dose over a few weeks or months. Stopping suddenly may cause unpleasant withdrawal symptoms or may worsen your medical problems. Pay careful attention to the instructions your doctor or other healthcare professional gives you about how much less to take and for how long.

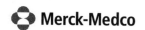
Effexor® (venlafaxine)

 ## How Will I Take *Effexor*® (venlafaxine)?

Effexor® (venlafaxine) is a pill that is usually taken 1 to 3 times a day with food. Be patient; like other antidepressants, it may take 2 to 6 weeks to start working.

To help prevent side effects, your doctor or other healthcare professional may start by giving you a low dose of this medication, increasing the amount slowly until it works well for you.

When a medication has initials after its name, such as XL, XR, SR, BID, DUR, and others, it usually means that the body absorbs the medication slowly over time, so you usually have to take it only once or twice a day. The body will absorb some medications of this type too fast if you crush or break them or dissolve them in liquid, and their effects will not last as long as they should. Check with your doctor or other healthcare professional before crushing or breaking your pills or dissolving your pills in liquid.

If you miss a dose of this medication, take the dose you missed as soon as possible. However, if it is almost time for your next dose, skip the missed dose and just take the next one. Do not double your dose. Take your medication exactly as directed by your doctor or other healthcare professional. Do not stop taking a prescription medication unless directed by your doctor or other healthcare professional.

 ## What Side Effects Can *Effexor*® (venlafaxine) Cause?

More Common

- Blurred vision

- Constipation

- Dizziness when standing up from a bed or a chair

- Drowsiness

- Dry mouth

- Ejaculation problems (erectile dysfunction)

- Headache

- Increased sweating

- Nausea

- Nervousness (anxiety)

- Trouble falling asleep or staying asleep (insomnia)

Less Common

- Fast heartbeat (palpitations)

- High blood pressure (hypertension)

- Rash (skin redness, bumps, itching, or irritation)

- Ringing in the ears (tinnitus)

- Seizures

- Trouble urinating or emptying the bladder

Tell your doctor or other healthcare professional if you have side effects that bother you, do not go away, make you worried about taking your medication, or make you want to stop taking your medication.

Do Other Medications Interact with *Effexor*® (venlafaxine)?

Effexor® (venlafaxine) is generally not prescribed for anyone who is taking MAO inhibitors, such as *Marplan*® (isocarboxazid), *Nardil*® (phenelzine), or *Parnate*® (tranylcypromine), because together they **may cause** serious or even fatal reactions. If your doctor or other healthcare professional wants you to stop taking one medication and start taking the other, you should wait at least 2 weeks between stopping one and starting the other.

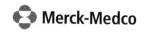

Effexor® (venlafaxine) is generally not prescribed for anyone who is taking triptans (migraine medications), such as *Imitrex®* (sumatriptan), *Zomig®* (zolmitriptan), and others (see Glossary), or *Meridia®* (sibutramine) and other appetite suppressants because together they ***may cause*** serious or even fatal reactions. Taken together, they ***may cause*** nervousness (anxiety), muscle weakness, confusion, and seizures.

Effexor® (venlafaxine) ***may increase*** the side effects of other medications that cause drowsiness, including anticholinergic medications, other antidepressants, antihistamines (allergy medications), antispasmodics, benzodiazepines (a type of tranquilizer), anxiety medications, narcotics (pain relievers), muscle relaxants, neuroleptic medications (a type of tranquilizer), seizure medications, or sleep medications. Avoid driving a car and other activities that need mental alertness, like using a knife or operating machinery, while taking these medications together.

Drinking alcoholic beverages (such as beer, wine, whiskey, and others) ***may increase*** the side effects.

Tell your doctor or other healthcare professional about all medications (both prescription and nonprescription [over-the-counter] medications) that you are taking.

 # Warning!

To give you the best care, your doctor or other healthcare professional needs to know about the diseases and medical conditions you have had—your full medical history. Tell your doctor or other healthcare professional if you have or have ever had, or presently take, any of the following:

- Allergy or previous reaction to *Effexor®* (venlafaxine)
- Changes in appetite or weight
- Heart problems
- High blood pressure (hypertension)

- Kidney problems

- Liver problems

- Manic depression

- MAO inhibitors such as *Marplan®* (isocarboxazid), *Nardil®* (phenelzine), or *Parnate®* (tranylcypromine)

- Nervousness (anxiety)

- Seizures (epilepsy)

- Trouble falling asleep or staying asleep (insomnia)

Effexor® (venlafaxine) may cause drowsiness. Avoid driving a car and other activities that need mental alertness, like using a knife or operating machinery, while taking this medication. Drinking alcoholic beverages (such as beer, wine, whiskey, and others) may increase the side effects.

Effexor® (venlafaxine) may make you unsteady on your feet, causing you to fall and possibly break a bone. If you have fallen recently, tell your doctor or other healthcare professional about it. Taking a different medication or a lower dose may make you less likely to fall. You should not stop taking this medication without first talking to your doctor or other healthcare professional.

Effexor® (venlafaxine) may raise blood pressure. People with high blood pressure (hypertension) taking *Effexor®* (venlafaxine) should have their blood pressure checked regularly.

Under certain circumstances, your doctor or other healthcare professional may decide that you should stop taking this medication. If you have taken it for more than a couple of weeks, he or she may want you to decrease it gradually, lowering the dose over a few weeks or months. Stopping suddenly may cause unpleasant withdrawal symptoms or may worsen your medical problems. Pay careful attention to the instructions your doctor or other healthcare professional gives you about how much less to take and for how long.

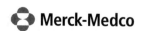
Desyrel® (trazodone) and *Serzone*® (nefazodone)

How Will I Take *Desyrel*® (trazodone) or *Serzone*® (nefazodone)?

Desyrel® (trazodone) is a pill that is usually taken 1 to 4 times a day with food. *Serzone*® (nefazodone) is a pill that is usually taken 2 times a day with or without food. Be patient; like other medications for depression, *Desyrel*® (trazodone) and *Serzone*® (nefazodone) may take 2 to 6 weeks to start working.

To help prevent side effects, your doctor or other healthcare professional may start by giving you a low dose of this medication, increasing the amount slowly until it works well for you.

If you miss a dose of this medication, take the dose you missed as soon as possible. However, if it is almost time for your next dose, skip the missed dose and just take the next one. Do not double your dose. Take your medication exactly as directed by your doctor or other healthcare professional. Do not stop taking a prescription medication unless directed by your doctor or other healthcare professional.

What Side Effects Can *Desyrel*® (trazodone) and *Serzone*® (nefazodone) Cause?

More Common

- Drowsiness

- Dry mouth

- Headache

- Nausea

- Nervousness (anxiety)

Less Common

- Constipation

- Dizziness when standing up from a bed or a chair

- Trouble falling asleep or staying asleep (insomnia) with *Serzone®* (nefazodone)

- Trouble urinating or emptying the bladder

Rare

- Lasting, painful erection (priapism)

- Seizures

Tell your doctor or other healthcare professional if you have side effects that bother you, do not go away, make you worried about taking your medication, or make you want to stop taking your medication.

Do Other Medications Interact with *Desyrel®* (trazodone) or *Serzone®* (nefazodone)?

Serzone® (nefazodone) ***may increase*** the side effects of these medications:

- *Baycol®* (cerivastatin)

- *Halcion®* (triazolam)

- *Lanoxin®* (digoxin)

- *Lipitor®* (atorvastatin)

- *Mevacor®* (lovastatin)

- *Neoral®* (cyclosporine)

- *Sandimmune®* (cyclosporine)

- *Xanax®* (alprazolam)

- *Zocor®* (simvastatin)

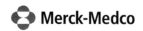

Desyrel® (trazodone) and *Serzone®* (nefazodone) are generally not prescribed for anyone who is taking MAO inhibitors, such as *Marplan®* (isocarboxazid), *Nardil®* (phenelzine), or *Parnate®* (tranylcypromine), because together they **may cause** serious or even fatal reactions. If your doctor or other healthcare professional wants you to stop taking one medication and start taking the other, you should wait at least 2 weeks between stopping one and starting the other.

Desyrel® (trazodone) and *Serzone®* (nefazodone) are generally not prescribed for anyone who is taking triptans (migraine medications) such as *Imitrex®* (sumatriptan), *Zomig®* (zolmitriptan), and others (see Glossary), or *Meridia®* (sibutramine) and other appetite suppressants, because together they **may cause** serious or even fatal reactions. Taken together, they **may cause** nervousness (anxiety), muscle weakness, confusion, and seizures.

Serzone® (nefazodone) is generally not prescribed for anyone who is taking *Propulsid®* (cisapride [withdrawn from general distribution; available only by special arrangement with the manufacturer]), *Seldane®* (terfenadine [no longer commercially available]), or *Hismanal®* (astemizole [no longer commercially available]), because together they **may cause** serious, sometimes fatal, heart problems.

Desyrel® (trazodone) and *Serzone®* (nefazodone) **may increase** the side effects of other medications that cause drowsiness, including anticholinergic medications, other antidepressants, antihistamines (allergy medications), antispasmodics, benzodiazepines (a type of tranquilizer), anxiety medications, narcotics (pain relievers), muscle relaxants, neuroleptic medications (a type of tranquilizer), seizure medications, or sleep medications. Avoid driving a car and other activities that need mental alertness, like using a knife or operating machinery, while taking these medications together.

Drinking alcoholic beverages (such as beer, wine, whiskey, and others) **may increase** the side effects of *Desyrel®* (trazodone) and *Serzone®* (nefazodone).

Tell your doctor or other healthcare professional about all medications (both prescription and nonprescription [over-the-counter] medications) that you are taking.

Warning!

To give you the best care, your doctor or other healthcare professional needs to know about the diseases and medical conditions you have had—your full medical history. Tell your doctor or other healthcare professional if you have or have ever had, or presently take, any of the following:

- Allergy or previous reaction to *Desyrel*® (trazodone) or *Serzone*® (nefazodone)

- Heart problems

- Liver problems

- Manic depression

- MAO inhibitors such as *Marplan*® (isocarboxazid), *Nardil*® (phenelzine), or *Parnate*® (tranylcypromine)

- Seizures (epilepsy)

Desyrel® (trazodone) and *Serzone*® (nefazodone) may make you unsteady on your feet, causing you to fall and possibly break a bone. If you have fallen recently, tell your doctor or other healthcare professional about it. Taking a different medication or a lower dose may make you less likely to fall. You should not stop taking this medication without first talking to your doctor or other healthcare professional.

Desyrel® (trazodone) and *Serzone*® (nefazodone) may cause drowsiness. Avoid driving a car and other activities that need mental alertness, like using a knife or operating machinery, while taking this medication. Drinking alcoholic beverages (such as beer, wine, whiskey, and others) may increase the side effects.

Note for men: Desyrel® (trazodone) or *Serzone*® (nefazodone) can cause a lasting, painful erection (priapism) which can be very serious if not treated. Call your doctor or other healthcare professional immediately if you develop an erection that hurts and will not go away.

Under certain circumstances, your doctor or other healthcare professional may decide that you should stop taking this medication. If you have taken it for more than a couple of weeks, he or she may want you to decrease it gradually, lowering the dose over a few weeks or months. Stopping suddenly may cause

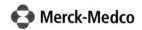

unpleasant withdrawal symptoms or may worsen your medical problems. Pay careful attention to the instructions your doctor or other healthcare professional gives you about how much less to take and for how long.

Remeron® (mirtazapine)

Remeron® (mirtazapine) is used to help relieve the symptoms of depression.

How Will I Take *Remeron*® (mirtazapine)?

Remeron® (mirtazapine) is a pill that is usually taken once a day at bedtime. It may be taken with or without food. Be patient; like other antidepressants, it may take 2 to 6 weeks to start working.

To help prevent side effects, your doctor or other healthcare professional may start by giving you a low dose of this medication, increasing the amount slowly until it works well for you.

If you miss a dose of this medication, take the dose you missed as soon as possible. However, if it is almost time for your next dose, skip the missed dose and just take the next one. Do not double your dose. Take your medication exactly as directed by your doctor or other healthcare professional. Do not stop taking a prescription medication unless directed by your doctor or other healthcare professional.

What Side Effects Can *Remeron*® (mirtazapine) Cause?

More Common

- Constipation
- Dizziness
- Drowsiness

- Dry mouth
- High cholesterol in your blood (hypercholesterolemia)

Less Common

- Abnormal dreams
- Back pain
- Confusion
- Fast heartbeat (palpitations)
- Frequent fever, sore throat, or flu-like symptoms that may be a sign of low white blood cells
- Frequent urination
- Headache
- Low blood pressure (hypotension)
- Muscle aches and pains
- Passing out or fainting
- Rash (skin redness, bumps, itching, or irritation)
- Shakiness or tremors

Rare

- Blurred vision
- Cardiac chest pain (angina)
- Seizures
- Trouble breathing or shortness of breath

Tell your doctor or other healthcare professional if you have side effects that bother you, do not go away, make you worried about taking your medication, or make you want to stop taking your medication.

241

Merck-Medco

Depression

Do Other Medications Interact with *Remeron®* (mirtazapine)?

Remeron® (mirtazapine) is generally not prescribed for anyone who is taking MAO inhibitors such as *Marplan®* (isocarboxazid), *Nardil®* (phenelzine), or *Parnate®* (tranylcypromine), because together they **may cause** serious or even fatal reactions. If your doctor or other healthcare professional wants you to stop taking one medication and start taking the other, you should wait at least 2 weeks between stopping one and starting the other.

Remeron® (mirtazapine) **may increase** the side effects of other medications that cause drowsiness, including anticholinergic medications, other antidepressants, antihistamines (allergy medications), antispasmodics, benzodiazepines (a type of tranquilizer), anxiety medications, narcotics (pain relievers), muscle relaxants, neuroleptic medications (a type of tranquilizer), seizure medications, or sleep medications. Avoid driving a car and other activities that need mental alertness, like using a knife or operating machinery, while taking these medications together.

Drinking alcoholic beverages (such as beer, wine, whiskey, and others) **may increase** the side effects.

Tell your doctor or other healthcare professional about all medications (both prescription and nonprescription [over-the-counter] medications) that you are taking.

 # Warning!

To give you the best care, your doctor or other healthcare professional needs to know about the diseases and medical conditions you have had—your full medical history. Tell your doctor or other healthcare professional if you have or have ever had, or presently take, any of the following:

- Allergy or previous reaction to *Remeron®* (mirtazapine)
- Heart problems

- High cholesterol (hypercholesterolemia)

- Kidney problems

- Liver problems

- Low blood pressure (hypotension)

- Manic depression

- MAO inhibitors such as *Marplan®* (isocarboxazid), *Nardil®* (phenelzine), or *Parnate®* (tranylcypromine)

- Seizures (epilepsy)

Remeron® (mirtazapine) may cause drowsiness. Avoid driving a car and other activities that need mental alertness, like using a knife or operating machinery, while taking this medication. Drinking alcoholic beverages (such as beer, wine, whiskey, and others) may increase the side effects.

Remeron® (mirtazapine) may make you unsteady on your feet, causing you to fall and possibly break a bone. If you have fallen recently, tell your doctor or other healthcare professional about it. Taking a different medication or a lower dose may make you less likely to fall. You should not stop taking this medication without first talking to your doctor or other healthcare professional.

Contact your doctor or other healthcare professional if you have frequent fevers, chills, sore throat, mouth sores, or flu-like symptoms. These may be signs of a serious blood problem that needs to be evaluated by your doctor or other healthcare professional.

Under certain circumstances, your doctor or other healthcare professional may decide that you should stop taking this medication. If you have taken it for more than a couple of weeks, he or she may want you to decrease it gradually, lowering the dose over a few weeks or months. Stopping suddenly may cause unpleasant withdrawal symptoms or may worsen your medical problems. Pay careful attention to the instructions your doctor or other healthcare professional gives you about how much less to take and for how long.

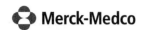

Wellbutrin® (bupropion)

 ## How Will I Take *Wellbutrin*® (bupropion)?

Wellbutrin® (bupropion) is a pill that is usually taken 1 to 4 times a day. It can be taken with or without food. Be patient; like other medications for depression, *Wellbutrin*® (bupropion) may take 2 to 6 weeks to start working.

To help prevent side effects, your doctor or other healthcare professional may start by giving you a low dose of this medication, increasing the amount slowly until it works well for you.

When a medication has initials after its name, such as XL, XR, SR, BID, DUR, and others, it usually means that the body absorbs the medication slowly over time, so you usually have to take it only once or twice a day. The body will absorb some medications of this type too fast if you crush or break them or dissolve them in liquid, and their effects will not last as long as they should. Check with your doctor or other healthcare professional before crushing or breaking your pills or dissolving your pills in liquid.

If you miss a dose of this medication, take the dose you missed as soon as possible. However, if it is almost time for your next dose, skip the missed dose and just take the next one. Do not double your dose. Take your medication exactly as directed by your doctor or other healthcare professional. Do not stop taking a prescription medication unless directed by your doctor or other healthcare professional.

 ## What Side Effects Can *Wellbutrin*® (bupropion) Cause?

More Common

- Constipation
- Dizziness when standing up from a bed or a chair

- Dry mouth

- Headache

- Increased sweating

- Nausea

- Nervousness (anxiety)

- Poor appetite

- Shakiness or tremors

Less Common

- Blurred vision

- Drowsiness

- Fast or irregular heartbeat (palpitations)

- Seizures

- Trouble falling asleep or staying asleep (insomnia)

Tell your doctor or other healthcare professional if you have side effects that bother you, do not go away, make you worried about taking your medication, or make you want to stop taking your medication.

Do Other Medications Interact with *Wellbutrin*® (bupropion)?

These medications ***may increase*** the side effects of *Wellbutrin*® (bupropion):

- *Norvir*® (ritonavir)

- *Tagamet*® (cimetidine)

Tegretol® (carbamazepine) ***may decrease*** how well *Wellbutrin*® (bupropion) works.

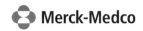
Wellbutrin® (bupropion) is generally not prescribed for anyone who is taking MAO inhibitors, such as *Marplan®* (isocarboxazid), *Nardil®* (phenelzine), or *Parnate®* (tranylcypromine), because together they ***may cause*** serious or even fatal reactions. If your doctor or other healthcare professional wants you to stop taking one medication and start taking the other, you should wait at least 2 weeks between stopping one and starting the other.

Tell your doctor or other healthcare professional about all medications (both prescription and nonprescription [over-the-counter] medications) that you are taking.

 # Warning!

To give you the best care, your doctor or other healthcare professional needs to know about the diseases and medical conditions you have had—your full medical history. Tell your doctor or other healthcare professional if you have or have ever had, or presently take, any of the following:

- Allergy or previous reaction to *Wellbutrin®* or *Zyban®* (bupropion)
- Bulimia or anorexia nervosa (eating disorders)
- Heart problems
- Liver problems
- Manic depression
- MAO inhibitors such as *Marplan®* (isocarboxazid), *Nardil®* (phenelzine), or *Parnate®* (tranylcypromine)
- Seizures (epilepsy)

Wellbutrin® (bupropion) may make you unsteady on your feet, causing you to fall and possibly break a bone. If you have fallen recently, tell your doctor or other healthcare professional about it. Taking a different medication or a lower dose may make you less likely to fall. You should not stop taking this medication without first talking to your doctor or other healthcare professional.

Wellbutrin® (bupropion) contains the same medication as *Zyban*® (bupropion). Do not take both medications unless directed by your doctor or other healthcare professional.

If you have had seizures in the past, tell your doctor or other healthcare professional because *Wellbutrin*® (bupropion) may cause seizures. Stopping this medication suddenly may also cause seizures. If your doctor or other healthcare professional decides that you should stop taking *Wellbutrin*® (bupropion), pay careful attention to the instructions he or she gives you about how much less to take and for how long.

Under certain circumstances, your doctor or other healthcare professional may decide that you should stop taking this medication. If you have taken it for more than a couple of weeks, he or she may want you to decrease it gradually, lowering the dose over a few weeks or months. Stopping suddenly may cause unpleasant withdrawal symptoms or may worsen your medical problems. Pay careful attention to the instructions your doctor or other healthcare professional gives you about how much less to take and for how long.

Ritalin® (methylphenidate)

Ritalin® (methylphenidate) is sometimes used to help relieve symptoms of depression.

How Will I Take *Ritalin*® (methylphenidate)?

Ritalin® (methylphenidate) is a pill that is usually taken 1 to 2 times a day. It is usually taken 30 to 45 minutes before breakfast and lunch because it can keep you from being able to fall asleep if taken later in the day or at bedtime. Unlike other medications used to treat depression, *Ritalin*® (methylphenidate) can help improve symptoms within 1 to 2 days.

When a medication has initials after its name, such as XL, XR, SR, BID, DUR, and others, it usually means that the body absorbs the medication slowly over time, so you usually have to take it only once or twice a day. The body will

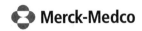

absorb some medications of this type too fast if you crush or break them or dissolve them in liquid, and their effects will not last as long as they should. Check with your doctor or other healthcare professional before crushing or breaking your pills or dissolving your pills in liquid.

If you miss a dose of this medication, take the dose you missed as soon as possible. However, if it is almost time for your next dose, skip the missed dose and just take the next one. Do not double your dose. Take your medication exactly as directed by your doctor or other healthcare professional. Do not stop taking a prescription medication unless directed by your doctor or other healthcare professional.

 ## What Side Effects Can *Ritalin*® (methylphenidate) Cause?

More Common

- Fast heartbeat (palpitations)
- High blood pressure (hypertension)
- Nervousness (anxiety)
- Poor appetite
- Trouble falling asleep or staying asleep (insomnia)

Less Common

- Cardiac chest pain (angina)

Tell your doctor or other healthcare professional if you have side effects that bother you, do not go away, make you worried about taking your medication, or make you want to stop taking your medication.

Do Other Medications Interact with *Ritalin®* (methylphenidate)?

Ritalin® (methylphenidate) ***may decrease*** how well *Ismelin®* (guanethidine) works.

Ritalin® (methylphenidate) ***may increase*** the side effects of these medications:

- *Cerebyx®* (fosphenytoin)
- *Coumadin®* (warfarin)
- *Dilantin®* (phenytoin)
- Tricyclic antidepressants such as *Elavil®* (amitriptyline), *Pamelor®* (nortriptyline), *Sinequan®* (doxepin), and others—see Glossary

Ritalin® (methylphenidate) is generally not prescribed for anyone who is taking MAO inhibitors, such as *Marplan®* (isocarboxazid), *Nardil®* (phenelzine), or *Parnate®* (tranylcypromine), because together they ***may cause*** serious or even fatal reactions. If your doctor or other healthcare professional wants you to stop taking one medication and start taking the other, you should wait at least 2 weeks between stopping one and starting the other.

Tell your doctor or other healthcare professional about all medications (both prescription and nonprescription [over-the-counter] medications) that you are taking.

Warning!

To give you the best care, your doctor or other healthcare professional needs to know about the diseases and medical conditions you have had—your full medical history. Tell your doctor or other healthcare professional if you have or have ever had, or presently take, any of the following:

- Allergy or previous reaction to *Ritalin®* (methylphenidate)
- Glaucoma (an eye disease)

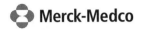
- Heart problems

- High blood pressure (hypertension)

- MAO inhibitors such as *Marplan*® (isocarboxazid), *Nardil*® (phenelzine), or *Parnate*® (tranylcypromine)

- Nervousness (anxiety)

- Seizures (epilepsy)

When *Ritalin*® (methylphenidate) is prescribed for someone who is depressed, it is usually prescribed for only a short time until other antidepressants begin to work. If you have been taking *Ritalin*® (methylphenidate) for more than 1 month, ask your doctor or other healthcare professional whether you still need it. Do not stop taking this medication unless directed by your doctor or other healthcare professional.

Under certain circumstances, your doctor or other healthcare professional may decide that you should stop taking this medication. If you have taken it for more than a couple of weeks, he or she may want you to decrease it gradually, lowering the dose over a few weeks or months. Stopping suddenly may cause unpleasant withdrawal symptoms or may worsen your medical problems. Pay careful attention to the instructions your doctor or other healthcare professional gives you about how much less to take and for how long.

Monoamine Oxidase (MAO) Inhibitors

Brand Name	Generic Name
Marplan®	isocarboxazid
Nardil®	phenelzine
Parnate®	tranylcypromine

How Will I Take MAO Inhibitors?

MAO inhibitors are pills that are usually taken 2 to 3 times a day. While you are taking MAO inhibitors, you must not eat certain foods (see Food Table on pages 255–256). Be patient; like other antidepressants, MAO inhibitors may take 2 to 6 weeks to start working.

To help prevent side effects, your doctor or other healthcare professional may start by giving you a low dose of this medication, increasing the amount slowly until it works well for you.

If you miss a dose of this medication, take the dose you missed as soon as possible. However, if it is almost time for your next dose, skip the missed dose and just take the next one. Do not double your dose. Take your medication exactly as directed by your doctor or other healthcare professional. Do not stop taking a prescription medication unless directed by your doctor or other healthcare professional.

What Side Effects Can MAO Inhibitors Cause?

More Common

- Dizziness when standing up from a bed or a chair
- Drowsiness
- Fast heartbeat (palpitations)

Less Common

- Blurred vision
- Constipation
- Dry mouth
- Weight gain

Rare

- Ejaculation problems (erectile dysfunction)

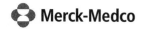
- Frequent fever, sore throat, or flu-like symptoms that may be a sign of low white blood cells

- High blood pressure (hypertension)

- Rash (skin redness, bumps, itching, or irritation)

- Shakiness or tremors

- Swelling or puffiness of the feet, ankles, or lower legs (edema)

- Trouble falling asleep or staying asleep (insomnia)

Tell your doctor or other healthcare professional if you have side effects that bother you, do not go away, make you worried about taking your medication, or make you want to stop taking your medication.

Do Other Medications Interact with MAO Inhibitors?

While you are taking MAO inhibitors, do not take these medications without talking to your doctor or other healthcare professional as the combination *may cause* extremely high blood pressure and even death:

- *Aldomet*® (methyldopa)

- *Alphagan*® (brimonidine)

- Beta-adrenergic bronchodilators such as *Proventil*® (albuterol), *Serevent*® (salmeterol), and others—see Glossary

- *BuSpar*® (buspirone)

- *Celexa*™ (citalopram)

- *Combivent*® (albuterol/ipratropium)

- *Comtan*® (entacapone)

- Decongestants that are frequently found in medications for coughs, colds, allergies, or asthma

- *Demerol*® (meperidine)

- *Desyrel*® (trazodone)

- Dextromethorphan, a cough suppressant that is frequently found in medications for coughs and colds
- *Effexor*® (venlafaxine)
- Epinephrine eyedrops
- *Ismelin*® (guanethidine)
- *Iopidine*® (apraclonidine)
- *Luvox*® (fluvoxamine)
- *Meridia*® (sibutramine) and other appetite suppressants—see Glossary
- Narcotics such as codeine, morphine, *Roxicet*™ (oxycodone), *Vicodin*® (hydromorphone), and others—see Glossary
- *Paxil*® (paroxetine)
- *Propine*® (dipivefrin)
- *Prozac*® (fluoxetine)
- *Reglan*® (metoclopramide)
- *Remeron*® (mirtazapine)
- *Ritalin*® (methylphenidate)
- *Serzone*® (nefazodone)
- *Sinemet*® (carbidopa/levodopa)
- *Tasmar*® (tolcapone)
- *Tegretol*® (carbamazepine)
- Tricyclic antidepressants such as *Elavil*® (amitriptyline), *Pamelor*® (nortriptyline), *Sinequan*® (doxepin), and others—see Glossary
- *Trileptal*® (oxcarbazepine)
- *Ultram*® (tramadol)
- *Wellbutrin*® (bupropion)
- *Zoloft*® (sertraline)
- *Zyban*® (bupropion)

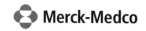

MAO inhibitors are generally not prescribed for anyone who is taking any other antidepressant because together they *may cause* serious or even fatal reactions. If your doctor or other healthcare professional wants you to stop taking one medication and start taking the other, you should wait at least 2 to 6 weeks between stopping one and starting the other, depending on which antidepressant medication you are taking.

MAO inhibitors *may increase* the side effects of these medications:

- Diabetes medications such as *DiaBeta®* (glyburide), *Glucophage®* (metformin), *Glucotrol®* (glipizide), and others—see Glossary

- Insulin

- Triptans (migraine medications) such as *Imitrex®* (sumatriptan), *Zomig®* (zolmitriptan), and others—see Glossary

Do not eat foods that contain tyramine or dopamine (natural substances that help support blood pressure) or tryptophan (a natural substance that aids in metabolism) while you are taking an MAO inhibitor. See Food Table on pages 255–256. Talk to your doctor or other healthcare professional if you have questions about diet.

Avoid drinking alcoholic beverages (such as beer, wine, whiskey, and others) or consuming caffeine (coffee, tea, colas, chocolate, and others) while you are taking an MAO inhibitor.

Do not take cold, hay fever, or weight-reduction medications while taking an MAO inhibitor. Talk to your doctor or other healthcare professional before taking any new prescription or over-the-counter medications.

Foods to Avoid when Taking MAO Inhibitors

Tyramine-Containing Foods		
Cheese and Dairy Products		
American Blue	Emmenthaler	Roquefort
Boursault	Gruyere	Sour cream
Brie	Mozzarella	Stilton
Camembert	Parmesan	Swiss
Cheddar	Romano	Yogurt
Meat / Fish		
Anchovies	Fermented sausages (such as bologna, pepperoni, salami, summer sausage, and others)	Meat extracts
Beef or chicken liver, other meats, fish (unrefrigerated, fermented, spoiled, smoked, pickled)		Meat prepared with tenderizer (such as Adolph's®)
	Dried fish (such as salted herring)	Herring (such as pickled, spoiled)
Caviar	Dried sausage	Shrimp paste
	Game meat	

Food list continued on next page.

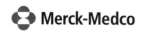

Foods to Avoid when Taking MAO Inhibitors (cont'd)

Alcoholic Beverages		
Beer	Red wine (especially Chianti)	Liquor
Fruits / Vegetables		
Bananas Bean curd Dried fruits (such as raisins, prunes, and others)	Avocados (especially overripe) Figs, canned (overripe) Miso soup Raspberries	Sauerkraut Soy sauce Yeast extracts (such as Marmite®)
Other Food and Beverages		
Broad beans (fava beans, overripe)	Caffeine (such as coffee, tea, colas, chocolate, and others) Nonalcoholic beer	Ginseng

Tell your doctor or other healthcare professional about all medications (both prescription and nonprescription [over-the-counter] medications) that you are taking.

What Else Should I Know about MAO Inhibitors?

Eat and drink exactly what your doctor or other healthcare professional has told you for the whole time that you are taking the MAO inhibitor and for 3 weeks after you stop taking it.

Talk with your doctor or other healthcare professional before starting to take any new prescription or nonprescription (over-the-counter) medications and before eating any foods that you haven't eaten before if they are not on your recommended diet.

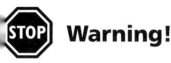 # Warning!

To give you the best care, your doctor or other healthcare professional needs to know about the diseases and medical conditions you have had—your full medical history. Tell your doctor or other healthcare professional if you have or have ever had, or presently take or do, any of the following:

- Allergy or previous reaction to MAO inhibitors
- Any prescription or nonprescription medications
- Diabetes
- Eat food or drink beverages containing caffeine (such as coffee, tea, colas, chocolate, and others)
- Heart problems
- High alcohol intake (drinking 3 or more alcoholic beverages, such as beer, wine, whiskey, and others, every day)
- Liver problems
- Seizures (epilepsy)

Taking MAO inhibitors at the same time as many other medications or when eating certain foods can be dangerous and even life-threatening. For example, eating certain foods while taking MAO inhibitors can cause blood pressure to suddenly rise to a very high level. If an MAO inhibitor is prescribed for you, ask your doctor or other healthcare professional for a complete list of foods and medications that you should not eat or take while taking your MAO inhibitor (see Food Table on pages 255–256).

Avoid drinking alcoholic beverages (such as beer, wine, whiskey, and others) or consuming caffeine (such as coffee, tea, colas, chocolate, and others), because they contain tyramines, which can be dangerous and even life-threatening when taking MAO inhibitors.

MAO inhibitors may make you unsteady on your feet, causing you to fall and possibly break a bone. If you have fallen recently, tell your doctor or other healthcare professional about it. Taking a different medication or a lower dose may make you less likely to fall. You should not stop taking this medication without first talking to your doctor or other healthcare professional.

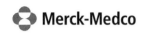

MAO inhibitors may cause drowsiness. Avoid driving a car and other activities that need mental alertness, like using a knife or operating machinery, while taking this medication.   Drinking alcoholic beverages (such as beer, wine, whiskey, and others) may increase the side effects.

See a doctor or other healthcare professional immediately if you get a severe or prolonged headache, feel that your heart is beating too slowly or too quickly, feel nauseated, start to vomit, or sweat more than usual for the weather and situation.

Tell your doctor or other healthcare professional if you are going to have surgery.

Under certain circumstances, your doctor or other healthcare professional may decide that you should stop taking this medication. If you have taken it for more than a couple of weeks, he or she may want you to decrease it gradually, lowering the dose over a few weeks or months. Stopping suddenly may cause unpleasant withdrawal symptoms or may worsen your medical problems. Pay careful attention to the instructions your doctor or other healthcare professional gives you about how much less to take and for how long.

Chapter 9

Diabetes

What Is Diabetes?

The body uses glucose (sugar) as fuel to create energy. Insulin, a hormone made by the pancreas (a gland near the stomach), controls blood sugar. It helps to move glucose out of the blood into the cells where it is stored or used for energy. People with diabetes have high blood sugar levels, a condition called hyperglycemia.

There are two common types of diabetes. When the pancreas does not make enough insulin it is called type 1 diabetes. When the pancreas makes insulin, but the body is resistant to the insulin that the pancreas makes, it is called type 2 diabetes. Both types of diabetes cause high blood sugar and can cause short-term and long-term problems that may be serious, even fatal. Untreated or poorly controlled diabetes may cause blindness, kidney failure, heart disease, stroke, nerve damage, foot amputations, and sexual problems.

Symptoms of Diabetes and High Blood Sugar (Glucose)

- Blurred vision
- Extreme hunger
- Frequent urination
- Frequent vaginal yeast infections
- Increased or excessive thirst
- Tiredness or sluggishness (fatigue)
- Unexplained weight loss
- Wounds or injuries that take a long time to heal

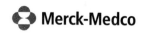

While some people with diabetes do not have any symptoms or have only very mild symptoms, others may have very severe symptoms and may even go into a coma. It is dangerous to ignore these symptoms or think they are normal signs of aging. If you have any of the symptoms listed above, tell your doctor or other healthcare professional.

Controlling Diabetes and High Blood Sugar (Glucose)

Keeping blood sugar (glucose) levels near normal may help prevent the problems caused by diabetes. Some people can control their blood sugar and diabetes with a healthy diet and exercise. Others will need medication or insulin to help control their blood sugar.

If you have diabetes, talk to your doctor or other healthcare professional before starting a new exercise plan or making any changes in what you eat. A change in your diet or exercise routine may affect your blood sugar and how much medication is needed to control it. Do not skip a meal or any dose of your medication unless directed by your doctor or other healthcare professional.

Checking blood sugar at home with a simple device called a glucose meter is a good way to know how well your blood sugar is controlled throughout the day. It also shows the effects of any changes in what you eat, the exercise you are getting, or the diabetes medications you are taking. Checking your blood sugar helps you and your doctor or other healthcare professional decide whether your treatment needs to be changed in any way.

If you have a home blood glucose meter, follow the instructions for use. Your doctor or other healthcare professional will tell you how often to check your blood sugar. Share the results with your doctor or other healthcare professional, so that he or she can change your medication and treatment plan, if necessary. People with diabetes who check their blood sugar at home may have more control over their diabetes and may have fewer symptoms than people who do not. If you do not have a glucose meter, ask your doctor or other healthcare professional if you should get one. You may benefit from checking your blood sugar levels even if you do not take insulin.

In addition to checking your blood sugar, other steps can be taken to check for early signs of complications from diabetes. People with diabetes are encouraged to have an eye examination once a year by an eye doctor (ophthalmologist or optometrist) to detect and help prevent vision loss from diabetes. Tell your doctor or other healthcare professional if you notice any sudden change in your vision.

Diabetes may increase the risk of developing foot sores, which may sometimes become serious. If left untreated, they may lead to the need for amputation. If you have any foot sores, call your doctor or other healthcare professional, so that your feet may be treated promptly. Ask your doctor or other healthcare professional to check your feet when you go for your regular appointments, and ask him or her to teach you how to check your own feet properly. Check your feet daily to find problems early on, before they become serious.

It is important to keep your blood pressure within a safe range. If you have diabetes, keeping your blood pressure under control is as important as keeping your blood sugar under control. If you take high blood pressure medication, make sure you take your medication as prescribed.

Diabetes may cause kidney problems. Protein in the urine could be a sign of early kidney disease. Your doctor or other healthcare professional will check the amount of protein in your urine regularly by asking you for a small sample of urine to be tested in a laboratory.

The risk of developing coronary artery disease is increased in people who have diabetes. High cholesterol is another risk for developing coronary artery disease. Talk to your doctor or other healthcare professional about how often you should have your cholesterol levels checked.

If you smoke, you should stop. Smoking increases the risk of developing complications of diabetes, such as problems with poor circulation and heart disease. Ask your doctor or other healthcare professional about ways to help you quit smoking.

If you get sick with a cold or flu or if you have surgery, you might not feel like taking your medication, or you might think you do not need to take as much medication because you are eating less. Actually, you may need as much or even more medication or insulin than usual when you are sick because illness

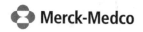

may increase your blood sugar. Ask your doctor or other healthcare professional for a plan for when you are sick so you know how to manage your medication.

Helping to prevent the flu (influenza) and pneumonia is important for people with diabetes. Ask your doctor or other healthcare professional about getting a flu shot every fall. Also, ask about getting a vaccination to help prevent pneumonia.

Warning about Hypoglycemia (Low Blood Sugar)

Low blood sugar (glucose), a condition called hypoglycemia, occurs when the amount of sugar in the blood falls to below normal levels. Low blood sugar may occur when there is too much insulin or other diabetes medication in your body. Missing a meal or not eating at the proper time may cause low blood sugar. Physical activity (such as cleaning the house, doing yard work, or exercising) may also lower your blood sugar. If low blood sugar is not corrected, it may cause serious symptoms or even a coma.

The symptoms of low blood sugar are:

- Blurred vision
- Confusion
- Dizziness
- Fast heartbeat (palpitations)
- Headache
- Hunger
- Increased or excessive sweating
- Irritability
- Nervousness (anxiety)
- Numbness or tingling in the hands or feet
- Passing out (fainting)
- Seizures

- Shakiness or tremors
- Tiredness or sluggishness (fatigue)

Your doctor or other healthcare professional will usually suggest that you drink or eat some form of sugar when your blood sugar is low if it is not yet time for a meal. Some typical choices are to drink 4 to 8 ounces of fruit juice, to swallow 2 to 4 glucose tablets, or to eat a few pieces of candy containing sugar. If you develop symptoms of low blood sugar, you should eat some sugar as soon as possible to help prevent more serious problems. Your symptoms should improve in about 10 minutes. Ask your doctor or other healthcare professional for a treatment plan for low blood sugar. Make sure your family and close friends know how to recognize the symptoms of low blood sugar. Always carry some form of sugar with you when you leave the house.

Talk to your doctor or other healthcare professional before drinking alcoholic beverages (such as beer, wine, whiskey, and others) because alcohol may cause problems with blood sugar control. Drinking alcoholic beverages may keep you from noticing that your blood sugar is low. Drinking alcoholic beverages may also cause reactions with some diabetes medications.

Medications for Diabetes

Several kinds of medications may be taken for diabetes. This chapter discusses these medications and/or categories of medications:

MEDICATIONS	See Page
Sulfonylureas	264
Actos® (pioglitazone) and *Avandia*® (rosiglitazone)	269
Glyset® (miglitol)	273
Precose® (acarbose)	276
Glucophage® (metformin)	280
Prandin™ (repaglinide)	284
Insulin	287

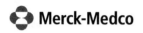

If you do not see the exact name of the medication that you take for diabetes listed above, check the Medication and Chapter Table to find out which category your medication falls under or check the Index.

Sulfonylureas

Sulfonylureas are pills that increase the amount of insulin in the body by helping the pancreas release the insulin that it makes. These medications are used for type 2 diabetes to help control blood sugar (glucose).

▲ Indicates medications that are more likely to cause unpleasant or dangerous side effects. These medications are generally not recommended for people over 65. The side effects may not be very obvious and may be mistaken for "just a part of getting older" but may be serious. If you are taking one of these medications, you might want to talk to your doctor or other healthcare professional to see if this medication is best for you. Safer medications may be available and lower dosages may be required. You should not stop taking these medications without first talking to your doctor or other healthcare professional.

See the WARNING section on page 268 for the specific safety problems associated with this medication ▲.

Brand Name	Generic Name
Amaryl®	glimepiride
DiaBeta®	glyburide
▲*Diabinese*®	chlorpropamide
Dymelor®	acetohexamide
Glucotrol®	glipizide
Glynase®	glyburide
Micronase®	glyburide
Orinase®	tolbutamide
Tolinase®	tolazamide

How Will I Take Sulfonylureas?

Sulfonylureas are usually taken 1 to 3 times a day. You can take this medication with or without food. Your doctor or other healthcare professional will tell you how many times a day to take your medication.

When a medication has initials after its name, such as XL, XR, SR, BID, DUR, and others, it usually means that the body absorbs the medication slowly over time, so you usually have to take it only once or twice a day. The body will absorb some medications of this type too fast if you crush or break them or dissolve them in liquid, and their effects will not last as long as they should. Check with your doctor or other healthcare professional before crushing or breaking your pills or dissolving your pills in liquid.

If you miss a dose of this medication, take the dose you missed as soon as possible. However, if it is almost time for your next dose, skip the missed dose and just take the next one. Do not double your dose. Take your medication exactly as directed by your doctor or other healthcare professional. Do not stop taking a prescription medication unless directed by your doctor or other healthcare professional.

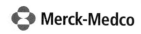

What Side Effects Can Sulfonylureas Cause?

More Common

- Decreased blood sugar (hypoglycemia)—see Warning about Hypoglycemia on page 262

- Increased sensitivity to the sun (bad sunburn)

- Nausea

- Reddening of the face (flushing) while drinking alcoholic beverages (such as beer, wine, whiskey, and others) and taking this medication

Less Common

- Diarrhea

- Dizziness

- Drowsiness

- Easy bruising ("black-and-blue" marks on the skin)

- Rash (skin redness, bumps, itching, or irritation)

- Swelling or puffiness of the feet, ankles, or lower legs (edema)

- Vomiting

Tell your doctor or other healthcare professional if you have side effects that bother you, do not go away, make you worried about taking your medication, or make you want to stop taking your medication.

Do Other Medications Interact with Sulfonylureas?

These medications *may increase* blood sugar (glucose) in people who have diabetes:

- Corticosteroids such as prednisone and others—see Glossary

- Diuretics (water pills) such as *HydroDIURIL®* (hydrochlorothiazide or HCTZ), *Lasix®* (furosemide), and others—see Glossary

- Thyroid medications such as *Cytomel*® (liothyronine), *Synthroid*® (levothyroxine), and others—see Glossary

These medications ***may decrease*** blood sugar (glucose) in people who have diabetes:

- *Marplan*® (isocarboxazid)
- *Nardil*® (phenelzine)
- *Parnate*® (tranylcypromine)

These medications ***may decrease*** how well sulfonylureas work and may result in high blood sugar (hyperglycemia):

- Isoniazid
- *Rifadin*® (rifampin)

These medications ***may increase*** the side effects of sulfonylureas and result in low blood sugar (hypoglycemia):

- Aspirin and medications that contain aspirin
- *Chloromycetin*® (chloramphenicol)
- *Diflucan*® (fluconazole)
- *Nizoral*® (ketoconazole)
- Nonsteroidal anti-inflammatory drugs (NSAIDs) such as *Motrin*® (ibuprofen), *Aleve*® (naproxen), *Vioxx*® (rofecoxib), *Celebrex*® (celecoxib), and others—see Glossary
- *Sporanox*® (itraconazole)
- Sulfa medications such as *Bactrim*™, *Septra*®, and others—see Glossary
- *Tagamet*® (cimetidine)

Beta blockers, such as *Inderal*® (propranolol), *Tenormin*® (atenolol), *Toprol*® (metoprolol), and others (see Glossary), ***may block*** the signs of low blood sugar (glucose) in your body.

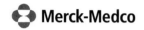

Drinking alcoholic beverages (such as beer, wine, whiskey, and others) *may increase* the side effects of sulfonylureas.

Bile acid binders such as *Questran*® (cholestyramine) or *Colestid*® (colestipol) or bulk-forming laxatives like *Metamucil*® (psyllium) *may decrease* the effects of sulfonylureas by preventing them from being absorbed completely. To help make sure they are absorbed so they can work properly, take sulfonylureas 1 hour before or 4 to 6 hours after taking a bile acid binder or a bulk-forming laxative.

Tell your doctor or other healthcare professional about all medications (both prescription and nonprescription [over-the-counter] medications) that you are taking.

 # Warning!

To give you the best care, your doctor or other healthcare professional needs to know about the diseases and medical conditions you have had—your full medical history. Tell your doctor or other healthcare professional if you have or have ever had any of the following:

- Allergy or previous reaction to any of the following:
    - Carbonic anhydrase inhibitors such as *Azopt*® (brinzolamide), *Diamox*® (acetazolamide), *Trusopt*® (dorzolamide), and others—see Glossary
    - Diabetes medications such as *Glucotrol*® (glipizide), *DiaBeta*® (glyburide), and others—see Glossary
    - Diuretics (water pills) such as *HydroDIURIL*® (hydrochlorothiazide or HCTZ), *Lasix*® (furosemide), and others—see Glossary
    - Sulfa medications such as *Bactrim*™, *Septra*®, and others—see Glossary
- Kidney problems
- Liver problems

Diabinese® (chlorpropamide) is a long-acting medication. Long-acting medications may cause long-lasting low blood sugar (glucose). *Diabinese*®

(chlorpropamide) is generally not recommended for people over 65 years old. Talk to your doctor or other healthcare professional to see if this medication is best for you. Safer medications may be available or a lower dose may be required. You should not stop taking this medication without first talking to your doctor or other healthcare professional.

Sulfonylureas may cause low blood sugar (glucose) which may be very serious. See Warning about Hypoglycemia (Low Blood Sugar) on page 262.

Since sulfonylureas may cause low blood sugar (glucose), they may make you unsteady on your feet, causing you to fall and possibly break a bone. If you have fallen recently, tell your doctor or other healthcare professional about it. Taking a different medication or a lower dose may make you less likely to fall. You should not stop taking this medication without first talking to your doctor or other healthcare professional.

If you are taking sulfonylureas, stay out of the sun as much as you can to avoid a serious sunburn. When you do go out in the sun, use sunblock or sunscreen, and wear protective clothing, such as a wide-brimmed hat and a long-sleeved shirt.

Actos® (pioglitazone) and *Avandia*® (rosiglitazone)

Actos® (pioglitazone) and *Avandia*® (rosiglitazone) help lower blood sugar (glucose) in type 2 diabetes by helping to improve the body's response to insulin.

How Will I Take *Actos*® (pioglitazone) and *Avandia*® (rosiglitazone)?

Actos® (pioglitazone) and *Avandia*® (rosiglitazone) are usually taken either 1 or 2 times a day. They can be taken with or without food. Your doctor or other healthcare professional will tell you how many times a day to take your medication.

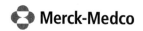

If you miss a dose of this medication, take the dose you missed as soon as possible. However, if it is almost time for your next dose, skip the missed dose and just take the next one. Do not double your dose. Take your medication exactly as directed by your doctor or other healthcare professional. Do not stop taking a prescription medication unless directed by your doctor or other healthcare professional.

 What Side Effects Can *Actos*® (pioglitazone) and *Avandia*® (rosiglitazone) Cause?

More Common

- Headache

- Muscle aches and pains

- Sinus infections and head colds

- Swelling or puffiness of the feet, ankles, or lower legs (edema)

- Weight gain

Less Common

- Decreased blood sugar (hypoglycemia)—see Warning about Hypoglycemia on page 262

Rare

- Liver problems that may cause yellowing of the skin or eyes (jaundice)

- Low red blood cells (anemia)

Tell your doctor or other healthcare professional if you have side effects that bother you, do not go away, make you worried about taking your medication, or make you want to stop taking your medication.

Do Other Medications Interact with *Actos*® (pioglitazone) and *Avandia*® (rosiglitazone)?

These medications *may increase* blood sugar (glucose) in people who have diabetes:

- Corticosteroids such as prednisone and others—see Glossary
- Diuretics (water pills) such as *HydroDIURIL*® (hydrochlorothiazide or HCTZ), *Lasix*® (furosemide), and others—see Glossary
- Isoniazid
- Thyroid medications such as *Cytomel*® (liothyronine), *Synthroid*® (levothyroxine), and others—see Glossary

These medications *may decrease* blood sugar (glucose) in people who have diabetes:

- *Marplan*® (isocarboxazid)
- *Nardil*® (phenelzine)
- *Parnate*® (tranylcypromine)

These medications *may increase* the side effects of *Actos*® (pioglitazone) or *Avandia*® (rosiglitazone) and result in a *decrease* in blood sugar (glucose):

- *Diflucan*® (fluconazole)
- *Nizoral*® (ketoconazole)
- *Sporanox*® (itraconazole)

Bile acid binders such as *Questran*® (cholestyramine) or *Colestid*® (colestipol) or bulk-forming laxatives like *Metamucil*® (psyllium) *may decrease* the effects of *Actos*® (pioglitazone) and *Avandia*® (rosiglitazone) by preventing them from being absorbed completely. To help make sure they are absorbed so they can work properly, take *Actos*® (pioglitazone) and *Avandia*® (rosiglitazone) 1 hour before or 4 to 6 hours after taking a bile acid binder or a bulk-forming laxative.

Beta blockers, such as *Inderal*® (propranolol), *Tenormin*® (atenolol), *Toprol*® (metoprolol), and others (see Glossary), *may block* the signs of low blood sugar (glucose) in your body.

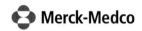

Tell your doctor or other healthcare professional about all medications (both prescription and nonprescription [over-the-counter] medications) that you are taking.

 # Warning!

To give you the best care, your doctor or other healthcare professional needs to know about the diseases and medical conditions you have had—your full medical history. Tell your doctor or other healthcare professional if you have or have ever had any of the following:

- Allergy or previous reaction to *Actos*® (pioglitazone) or *Avandia*® (rosiglitazone)

- Congestive heart failure

- High alcohol intake (drinking 3 or more alcoholic beverages, such as beer, wine, whiskey, and others, every day)

- Liver problems

- Low red blood cells (anemia)

Since *Actos*® (pioglitazone) and *Avandia*® (rosiglitazone) may cause damage to your liver, your doctor or other healthcare professional may order blood tests to find out early on if the medication is causing liver problems, before they become serious.

Since *Actos*® (pioglitazone) and *Avandia*® (rosiglitazone) may cause low blood sugar (glucose), they may make you unsteady on your feet, causing you to fall and possibly break a bone. If you have fallen recently, tell your doctor or other healthcare professional about it. Taking a different medication or a lower dose may make you less likely to fall. You should not stop taking this medication without first talking to your doctor or other healthcare professional.

These medications may cause low blood sugar (glucose) which may be very serious. See Warning about Hypoglycemia (Low Blood Sugar) on page 262.

Glyset® (miglitol)

Glyset® (miglitol) helps to slow the breakdown of carbohydrates from food into glucose. It helps prevent the glucose from being released into the blood all at once after a meal. This helps to keep blood sugar (glucose) from rising too high after eating. This medication is used for type 2 diabetes to help lower blood sugar.

How Will I Take *Glyset*® (miglitol)?

Glyset® (miglitol) is usually taken 3 times a day. It should be taken with the first bite of a meal. Your doctor or other healthcare professional will tell you how many times a day to take your medication.

To help prevent side effects, your doctor or other healthcare professional may start by giving you a low dose of this medication, increasing the amount slowly until it works well for you.

If you miss a dose of this medication, do not take the dose you missed or double your dose; take your regular dose at your next meal. Take your medication exactly as directed by your doctor or other healthcare professional. Do not stop taking a prescription medication unless directed by your doctor or other healthcare professional.

What Side Effects Can *Glyset*® (miglitol) Cause?

More Common

- Diarrhea

- Gas or bloating

- Rash (skin redness, bumps, itching, or irritation)

- Stomach pain

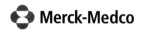

Less Common

- Decreased blood sugar (hypoglycemia)—see Warning about Hypoglycemia on page 262

Tell your doctor or other healthcare professional if you have side effects that bother you, do not go away, make you worried about taking your medication, or make you want to stop taking your medication.

Do Other Medications Interact with *Glyset®* (miglitol)?

These medications *may increase* blood sugar (glucose) in people who have diabetes:

- Corticosteroids such as prednisone and others—see Glossary

- Diuretics (water pills) such as *HydroDIURIL®* (hydrochlorothiazide or HCTZ), *Lasix®* (furosemide), and others—see Glossary

- Isoniazid

- Thyroid medications such as *Cytomel®* (liothyronine), *Synthroid®* (levothyroxine), and others—see Glossary

These medications *may decrease* blood sugar (glucose) in people who have diabetes:

- *Marplan®* (isocarboxazid)

- *Nardil®* (phenelzine)

- *Parnate®* (tranylcypromine)

Digestive enzyme medications such as *Creon®* (pancrelipase), *Pancrease®* (pancrelipase), or *Viokase®* (pancreatin) *may decrease* how well *Glyset®* (miglitol) works.

Beta blockers, such as *Inderal®* (propranolol), *Tenormin®* (atenolol), *Toprol®* (metoprolol), and others (see Glossary), *may block* the signs of low blood sugar (glucose) in your body.

Tell your doctor or other healthcare professional about all medications (both prescription and nonprescription [over-the-counter] medications) that you are taking.

What Else Should I Know about *Glyset*® (miglitol)?

Gastrointestinal symptoms (such as gas, diarrhea, and stomach pain) are the most common side effects. Many people do not get these symptoms, and for most of those who get them, the pain and discomfort become less after the medication is taken for a few weeks.

 # Warning!

To give you the best care, your doctor or other healthcare professional needs to know about the diseases and medical conditions you have had—your full medical history. Tell your doctor or other healthcare professional if you have or have ever had any of the following:

- Allergy or previous reaction to *Glyset*® (miglitol)

- Bowel obstruction (blockage)

- Inflammatory bowel disease (ulcerative colitis or Crohn's disease)

- Kidney problems

This medication may cause low blood sugar (glucose) which may be very serious. See Warning about Hypoglycemia (Low Blood Sugar) on page 262.

If you develop low blood sugar (glucose) while taking *Glyset*® (miglitol), eating some ordinary table sugar, drinking juice, or eating candy will not raise your blood sugar to a safe level. You will have to take a glucose gel or glucose tablets made specifically for people who have diabetes. Ask your doctor or other healthcare professional which type of glucose you should keep on hand.

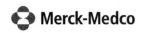

Since *Glyset*® (miglitol) may cause low blood sugar (glucose), it may make you unsteady on your feet, causing you to fall and possibly break a bone. If you have fallen recently, tell your doctor or other healthcare professional about it. Taking a different medication or a lower dose may make you less likely to fall. You should not stop taking this medication without first talking to your doctor or other healthcare professional.

Precose® (acarbose)

Precose® (acarbose) helps to slow the breakdown of carbohydrates into glucose. It helps prevent the glucose in food from being released into the blood all at once after a meal. It helps to keep blood sugar (glucose) from rising too high after eating. This medication is used for type 2 diabetes to help lower blood sugar.

 ## How Will I Take *Precose*® (acarbose)?

Precose® (acarbose) is usually taken 3 times a day. It should be taken with the first bite of a meal. Your doctor or other healthcare professional will tell you how many times a day to take your medication.

To help prevent side effects, your doctor or other healthcare professional may start by giving you a low dose of this medication, increasing the amount slowly until it works well for you.

If you miss a dose of this medication, do not take the dose you missed or double your dose; take your regular dose at your next meal. Take your medication exactly as directed by your doctor or other healthcare professional. Do not stop taking a prescription medication unless directed by your doctor or other healthcare professional.

What Side Effects Can *Precose*® (acarbose) Cause?

More Common

- Diarrhea

- Gas or bloating

- Stomach pain

Less Common

- Decreased blood sugar (hypoglycemia)—see Warning about Hypoglycemia on page 262

- Liver problems that may cause yellowing of the skin or eyes (jaundice)

- Low red blood cells (anemia)

- Rash (skin redness, bumps, itching, or irritation)

Tell your doctor or other healthcare professional if you have side effects that bother you, do not go away, make you worried about taking your medication, or make you want to stop taking your medication.

Do Other Medications Interact with *Precose*® (acarbose)?

These medications ***may increase*** blood sugar (glucose) in people who have diabetes:

- Corticosteroids such as prednisone and others—see Glossary

- Diuretics (water pills) such as *HydroDIURIL*® (hydrochlorothiazide or HCTZ), *Lasix*® (furosemide), and others—see Glossary

- Isoniazid

- Thyroid medications such as *Cytomel*® (liothyronine), *Synthroid*® (levothyroxine), and others—see Glossary

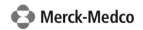

These medications *may decrease* blood sugar (glucose) in people who have diabetes:

- *Marplan*® (isocarboxazid)
- *Nardil*® (phenelzine)
- *Parnate*® (tranylcypromine)

Precose® (acarbose) *may decrease* how well *Lanoxin*® (digoxin) works.

Digestive enzyme medications, such as *Creon*® (pancrelipase), *Pancrease*® (pancrelipase), or *Viokase*® (pancrelipase), *may decrease* how well *Precose*® (acarbose) works.

Beta blockers, such as *Inderal*® (propranolol), *Tenormin*® (atenolol), *Toprol*® (metoprolol), and others (see Glossary), *may block* the signs of low blood sugar (glucose) in your body.

Tell your doctor or other healthcare professional about all medications (both prescription and nonprescription [over-the-counter] medications) that you are taking.

What Else Should I Know about *Precose*® (acarbose)?

Gastrointestinal symptoms (such as gas, diarrhea, and stomach pain) are the most common side effects that people get during the first week of taking these medications. Many people do not get these symptoms, and for most of those who get them, the pain and discomfort become less after the medication is taken for a few weeks.

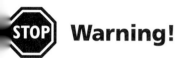 **Warning!**

To give you the best care, your doctor or other healthcare professional needs to know about the diseases and medical conditions you have had—your full medical history. Tell your doctor or other healthcare professional if you have or have ever had any of the following:

- Allergy or previous reaction to *Precose*® (acarbose)
- Bowel obstruction (blockage)
- Inflammatory bowel disease (ulcerative colitis or Crohn's disease)
- Kidney problems
- Liver problems

This medication may cause low blood sugar (glucose), which may be very serious. See Warning about Hypoglycemia (Low Blood Sugar) on page 262.

If you develop low blood sugar (glucose) while taking *Precose*® (acarbose), eating some ordinary table sugar, drinking juice, or eating candy will not raise your blood sugar to a safe level. You will have to take a glucose gel or glucose tablets made specifically for people who have diabetes. Ask your doctor or other healthcare professional which type of glucose you should keep on hand.

Since *Precose*® (acarbose) may cause low blood sugar (glucose), it may make you unsteady on your feet, causing you to fall and possibly break a bone. If you have fallen recently, tell your doctor or other healthcare professional about it. Taking a different medication or a lower dose may make you less likely to fall. You should not stop taking this medication without first talking to your doctor or other healthcare professional.

Since *Precose*® (acarbose) may cause damage to your liver, your doctor or other healthcare professional may order blood tests to find out early on if the medication is causing liver problems, before they become serious.

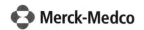

Glucophage® (metformin)

Glucophage® (metformin) helps to lower blood sugar (glucose) by helping to improve the body's response to insulin and helping to lower production of glucose in the liver. This medication is used for type 2 diabetes to help lower blood sugar.

How Will I Take *Glucophage*® (metformin)?

Glucophage® (metformin) is usually taken 1 to 3 times a day. It may be taken with food to help prevent stomach upset. Your doctor or other healthcare professional will tell you how often to take this medication.

To help prevent side effects, your doctor or other healthcare professional may start by giving you a low dose of this medication, increasing the amount slowly until it works well for you.

If you miss a dose of this medication, take the dose you missed as soon as possible. However, if it is almost time for your next dose, skip the missed dose and just take the next one. Do not double your dose. Take your medication exactly as directed by your doctor or other healthcare professional. Do not stop taking a prescription medication unless directed by your doctor or other healthcare professional.

What Side Effects Can *Glucophage*® (metformin) Cause?

More Common

- Diarrhea

- Gas or bloating

- Nausea

- Poor appetite

- Vomiting

Less Common

- Decreased blood sugar (hypoglycemia)—See Warning about Hypoglycemia on page 262
- Low vitamin B$_{12}$ in the blood
- Metallic or unpleasant taste in mouth

Rare

Abnormal buildup of acid in the body (lactic acidosis). This can be serious, possibly even fatal. Call your doctor or other healthcare professional right away if you have the following symptoms of lactic acidosis:

- A strong odor to your breath
- Drowsiness
- Muscle aches and spasms
- Nausea
- Slow heartbeat (palpitations)
- Stomach pain (except at the beginning of treatment)
- Tiredness or sluggishness (fatigue)
- Trouble breathing or shortness of breath

Tell your doctor or other healthcare professional if you have side effects that bother you, do not go away, make you worried about taking your medication, or make you want to stop taking your medication.

 Do Other Medications Interact with *Glucophage*® (metformin)?

These medications ***may increase*** blood sugar (glucose) in people who have diabetes:

- Corticosteroids such as prednisone and others—see Glossary

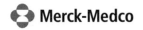

- Diuretics (water pills) such as *HydroDIURIL*® (hydrochlorothiazide or HCTZ), *Lasix*® (furosemide), and others—see Glossary
- Thyroid medications such as *Cytomel*® (liothyronine), *Synthroid*® (levothyroxine), and others—see Glossary

These medications ***may decrease*** blood sugar (glucose) in people who have diabetes:

- *Marplan*® (isocarboxazid)
- *Nardil*® (phenelzine)
- *Parnate*® (tranylcypromine)

These medications ***may increase*** the side effects of *Glucophage*® (metformin) and ***may decrease*** blood sugar (glucose) or ***may increase*** the risk of lactic acidosis:

- *Lanoxin*® (digoxin)
- Morphine
- Quinidine such as *Cardioquin*®, *Quinaglute*®, and others—see Glossary
- Procainamide such as *Procanbid*® or *Pronestyl*®
- *Tagamet*® (cimetidine)

Drinking alcoholic beverages (such as beer, wine, whiskey, and others) ***may increase*** the side effects of *Glucophage*® (metformin).

Beta blockers, such as *Inderal*® (propranolol), *Tenormin*® (atenolol), *Toprol*® (metoprolol), and others (see Glossary), ***may block*** the signs of low blood sugar (glucose) in your body.

Tell your doctor or other healthcare professional about all medications (both prescription and nonprescription [over-the-counter] medications) that you are taking.

Warning!

To give you the best care, your doctor or other healthcare professional needs to know about the diseases and medical conditions you have had—your full medical history. Tell your doctor or other healthcare professional if you have or have ever had any of the following:

- Allergy or previous reaction to *Glucophage®* (metformin)

- Congestive heart failure

- High alcohol intake (drinking 3 or more alcoholic beverages, such as beer, wine, whiskey, and others, every day)

- Kidney problems

- Liver problems

This medication may cause low blood sugar (glucose) which may be very serious. See Warning about Hypoglycemia (Low Blood Sugar) on page 262.

Since *Glucophage®* (metformin) may cause low blood sugar (glucose), it may make you unsteady on your feet, causing you to fall and possibly break a bone. If you have fallen recently, tell your doctor or other healthcare professional about it. Taking a different medication or a lower dose may make you less likely to fall. You should not stop taking this medication without first talking to your doctor or other healthcare professional.

Surgery or some x-ray tests that use a dye injected into your veins through an intravenous (IV) tube may increase your risk of developing lactic acidosis. This is an abnormal buildup of acid in the body that can be serious, possibly even fatal. Talk to your doctor or other healthcare professional before you have surgery or other laboratory tests. You may be directed to stop taking *Glucophage®* (metformin) 2 days before the surgery or test or for a while after it.

Talk to your doctor or other healthcare professional before drinking alcoholic beverages (such as beer, wine, whiskey, and others) while taking *Glucophage®* (metformin). Alcohol increases your risk of developing lactic acidosis. This is an abnormal buildup of acid in the body that can be serious, possibly even fatal.

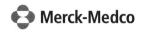

Prandin™ (repaglinide)

Prandin™ (repaglinide) helps the pancreas release insulin into the body. This medication is used for type 2 diabetes to help lower blood sugar (glucose).

How Will I Take *Prandin*™ (repaglinide)?

Prandin™ (repaglinide) is usually taken 2 to 4 times a day, 15 to 30 minutes before meals. If you miss a meal, skip the dose of *Prandin*™ (repaglinide) that you would have taken before that meal. Ask your doctor or other healthcare professional about taking an extra dose of *Prandin*™ (repaglinide) if you plan to eat an extra meal. Your doctor or other healthcare professional will tell you how often to take this medication.

If you miss a dose of this medication, do not take the dose you missed or double your dose; take your regular dose at your next meal. Take your medication exactly as directed by your doctor or other healthcare professional. Do not stop taking a prescription medication unless directed by your doctor or other healthcare professional.

What Side Effects Can *Prandin*™ (repaglinide) Cause?

More Common

- Diarrhea

- Nausea

- Stomach pain

- Vomiting

Less Common

- Constipation

- Decreased blood sugar (hypoglycemia)—see Warning about Hypoglycemia on page 262

Tell your doctor or other healthcare professional if you have side effects that bother you, do not go away, make you worried about taking your medication, or make you want to stop taking your medication.

Do Other Medications Interact with *Prandin*™ (repaglinide)?

These medications *may increase* blood sugar (glucose) in people who have diabetes:

- Corticosteroids such as prednisone and others—see Glossary
- Diuretics (water pills) such as *HydroDIURIL*® (hydrochlorothiazide or HCTZ), *Lasix*® (furosemide), and others—see Glossary
- Thyroid medications such as *Cytomel*® (liothyronine), *Synthroid*® (levothyroxine), and others—see Glossary

These medications *may decrease* blood sugar (glucose) in people who have diabetes:

- *Marplan*® (isocarboxazid)
- *Nardil*® (phenelzine)
- *Parnate*® (tranylcypromine)

These medications *may decrease* how well *Prandin*™ (repaglinide) works:

- Barbiturates such as *Luminal*® (phenobarbital), *Seconal*® (secobarbital), and others—see Glossary
- *Rifadin*® (rifampin)

These medications *may increase* the side effects of *Prandin*™ (repaglinide):

- *Biaxin*® (clarithromycin)
- *Diflucan*® (fluconazole)
- Erythromycin such as *Ery-Tab*®, *Erythrocin*®, and others—see Glossary
- *Nizoral*® (ketoconazole)

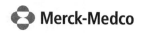

• *Sporanox*® (itraconazole)

Beta blockers, such as *Inderal*® (propranolol), *Tenormin*® (atenolol), *Toprol*® (metoprolol), and others (see Glossary), ***may block*** the signs of low blood sugar (glucose) in your body.

Tell your doctor or other healthcare professional about all medications (both prescription and nonprescription [over-the-counter] medications) that you are taking.

 # Warning!

To give you the best care, your doctor or other healthcare professional needs to know about the diseases and medical conditions you have had—your full medical history. Tell your doctor or other healthcare professional if you have or have ever had any of the following:

- Allergy or previous reaction to *Prandin*™ (repaglinide)

- Heart problems

- Liver problems

This medication may cause low blood sugar (glucose), which may be very serious. See Warning about Hypoglycemia (Low Blood Sugar) on page 262.

Since *Prandin*™ (repaglinide) may cause low blood sugar (glucose), it may make you unsteady on your feet, causing you to fall and possibly break a bone. If you have fallen recently, tell your doctor or other healthcare professional about it. Taking a different medication or a lower dose may make you less likely to fall. You should not stop taking this medication without first talking to your doctor or other healthcare professional.

Insulin

Insulin is used for type 1 diabetes to help lower blood sugar (glucose). When diet, exercise, weight reduction, and oral diabetes medications do not control blood sugar in people with type 2 diabetes, they may have to take insulin.

Insulin comes in different types. Some work quickly but do not last for a long time. Others take longer to start working but last longer. The chart below describes the differences among the various types of insulin.

Type of Insulin	When It Starts to Work	How Long It Lasts
Humalog®	15 to 20 minutes	6 to 8 hours
Regular	30 to 60 minutes	8 to 12 hours
NPH	60 to 90 minutes	24 hours
Lente	1 to 2.5 hours	24 hours
Ultra-lente	4 to 8 hours	More than 36 hours

How Will I Take Insulin?

Your doctor or other healthcare professional will decide which type or types of insulin, the amount to be injected, how often to inject your insulin, and at what time of day to inject your insulin. Insulin is usually taken 1 to 4 times a day. You may have to use more than one type of insulin. Insulin is usually injected 30 minutes before meals; the long-acting form is usually taken 30 minutes before breakfast.

Insulin is usually injected just under the skin of the thigh, stomach, or upper arm. Changing the place where you inject from day to day will help prevent irritation or other skin problems where you inject the needle. For more instruction on how and where to inject the insulin, talk to your doctor or other healthcare professional.

There are several devices that may help you measure and inject your insulin such as magnifiers, insulin pens, cartridges, and others. Ask your doctor or other healthcare professional for advice about these devices.

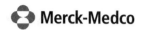

Talk to your doctor or other healthcare professional to find out what to do if you forget a dose of this medication.

 ## What Side Effects Can Insulin Cause?

More Common

- Decreased blood sugar (hypoglycemia)—see Warning about Hypoglycemia on page 262

- Redness or swelling where the shot is given

- Weight gain

Rare

- Allergic reactions such as rash (skin redness, bumps, itching, or irritation), swelling of the face and throat, or trouble breathing. This usually does not occur when human insulin is used.

Tell your doctor or other healthcare professional if you have side effects that bother you, do not go away, make you worried about taking your medication, or make you want to stop taking your medication.

 ## Do Other Medications Interact with Insulin?

These medications *may increase* blood sugar (glucose) in people who have diabetes:

- Corticosteroids such as prednisone and others—see Glossary

- Diuretics (water pills) such as *HydroDIURIL®* (hydrochlorothiazide or HCTZ), *Lasix®* (furosemide), and others—see Glossary

- Thyroid medications such as *Cytomel®* (liothyronine), *Synthroid®* (levothyroxine), and others—see Glossary

These medications *may decrease* blood sugar (glucose) in people who have diabetes:

- *Marplan*® (isocarboxazid)
- *Nardil*® (phenelzine)
- *Parnate*® (tranylcypromine)

Drinking alcoholic beverages (such as beer, wine, whiskey, and others) *may increase* the side effects of insulin.

Aspirin and medications that contain aspirin *may increase* the side effects of insulin.

Beta blockers, such as *Inderal*® (propranolol), *Tenormin*® (atenolol), *Toprol*® (metoprolol), and others (see Glossary), *may block* the signs of low blood sugar (glucose) in your body.

Tell your doctor or other healthcare professional about all medications (both prescription and nonprescription [over-the-counter] medications) that you are taking.

What Else Should I Know about Insulin?

Use a different place for injecting your insulin from one day to the next to help prevent irritation or other skin problems where you inject the needle. Your doctor or other healthcare professional will help you make a plan for rotating injection sites.

If there is a change in color or clarity (clearness) of the insulin, frosting (coating) of the bottle, or if unusual clumping or specks are floating in the insulin, it should not be used. It is important to store insulin correctly, since you might not be able to see changes in potency (strength) or purity of insulin. So if you note changes in your blood sugar (glucose) level that you cannot explain by changes in your diet, exercise, or medication, your insulin may be causing the problem. You should try a new bottle of insulin.

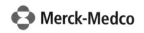

Insulin products are usually stored in a refrigerator (not in a freezer), or they may be kept at room temperature (59°F to 86°F). The potency of insulin depends on what type of product, what type of container (vial or cartridge), whether it is opened or unopened, and how it is stored. Read the package information for specific storage information and expiration times.

 # Warning!

To give you the best care, your doctor or other healthcare professional needs to know about the diseases and medical conditions you have had—your full medical history. Tell your doctor or other healthcare professional if you have or have ever had any of the following:

- Allergy or previous reaction to insulin

- Kidney problems

- Liver problems

- Overactive thyroid (hyperthyroidism)

- Underactive thyroid (hypothyroidism)

Do not change the kind or the dose of insulin you use unless directed by your doctor or other healthcare professional.

Insulin may cause low blood sugar (glucose) which may be very serious. See Warning about Hypoglycemia (Low Blood Sugar) on page 262.

Since insulin may cause low blood sugar (glucose), it may make you unsteady on your feet, causing you to fall and possibly break a bone. If you have fallen recently, tell your doctor or other healthcare professional about it. Taking a different medication or a lower dose may make you less likely to fall. You should not stop taking this medication without first talking to your doctor or other healthcare professional.

Glaucoma

What Is Glaucoma?

Glaucoma is a serious eye disease and one of the leading causes of blindness in older adults. With glaucoma, fluid builds up inside the eye, and this fluid buildup puts pressure on the eye. The increased pressure can damage the optic nerve, the important nerve that sends images from the eye to the brain. There are different types of glaucoma, all of which can cause visual damage. The two main types of glaucoma are called "open-angle" and "closed-angle" glaucoma.

Closed-angle glaucoma, also called acute glaucoma or narrow-angle glaucoma, is not common. In this type of glaucoma, fluid buildup occurs quickly, causing a serious increase in eye pressure. The symptoms are usually very noticeable and include severe headaches, eye pain, nausea, rainbows around lights at night, and very blurred vision. If these symptoms occur, immediate medical treatment is needed because a fast increase in eye pressure can lead to serious and permanent eye damage.

Open-angle glaucoma is also called chronic or wide-angle glaucoma. It is the most common form of glaucoma. Open-angle glaucoma usually responds well to medication, especially if diagnosed and treated early. Early open-angle glaucoma does not have symptoms, so you do not know you have an eye problem. If glaucoma is left untreated or not treated early enough, it can lead to blindness. For this reason, and because glaucoma becomes more common as you get older, it is important for older adults to have regular eye exams to check for glaucoma. Ask your doctor or other healthcare professional how often you should have your eyes checked for glaucoma.

Since there are few symptoms in early open-angle glaucoma, you will not be able to tell if your treatment is working without being tested. If you already are using medication for glaucoma, it is important for you to keep your regular eye appointments so your doctor or other healthcare professional can tell how

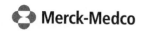

well your treatment is working and make changes in your medication when necessary.

Several kinds of medications may be used to treat glaucoma. These include eyedrops, ointments, gels, and pills. Like all medication, eyedrops, ointments, and gels must be stored properly and applied correctly to get the most benefit from the medication. Check the instructions that come with your prescriptions for directions on proper storage and use of your eye medications. Also read the general instructions below on using eyedrops, eye ointments, and gels.

How Should I Use Eyedrops?

1. Wash and dry your hands to help prevent contamination of the eyedrops and eye infections.

2. Do not let the dropper or bottle top touch anything, and do not rinse the dropper or the top of the bottle with water.

3. If you notice any change in the color of the eyedrops, you should get a new bottle.

4. Sit down and tilt your head back or lie down so that you do not lose your balance when putting in the eyedrops.

5. With one hand, gently pull down the lower lid of the eye to form a small pocket under your eye.

6. Holding the dropper or the tip of the bottle above your eye, look up toward the ceiling. Drop 1 drop of the medication inside the lower lid. Be careful not to let the dropper or tip of the bottle touch your eye, eyelid, or finger.

7. Gently close your eye and then look down.

8. Immediately press the padded tip of your index finger (forefinger) against the inside corner of your closed eye. This will keep the medication from entering the tear duct next to that eye. Firmly but gently hold your finger there for 1 minute. Doing this will help keep the medication in contact

with your eye and help prevent it from being absorbed into your bloodstream.

9. Wait 5 minutes between drops of the same medication to allow time for the medication to be absorbed into the eye. The eye can usually hold 1 drop at a time. Adding a couple of drops at the same time usually causes some of the medication to drip out of the eye.

10. Wait 10 minutes between drops of other medication to help prevent medication interactions. If you are using both drops and ointments, use drops before ointments.

11. Replace the dropper or cap tightly, store your medication as directed, and wash your hands and face to remove any medication that has dripped on them.

How Should I Use Eye Ointments and Gels?

1. If you use eyedrops too, use the eyedrops 10 minutes before your ointment or gel.

2. Wash and dry your hands, and sit or lie down to apply eye ointments and gels so that you do not lose your balance.

3. Hold the tube in your hand for a few minutes to warm the ointment. Doing this will help the ointment flow more easily.

4. Remove the cap from the tube. Put the cap down, with the outside part facing down, on a clean, dry surface. Never let the tip of the open tube touch any surface. If it does, you may want to get a new tube.

5. If using a new tube for the first time, squeeze out the first 1/4 inch of medication and throw it away because it may be too dry to use.

6. Tilt your head back or lie on your back. With one hand, gently pull down the lower lid of the eye you are about to treat.

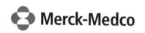

7. While looking up, squeeze a small amount of ointment (about 1/4 inch to 1/2 inch) directly from the tube inside the lower lid of your eye in a sweeping motion. Be careful not to let the tip of the tube touch your eye, eyelid, or finger.

8. Gently close the eye. Keeping it closed, roll your eyeball around in all directions. Your eyesight may blur for a few minutes.

9. Put the cap back on the tube. Store the tube as directed.

10. Wash your hands and face to remove any medication.

Medications for Glaucoma

Several kinds of medications may be used or taken for glaucoma. This chapter discusses these medications and/or categories of medications:

MEDICATIONS	See Page
Miotic Medications	295
Epinephrine and *Propine*® (dipivefrin)	299
Alphagan® (brimonidine)	303
Iopidine® (apraclonidine)	307
Beta Blocker Eyedrops	310
Carbonic Anhydrase Inhibitors	315
Xalatan® (latanoprost)	320

If you do not see the exact name of the medication that you take or use for glaucoma listed above, check the Medication and Chapter Table to find out which category your medication falls under or check the Index.

Miotic Medications

Miotic medications reduce the pressure in the eye caused from the fluid buildup by increasing the flow of fluid out of the eye. This type of medication is called miotic medication because it causes the pupil to contract (become smaller).

Brand Name	Generic Name
Adsorbocarpine™	pilocarpine
E-Pilo®†	pilocarpine/epinephrine
Humorsol®	demecarium
Isopto® Carbachol	carbachol
Isopto® Carpine	pilocarpine
Ocusert®	pilocarpine
P_1E_1®, P_2E_1®, P_4E_1®, P_6E_1®†	pilocarpine/epinephrine
Phospholine Iodide®	echothiophate
Pilocar®	pilocarpine
Pilostat®	pilocarpine

†For combination products see both this section and the epinephrine information section on pages 299–303.

How Will I Use Miotic Medications?

Miotic medications may come as eyedrops and gels to be put in the eye or discs to put under the eyelid. Miotic eyedrops are usually used 2 to 4 times a day. The gel is usually put in the eye once daily at bedtime. *Ocusert®* (pilocarpine) is a miotic medication disc that is placed under the eyelid and left there for up to a week. Your doctor or other healthcare professional will tell you how often to use your medication. Please read the instructions for using eyedrops, ointments, and gels on pages 292–294.

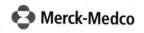
Pilocarpine eyedrops should usually be kept at room temperature (59°F to 86°F) and protected from light. Pilocarpine gel should be kept refrigerated (36°F to 46°F) until it is opened. Once opened, it should be kept at room temperature and thrown away after 8 weeks. *Ocusert®* (pilocarpine) discs should be kept refrigerated until used. *Phospholine Iodide®* (echothiophate) eyedrops come in a powder that must be mixed with the liquid that comes in the package. Before mixing, the bottles should be kept at room temperature. After mixing, the bottle may be kept at room temperature for 1 month or refrigerated for 6 months. Always check the package for specific storage instructions.

If you miss a dose of this medication, apply the dose you missed as soon as possible. However, if it is almost time for your next dose, skip the missed dose and just apply the next one. Do not double your dose. Apply your medication exactly as directed by your doctor or other healthcare professional. Do not stop using a prescription medication unless directed by your doctor or other healthcare professional.

 ## What Side Effects Can Miotic Medications Cause?

More Common

- Blurred vision

- Eye burning and irritation

- Narrowing (constriction) of the pupil of the eye

- Trouble with night vision

Less Common

- Brow ache (aching behind the eyebrows)

- Cataracts

- Eye pain

- Eyelid twitching

- Headache

- Increased tearing (watery eyes)
- Redness of the eye
- Stuffy nose (nasal congestion)
- Unpleasant taste

Rare

- Decreased bladder control (incontinence)
- Diarrhea
- Fast, slow, or irregular heartbeat (palpitations)
- Increased mouth watering (salivation)
- Increased or excessive sweating (perspiration)
- Nausea
- Seeing sparks or flashing light, which could be a sign of a serious problem (retinal detachment). Call your doctor or other healthcare professional right away.
- Shakiness or tremors
- Trouble breathing or shortness of breath
- Vomiting

Tell your doctor or other healthcare professional if you have side effects that bother you, do not go away, make you worried about using your medication, or make you want to stop using your medication.

 Do Other Medications Interact with Miotic Medications?

Medication interactions do not frequently occur with these eye medications. Sometimes using different eye medications too close together may cause an interaction. To help prevent interactions, wait at least 10 minutes between using different eyedrops.

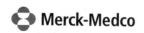

What Else Should I Know about Miotic Medications?

Miotic medications reduce vision in dim light or darkness. Avoid driving at night if you have decreased night vision from your medication.

If you wear eyeglasses or contact lenses, you may have to have your lens prescription changed when you start or stop using miotic medications.

For convenience, some eyedrops contain more than one medication. You should read the section in this chapter on each ingredient contained in your combination eyedrop.

 # Warning!

To give you the best care, your doctor or other healthcare professional needs to know about the diseases and medical conditions you have had—your full medical history. Tell your doctor or other healthcare professional if you have or have ever had any of the following:

- Allergy or previous reaction to miotic medications
- Breathing problems (asthma and COPD, including emphysema or chronic bronchitis)
- Enlarged prostate (benign prostatic hypertrophy)
- Heart attack (myocardial infarction)
- Heart problems
- Myasthenia gravis
- Narrow-angle glaucoma
- Overactive thyroid (hyperthyroidism)
- Parkinson's disease
- Retinal detachments
- Scratched cornea of the eye (corneal abrasion)
- Stomach problems (ulcers)
- Trouble urinating or emptying the bladder

Most eyedrops may cause some blurring of vision immediately after putting them in your eye. Avoid driving a car and such activities as using a knife or operating machinery immediately after using this medication.

Miotic medications may cause problems with anesthesia for surgery. Tell your doctor or other healthcare professional if you will be having surgery or major dental work in case he or she wants you to stop your medication for a few days.

Epinephrine and *Propine*® (dipivefrin)

Epinephrine and *Propine*® (dipivefrin) reduce the pressure in the eye caused from fluid buildup by increasing the flow of fluid out of the eye and decreasing the amount of fluid produced in the eye. These medications are called mydriatic medications because they cause the pupil to dilate (become wider or larger).

Brand Name	Generic Name
Epifrin®	epinephrine
E-Pilo®†	epinephrine/pilocarpine
Glaucon®	epinephrine
P_1E_1®, P_2E_1®, P_4E_1®, P_6E_1®†	epinephrine/pilocarpine
Propine®	dipivefrin

†For combination products, see both this section and the miotic medication information section on pages 295–299.

How Will I Use Epinephrine and *Propine*® (dipivefrin)?

Epinephrine and *Propine*® (dipivefrin) come as eyedrops that are usually used 1 to 3 times a day. Your doctor or other healthcare professional will tell you how often to use your medication. Please read the instructions for using eyedrops on pages 292–293.

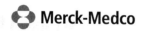
If you miss a dose of this medication, apply the dose you missed as soon as possible. However, if it is almost time for your next dose, skip the missed dose and just apply the next one. Do not double your dose. Apply your medication exactly as directed by your doctor or other healthcare professional. Do not stop using a prescription medication unless directed by your doctor or other healthcare professional.

What Side Effects Can Epinephrine and *Propine*® (dipivefrin) Cause?

More Common

- Brow ache (aching behind the eyebrows)
- Eye burning and irritation
- Headache
- Redness of the eyes or eyelids
- Widening (dilation) of the pupil in the eye

Less Common

- Staining or color change in the eyes after prolonged use of epinephrine

Rare

- Fast or irregular heartbeat (palpitations)
- High blood pressure (hypertension)

Tell your doctor or other healthcare professional if you have side effects that bother you, do not go away, make you worried about using your medication, or make you want to stop using your medication.

Do Other Medications Interact with Epinephrine and *Propine*® (dipivefrin)?

Epinephrine and *Propine*® (dipivefrin) ***may decrease*** how well high blood pressure (hypertension) medications (see Glossary) work.

Epinephrine and *Propine*® (dipivefrin) are generally not prescribed for anyone who is taking MAO inhibitors, such as *Marplan*® (isocarboxazid), *Nardil*® (phenelzine), or *Parnate*® (tranylcypromine), because together they ***may cause*** serious or even fatal reactions. If your doctor or other healthcare professional wants you to stop taking one medication and start taking the other, you should wait at least 2 weeks between stopping one and starting the other.

Medication interactions do not frequently occur with these eye medications. Sometimes using different eye medications too close together may cause an interaction. To help prevent interactions, wait at least 10 minutes between using different eyedrops.

Tell your doctor or other healthcare professional about all medications (both prescription and nonprescription [over-the-counter] medications) that you are taking.

Why Else Do People Use Epinephrine?

Epinephrine injections may be used for severe allergic reactions such as allergies to bee stings.

What Else Should I Know about Epinephrine and *Propine*® (dipivefrin)?

Keep these medications away from heat and light. The eyedrops should be stored between 36°F and 75°F to avoid overheating and to keep from freezing. Throw away the medication if the liquid turns brown.

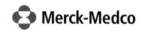

For convenience, some eyedrops contain more than one medication. You should read the section in this chapter on each ingredient contained in your combination eyedrop.

 # Warning!

To give you the best care, your doctor or other healthcare professional needs to know about the diseases and medical conditions you have had—your full medical history. Tell your doctor or other healthcare professional if you have or have ever had, or presently take, any of the following:

- Allergy or previous reaction to epinephrine or *Propine*® (dipivefrin)
- Breathing problems (asthma and COPD, including emphysema or chronic bronchitis)
- Coronary artery disease
- Diabetes
- Heart attack (myocardial infarction)
- Heart rhythm problems (arrhythmias)
- High blood pressure (hypertension)
- MAO inhibitors such as *Marplan*® (isocarboxazid), *Nardil*® (phenelzine), or *Parnate*® (tranylcypromine)
- Narrow-angle glaucoma
- Overactive thyroid (hyperthyroidism)

Epinephrine may cause problems with anesthesia for surgery. Tell your doctor or other healthcare professional if you will be having surgery or major dental work in case he or she wants you to stop your medication for a few days.

Most eyedrops may cause blurred vision immediately after putting them in your eye. Avoid driving a car and such activities as using a knife or operating machinery immediately after using this medication.

If you wear contact lenses, take out your lenses before using the medication. You may put your contact lenses in your eyes 15 minutes after using your eyedrops.

Alphagan® (brimonidine)

Alphagan® (brimonidine) reduces the pressure in the eye caused from fluid buildup by decreasing the amount of fluid produced in the eye.

How Will I Use *Alphagan*® (brimonidine)?

Alphagan® (brimonidine) comes as eyedrops that are usually used 1 to 3 times a day. Your doctor or other healthcare professional will tell you how often to use your medication. Please read the instructions for using eyedrops on pages 292–293.

Alphagan® (brimonidine) should be stored at or below 77°F and protected from light.

If you miss a dose of this medication, apply the dose you missed as soon as possible. However, if it is almost time for your next dose, skip the missed dose and just apply the next one. Do not double your dose. Apply your medication exactly as directed by your doctor or other healthcare professional. Do not stop using a prescription medication unless directed by your doctor or other healthcare professional.

What Side Effects Can *Alphagan*® (brimonidine) Cause?

More Common

- Allergic reactions such as rash (skin redness, bumps, itching, or irritation), swelling of the face and throat, or trouble breathing

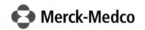
- Brow ache (aching behind the eyebrows)
- Dry mouth
- Eye burning and irritation
- Headache
- Redness of the eyes or eyelids
- Tiredness or sluggishness (fatigue)

Less Common

- Drowsiness
- Dry eyes
- Muscle aches and pain
- Nausea
- Staining or color change in the eyes after prolonged use
- Vision changes

Rare

- Fast or irregular heartbeat (palpitations)
- High blood pressure (hypertension)
- Nervousness (anxiety)
- Passing out or fainting
- Taste changes
- Trouble falling asleep or staying asleep (insomnia)

Tell your doctor or other healthcare professional if you have side effects that bother you, do not go away, make you worried about using your medication, or make you want to stop using your medication.

Do Other Medications Interact with *Alphagan®* (brimonidine)?

Alphagan® (brimonidine) ***may increase*** the side effects of high blood pressure (hypertension) medications—see Glossary.

Alphagan® (brimonidine) ***may increase*** the side effects of other medications that cause drowsiness, including anticholinergic medications, antidepressants, antihistamines (allergy medications), antispasmodics, benzodiazepines (a type of tranquilizer), anxiety medications, narcotics (pain relievers), muscle relaxants, neuroleptic medications (a type of tranquilizer), seizure medications, or sleep medications. Avoid driving a car and other activities that need mental alertness, like using a knife or operating machinery, while taking these medications together.

Drinking alcoholic beverages (such as beer, wine, whiskey, and others) ***may increase*** the side effects of *Alphagan®* (brimonidine).

Alphagan® (brimonidine) is generally not prescribed for anyone who is taking MAO inhibitors, such as *Marplan®* (isocarboxazid), *Nardil®* (phenelzine), or *Parnate®* (tranylcypromine), because together they ***may cause*** serious or even fatal reactions. If your doctor or other healthcare professional wants you to stop taking one medication and start taking the other, you should wait at least 2 weeks between stopping one and starting the other.

Medication interactions do not frequently occur with these eye medications. Sometimes using different eye medications too close together may cause an interaction. To help prevent interactions, wait at least 10 minutes between using different eyedrops.

Tell your doctor or other healthcare professional about all medications (both prescription and nonprescription [over-the-counter] medications) that you are taking.

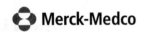
(STOP) Warning!

To give you the best care, your doctor or other healthcare professional needs to know about the diseases and medical conditions you have had—your full medical history. Tell your doctor or other healthcare professional if you have or have ever had, or presently take, any of the following:

- Allergy or previous reaction to *Alphagan®* (brimonidine) or benzalkonium chloride

- Heart problems

- Kidney problems

- Liver problems

- Low blood pressure (hypotension)

- MAO inhibitors such as *Marplan®* (isocarboxazid), *Nardil®* (phenelzine), or *Parnate®* (tranylcypromine)

- Narrow-angle glaucoma

- Poor circulation

- Sadness, feeling blue or down, depressed mood (depression)

- Soft contact lenses

Alphagan® (brimonidine) may cause drowsiness. Avoid driving a car and other activities that require mental alertness, like using a knife or operating machinery, while using this medication. Drinking alcoholic beverages (such as beer, wine, whiskey, and others) may increase the side effects.

If you wear soft contact lenses, take out your lenses before using this medication. You may put your contact lenses in your eyes 15 minutes after using your medication.

Iopidine® (apraclonidine)

Iopidine® (apraclonidine) reduces the pressure in the eye caused from fluid buildup by decreasing the amount of fluid produced in the eye.

How Will I Use *Iopidine*® (apraclonidine)?

Iopidine® (apraclonidine) comes as eyedrops that are usually used 1 to 3 times a day. Your doctor or other healthcare professional will tell you how often to use your medication. Please read the instructions for using eyedrops on pages 292–293.

Iopidine® (apraclonidine) should be stored at room temperature (59°F to 86°F) and protected from light.

If you miss a dose of this medication, apply the dose you missed as soon as possible. However, if it is almost time for your next dose, skip the missed dose and just apply the next one. Do not double your dose. Apply your medication exactly as directed by your doctor or other healthcare professional. Do not stop using a prescription medication unless directed by your doctor or other healthcare professional.

What Side Effects Can *Iopidine*® (apraclonidine) Cause?

More Common

- Brow ache (aching behind the eyebrows)

- Eye burning and irritation

- Headache

- Increased tearing (watery eyes)

- Redness of the eyes or eyelids

- Tiredness or sluggishness (fatigue)

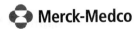

Less Common

- Constipation
- Dizziness
- Drowsiness
- Dry mouth, eyes, and nose
- Nausea
- Nervousness (anxiety)
- Taste changes

Rare

- Cardiac chest pain
- Sadness, feeling blue or down, depressed mood (depression)

Tell your doctor or other healthcare professional if you have side effects that bother you, do not go away, make you worried about using your medication, or make you want to stop using your medication.

Do Other Medications Interact with *Iopidine®* (apraclonidine)?

Iopidine® (apraclonidine) ***may increase*** the side effects of high blood pressure (hypertension) medications (see Glossary).

Iopidine® (apraclonidine) ***may increase*** the side effects of other medications that cause drowsiness, including anticholinergic medications, antidepressants, antihistamines (allergy medications), antispasmodics, benzodiazepines (a type of tranquilizer), anxiety medications, narcotics (pain relievers), muscle relaxants, neuroleptic medications (a type of tranquilizer), seizure medications, or sleep medications. Avoid driving a car and other activities that need mental alertness, like using a knife or operating machinery, while taking these medications together.

Drinking alcoholic beverages (such as beer, wine, whiskey, and others) *may increase* the side effects of *Iopidine*® (apraclonidine).

Iopidine® (apraclonidine) is generally not prescribed for anyone who is taking MAO inhibitors, such as *Marplan*® (isocarboxazid), *Nardil*® (phenelzine), or *Parnate*® (tranylcypromine), because together they *may cause* serious or even fatal reactions. If your doctor or other healthcare professional wants you to stop taking one medication and start taking the other, you should wait at least 2 weeks between stopping one and starting the other.

Medication interactions do not frequently occur with these eye medications. Sometimes using different eye medications too close together may cause an interaction. To help prevent interactions, wait at least 10 minutes between using different eyedrops.

Tell your doctor or other healthcare professional about all medications (both prescription and nonprescription [over-the-counter] medications) that you are taking.

 # Warning!

To give you the best care, your doctor or other healthcare professional needs to know about the diseases and medical conditions you have had—your full medical history. Tell your doctor or other healthcare professional if you have or have ever had, or presently take, any of the following:

- Allergy or previous reaction to *Iopidine*® (apraclonidine) or *Catapres*® (clonidine)

- Heart problems

- Kidney problems

- Liver problems

- MAO inhibitors such as *Marplan*® (isocarboxazid), *Nardil*® (phenelzine), or *Parnate*® (tranylcypromine)

- Narrow-angle glaucoma

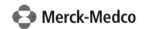

- Overactive thyroid (hyperthyroidism)

- Poor circulation

- Sadness, feeling blue or down, depressed mood (depression)

Iopidine® (apraclonidine) may cause problems with anesthesia. Tell your doctor or other healthcare professional if you will be having surgery or major dental work in case he or she wants you to stop your medication for a few days.

Iopidine® (apraclonidine) may cause drowsiness. Avoid driving a car and other activities that require mental alertness, like using a knife or operating machinery, while using this medication. Drinking alcoholic beverages (such as beer, wine, whiskey, and others) may increase the side effects.

Beta Blocker Eyedrops

Beta blocker eyedrops help reduce the pressure in the eye caused from fluid buildup by decreasing the amount of fluid produced in the eye.

Brand Name	Generic Name
Betagan®	levobunolol
Betoptic®	betaxolol
Cosopt®†	timolol/dorzolamide
Ocupress®	carteolol
OptiPranolol®	metipranolol
Timoptic®	timolol

†For combination products, see both this section and the carbonic anhydrase inhibitor information section on pages 315–320.

How Will I Use Beta Blocker Eyedrops?

Beta blocker eyedrops are usually used once or twice a day. Your doctor or other healthcare professional will tell you how many times a day to use your medication. Please read the instructions for using eyedrops on pages 292–293.

All beta blocker eyedrops should be kept at room temperature (59°F to 86°F) and protected from light, except *Ocupress*® (carteolol) which should be kept between 59°F and 77°F. *Betoptic S*® (betaxolol suspension) should be shaken well before each time you use it. The *Timoptic-XE*® bottle should be turned upside down once each time before you use it.

If you miss a dose of this medication, apply the dose you missed as soon as possible. However, if it is almost time for your next dose, skip the missed dose and just apply the next one. Do not double your dose. Apply your medication exactly as directed by your doctor or other healthcare professional. Do not stop using a prescription medication unless directed by your doctor or other healthcare professional.

What Side Effects Can Beta Blocker Eyedrops Cause?

More Common

- Blurred vision

- Double vision

- Drooping eyelids

- Eye irritation with redness and swelling

- Headache

- Increased tearing (watery eyes)

- Staining or color change in the eyes after prolonged use

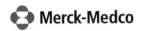

Less Common

- Congestive heart failure
- Dizziness when standing up from a bed or a chair
- Erection problems (erectile dysfunction)
- Loss of interest in sex (decreased libido)
- Low blood pressure (hypotension)
- Nausea
- Nervousness (anxiety)
- Passing out or fainting
- Rash (skin redness, bumps, itching, or irritation)
- Sadness, feeling blue or down, depressed mood (depression)
- Slow heartbeat (palpitations)
- Tiredness or sluggishness (fatigue)
- Trouble breathing or shortness of breath with asthma and COPD, including emphysema or chronic bronchitis
- Weakness

Tell your doctor or other healthcare professional if you have side effects that bother you, do not go away, make you worried about using your medication, or make you want to stop using your medication.

 Do Other Medications Interact with Beta Blocker Eyedrops?

Beta blocker eyedrops *may increase* the side effects of these medications:

- High blood pressure (hypertension) medications—see Glossary
- Heart rhythm problem (arrhythmia) medications—see Glossary

Medication interactions do not frequently occur with these eye medications. Sometimes using different eye medications too close together may cause an interaction. To help prevent interactions, wait at least 10 minutes between using different eyedrops.

Tell your doctor or other healthcare professional about all medications (both prescription and nonprescription [over-the-counter] medications) that you are taking.

Why Else Do People Take Beta Blockers?

In tablet form, beta blockers may be taken for high blood pressure (hypertension), cardiac chest pain (angina), congestive heart failure, migraine headaches, and many other conditions.

What Else Should I Know about Beta Blocker Eyedrops?

For convenience some eyedrops contain more than one medication. You should read the section in this chapter on each ingredient contained in your combination eyedrop.

 # Warning!

To give you the best care, your doctor or other healthcare professional needs to know about the diseases and medical conditions you have had—your full medical history. Tell your doctor or other healthcare professional if you have or have ever had any of the following:

- Allergy or previous reaction to beta blockers

- Breathing problems (asthma and COPD, including emphysema or chronic bronchitis)

- Congestive heart failure

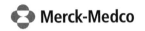
- Depression

- Diabetes

- Heart rhythm problems (arrhythmias)

- Myasthenia gravis

- Narrow-angle glaucoma

- Overactive thyroid (hyperthyroidism)

Most eyedrops can cause some blurring of vision immediately after putting them in your eye. Avoid driving a car and such activities as using a knife or operating machinery immediately after using this medication.

Beta blockers may worsen the symptoms of some lung problems, especially asthma and COPD, including emphysema and chronic bronchitis. Tell your doctor or other healthcare professional if you have trouble breathing or shortness of breath.

Beta blockers may hide the symptoms of low blood sugar (hypoglycemia). This can cause problems for people with diabetes. Ask your doctor or other healthcare professional how often you should check your blood sugar (glucose).

Beta blockers may worsen the symptoms of poor circulation (peripheral vascular disease). Tell your doctor or other healthcare professional if you develop symptoms of poor circulation such as pain, numbness, or coldness of your legs, feet, and hands.

Beta blockers may make you unsteady on your feet, causing you to fall and possibly break a bone. If you have fallen recently, tell your doctor or other healthcare professional about it. Taking a different medication or a lower dose may make you less likely to fall. You should not stop taking this medication without first talking to your doctor or other healthcare professional.

Carbonic Anhydrase Inhibitors

Carbonic anhydrase inhibitors reduce the pressure in the eye caused by fluid buildup by decreasing the amount of fluid produced in the eye. They come in eyedrops and pills. The eyedrops often have fewer side effects because lower doses may be used when the medication is put right in the eye where it needs to work.

Brand Name	Generic Name
Azopt® Eyedrops	brinzolamide
Cosopt® Eyedrops†	dorzolamide/timolol
Daranide® Pills	dichlorphenamide
Diamox® Pills	acetazolamide
Neptazane® Pills	methazolamide
Trusopt® Eyedrops	dorzolamide

†For combination products, see both this section and the beta blocker eyedrops information section on pages 310–314.

How Will I Use Carbonic Anhydrase Inhibitors?

The eyedrops are usually used 3 times a day. The pills are usually taken 1 to 4 times a day. Taking the pills with food may help prevent stomach upset. Your doctor or other healthcare professional will tell you how many times a day to use your medication. If you are using the eyedrops, please read pages 292–293 for instructions on using eyedrops.

When a medication has the word "sequel" after its name, it usually means that the body absorbs the medication slowly over time, so you usually have to take it only once or twice a day. The body will absorb some medications of this type too fast if you crush or break them or dissolve them in liquid, and their effects will not last as long as they should. Check with your doctor or other healthcare professional before crushing or breaking your pills or dissolving your pills in liquid.

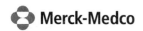
If you miss a dose of this medication, take the dose you missed as soon as possible. However, if it is almost time for your next dose, skip the missed dose and just take the next one. Do not double your dose. Take your medication exactly as directed by your doctor or other healthcare professional. Do not stop taking a prescription medication unless directed by your doctor or other healthcare professional.

What Side Effects Can Carbonic Anhydrase Inhibitors Cause?

Eyedrops

More Common

- Bitter taste
- Blurred vision
- Eye burning and irritation
- Increased sensitivity of eyes to light

Less Common

- Dry eyes
- Headache
- Nausea
- Tiredness or sluggishness (fatigue)
- Weakness

Rare

- Allergic reactions such as rash (skin redness, bumps, itching, or irritation), swelling of the face and throat, or trouble breathing
- Double vision
- Increased tearing (watery eyes)
- Nausea

Pills

More Common

- Drowsiness

- Erection problems (erectile dysfunction)

- Loss of interest in sex (decreased libido)

- Poor appetite

- Taste changes

- Tingling, numbness, or pain of the hands and legs

- Weight loss

- Worsening of gout (very painful, swollen joints)

Less Common

- Allergic reactions such as rash (skin redness, bumps, itching, or irritation), swelling of the face and throat, or trouble breathing

- Bleeding that may not stop easily (nose bleeds, bleeding while brushing your teeth, and cuts)

- Confusion

- Easy bruising ("black-and-blue" marks on the skin)

- Frequent fever, sore throat, or flu-like symptoms that may be a sign of low white blood cells

- Kidney problems

- Kidney stones

- Low blood pressure (hypotension)

- Low red blood cells (anemia)

Tell your doctor or other healthcare professional if you have side effects that bother you, do not go away, make you worried about taking your medication, or make you want to stop taking your medication.

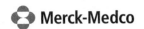 Glaucoma

 Do Other Medications Interact with Carbonic Anhydrase Inhibitors?

Carbonic anhydrase inhibitors *may increase* the side effects of aspirin and medications that contain aspirin.

Carbonic anhydrase inhibitors *may increase* the side effects of these medications:

- Diuretics (water pills) such as *HydroDIURIL*® (hydrochlorothiazide or HCTZ), *Lasix*® (furosemide), and others—see Glossary
- *Neoral*® (cyclosporine)
- Quinidine such as *Quinaglute*®, *Quinidex*®, and others—see Glossary
- *Sandimmune*® (cyclosporine)

Oral carbonic anhydrase inhibitors *may decrease* how well lithium, such as *Eskalith*®, *Lithobid*®, and others (see Glossary), works.

Taking *Topamax*® (topiramate) together with an oral carbonic anhydrase inhibitor *may increase* the chance of developing kidney stones.

Medication interactions do not frequently occur with these eyedrops. Sometimes using different eye medications too close together may cause an interaction. To help prevent interactions, wait at least 10 minutes between using different eyedrops.

Carbonic anhydrase inhibitors must be used carefully if prescribed for anyone who is taking *Propulsid*® (cisapride [withdrawn from general distribution; available only by special arrangement with the manufacturer]), *Seldane*® (terfenadine [no longer commercially available]), or *Hismanal*® (astemizole [no longer commercially available]), because together they *may cause* serious, sometimes fatal, heart problems.

Tell your doctor or other healthcare professional about all medications (both prescription and nonprescription [over-the-counter] medications) that you are taking.

Why Else Do People Take Carbonic Anhydrase Inhibitors?

Diamox® (acetazolamide) may also be used as a diuretic and to help prevent seizures from epilepsy.

 # Warning!

To give you the best care, your doctor or other healthcare professional needs to know about the diseases and medical conditions you have had—your full medical history. Tell your doctor or other healthcare professional if you have or have ever had any of the following:

- Allergy or previous reaction to any of the following:
    - ◆ Carbonic anhydrase inhibitors such as *Azopt®* (brinzolamide), *Diamox®* (acetazolamide), *Trusopt®* (dorzolamide), and others—see Glossary
    - ◆ Diabetes medications such as *DiaBeta®* (glyburide), *Glucophage®* (metformin), *Glucotrol®* (glipizide), and others—see Glossary
    - ◆ Diuretics (water pills) such as *HydroDIURIL®* (hydrochlorothiazide or HCTZ), *Lasix®* (furosemide), and others—see Glossary
    - ◆ Sulfa medications such as *Bactrim™*, *Septra®*, and others—see Glossary
- Kidney problems
- Kidney stones
- Liver problems
- Low potassium in the blood (hypokalemia)
- Narrow-angle glaucoma
- Soft contact lenses

If you wear contact lenses, take out your lenses before using the medication. You may put your contact lenses in your eyes 15 minutes after using your medication.

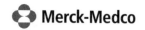

Most eyedrops may cause some blurring of vision immediately after putting them in your eye. Avoid driving a car and such activities like using a knife or operating machinery immediately after using this medication.

Xalatan® (latanoprost)

How Will I Use *Xalatan*® (latanoprost)?

Xalatan® (latanoprost) is usually used once a day, usually at bedtime. Your doctor or other healthcare professional will tell you how often to use your medication. Please read pages 292–293 for instructions on using eyedrops.

Before opening *Xalatan*® (latanoprost), the bottle should be kept refrigerated (36°F to 46°F). Once opened, the bottle may be kept at room temperature (59°F to 86°F) for up to 6 weeks and then thrown away.

If you miss a dose of this medication, apply the dose you missed as soon as possible. However, if it is almost time for your next dose, skip the missed dose and just apply the next one. Do not double your dose. Apply your medication exactly as directed by your doctor or other healthcare professional. Do not stop using a prescription medication unless directed by your doctor or other healthcare professional.

What Side Effects Can *Xalatan*® (latanoprost) Cause?

More Common

- Blurred vision
- Change in color and length of eyelashes
- Change in color of eyelid
- Change in eye color to a shade that is browner than it was

- Eye burning and irritation
- Headache
- Itching

Less Common

- Double vision
- Dry eyes
- Eyelid swelling
- Increased head colds and flu
- Muscle aches and pain
- Rash (skin redness, bumps, itching, or irritation)
- Sensitivity of the eye to light
- Watery eyes

Rare

- Seeing sparks or flashing light which could be a sign of a serious problem (retinal detachment). Call your doctor or other healthcare professional right away.

Tell your doctor or other healthcare professional if you have side effects that bother you, do not go away, make you worried about using your medication, or make you want to stop using your medication.

Do Other Medications Interact with *Xalatan*® (latanoprost)?

Medication interactions do not frequently occur with these eye medications. Sometimes using different eye medications too close together may cause an interaction. To help prevent interactions, wait at least 10 minutes between using different eyedrops.

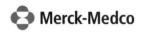

Tell your doctor or other healthcare professional about all medications (both prescription and nonprescription [over-the-counter] medications) that you are taking.

 # Warning!

To give you the best care, your doctor or other healthcare professional needs to know about the diseases and medical conditions you have had—your full medical history. Tell your doctor or other healthcare professional if you have or have ever had any of the following:

- Allergy or previous reaction to *Xalatan®* (latanoprost) or benzalkonium chloride
- Contact lenses
- Eye infection in the last 3 months
- Kidney problems
- Liver problems
- Narrow-angle glaucoma

If you wear contact lenses, take out your lenses before using the medication. You may put your contact lenses in your eyes 15 minutes after using your medication.

Most eyedrops may cause some blurring of vision immediately after putting them in your eye. Avoid driving a car and such activities as using a knife or operating machinery immediately after using this medication.

Xalatan® (latanoprost) may gradually make your eyes browner. This may happen over several months to years. Talk to your doctor or other healthcare professional if you notice a change in your eye color, and keep your scheduled appointments so he or she can follow your eye changes.

Chapter 11

Heartburn, Ulcers, and Indigestion

What Is Heartburn?

Heartburn, often called gastroesophageal reflux or GERD, is a condition in which small amounts of food and acid from the stomach come up into the swallowing tube (esophagus). A person who has heartburn usually has a burning feeling in the middle of the upper chest. This can happen after eating or after lying down. For some people, caffeine (such as in coffee, tea, colas, chocolate, and others), fried food, carbonated beverages, tomatoes, citrus fruits, and other kinds of food may cause heartburn. Smoking cigarettes and/or drinking alcoholic beverages (such as beer, wine, whiskey, and others) may also cause heartburn.

What Are Ulcers?

Ulcers, often called peptic ulcer disease or PUD, are irritations in the lining of the stomach or small intestine. Ulcers are formed when the lining of the stomach or small intestine is damaged, creating a small hole in the stomach lining.

Common symptoms of ulcers are gnawing pain, burning, soreness, and an empty feeling in the stomach. Most ulcers are the result of infection with the bacteria called *Helicobacter pylori*. Other causes are medications, such as aspirin, corticosteroids, and nonsteroidal anti-inflammatory drugs (NSAIDs)—see Glossary. A possible complication of ulcers is internal bleeding from the wall of the stomach or intestines. A bleeding ulcer can be serious, and sometimes fatal, if not treated.

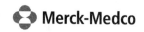

Some people may have some of the symptoms above but may not have an ulcer or irritation in the stomach. These symptoms are real, despite the fact that a cause may not be found. People with these symptoms may be having indigestion, which is described below.

What Is Indigestion?

Indigestion, also known as dyspepsia, is pain, discomfort, nausea, uncomfortable fullness, or bloating in the stomach soon after eating. To some people, indigestion describes their symptoms of heartburn. To others, indigestion refers to the pain of ulcers. However, many people with indigestion do not have a serious medical condition, even though they may be quite uncomfortable. Although sometimes caused by stomach acid, in some people indigestion may be caused by particular foods, certain medications, and eating too much. It can also be caused by stress. Talk to your doctor or other healthcare professional to better understand the cause of your symptoms of indigestion.

If you have problems with heartburn, ulcer, or indigestion, you may have to change your eating habits by eating smaller portions more frequently and avoiding foods known to aggravate your condition. You can also make other changes to help reduce your symptoms, such as raising the head of your bed if you have had heartburn at night, avoiding eating 2 hours before bedtime, limiting alcoholic beverages (such as beer, wine, whiskey, and others), and stopping smoking. Medications can also be used when these changes do not relieve your symptoms.

Several kinds of medications may be taken to relieve heartburn, ulcer, or indigestion. This chapter discusses these medications and/or categories of medications:

MEDICATIONS	See Page
H$_2$-Blockers	325
Proton Pump Inhibitors	330
Carafate® (sucralfate)	333
Cytotec® (misoprostol)	336
Antacids	339
Tetracycline	344
Amoxicillin	348
Biaxin® (clarithromycin)	350
Flagyl® (metronidazole)	354
Pepto-Bismol® (bismuth subsalicylate)	359
Reglan® (metoclopramide)	363
Propulsid® (cisapride)	367

If you do not see the exact name of the medication that you take for heartburn, ulcer, or indigestion listed above, check the Medication and Chapter Table to find out which category your medication falls under or check the Index.

H$_2$-Blockers

Histamine$_2$ (H$_2$) is a natural substance found in the body that stimulates cells in the stomach to produce acid, which helps digest food. H$_2$-blockers are used to block histamine$_2$ to help reduce stomach acid. H$_2$-blockers may be used to treat heartburn, ulcer, or indigestion. These medications may be obtained by prescription or purchased over-the-counter (OTC). In peptic ulcer disease caused by *Helicobacter pylori (H. pylori)*, you may also be prescribed antibiotics or *Pepto-Bismol*® (bismuth subsalicylate).

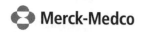

Brand Name	Generic Name
Axid®	nizatidine
Pepcid®	famotidine
Tagamet®	cimetidine
Zantac®	ranitidine

How Will I Take H₂-Blockers?

For an ulcer, H_2-blockers are usually taken as pills once or twice a day every day for 6 to 8 weeks. Sometimes, they are taken in low doses for a longer period to help prevent an ulcer from coming back. For heartburn, H_2-blockers are usually taken 1 to 2 times a day. If you take an H_2-blocker just once a day, it is usually taken at bedtime. Follow the directions on the package, or ask your doctor or other healthcare professional to tell you how often and for how long to take this medication.

If you miss a dose of this medication, take the dose you missed as soon as possible. However, if it is almost time for your next dose, skip the missed dose and just take the next one. Do not double your dose. Take your medication exactly as directed by your doctor or other healthcare professional. Do not stop taking a prescription medication unless directed by your doctor or other healthcare professional.

What Side Effects Can H₂-Blockers Cause?

More Common

- Diarrhea

- Dizziness

- Rash (skin redness, bumps, itching, or irritation)

Less Common

- Confusion

- Increased breast size in men

- Loss of interest in sex (decreased libido)

- Muscle aches and spasms

Rare

- Frequent fever, sore throat, or flu-like symptoms that may be a sign of low white blood cells

- Low red blood cells (anemia)

Tell your doctor or other healthcare professional if you have side effects that bother you, do not go away, make you worried about taking your medication, or make you want to stop taking your medication.

Do Other Medications Interact with H$_2$-Blockers?

H$_2$-blockers* **may increase** the side effects of:

- Benzodiazepines such as *Ativan*® (lorazepam), *Klonopin*® (clonazepam), *Xanax*® (alprazolam), and others—see Glossary

- Beta blockers such as *Inderal*® (propranolol), *Tenormin*® (atenolol), *Toprol*® (metoprolol), and others—see Glossary

- Calcium channel blockers such as *Cardizem*® (diltiazem), *Norvasc*® (amlodipine), *Procardia*® (nifedipine), and others—see Glossary

- *Coumadin*® (warfarin)

- *Ethmozine*® (moricizine)

- *Glucophage*® (metformin)

*These interactions most commonly occur with *Tagamet*® (cimetidine) but may occur with any of the H$_2$-blockers. Talk to your doctor or other healthcare professional if you have questions about these medications.

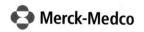

- *Mirapex®* (pramipexole)
- Procainamide such as *Procanbid®* or *Pronestyl®*
- Quinidine such as *Quinaglute®*, *Quinidex®*, and others—see Glossary
- *Rythmol®* (propafenone)
- Seizure medications such as *Dilantin®* (phenytoin), *Depakote®* (valproic acid), *Neurontin®* (gabapentin), *Tegretol®* (carbamazepine), and others—see Glossary
- *Tambocor®* (flecainide)
- Theophylline such as *Theo-Dur®*, *Uniphyl®*, and others—see Glossary
- Tricyclic antidepressants such as *Elavil®* (amitriptyline), *Pamelor®* (nortriptyline), *Sinequan®* (doxepin), and others—see Glossary
- *Wellbutrin®* (bupropion)
- *Zyban®* (bupropion)

H_2-blockers ***may decrease*** how well these medications work:

- *Diflucan®* (fluconazole)
- *Nizoral®* (ketoconazole)
- *Sporanox®* (itraconazole)

Many nonprescription (over-the-counter [OTC]) medications such as pain, cough, cold, allergy, and sleep medications contain aspirin or nonsteroidal anti-inflammatory drugs (NSAIDs) that can cause indigestion, heartburn, or ulcers. You should talk to your doctor or other healthcare professional before taking any new OTC medications.

These medications may make heartburn, ulcers, or indigestion worse:

- Aspirin, medications that contain aspirin, and aspirin-like medications (salicylates)—see Glossary
- Corticosteroids such as prednisone and others—see Glossary
- Nonsteroidal anti-inflammatory drugs (NSAIDs) such as *Motrin®* (ibuprofen), *Aleve®* (naproxen), *Vioxx®* (rofecoxib), *Celebrex®* (celecoxib), and others—see Glossary

Drinking alcoholic beverages (such as beer, wine, whiskey, and others) may make heartburn, ulcers, or indigestion worse.

Antacids such as *Maalox®* or *Mylanta®* (aluminum hydroxide/magnesium hydroxide), *Rolaids®* or *Tums®* (calcium carbonate), or *Amphojel®* (aluminum hydroxide) *may decrease* the effects of H_2-blockers when taken at the same time. If you are using antacids, take an H_2-blocker 1 hour before or 2 hours after taking your antacid.

Tell your doctor or other healthcare professional about all medications (both prescription and nonprescription [over-the-counter] medications) that you are taking.

What Else Should I Know about H_2-Blockers?

It may take as long as 8 weeks for an ulcer to heal. Do not stop taking this medication unless directed by your doctor or other healthcare professional.

 # Warning!

To give you the best care, your doctor or other healthcare professional needs to know about the diseases and medical conditions you have had—your full medical history. Tell your doctor or other healthcare professional if you have or have ever had any of the following:

- Allergy or previous reaction to an H_2-blocker
- Kidney problems
- Liver problems

H_2-blockers are available over-the-counter and do not require a prescription. If you need H_2-blockers regularly, it may be a sign of a medical problem that needs other treatment. Ask your doctor or other healthcare professional to evaluate your symptoms if you need to use H_2-blockers regularly.

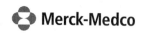

Stomach pain may be a sign of an ulcer. However, you may have an ulcer without feeling any pain at all. If ulcers are not treated, they may cause serious stomach or intestinal bleeding. Tell your doctor or other healthcare professional if you have severe stomach pain or stomach pain that keeps returning. Call your doctor or other healthcare professional right away if you have black, tarry-looking bowel movements (stools), if you vomit dark material that looks like coffee grounds, or if you notice any blood in your bowel movements. Any of these symptoms may be a sign of a bleeding ulcer.

Proton Pump Inhibitors

Proton pump inhibitors (PPIs) help prevent the stomach from making acid. Proton pump inhibitors are usually prescribed for heartburn and peptic ulcer disease. With peptic ulcer disease caused by *H. pylori*, you may also be prescribed antibiotics or *Pepto-Bismol®* (bismuth subsalicylate). Proton pump inhibitors may also help to prevent ulcers in a person who is taking nonsteroidal anti-inflammatory drugs (NSAIDs) such as *Motrin®* (ibuprofen), *Aleve®* (naproxen), *Vioxx®* (rofecoxib), *Celebrex®* (celecoxib), and others—see Glossary.

Brand Name	Generic Name
Aciphex®	rabeprazole
Prevacid®	lansoprazole
Prilosec®	omeprazole
Protonix®	pantoprazole

 ## How Will I Take Proton Pump Inhibitors?

Proton pump inhibitors are available in pill form. *Aciphex®* (rabeprazole) is usually taken 30 minutes after breakfast. Other proton pump inhibitors are usually taken 1 to 2 times a day before meals. Your doctor or other healthcare professional will tell you how many times a day to take your medication.

Most of these medications are usually swallowed whole and are not to be crushed, opened, or chewed. However, if you have difficulty swallowing, *Prevacid®* (lansoprazole) capsules may be opened and the contents may be mixed in with a tablespoon of soft food such as applesauce and swallowed right away. The granules should not be crushed or chewed.

If you miss a dose of this medication, take the dose you missed as soon as possible. However, if it is almost time for your next dose, skip the missed dose and just take the next one. Do not double your dose. Take your medication exactly as directed by your doctor or other healthcare professional. Do not stop taking a prescription medication unless directed by your doctor or other healthcare professional.

What Side Effects Can Proton Pump Inhibitors Cause?

Less Common

- Constipation
- Cough
- Diarrhea
- Headache
- Nausea
- Vomiting

Rare

- Dizziness
- Rash (skin redness, bumps, itching, or irritation)

Tell your doctor or other healthcare professional if you have side effects that bother you, do not go away, make you worried about taking your medication, or make you want to stop taking your medication.

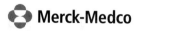

Do Other Medications Interact with Proton Pump Inhibitors?

Proton pump inhibitors *may increase* the side effects of these medications:

- Benzodiazepines such as *Ativan®* (lorazepam), *Klonopin®* (clonazepam), *Xanax®* (alprazolam), and others—see Glossary
- *Coumadin®* (warfarin)
- *Dilantin®* (phenytoin)
- *Neoral®* (cyclosporine)
- *Sandimmune®* (cyclosporine)
- Theophylline such as *Theo-Dur®*, *Uniphyl®*, and others—see Glossary

Proton pump inhibitors *may decrease* how well these medications work:

- *Diflucan®* (fluconazole)
- Iron supplements (ferrous sulfate, ferrous gluconate, and ferrous fumarate)
- *Nizoral®* (ketoconazole)
- *Sporanox®* (itraconazole)

Many nonprescription (over-the-counter [OTC]) medications such as pain, cough, cold, allergy, and sleep medications contain aspirin or nonsteroidal anti-inflammatory drugs (NSAIDs) that can cause indigestion, heartburn, or ulcers. You should talk to your doctor or other healthcare professional before taking any new OTC medications.

These medications may make heartburn, ulcers, or indigestion worse:

- Aspirin, medications that contain aspirin, and aspirin-like medications (salicylates)—see Glossary
- Corticosteroids such as prednisone and others—see Glossary
- Nonsteroidal anti-inflammatory drugs (NSAIDs) such as *Motrin®* (ibuprofen), *Aleve®* (naproxen), *Vioxx®* (rofecoxib), *Celebrex®* (celecoxib), and others—see Glossary

Drinking alcoholic beverages (such as beer, wine, whiskey, and others) may make indigestion, heartburn, or ulcers worse.

Tell your doctor or other healthcare professional about all medications (both prescription and nonprescription [over-the-counter] medications) that you are taking.

 # Warning!

To give you the best care, your doctor or other healthcare professional needs to know about the diseases and medical conditions you have had—your full medical history. Tell your doctor or other healthcare professional if you have or have ever had an allergy or previous reaction to a proton pump inhibitor and/or liver problems.

Stomach pain may be a sign of an ulcer. However, you may have an ulcer without feeling any pain at all. If ulcers are not treated, they may cause serious stomach or intestinal bleeding. Tell your doctor or other healthcare professional if you have severe stomach pain or stomach pain that keeps returning. Call your doctor or other healthcare professional right away if you have black, tarry-looking bowel movements (stools), if you vomit dark material that looks like coffee grounds, or if you notice any blood in your bowel movements. Any of these symptoms may be a sign of a bleeding ulcer.

Carafate® (sucralfate)

Carafate® (sucralfate) forms a protective coating over an ulcer in the lining of the stomach and helps to allow it to heal.

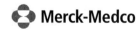

How Will I Take *Carafate*® (sucralfate)?

Carafate® (sucralfate) is usually taken as a pill 2 to 4 times a day, 1 hour before meals and at bedtime. Your doctor or other healthcare professional will tell you how often to take this medication.

If you miss a dose of this medication, take the dose you missed as soon as possible. However, if it is almost time for your next dose, skip the missed dose and just take the next one. Do not double your dose. Take your medication exactly as directed by your doctor or other healthcare professional. Do not stop taking a prescription medication unless directed by your doctor or other healthcare professional.

What Side Effects Can *Carafate*® (sucralfate) Cause?

More Common

- Constipation

Tell your doctor or other healthcare professional if you have side effects that bother you, do not go away, make you worried about taking your medication, or make you want to stop taking your medication.

Do Other Medications Interact with *Carafate*® (sucralfate)?

Carafate® (sucralfate) *may decrease* the absorption of other medications. If you are taking other medications, you should take *Carafate*® (sucralfate) 2 hours before or 1 hour after taking your other medications.

Antacids such as *Maalox*® or *Mylanta*® (aluminum hydroxide/magnesium hydroxide), *Rolaids*® or *Tums*® (calcium carbonate), or *Amphojel*® (aluminum hydroxide) *may decrease* the effects of *Carafate*® (sucralfate) when taken at the same time. If you are using antacids, take *Carafate*® (sucralfate) 1 hour before or 2 hours after taking your antacid.

Many nonprescription (over-the-counter [OTC]) medications such as pain, cough, cold, allergy, and sleep medications contain aspirin or nonsteroidal anti-inflammatory drugs (NSAIDs) that can cause indigestion, heartburn, or ulcers. You should talk to your doctor or other healthcare professional before taking any new OTC medications.

These medications may make indigestion, heartburn, or ulcers worse:

- Aspirin, medications that contain aspirin, and aspirin-like medications (salicylates)—see Glossary

- Corticosteroids such as prednisone and others—see Glossary

- Nonsteroidal anti-inflammatory drugs (NSAIDs) such as *Motrin*® (ibuprofen), *Aleve*® (naproxen), *Vioxx*® (rofecoxib), *Celebrex*® (celecoxib), and others—see Glossary

Drinking alcoholic beverages (such as beer, wine, whiskey, and others) may make indigestion, heartburn, or ulcers worse.

Tell your doctor or other healthcare professional about all medications (both prescription and nonprescription [over-the-counter] medications) that you are taking.

Why Else Do People Take *Carafate*® (sucralfate)?

Carafate® (sucralfate) may be mixed in with water and applied to sores in the mouth caused by chemotherapy for cancer.

 # Warning!

To give you the best care, your doctor or other healthcare professional needs to know about the diseases and medical conditions you have had—your full medical history. Tell your doctor or other healthcare professional if you have or have ever had kidney problems.

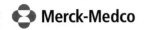

Stomach pain may be a sign of an ulcer. However, you may have an ulcer without feeling any pain at all. If ulcers are not treated, they may cause serious stomach or intestinal bleeding. Tell your doctor or other healthcare professional if you have severe stomach pain or stomach pain that keeps returning. Call your doctor or other healthcare professional right away if you have black, tarry-looking bowel movements (stools), if you vomit dark material that looks like coffee grounds, or if you notice any blood in your bowel movements. Any of these symptoms may be a sign of a bleeding ulcer.

Cytotec® (misoprostol)

Cytotec® (misoprostol) helps to protect the lining of the stomach from the side effects of aspirin and nonsteroidal anti-inflammatory drugs (NSAIDs) such as *Motrin*® (ibuprofen), *Aleve*® (naproxen), and others (see Glossary), and helps reduce the likelihood of developing ulcers.

How Will I Take *Cytotec*® (misoprostol)?

Cytotec® (misoprostol) is usually taken 2 to 4 times a day with meals or after meals and at bedtime. Your doctor or other healthcare professional will tell you how many times a day to take your medication.

If you miss a dose of this medication, take the dose you missed as soon as possible. However, if it is almost time for your next dose, skip the missed dose and just take the next one. Do not double your dose. Take your medication exactly as directed by your doctor or other healthcare professional. Do not stop taking a prescription medication unless directed by your doctor or other healthcare professional.

What Side Effects Can *Cytotec*® (misoprostol) Cause?

More Common

- Diarrhea

- Gas or bloating

- Headache

- Nausea

- Stomach pain

Rare

- Return of periods (menstrual bleeding) after menopause

Tell your doctor or other healthcare professional if you have side effects that bother you, do not go away, make you worried about taking your medication, or make you want to stop taking your medication.

Do Other Medications Interact with *Cytotec*® (misoprostol)?

Antacids that contain magnesium like *Maalox*® and *Mylanta*® (aluminum hydroxide/magnesium hydroxide) ***may increase*** the side effects of *Cytotec*® (misoprostol).

Many nonprescription (over-the-counter [OTC]) medications such as pain, cough, cold, allergy, and sleep medications contain aspirin or nonsteroidal anti-inflammatory drugs (NSAIDs) that can cause indigestion, heartburn, or ulcers. You should talk to your doctor or other healthcare professional before taking any new OTC medications.

These medications may make indigestion, heartburn, or ulcers worse:

- Aspirin, medications that contain aspirin, and aspirin-like medications (salicylates)—see Glossary

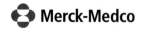
- Corticosteroids such as prednisone and others—see Glossary

- Nonsteroidal anti-inflammatory drugs (NSAIDs) such as *Motrin*® (ibuprofen), *Aleve*® (naproxen), *Vioxx*® (rofecoxib), *Celebrex*® (celecoxib), and others—see Glossary

Drinking alcoholic beverages (such as beer, wine, whiskey, and others) may make indigestion, heartburn, or ulcers worse.

Tell your doctor or other healthcare professional about all medications (both prescription and nonprescription [over-the-counter] medications) that you are taking.

What Else Should I Know about *Cytotec*® (misoprostol)?

Taking *Cytotec*® (misoprostol) with a snack, meal, or milk may help reduce side effects. If diarrhea is a particular problem for you when you take *Cytotec*® (misoprostol), tell your doctor or other healthcare professional about it. Taking a different medication or a lower dose may decrease your side effects. You should not stop taking this medication without first talking to your doctor or other healthcare professional.

 # Warning!

To give you the best care, your doctor or other healthcare professional needs to know about the diseases and medical conditions you have had—your full medical history. Tell your doctor or other healthcare professional if you have or have ever had any of the following:

- Allergy or previous reaction to *Cytotec*® (misoprostol)

- Inflammatory bowel disease (ulcerative colitis or Crohn's disease)

- Kidney problems

- Seizure (epilepsy)

Stomach pain may be a sign of an ulcer. However, you may have an ulcer without feeling any pain at all. If ulcers are not treated, they may cause serious stomach or intestinal bleeding. Tell your doctor or other healthcare professional if you have severe stomach pain or stomach pain that keeps returning. Call your doctor or other healthcare professional right away if you have black, tarry-looking bowel movements (stools), if you vomit dark material that looks like coffee grounds, or if you notice any blood in your bowel movements. Any of these symptoms may be a sign of a bleeding ulcer.

Antacids

Antacids are medications that help to lower or neutralize stomach acid. Most antacids contain aluminum, calcium, or magnesium. While liquid forms of antacids are usually preferred because they start working faster, tablets are more convenient to carry and use. Simethicone is added to some antacids to reduce gas or bloating. If you do not see the name of the antacid you are taking listed below, check the ingredients listed on the label of your medication bottle for whether they contain magnesium, aluminum, calcium, or other ingredients.

Aluminum-Containing Antacids	
Brand Name	**Generic Name**
Alamag™	aluminum/magnesium
AlternaGEL®	aluminum
Amphojel®	aluminum
Basaljel®	aluminum
Di-Gel®	aluminum/magnesium/simethicone
Gaviscon®	aluminum/sodium bicarbonate/calcium/alginic acid
Maalox®	aluminum/magnesium
Riopan®	aluminum/magnesium

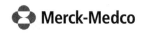
Calcium-Containing Antacids

Brand Name	Generic Name
Alka-Mints®	calcium
Alkets®	calcium/magnesium
Amitone®	calcium
Chooz®	calcium
Dicarbosil®	calcium
Equilet®	calcium
Mallamint™ (sugar-free)	calcium
Rolaids®	calcium/magnesium
Titralac®	calcium
Titralac® Plus	calcium/simethicone
Tums®	calcium

Magnesium-Containing Antacids

Brand Name	Generic Name
Alamag™	aluminum/magnesium
Alkets®	calcium/magnesium
Di-Gel®	aluminum/magnesium/simethicone
Gelusil®	aluminum/magnesium/simethicone
Kudrox®	aluminum/magnesium/simethicone
Maalox®	aluminum/magnesium
Magnalox™	magnesium
Mylanta®	aluminum/magnesium/simethicone
Phillips'® Milk of Magnesia	magnesium
Riopan®	aluminum/magnesium
Riopan Plus®	aluminum/magnesium/simethicone
Rolaids®	calcium/magnesium
Simaal™	aluminum/magnesium/simethicone

Sodium Bicarbonate-Containing Antacids	
Brand Name	**Generic Name**
Bell/ans™	sodium bicarbonate
Bromo-Seltzer®	sodium bicarbonate
Citrocarbonate®	sodium bicarbonate/sodium citrate
Gaviscon®	aluminum/sodium bicarbonate/ calcium/alginic acid, magnesium

How Will I Take Antacids?

Antacids usually come in tablet or liquid form. They are best taken on an empty stomach, 1 hour before or 2 hours after meals. Liquid products provide faster relief than pills or chewable tablets. Antacid tablets should be chewed completely. Pills may be swallowed with milk or water. Antacids are usually taken 1 hour before or 2 hours after taking other medications. Antacids are available without prescription. Follow the instructions given on the package or ask your doctor or other healthcare professional how often to use this medication.

This medication is often used "as needed," so missing a dose should not be a problem. If you miss a dose and it is almost time for the next dose, you should skip the forgotten dose. Do not double the dose. Take your medication as directed by your doctor or other healthcare professional.

What Side Effects Can Antacids Cause?

More Common

- Constipation from antacids that contain aluminum or calcium
- Diarrhea from antacids that contain magnesium

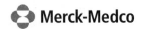

Less Common

- High calcium in your blood (hypercalcemia) from antacids that contain calcium

- High magnesium in your blood from antacids that contain magnesium

- Stomach pain

Tell your doctor or other healthcare professional if you have side effects that bother you, do not go away, make you worried about taking your medication, or make you want to stop taking your medication.

Do Other Medications Interact with Antacids?

Antacids *may decrease* how well many other medications work. If you take an antacid and are also taking any other medication, take the other medication 1 hour before or 2 hours after taking the antacid.

Many nonprescription (over-the-counter [OTC]) medications such as pain, cough, cold, allergy, and sleep medications contain aspirin or nonsteroidal anti-inflammatory drugs (NSAIDs) that can cause indigestion, heartburn, or ulcers. You should talk to your doctor or other healthcare professional before taking any new OTC medications.

These medications may make indigestion, heartburn, or ulcers worse:

- Aspirin, medications that contain aspirin, and aspirin-like medications (salicylates)—see Glossary

- Corticosteroids such as prednisone and others—see Glossary

- Nonsteroidal anti-inflammatory drugs (NSAIDs) such as *Motrin®* (ibuprofen), *Aleve®* (naproxen), *Vioxx®* (rofecoxib), *Celebrex®* (celecoxib), and others—see Glossary

Drinking alcoholic beverages (such as beer, wine, whiskey, and others) may make indigestion, heartburn, or ulcers worse.

Tell your doctor or other healthcare professional about all medications (both prescription and nonprescription [over-the-counter] medications) that you are taking.

 # Warning!

To give you the best care, your doctor or other healthcare professional needs to know about the diseases and medical conditions you have had—your full medical history. Tell your doctor or other healthcare professional if you have or have ever had any of the following:

- Congestive heart failure

- High blood pressure (hypertension)

- Kidney problems

Many antacids, like sodium bicarbonate, contain high levels of salt (sodium). Antacids with a high sodium content can cause you to retain water and may worsen high blood pressure and congestive heart failure. If you have high blood pressure or congestive heart failure, or if you are on a low salt diet, talk to your doctor or other healthcare professional before taking any antacids.

Many antacids contain magnesium that is removed from your body by the kidneys. If you have kidney problems, your kidneys may not be able to remove the magnesium in the antacid from your body, and this may increase magnesium levels in your blood. If you have kidney problems, talk to your doctor or other healthcare professional before taking any antacids.

Antacids are available over-the-counter and do not require a prescription. If you need antacids regularly, you might have a medical problem that needs other treatment. Ask your doctor or other healthcare professional to evaluate your symptoms if you need to use antacids regularly.

Stomach pain may be a sign of an ulcer. However, you may have an ulcer without feeling any pain at all. If ulcers are not treated, they may cause serious stomach or intestinal bleeding. Tell your doctor or other healthcare professional

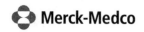

if you have severe stomach pain or stomach pain that keeps returning. Call your doctor or other healthcare professional right away if you have black, tarry-looking bowel movements (stools), if you vomit dark material that looks like coffee grounds, or if you notice any blood in your bowel movements. Any of these symptoms may be a sign of a bleeding ulcer.

Tetracycline

A bacteria called *Helicobacter pylori (H. pylori)* causes most cases of peptic ulcer disease. Tetracycline is an antibiotic that helps fight this bacteria. Taken together with other types of ulcer treatment, it can help kill the bacteria and help keep ulcers from coming back.

 ## How Will I Take Tetracycline?

Tetracycline is usually taken 2 to 4 times a day for 10 to 14 days. It should be taken on an empty stomach, 1 hour before or 2 hours after a meal. Tetracycline should be taken with a full glass of water. Your doctor or other healthcare professional will tell you how many times a day to take your medication.

Tetracycline may be taken along with other antibiotics and an H_2-blocker or a proton pump inhibitor. You may also be told to take *Pepto-Bismol*® (bismuth subsalicylate) along with your antibiotic. Even if you start feeling better, you need to finish the whole prescription to make sure that the infection is completely treated and does not come back.

If you miss a dose of this medication, take the dose you missed as soon as possible. However, if it is almost time for your next dose, skip the missed dose and just take the next one. Do not double your dose. Take your medication exactly as directed by your doctor or other healthcare professional. Do not stop taking a prescription medication unless directed by your doctor or other healthcare professional.

What Side Effects Can Tetracycline Cause?

More Common
- Diarrhea
- Increased sensitivity to the sun (bad sunburn)
- Nausea

Less Common
- Heartburn
- Kidney problems
- Liver problems that may cause yellowing of the skin or eyes (jaundice)
- Peeling of the skin and severe skin rash
- Trouble swallowing
- Vomiting
- Yeast (*Candida*) infection of the vagina

Tell your doctor or other healthcare professional if you have side effects that bother you, do not go away, make you worried about taking your medication, or make you want to stop taking your medication.

Do Other Medications Interact with Tetracycline?

Tetracycline *may increase* the side effects of *Coumadin*® (warfarin) and *Lanoxin*® (digoxin).

The following medications *may decrease* how well tetracycline works:
- Calcium supplements or products that contain calcium such as *Tums*® (calcium carbonate), *Os-Cal*® (calcium carbonate), *Citracal*® (calcium citrate), and others—see Glossary
- Foods that are rich in calcium like milk, cheese, yogurt, and ice cream

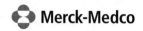

- Iron supplements such as ferrous gluconate and ferrous sulfate and multivitamins or other products that contain iron

Bile acid binders such as *Questran*® (cholestyramine) or *Colestid*® (colestipol) or bulk-forming laxatives like *Metamucil*® (psyllium) ***may decrease*** the effects of tetracycline by preventing it from being absorbed completely. To help make sure it is absorbed so it can work properly, take tetracycline 1 hour before or 4 to 6 hours after taking a bile acid binder or a bulk-forming laxative.

Antacids such as *Maalox*® or *Mylanta*® (aluminum hydroxide/magnesium hydroxide), *Rolaids*® or *Tums*® (calcium carbonate), or *Amphojel*® (aluminum hydroxide) ***may decrease*** the effects of tetracycline when taken at the same time. If you are using antacids, take tetracycline 1 hour before or 2 hours after taking your antacid.

Many nonprescription (over-the-counter [OTC]) medications such as pain, cough, cold, allergy, and sleep medications contain aspirin or nonsteroidal anti-inflammatory drugs (NSAIDs) that can cause indigestion, heartburn, or ulcers. You should talk to your doctor or other healthcare professional before taking any new OTC medications.

These medications may make indigestion, heartburn, or ulcers worse:

- Aspirin, medications that contain aspirin, and aspirin-like medications (salicylates)—see Glossary

- Corticosteroids such as prednisone and others—see Glossary

- Nonsteroidal anti-inflammatory drugs (NSAIDs) such as *Motrin*® (ibuprofen), *Aleve*® (naproxen), *Vioxx*® (rofecoxib), *Celebrex*® (celecoxib), and others—see Glossary

Drinking alcoholic beverages (such as beer, wine, whiskey, and others) may make indigestion, heartburn, or ulcers worse.

Tell your doctor or other healthcare professional about all medications (both prescription and nonprescription [over-the-counter] medications) that you are taking.

Warning!

To give you the best care, your doctor or other healthcare professional needs to know about the diseases and medical conditions you have had—your full medical history. Tell your doctor or other healthcare professional if you have or have ever had any of the following:

- Allergy or previous reaction to any tetracycline antibiotic
- Kidney problems
- Liver problems

If you have diarrhea that is very bad or does not stop, call your doctor or other healthcare professional. This could mean that you have a serious problem that needs medical attention.

Tetracycline can be harmful when it is old and its chemical ingredients break down. Do not take tetracycline after its expiration date. Throw away any tetracycline that is left after your doctor or other healthcare professional has told you to stop taking it.

If you are taking tetracycline, stay out of the sun as much as you can to avoid a serious sunburn. When you do go out in the sun, use sunblock or sunscreen and wear protective clothing such as a wide-brimmed hat and a long-sleeved shirt.

Stomach pain may be a sign of an ulcer. However, you may have an ulcer without feeling any pain at all. If ulcers are not treated, they may cause serious stomach or intestinal bleeding. Tell your doctor or other healthcare professional if you have severe stomach pain or stomach pain that keeps returning. Call your doctor or other healthcare professional right away if you have black, tarry-looking bowel movements (stools), if you vomit dark material that looks like coffee grounds, or if you notice any blood in your bowel movements. Any of these symptoms may be a sign of a bleeding ulcer.

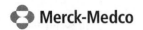

Amoxicillin

A bacteria called *Helicobacter pylori (H. pylori)* causes most cases of peptic ulcer disease. Amoxicillin is an antibiotic that helps fight this bacteria. Taken together with other types of ulcer treatment, it can help kill the bacteria and help keep ulcers from coming back.

How Will I Take Amoxicillin?

Amoxicillin is usually taken 2 to 4 times a day for 10 to 14 days. Amoxicillin may be taken with or without food. Your doctor or other healthcare professional will tell you how many times a day to take your medication.

Amoxicillin may be taken along with other antibiotics and an H_2-blocker or a proton pump inhibitor. You may also be told to take *Pepto-Bismol®* (bismuth subsalicylate) along with your antibiotic. Even if you start feeling better, you need to finish the whole prescription to make sure that the infection is completely treated and does not come back.

If you miss a dose of this medication, take the dose you missed as soon as possible. However, if it is almost time for your next dose, skip the missed dose and just take the next one. Do not double your dose. Take your medication exactly as directed by your doctor or other healthcare professional. Do not stop taking a prescription medication unless directed by your doctor or other healthcare professional.

What Side Effects Can Amoxicillin Cause?

More Common

- Diarrhea
- Nausea
- Vomiting

Less Common

- Allergic reactions such as rash (skin redness, bumps, itching, or irritation), swelling of the face and throat, or trouble breathing

- Yeast (*Candida*) infection of the vagina

Tell your doctor or other healthcare professional if you have side effects that bother you, do not go away, make you worried about taking your medication, or make you want to stop taking your medication.

Do Other Medications Interact with Amoxicillin?

Amoxicillin **may increase** the side effects of *Rheumatrex®* (methotrexate).

Benemid® (probenecid) **may increase** the side effects of amoxicillin.

Bile acid binders such as *Questran®* (cholestyramine) or *Colestid®* (colestipol) or bulk-forming laxatives like *Metamucil®* (psyllium) **may decrease** the effects of amoxicillin by preventing it from being absorbed completely. To help make sure it is absorbed so it can work properly, take amoxicillin 1 hour before or 4 to 6 hours after taking a bile acid binder or a bulk-forming laxative.

Many nonprescription (over-the-counter [OTC]) medications such as pain, cough, cold, allergy, and sleep medications contain aspirin or nonsteroidal anti-inflammatory drugs (NSAIDs) that can cause indigestion, heartburn, or ulcers. You should talk to your doctor or other healthcare professional before taking any new OTC medications.

These medications may make indigestion, heartburn, or ulcers worse:

- Aspirin, medications that contain aspirin, and aspirin-like medications (salicylates)—see Glossary

- Corticosteroids such as prednisone and others—see Glossary

- Nonsteroidal anti-inflammatory drugs (NSAIDs) such as *Motrin®* (ibuprofen), *Aleve®* (naproxen), *Vioxx®* (rofecoxib), *Celebrex®* (celecoxib), and others—see Glossary

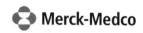

Drinking alcoholic beverages (such as beer, wine, whiskey, and others) may make indigestion, heartburn, or ulcers worse.

Tell your doctor or other healthcare professional about all medications (both prescription and nonprescription [over-the-counter] medications) that you are taking.

Warning!

To give you the best care, your doctor or other healthcare professional needs to know about the diseases and medical conditions you have had—your full medical history. Tell your doctor or other healthcare professional if you have or have ever had an allergy or previous reaction to penicillin, amoxicillin, or other antibiotics and/or kidney problems.

If you have diarrhea that is very bad or does not stop, call your doctor or other healthcare professional. This could mean that you have a serious problem that needs medical attention.

Stomach pain may be a sign of an ulcer. However, you may have an ulcer without feeling any pain at all. If ulcers are not treated, they may cause serious stomach or intestinal bleeding. Tell your doctor or other healthcare professional if you have severe stomach pain or stomach pain that keeps returning. Call your doctor or other healthcare professional right away if you have black, tarry-looking bowel movements (stools), if you vomit dark material that looks like coffee grounds, or if you notice any blood in your bowel movements. Any of these symptoms may be a sign of a bleeding ulcer.

Biaxin® (clarithromycin)

A bacteria called *Helicobacter pylori (H. pylori)* causes most cases of peptic ulcer disease. *Biaxin*® (clarithromycin) is an antibiotic that helps fight this bacteria. Taken together with other types of ulcer treatment, it can help kill the bacteria and help keep ulcers from coming back.

How Will I Take *Biaxin*® (clarithromycin)?

Biaxin® (clarithromycin) is usually taken 1 to 2 times a day for 10 to 14 days. It may be taken with food to help prevent stomach upset. Your doctor or other healthcare professional will tell you how many times a day to take your medication.

Biaxin® (clarithromycin) may be taken along with an H_2-blocker or a proton pump inhibitor. You may also be told to take *Pepto-Bismol*® (bismuth subsalicylate) along with your antibiotic. Even if you start feeling better, you need to finish the whole prescription to make sure that the infection is completely treated and does not come back.

If you miss a dose of this medication, take the dose you missed as soon as possible. However, if it is almost time for your next dose, skip the missed dose and just take the next one. Do not double your dose. Take your medication exactly as directed by your doctor or other healthcare professional. Do not stop taking a prescription medication unless directed by your doctor or other healthcare professional.

What Side Effects Can *Biaxin*® (clarithromycin) Cause?

More Common

- Changes in taste

- Diarrhea

- Headache

- Nausea

- Stomach pain

Less Common

- Allergic reactions such as rash (skin redness, bumps, itching, or irritation), swelling of the face and throat, or trouble breathing

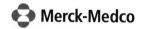

- Fast or irregular heartbeat (palpitations)

- Liver problems that may cause yellowing of the skin or eyes (jaundice)

Rare

- Frequent fever, sore throat, or flu-like symptoms that may be a sign of low white blood cells

---

Tell your doctor or other healthcare professional if you have side effects that bother you, do not go away, make you worried about taking your medication, or make you want to stop taking your medication.

 ## Do Other Medications Interact with *Biaxin*® (clarithromycin)?

Biaxin® (clarithromycin) *may increase* the side effects of these medications:

- Benzodiazepines such as *Ativan*® (lorazepam), *Klonopin*® (clonazepam), *Xanax*® (alprazolam), and others—see Glossary

- *BuSpar*® (buspirone)

- *Cafergot*® (ergotamine)

- *Coumadin*® (warfarin)

- *Ergomar*® (ergotamine)

- *Lanoxin*® (digoxin)

- *Neoral*® (cyclosporine)

- *Norpace*® (disopyramide)

- *Orap*® (pimozide)

- *Rifadin*® (rifampin)

- *Sandimmune*® (cyclosporine)

- Statins such as *Lipitor*® (atorvastatin), *Pravachol*® (pravastatin), *Zocor*® (simvastatin), and others—see Glossary

- *Tegretol*® (carbamazepine)

- Theophylline such as *Theo-Dur*®, *Uniphyl*®, and others—see Glossary

- *Wigraine*® (ergotamine)

Biaxin® (clarithromycin) is generally not prescribed for anyone who is taking *Propulsid*® (cisapride [withdrawn from general distribution; available only by special arrangement with the manufacturer]), *Seldane*® (terfenadine [no longer commercially available]), or *Hismanal*® (astemizole [no longer commercially available]), because together they ***may cause*** serious, sometimes fatal, heart problems.

Many nonprescription (over-the-counter [OTC]) medications such as pain, cough, cold, allergy, and sleep medications contain aspirin or nonsteroidal anti-inflammatory drugs (NSAIDs) that can cause indigestion, heartburn, or ulcers. You should talk to your doctor or other healthcare professional before taking any new OTC medications.

These medications may make indigestion, heartburn, or ulcers worse:

- Aspirin, medications that contain aspirin, and aspirin-like medications (salicylates)—see Glossary

- Corticosteroids such as prednisone and others—see Glossary

- Nonsteroidal anti-inflammatory drugs (NSAIDs) such as *Motrin*® (ibuprofen), *Aleve*® (naproxen), *Vioxx*® (rofecoxib), *Celebrex*® (celecoxib), and others—see Glossary

Drinking alcoholic beverages (such as beer, wine, whiskey, and others) may make indigestion, heartburn, or ulcers worse.

Tell your doctor or other healthcare professional about all medications (both prescription and nonprescription [over-the-counter] medications) that you are taking.

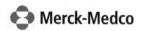

(STOP) **Warning!**

To give you the best care, your doctor or other healthcare professional needs to know about the diseases and medical conditions you have had—your full medical history. Tell your doctor or other healthcare professional if you have or have ever had any of the following:

- Allergy or previous reaction to *Biaxin*® (clarithromycin) or erythromycin such as *Ery-Tab*®, *Erythrocin*®, and others—see Glossary

- Heart rhythm problems (arrhythmia)

- Kidney problems

- Liver problems

If you have diarrhea that is very bad or does not stop, call your doctor or other healthcare professional. This could mean that you have a serious problem that needs medical attention.

Stomach pain may be a sign of an ulcer. However, you may have an ulcer without feeling any pain at all. If ulcers are not treated, they may cause serious stomach or intestinal bleeding. Tell your doctor or other healthcare professional if you have severe stomach pain or stomach pain that keeps returning. Call your doctor or other healthcare professional right away if you have black, tarry-looking bowel movements (stools), if you vomit dark material that looks like coffee grounds, or if you notice any blood in your bowel movements. Any of these symptoms may be a sign of a bleeding ulcer.

Flagyl® (metronidazole)

A bacteria called *Helicobacter pylori (H. pylori)* causes most cases of peptic ulcer disease. *Flagyl*® (metronidazole) is an antibiotic that helps fight this bacteria. Taken together with other types of ulcer treatment, it can help kill the bacteria and help keep ulcers from coming back.

How Will I Take *Flagyl®* (metronidazole)?

Flagyl® (metronidazole) is usually taken 3 to 4 times a day for 10 to 14 days. It may be taken with food to help prevent stomach upset. Your doctor or other healthcare professional will tell you how many times a day to take your medication.

Flagyl® (metronidazole) may be taken along with other antibiotics and an H$_2$-blocker or a proton pump inhibitor. You may also be told to take *Pepto-Bismol®* (bismuth subsalicylate) along with your antibiotic. Even if you start feeling better, you need to finish the whole prescription to make sure that the infection is completely treated and does not come back.

If you miss a dose of this medication, take the dose you missed as soon as possible. However, if it is almost time for your next dose, skip the missed dose and just take the next one. Do not double your dose. Take your medication exactly as directed by your doctor or other healthcare professional. Do not stop taking a prescription medication unless directed by your doctor or other healthcare professional.

What Side Effects Can *Flagyl®* (metronidazole) Cause?

More Common

- Diarrhea
- Dizziness
- Headache
- Nausea
- Poor appetite
- Vomiting

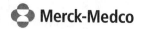

Less Common

- Allergic reactions such as rash (skin redness, bumps, itching, or irritation), swelling of the face and throat, or trouble breathing

- Change in taste

- Frequent fever, sore throat, or flu-like symptoms that may be a sign of low white blood cells

- Low red blood cells (anemia)

- Seizures

- Tingling, pain, or weakness in hands and feet

- Yeast (*Candida*) infection of the vagina

Tell your doctor or other healthcare professional if you have side effects that bother you, do not go away, make you worried about taking your medication, or make you want to stop taking your medication.

Do Other Medications Interact with *Flagyl*® (metronidazole)?

Flagyl® (metronidazole) *may increase* the side effects of these medications:

- *Antabuse*® (disulfiram)

- *Coumadin*® (warfarin)

- *Dilantin*® (phenytoin)

- Lithium such as *Eskalith*®, *Lithobid*®, and others—see Glossary

Barbiturates, such as *Butisol*® (butabarbital), *Luminal*® (phenobarbital), *Mebaral*® (mephobarbital), and others (see Glossary), *may decrease* how well *Flagyl*® (metronidazole) works.

Flagyl® (metronidazole) may make you feel sick to your stomach, cause reddening of the face (flushing), or cause headaches if you also take or use the following:

- Alcoholic beverages (such as beer, wine, whiskey, and others)

- Elixirs or other liquid medications that contain alcohol

- Mouthwash and throat sprays that contain alcohol

Many nonprescription (over-the-counter [OTC]) medications such as pain, cough, cold, allergy, and sleep medications contain aspirin or nonsteroidal anti-inflammatory drugs (NSAIDs) that can cause indigestion, heartburn, or ulcers. You should talk to your doctor or other healthcare professional before taking any new OTC medications.

These medications may make indigestion, heartburn, or ulcers worse:

- Aspirin, medications that contain aspirin, and aspirin-like medications (salicylates)—see Glossary

- Corticosteroids such as prednisone and others—see Glossary

- Nonsteroidal anti-inflammatory drugs (NSAIDs) such as *Motrin®* (ibuprofen), *Aleve®* (naproxen), *Vioxx®* (rofecoxib), *Celebrex®* (celecoxib), and others—see Glossary

Drinking alcoholic beverages (such as beer, wine, whiskey, and others) may make indigestion, heartburn, or ulcers worse.

Tell your doctor or other healthcare professional about all medications (both prescription and nonprescription [over-the-counter] medications) that you are taking.

 # Warning!

To give you the best care, your doctor or other healthcare professional needs to know about the diseases and medical conditions you have had—your full medical history. Tell your doctor or other healthcare professional if you have or have ever had any of the following:

- Allergy or previous reaction to *Flagyl®* (metronidazole)

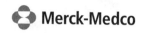

- High alcohol intake (drinking 3 or more alcoholic beverages, such as beer, wine, whiskey, and others, every day)

- Liver problems

- Low red blood cells (anemia)

- Seizures (epilepsy)

Do not drink any alcoholic beverage (such as beer, wine, whiskey, and others) while you are taking *Flagyl®* (metronidazole) or for 3 days after you have stopped taking *Flagyl®* (metronidazole). The combination of *Flagyl®* (metronidazole) and alcohol may cause stomach pain, nausea, vomiting, headaches, and reddening of the face (flushing).

Do not take *Flagyl®* (metronidazole) if you have taken *Antabuse®* (disulfiram) within 2 weeks.

If you have diarrhea that is very bad or does not stop, call your doctor or other healthcare professional. This could mean that you have a serious problem that needs medical attention.

Stomach pain may be a sign of an ulcer. However, you may have an ulcer without feeling any pain at all. If ulcers are not treated, they may cause serious stomach or intestinal bleeding. Tell your doctor or other healthcare professional if you have severe stomach pain or stomach pain that keeps returning. Call your doctor or other healthcare professional right away if you have black, tarry-looking bowel movements (stools), if you vomit dark material that looks like coffee grounds, or if you notice any blood in your bowel movements. Any of these symptoms may be a sign of a bleeding ulcer.

If you have had seizures in the past, tell your doctor or other healthcare professional because *Flagyl®* (metronidazole) may cause seizures. Stopping this medication suddenly may also cause seizures. If your doctor or other healthcare professional decides that you should stop taking *Flagyl®* (metronidazole), pay careful attention to the instructions he or she gives you about how much less to take and for how long.

Pepto-Bismol® (bismuth subsalicylate)

How Will I Take *Pepto-Bismol®* (bismuth subsalicylate)?

Pepto-Bismol® (bismuth subsalicylate) is usually taken 4 times a day for peptic ulcer disease. It may be used "as needed" for indigestion. Your doctor or other healthcare professional will tell you how many times a day to take your medication.

If you miss a dose of this medication, take the dose you missed as soon as possible. However, if it is almost time for your next dose, skip the missed dose and just take the next one. Do not double your dose. Take your medication exactly as directed by your doctor or other healthcare professional. Do not stop taking a prescription medication unless directed by your doctor or other healthcare professional.

What Side Effects Can *Pepto-Bismol®* (bismuth subsalicylate) Cause?

More Common

- Darkening of the tongue and bowel movements (harmless and temporary)

Less Common

- Constipation
- Dizziness
- Headache
- Ringing in the ears (tinnitus)

Rare

- Blurred vision
- Confusion

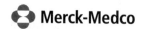

- Increased thirst
- Rapid breathing

Tell your doctor or other healthcare professional if you have side effects that bother you, do not go away, make you worried about taking your medication, or make you want to stop taking your medication.

 ## Do Other Medications Interact with *Pepto-Bismol*® (bismuth subsalicylate)?

Pepto-Bismol® (bismuth subsalicylate) ***may increase*** the side effects of these medications:

- *Coumadin*® (warfarin)
- *Depakene*® (valproic acid)
- Diabetes medications such as *DiaBeta*® (glyburide), *Glucophage*® (metformin), *Glucotrol*® (glipizide), and others—see Glossary
- Insulin
- Nonsteroidal anti-inflammatory drugs (NSAIDs) such as *Motrin*® (ibuprofen), *Aleve*® (naproxen), *Vioxx*® (rofecoxib), *Celebrex*® (celecoxib), and others—see Glossary
- *Rheumatrex*® (methotrexate)

Pepto-Bismol® (bismuth subsalicylate) ***may decrease*** how well these medications work:

- *Anturane*® (sulfinpyrazone)
- *Benemid*® (probenecid)
- High blood pressure (hypertension) medications and diuretics (water pills)—see Glossary

Corticosteroids such as prednisone and others (see Glossary) *may decrease* how well *Pepto-Bismol®* (bismuth subsalicylate) works.

Many nonprescription (over-the-counter [OTC]) medications such as pain, cough, cold, allergy, and sleep medications contain aspirin or nonsteroidal anti-inflammatory drugs (NSAIDs) that can cause indigestion, heartburn, or ulcers. You should talk to your doctor or other healthcare professional before taking any new OTC medications.

These medications may make indigestion, heartburn, or ulcers worse:

- Aspirin, medications that contain aspirin, and aspirin-like medications (salicylates)—see Glossary

- Corticosteroids such as prednisone and others—see Glossary

- Nonsteroidal anti-inflammatory drugs (NSAIDs) such as *Motrin®* (ibuprofen), *Aleve®* (naproxen), *Vioxx®* (rofecoxib), *Celebrex®* (celecoxib), and others—see Glossary

Drinking alcoholic beverages (such as beer, wine, whiskey, and others) may make indigestion, heartburn, or ulcers worse.

Antacids such as *Maalox®* or *Mylanta®* (aluminum hydroxide/magnesium hydroxide), *Rolaids®* or *Tums®* (calcium carbonate), or *Amphojel®* (aluminum hydroxide) *may decrease* the effects of *Pepto-Bismol®* (bismuth subsalicylate) when taken at the same time. If you are using antacids, take *Pepto-Bismol®* (bismuth subsalicylate) 1 hour before or 2 hours after taking your antacid.

Tell your doctor or other healthcare professional about all medications (both prescription and nonprescription [over-the-counter] medications) that you are taking.

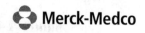

(STOP) **Warning!**

To give you the best care, your doctor or other healthcare professional needs to know about the diseases and medical conditions you have had—your full medical history. Tell your doctor or other healthcare professional if you have or have ever had any of the following:

- Allergy or previous reaction to *Pepto-Bismol*® (bismuth subsalicylate), aspirin, or nonsteroidal anti-inflammatory drugs (NSAIDs) such as *Motrin*® (ibuprofen), *Aleve*® (naproxen), *Vioxx*® (rofecoxib), *Celebrex*® (celecoxib), and others—see Glossary

- Asthma or nasal polyps (overgrowth of tissue in the nasal lining)

- Bleeding problems

- Diabetes

- High alcohol intake (drinking 3 or more alcoholic beverages such as beer, wine, whiskey, and others, every day)

- Kidney problems

- Liver problems

- Seizures (epilepsy)

- Stomach problems (ulcer)

Stomach pain may be a sign of an ulcer. However, you may have an ulcer without feeling any pain at all. If ulcers are not treated, they may cause serious stomach or intestinal bleeding. Tell your doctor or other healthcare professional if you have severe stomach pain or stomach pain that keeps returning. Call your doctor or other healthcare professional right away if you have black, tarry-looking bowel movements (stools), if you vomit dark material that looks like coffee grounds, or if you notice any blood in your bowel movements. Any of these symptoms may be a sign of a bleeding ulcer.

Aspirin may cause a serious, even fatal illness called Reye's syndrome when given to children with flu-like symptoms. *Pepto-Bismol*® (bismuth subsalicylate) is aspirin-like medication. Do not give *Pepto-Bismol*® (bismuth subsalicylate) to children without talking to a doctor or other healthcare professional.

Reglan® (metoclopramide)

Reglan® (metoclopramide) may be used for heartburn. It helps to move the food through the stomach and helps to prevent acid from flowing back up into the tube that connects the mouth to the stomach (esophagus).

How Will I Take *Reglan*® (metoclopramide)?

Reglan® (metoclopramide) is available as a pill or liquid. It is usually taken 4 times a day, 30 minutes before each meal and at bedtime. Your doctor or other healthcare professional will tell you how many times a day to take your medication.

If you miss a dose of this medication, take the dose you missed as soon as possible. However, if it is almost time for your next dose, skip the missed dose and just take the next one. Do not double your dose. Take your medication exactly as directed by your doctor or other healthcare professional. Do not stop taking a prescription medication unless directed by your doctor or other healthcare professional.

What Side Effects Can *Reglan*® (metoclopramide) Cause?

More Common

- Diarrhea

- Drowsiness

- Nausea

- Nervousness (anxiety)

- Tiredness or sluggishness (fatigue)

- Weakness

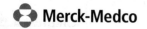

Less Common

- Dizziness

- Jerking motions, uncontrollable, repetitive movements of the face, neck, and arms (tics)

- Sadness, feeling blue or down, depressed mood (depression)

- Seizures

- Shakiness or tremors

Rare

- Breast swelling or discharge

- Fast heartbeat (palpitations)

- Fever

- High blood pressure (hypertension)

- Rash (skin redness, bumps, itching, or irritation)

Tell your doctor or other healthcare professional if you have side effects that bother you, do not go away, make you worried about taking your medication, or make you want to stop taking your medication.

 Do Other Medications Interact with *Reglan*® (metoclopramide)?

The following medications ***may decrease*** how well *Reglan*® (metoclopramide) works:

- Anticholinergic medications such as *Artane*® (trihexyphenidyl), *Cogentin*® (benztropine), and others—see Glossary

- *Sinemet*® (levodopa/carbidopa)

Reglan® (metoclopramide) ***may decrease*** how well these medications work:

- *Lanoxin*® (digoxin)
- Tetracycline antibiotics such as *Dynacin*® (minocycline), *Sumycin*® (tetracycline), *Vibramycin*® (doxycycline), and others—see Glossary

Reglan® (metoclopramide) ***may increase*** the side effects of these medications:

- *Neoral*® (cyclosporine)
- *Sandimmune*® (cyclosporine)

Reglan® (metoclopramide) ***may increase*** the side effects of other medications that cause drowsiness, including antidepressants, antihistamines (allergy medications), benzodiazepines (a type of tranquilizer), anxiety medications, narcotics (pain relievers), muscle relaxants, neuroleptic medications (a type of tranquilizer), seizure medications, or sleep medications. Avoid driving a car and other activities that need mental alertness, like using a knife or operating machinery, while taking this medication.

Reglan® (metoclopramide) is generally not prescribed for anyone who is taking MAO inhibitors, such as *Marplan*® (isocarboxazid), *Nardil*® (phenelzine), or *Parnate*® (tranylcypromine), because together they ***may cause*** serious or even fatal reactions. If your doctor or other healthcare professional wants you to stop taking one medication and start taking the other, you should wait at least 2 weeks between stopping one and starting the other.

Many nonprescription (over-the-counter [OTC]) medications such as pain, cough, cold, allergy, and sleep medications contain aspirin or nonsteroidal anti-inflammatory drugs (NSAIDs) that can cause indigestion, heartburn, or ulcers. You should talk to your doctor or other healthcare professional before taking any new OTC medications.

These medications may make indigestion, heartburn, or ulcers worse:

- Aspirin, medications that contain aspirin, and aspirin-like medications (salicylates)—see Glossary

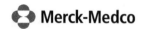

- Corticosteroids such as prednisone and others—see Glossary

- Nonsteroidal anti-inflammatory drugs (NSAIDs) such as *Motrin*®
  (ibuprofen), *Aleve*® (naproxen), *Vioxx*® (rofecoxib), *Celebrex*® (celecoxib),
  and others—see Glossary

Drinking alcoholic beverages (such as beer, wine, whiskey, and others) **may
increase** the side effects of *Reglan*® (metoclopramide). It may also make
indigestion, heartburn, or ulcers worse.

Tell your doctor or other healthcare professional about all medications (both
prescription and nonprescription [over-the-counter] medications) that you are
taking.

Why Else Do People Take *Reglan*® (metoclopramide)?

Reglan® (metoclopramide) may be taken by people who have a problem with
slow digestion (gastroparesis) to help move food from the stomach to the
intestines. *Reglan*® (metoclopramide) can also be used to help prevent nausea
and vomiting in people who are getting treatment for cancer.

 # Warning!

To give you the best care, your doctor or other healthcare professional needs
to know about the diseases and medical conditions you have had—your full
medical history. Tell your doctor or other healthcare professional if you have,
or have ever had, or presently take, any of the following:

- Allergy or previous reaction to *Reglan*® (metoclopramide) or neuroleptic
  medications such as *Risperdal*® (risperidone), *Thorazine*®
  (chlorpromazine), *Zyprexa*® (olanzapine), and others—see Glossary

- High blood pressure (hypertension)

- Kidney problems

- MAO inhibitors such as *Marplan*® (isocarboxazid), *Nardil*® (phenelzine), or *Parnate*® (tranylcypromine)

- Parkinson's disease

- Sadness, feeling blue or down, depressed mood (depression)

- Seizures (epilepsy)

If you have had seizures in the past, tell your doctor or other healthcare professional because *Reglan*® (metoclopramide) may cause seizures. Stopping this medication suddenly may also cause seizures. If your doctor or other healthcare professional decides that you should stop taking *Reglan*® (metoclopramide), pay careful attention to the instructions he or she gives you about how much less to take and for how long.

Stomach pain may be a sign of an ulcer. However, you may have an ulcer without feeling any pain at all. If ulcers are not treated, they may cause serious stomach or intestinal bleeding. Tell your doctor or other healthcare professional if you have severe stomach pain or stomach pain that keeps returning. Call your doctor or other healthcare professional right away if you have black, tarry-looking bowel movements (stools), if you vomit dark material that looks like coffee grounds, or if you notice any blood in your bowel movements. Any of these symptoms may be a sign of a bleeding ulcer.

Reglan® (metoclopramide) may cause drowsiness. Avoid driving a car and other activities that need mental alertness, like using a knife or operating machinery, while taking this medication. Drinking alcoholic beverages (such as beer, wine, whiskey, and others) may increase the side effects.

Propulsid® (cisapride)

Propulsid® (cisapride) helps to move food through your stomach. It is sometimes used for heartburn. Recently, it has been withdrawn from general distribution because of heart rhythm problems that may occur when this medication is taken. It is now available only by special arrangement with the manufacturer.

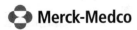

How Will I Take *Propulsid*® (cisapride)?

Propulsid® (cisapride) is available in a pill and a liquid form. It is usually taken 4 times a day, 30 minutes before each meal and at bedtime. Your doctor or other healthcare professional will tell you how many times a day to take your medication.

If you miss a dose of this medication, take the dose you missed as soon as possible. However, if it is almost time for your next dose, skip the missed dose and just take the next one. Do not double your dose. Take your medication exactly as directed by your doctor or other healthcare professional. Do not stop taking a prescription medication unless directed by your doctor or other healthcare professional.

What Side Effects Can *Propulsid*® (cisapride) Cause?

More Common

- Diarrhea
- Gas and bloating
- Nausea
- Stomach pain

Less Common

- Constipation
- Dizziness
- Fast or irregular heartbeat (palpitations) which may be serious or even fatal
- Headache
- Muscle aches and spasms
- Rash (skin redness, bumps, itching, or irritation)

- Trouble falling asleep or staying asleep (insomnia)
- Vision problems

Do Other Medications Interact with *Propulsid*® (cisapride)?

Propulsid® (cisapride) ***may increase*** the side effects of the following medications:

- Benzodiazepines such as *Ativan*® (lorazepam), *Klonopin*® (clonazepam), *Xanax*® (alprazolam), and others—see Glossary
- *Coumadin*® (warfarin)
- *Procardia*® (nifedipine)

The following medications ***may increase*** the side effects of *Propulsid*® (cisapride) and may cause serious, even fatal reactions:

- *Biaxin*® (clarithromycin)
- *Diamox*® (acetazolamide)
- *Diflucan*® (fluconazole)
- Diuretics (water pills) such as *HydroDIURIL*® (hydrochlorothiazide or HCTZ), *Lasix*® (furosemide), and others—see Glossary
- Erythromycin such as *Ery-Tab*®, *Erythrocin*®, and others—see Glossary
- *Flexeril*® (cyclobenzaprine)
- Heart rhythm problem (arrhythmia) medications—see Glossary
- *Hismanal*® (astemizole [no longer commercially available])
- *Ludiomil*® (maprotiline)
- *Luvox*® (fluvoxamine)
- *Neptazane*® (methazolamide)
- Neuroleptic medications such as *Risperdal*® (risperidone), *Thorazine*® (chlorpromazine), *Zyprexa*® (olanzapine), and others—see Glossary
- *Nizoral*® (ketoconazole)

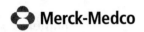

- Protease inhibitors such as *Crixivan®* (indinavir), *Norvir®* (ritonavir), and others—see Glossary

- Quinidine such as *Quinaglute®*, *Quinidex®*, and others—see Glossary

- *Reglan®* (metoclopramide)

- *Rescriptor®* (delavirdine)

- *Seldane®* (terfenadine [no longer commercially available])

- *Serzone®* (nefazodone)

- *Sporanox®* (itraconazole)

- *Sustiva®* (efavirenz)

- Tricyclic antidepressants such as *Elavil®* (amitriptyline), *Pamelor®* (nortriptyline), *Sinequan®* (doxepin), and others—see Glossary

- *Vascor®* (bepridil)

- *Zagam®* (sparfloxacin)

Antispasmodic (see Glossary) medications **may decrease** how well *Propulsid®* (cisapride) works.

Propulsid® (cisapride) **may increase** the side effects of alcoholic beverages (such as beer, wine, whiskey, and others). Drinking alcoholic beverages may also make indigestion, heartburn, or ulcers worse.

Many medications interact with *Propulsid®* (cisapride) and **may cause** serious, even fatal, problems. Talk to your doctor or other healthcare professional before taking any medication while taking *Propulsid®* (cisapride).

Many nonprescription (over-the-counter [OTC]) medications such as pain, cough, cold, allergy, and sleep medications contain aspirin or nonsteroidal anti-inflammatory drugs (NSAIDs) that can cause indigestion, heartburn, or ulcers. You should talk to your doctor or other healthcare professional before taking any new OTC medications.

These medications may make indigestion, heartburn, or ulcers worse:

- Aspirin, medications that contain aspirin, and aspirin-like medications (salicylates)—see Glossary

- Corticosteroids such as prednisone and others—see Glossary

- Nonsteroidal anti-inflammatory drugs (NSAIDs) such as *Motrin*®
(ibuprofen), *Aleve*® (naproxen), *Vioxx*® (rofecoxib), *Celebrex*® (celecoxib),
and others—see Glossary

Grapefruit and grapefruit juice *may increase* the side effects of *Propulsid*®
(cisapride). This interaction can happen whether you eat the grapefruit or drink
the grapefruit juice at the same time as you take your medication or if you take
the medication separately from the grapefruit or grapefruit juice. Talk to your
doctor or other healthcare professional before eating grapefruit or drinking
grapefruit juice if you are taking this medication. Please also read the discussion
on A Warning about Grapefruit and Grapefruit Juice on pages i-ii.

Tell your doctor or other healthcare professional about all medications (both
prescription and nonprescription [over-the-counter] medications) that you are
taking.

 # Warning!

To give you the best care, your doctor or other healthcare professional needs
to know about the diseases and medical conditions you have had—your full
medical history. Tell your doctor or other healthcare professional if you have
or have ever had any of the following:

- Allergy or previous reaction to *Propulsid*® (cisapride)

- Congestive heart failure

- Heart rhythm problems (arrhythmia)

- Kidney problems

- Liver problems

Stomach pain may be a sign of an ulcer. However, you may have an ulcer
without feeling any pain at all. If ulcers are not treated, they may cause serious
stomach or intestinal bleeding. Tell your doctor or other healthcare professional

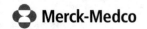

if you have severe stomach pain or stomach pain that keeps returning. Call your doctor or other healthcare professional right away if you have black, tarry-looking bowel movements (stools), if you vomit dark material that looks like coffee grounds, or if you notice any blood in your bowel movements. Any of these symptoms may be a sign of a bleeding ulcer.

Propulsid® (cisapride) increases the effects of alcoholic beverages (such as beer, wine, whiskey, and others) and may cause more drowsiness. Avoid driving a car and other activities that need mental alertness, like using a knife or operating machinery, while taking this medication and drinking alcoholic beverages (such as beer, wine, whiskey, and others).

Chapter 12

High Blood Pressure

What Is High Blood Pressure (Hypertension)?

The heart pumps blood through blood vessels to carry oxygen and nutrients throughout the body. As blood flows through the vessels, it puts pressure on the walls of the blood vessels. Blood pressure is the measurement of the pressure against the walls of the blood vessels. The higher the pressure, the harder the heart has to work.

Blood pressure is measured in millimeters of mercury (mm Hg). Measuring your blood pressure results in two numbers. The top number, systolic pressure, is the pressure each time the heart beats. The bottom number, diastolic pressure, is the pressure between beats. A normal blood pressure reading is 120/80 mm Hg.

If you have high blood pressure (hypertension), it means that your pressure is higher than normal. High blood pressure is most often defined as having a systolic pressure above 140 mm Hg, a diastolic pressure above 90 mm Hg, or both.

While high blood pressure is one of the most common medical problems and occurs in about one quarter of people in the United States, it is not a normal part of getting older. It is common for older adults to have a high systolic (top number) with a normal diastolic (low number) blood pressure. This is called isolated systolic hypertension. Having isolated systolic hypertension is just as serious as having both numbers high.

High blood pressure is sometimes called a "silent killer" because it often does not cause any obvious symptoms. If high blood pressure is not treated, it may lead to complications, such as heart attack (myocardial infarction), stroke, congestive heart failure, or kidney problems. Treatment of high blood pressure has been shown to help reduce the risk of stroke, heart attack, and death in both younger and older adults.

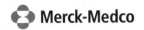

Factors that increase your risk of developing high blood pressure include:

- Being overweight
- Drinking more than 2 alcoholic beverages (such as beer, wine, whiskey, and others) every day
- A high-salt (sodium) diet
- Not getting enough exercise

Have your blood pressure checked regularly. If you have high blood pressure, there are a number of things that you and your doctor or other healthcare professional can do to help improve your blood pressure. For example, you may lower the amount of salt (sodium) you eat, lose weight, get regular exercise, quit smoking, drink fewer alcoholic beverages (such as beer, wine, whiskey, and others), and take blood pressure medication. Check with your doctor or other healthcare professional before starting an exercise program.

Medications for High Blood Pressure

Several kinds of medications may be taken for high blood pressure. This chapter discusses these medications and/or categories of medications:

MEDICATIONS	See Page
Thiazide and Loop Diuretics (Water Pills)	375
Potassium-Sparing Diuretics (Water Pills)	382
Beta Blockers	386
Angiotensin-Converting Enzyme (ACE) Inhibitors	392
Angiotensin II (A-II) Blockers	397
Calcium Channel Blockers	401
Aldomet® (methyldopa)	408
Catapres® (clonidine)	413
Alpha Blockers	417
Apresoline® (hydralazine)	421
Loniten® (minoxidil)	426

If you do not see the exact name of the medication that you take for high blood pressure listed above, check the Medication and Chapter Table to find out which category your medication falls under or check the Index.

Thiazide and Loop Diuretics (Water Pills)

Thiazide and loop diuretics (water pills) are used to help reduce high blood pressure. They increase the amount of urine that your body makes, which helps your kidneys to remove salt (sodium) and water from the body. Thiazides are most often used for high blood pressure. Loop diuretics may be used when a person has high blood pressure and congestive heart failure or kidney problems.

Thiazide and loop diuretics cause potassium to leave the body with sodium and water. Other diuretics, called potassium-sparing diuretics, do not cause potassium to leave the body. In order to help keep potassium blood levels normal, some diuretic medications contain both a thiazide diuretic and a potassium-sparing diuretic. Sometimes diuretics are also combined with other types of blood pressure medications for the convenience of having to take only one pill.

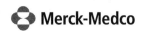

Names of combination blood pressure medications are not listed below. This section only contains information on thiazide and loop diuretics. Check the Medication and Chapter Table if you have questions about which other section to review.

Brand Name	Generic Name	Type of Diuretic
Aldactazide®*	spironolactone/ hydrochlorothiazide	Potassium-Sparing/Thiazide*
Aldactone®	spironolactone	Potassium-Sparing
Aquatensen®	methyclothiazide	Thiazide
Bumex®	bumetanide	Loop
Demadex®	torsemide	Loop
Diucardin®	hydroflumethiazide	Thiazide
Diurese™	trichlormethiazide	Thiazide
Diuril®	chlorothiazide	Thiazide
Dyazide®*	triamterene/ hydrochlorothiazide	Potassium-Sparing/Thiazide*
Dyrenium®	triamterene	Potassium-Sparing
Edecrin®	ethacrynic acid	Loop
Enduron®	methyclothiazide	Thiazide
Exna®	benzthiazide	Thiazide
HydroDIURIL®	hydrochlorothiazide (HCTZ)	Thiazide
Hydromox®	quinethazone	Thiazide
Hygroton®	chlorthalidone	Thiazide

*For convenience, thiazide diuretics are combined with potassium-sparing diuretics for people who need both medications. Please also read the section about Potassium-Sparing Diuretics on pages 382–386. Also, note that diuretics may be combined with other high blood pressure medications. Check the Medication and Chapter Table to find the other medication sections you should read if you are taking a combination medication.

Brand Name	Generic Name	Type of Diuretic
Lasix®	furosemide	Loop
Lozol®	indapamide	Thiazide
Maxzide®*	triamterene/ hydrochlorothiazide	Potassium-Sparing/Thiazide*
Midamor®	amiloride	Potassium-Sparing
Moduretic®*	amiloride/ hydrochlorothiazide	Potassium-Sparing/Thiazide*
Naqua®	trichlormethiazide	Thiazide
Naturetin®	bendroflumethiazide	Thiazide
Renese®	polythiazide	Thiazide
Zaroxolyn®	metolazone	Thiazide

*For convenience, thiazide diuretics are combined with potassium-sparing diuretics for people who need both medications. Please also read the section about Potassium-Sparing Diuretics on pages 382–386. Also, note that diuretics may be combined with other high blood pressure medications. Check the Medication and Chapter Table to find the other medication sections you should read if you are taking a combination medication.

How Will I Take Thiazide and Loop Diuretics?

Thiazide and loop diuretics are usually taken 1 to 2 times daily. If taken only once a day, they are usually taken in the morning. If you need to take them twice a day, do not wait to take the second dose until the evening since it may keep you up at night with frequent urination. If they cause you to have to urinate frequently, you may want to take them after you get back from activities outside your home. Your doctor or other healthcare professional will tell you how many times a day to take your medication.

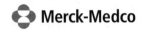

If you miss a dose of this medication, take the dose you missed as soon as possible. However, if it is almost time for your next dose, skip the missed dose and just take the next one. Do not double your dose. Take your medication exactly as directed by your doctor or other healthcare professional. Do not stop taking a prescription medication unless directed by your doctor or other healthcare professional.

What Side Effects Can Thiazide and Loop Diuretics Cause?

More Common

- Gout (very painful, swollen joints)

- Headache

- Increased sensitivity to the sun (bad sunburn)

- Tiredness or sluggishness (fatigue)

- Weakness or muscle cramps that may be a sign of low potassium in your blood (hypokalemia)

Less Common

- Dizziness when standing up from a bed or a chair

- Erection problems (erectile dysfunction)

- Increased thirst and dry mouth with dizziness when standing that may be a sign of excessive water loss (dehydration)

- Increased blood sugar (hyperglycemia)

Rare

- Allergic reactions such as rash (skin redness, bumps, itching, or irritation), swelling of the face and throat, or trouble breathing

- Easy bruising ("black-and-blue" marks on the skin)

- Skin rash with fever and joint pain or swelling that may be a sign of lupus

Tell your doctor or other healthcare professional if you have side effects that bother you, do not go away, make you worried about taking your medication, or make you want to stop taking your medication.

 ## Do Other Medications Interact with Thiazide and Loop Diuretics?

Thiazide and loop diuretics **may cause** low potassium blood levels (hypokalemia), which **may increase** the side effects of *Lanoxin*® (digoxin).

Nonsteroidal anti-inflammatory drugs (NSAIDs), such as *Motrin*® (ibuprofen), *Aleve*® (naproxen), *Vioxx*® (rofecoxib), *Celebrex*® (celecoxib), and others (see Glossary), **may decrease** how well thiazide and loop diuretics work.

Many nonprescription (over-the-counter [OTC]) medications such as antacids, laxatives, pain, cough, cold, and allergy medications contain medications that **may increase** blood pressure. If you are taking blood pressure medication, you should talk to your doctor or other healthcare professional before taking any new OTC medications.

Thiazide and loop diuretics **may increase** the side effects of lithium such as *Eskalith*®, *Lithobid*®, and others—see Glossary.

Other high blood pressure medications (see Glossary) **may increase** the effects of thiazide and loop diuretics.

Bile acid binders such as *Questran*® (cholestyramine) or *Colestid*® (colestipol) or bulk-forming laxatives like *Metamucil*® (psyllium) **may decrease** the effects of thiazide and loop diuretics by preventing them from being absorbed completely. To help make sure they are absorbed so they can work properly, take your thiazide or loop diuretic 1 hour before or 4 to 6 hours after taking a bile acid binder or a bulk-forming laxative.

Thiazide or loop diuretics **may decrease** how well diabetes medications such as *Glynase*® (glyburide), *Glucotrol*® (glipizide), and others (see Glossary) work.

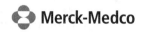

Thiazide and loop diuretics must be used carefully if prescribed for anyone who is taking *Propulsid®* (cisapride [withdrawn from general distribution; available only by special arrangement with the manufacturer]), *Seldane®* (terfenadine [no longer commercially available]), or *Hismanal®* (astemizole [no longer commercially available]), because the low potassium blood levels that may be caused by diuretics ***may cause*** serious, sometimes fatal, heart problems when taken with these medications.

Tell your doctor or other healthcare professional about all medications (both prescription and nonprescription [over-the-counter] medications) that you are taking.

Why Else Do People Take Thiazide and Loop Diuretics?

Thiazide and loop diuretics are sometimes used to help reduce puffiness or swelling of the legs and ankles (edema) and to help treat kidney problems, congestive heart failure, and liver problems.

What Else Should I Know about Thiazide and Loop Diuretics?

Medications cannot cure high blood pressure, but they can help control it and help reduce the chance of stroke, heart attack (myocardial infarction), congestive heart failure, kidney failure, and death. It is important to take your blood pressure medication daily as prescribed to help reduce your risks. Keeping your weight down, eating a healthy diet that is low in salt (sodium), and exercising regularly will also help control your blood pressure. Ask your doctor or other healthcare professional for a diet and exercise plan.

Have your blood pressure checked regularly as directed by your doctor or other healthcare professional.

Warning!

To give you the best care, your doctor or other healthcare professional needs to know about the diseases and medical conditions you have had—your full medical history. Tell your doctor or other healthcare professional if you have or have ever had any of the following:

- Allergy or previous reaction to any of the following:

  ◆ Carbonic anhydrase inhibitors such as *Azopt*® (brinzolamide), *Diamox*® (acetazolamide), *Trusopt*® (dorzolamide), and others—see Glossary

  ◆ Diabetes medications such as *DiaBeta*® (glyburide), *Glucophage*® (metformin), *Glucotrol*® (glipizide), and others—see Glossary

  ◆ Diuretics (water pills) such as *HydroDIURIL*® (hydrochlorothiazide or HCTZ), *Lasix*® (furosemide), and others—see Glossary

  ◆ Sulfa medications such as *Bactrim*™, *Septra*®, and others—see Glossary

- Diabetes

- Gout

- Kidney problems

- Liver problems

- Lupus

Because diuretics can cause low potassium blood levels (hypokalemia) and high blood sugar (hyperglycemia), your doctor or other healthcare professional may order blood tests to check your potassium levels and blood sugar (glucose).

Dehydration (excessive water loss) can be a problem for older adults. Increased thirst, dry mouth, weakness or dizziness when standing up from a bed or a chair, and dark or decreased urine may be signs of dehydration. Diuretics may cause dehydration by themselves, but it is more likely to occur during very hot weather, after vigorous exercise, or when you have severe diarrhea or vomiting. If not treated, this can be serious. Call your doctor or other healthcare professional if you develop these symptoms.

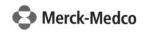

If you are taking diuretics, stay out of the sun as much as you can to avoid a serious sunburn. When you do go out in the sun, use sunblock or sunscreen, and wear protective clothing, such as a wide-brimmed hat and a long-sleeved shirt.

Potassium-Sparing Diuretics (Water Pills)

Potassium-sparing diuretics (water pills) are used to help reduce high blood pressure. They increase the amount of urine that your body makes, which helps your kidneys to remove salt (sodium) and water from your body.

Unlike thiazide and loop diuretics that cause potassium to leave the body with sodium and water, potassium-sparing diuretics prevent potassium from leaving the body. Potassium-sparing diuretics are often used with thiazide diuretics for high blood pressure. In order to help keep potassium blood levels normal, some diuretic medications contain both a thiazide diuretic and a potassium-sparing diuretic.

Brand Name	Generic Name	Type of Diuretic
Aldactazide®*	spironolactone/ hydrochlorothiazide	Potassium-Sparing/Thiazide*
Aldactone®	spironolactone	Potassium-Sparing
Dyazide®*	triamterene/ hydrochlorothiazide	Potassium-Sparing/Thiazide*
Dyrenium®	triamterene	Potassium-Sparing
Maxzide®*	triamterene/ hydrochlorothiazide	Potassium-Sparing/Thiazide*
Midamor®	amiloride	Potassium-Sparing
Moduretic®*	amiloride/ hydrochlorothiazide	Potassium-Sparing/Thiazide*

*For convenience, potassium-sparing diuretics are combined with thiazide diuretics for people who need both medications. Diuretics may also be combined with other high blood pressure medications. Check the Medication and Chapter Table to find the other medication sections you should read if you are taking a combination medication.

How Will I Take Potassium-Sparing Diuretics?

Potassium-sparing diuretics are usually taken 1 to 2 times a day. If taken only once a day, they are usually taken in the morning. If you need to take them twice a day, do not wait to take the second dose until the evening since it may keep you up at night with frequent urination. If they cause you to have to urinate frequently, you may want to take them after you get back from activities outside your home. Your doctor or other healthcare professional will tell you how many times a day to take your medication.

If you miss a dose of this medication, take the dose you missed as soon as possible. However, if it is almost time for your next dose, skip the missed dose and just take the next one. Do not double your dose. Take your medication exactly as directed by your doctor or other healthcare professional. Do not stop taking a prescription medication unless directed by your doctor or other healthcare professional.

What Side Effects Can Potassium-Sparing Diuretics Cause?

More Common

- High potassium in the blood (hyperkalemia)

- Nausea

- Poor appetite

Less Common

- Diarrhea

- Dizziness

- Erection problems (erectile dysfunction)

- Increased breast size in men with *Aldactone*® (spironolactone)

- Loss of interest in sex (decreased libido)

- Tingling, pain, or weakness in hands and feet

- Vomiting

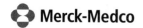
Rare

- Increased sensitivity to the sun (bad sunburn)

- Rash (skin redness, bumps, itching, or irritation)

Tell your doctor or other healthcare professional if you have side effects that bother you, do not go away, make you worried about taking your medication, or make you want to stop taking your medication.

 ## Do Other Medications Interact with Potassium-Sparing Diuretics?

Nonsteroidal anti-inflammatory medications (NSAIDs), such as *Motrin®* (ibuprofen), *Aleve®* (naproxen), *Vioxx®* (rofecoxib), *Celebrex®* (celecoxib), and others (see Glossary), *may decrease* how well potassium-sparing diuretics work.

Many nonprescription (over-the-counter [OTC]) medications such as antacids, laxatives, pain, cough, cold, and allergy medications contain medications that *may increase* blood pressure. If you are taking blood pressure medication, you should talk to your doctor or other healthcare professional before taking any new OTC medications.

The following *may increase* potassium blood levels and *may increase* the side effects of potassium-sparing diuretics:

- ACE inhibitors such as *Accupril®* (quinapril), *Vasotec®* (enalapril), *Zestril®* (lisinopril), and others—see Glossary

- Potassium supplements such as *K-Dur®*, *Klor-Con®*, *Slow K®*, and others—see Glossary

- Salt substitutes

Tell your doctor or other healthcare professional about all medications (both prescription and nonprescription [over-the-counter] medications) that you are taking.

Why Else Do People Take Potassium-Sparing Diuretics?

Aldactone® (spironolactone) may sometimes be used for severe liver problems or congestive heart failure.

What Else Should I Know about Potassium-Sparing Diuretics?

Medications cannot cure high blood pressure, but they can help control it and help reduce the chance of stroke, heart attack (myocardial infarction), congestive heart failure, kidney failure, and death. It is important to take your blood pressure medication daily as prescribed to reduce your risks. Keeping your weight down, eating a healthy diet that is low in salt (sodium), and exercising regularly will also help control your blood pressure. Ask your doctor or other healthcare professional for a diet and exercise plan.

Have your blood pressure checked regularly as directed by your doctor or other healthcare professional.

 # Warning!

To give you the best care, your doctor or other healthcare professional needs to know about the diseases and medical conditions you have had—your full medical history. Tell your doctor or other healthcare professional if you have or have ever had, or presently take, any of the following:

- ACE inhibitors such as *Accupril*® (quinapril), *Vasotec*® (enalapril), *Zestril*® (lisinopril), and others—see Glossary

- Allergy or previous reaction to potassium-sparing diuretics

- Diabetes

- High potassium in your blood (hyperkalemia)

- Kidney problems

- Low potassium in your blood (hypokalemia)

385

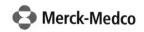

- Potassium supplements such as *K-Dur®*, *Klor-Con®*, *Slow K®*, and others—see Glossary

Kidney problems or diabetes may increase the amount of potassium in the blood. Your doctor or other healthcare professional may order blood tests to make sure your potassium blood levels do not get too high while taking a potassium-sparing diuretic.

Ask your doctor or other healthcare professional before using salt substitutes because many contain potassium that could increase your potassium blood levels.

If you are taking potassium-sparing diuretics, stay out of the sun as much as you can to avoid a serious sunburn. When you do go out in the sun, use sunblock or sunscreen, and wear protective clothing, such as a wide-brimmed hat and a long-sleeved shirt.

Beta Blockers

Beta blockers slow the heartbeat and help to lower blood pressure.

Many blood pressure pills contain two different medications in one pill. Names of combination medications are not listed below. This section only contains information on beta blockers. Check the Medication and Chapter Table to find out which other sections to review for more information on your second medication.

Brand Name	Generic Name
Blocadren®	timolol
Cartrol®	carteolol
Coreg®	carvedilol
Corgard®	nadolol
Inderal®	propranolol
Kerlone®	betaxolol
Levatol®	penbutolol
Lopressor®	metoprolol
Normodyne®	labetalol
Sectral®	acebutolol
Tenormin®	atenolol
Toprol®	metoprolol
Trandate®	labetalol
Visken®	pindolol
Zebeta®	bisoprolol

How Will I Take Beta Blockers?

Beta blockers are usually taken 1 to 3 times a day. They may be taken with or without food. However, the way you take most of them should be consistent. They should either always be taken with food or always be taken without food. Your doctor or other healthcare professional will tell you how often to take your medication.

When a medication has initials after its name, such as XL, XR, SR, BID, DUR, and others, it usually means that the body absorbs the medication slowly over time, so you usually have to take it only once or twice a day. The body will absorb some medications of this type too fast if you crush or break them or dissolve them in liquid, and their effects will not last as long as they should.

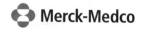

Check with your doctor or other healthcare professional before crushing or breaking your pills or dissolving your pills in liquid.

If you miss a dose of this medication, take the dose you missed as soon as possible. However, if it is almost time for your next dose, skip the missed dose and just take the next one. Do not double your dose. Take your medication exactly as directed by your doctor or other healthcare professional. Do not stop taking a prescription medication unless directed by your doctor or other healthcare professional.

What Side Effects Can Beta Blockers Cause?

More Common

- Dizziness when standing up from a bed or a chair
- Erection problems (erectile dysfunction)
- Loss of interest in sex (decreased libido)
- Tiredness or sluggishness (fatigue)
- Weakness

Less Common

- Change in blood sugar
- Congestive heart failure
- Heartburn
- Leg pain when walking
- Rash (skin redness, bumps, itching, or irritation)
- Sadness, feeling blue or down, depressed mood (depression)
- Slow or irregular heartbeat (palpitations)
- Strange dreams and nightmares

- Trouble breathing or shortness of breath in asthma and COPD, including emphysema and chronic bronchitis

---

Tell your doctor or other healthcare professional if you have side effects that bother you, do not go away, make you worried about taking your medication, or make you want to stop taking your medication.

Do Other Medications Interact with Beta Blockers?

Many nonprescription (over-the-counter [OTC]) medications such as antacids, laxatives, pain, cough, cold, and allergy medications contain medications that **may increase** blood pressure. If you are taking blood pressure medication, you should talk to your doctor or other healthcare professional before taking any new OTC medications.

Beta blockers **may decrease** how well diabetes medications, such as *DiaBeta®* (glyburide), *Glucophage®* (metformin), *Glucotrol®* (glipizide), and others (see Glossary), work.

These medications **may increase** the side effects of beta blockers:

- Heart rhythm problem (arrhythmia) medications—see Glossary

- High blood pressure medications and diuretics (water pills)—see Glossary

- *Lanoxin®* (digoxin)

- Neuroleptic medications such as *Risperdal®* (risperidone), *Thorazine®* (chlorpromazine), *Zyprexa®* (olanzapine), and others—see Glossary

- Propylthiouracil or PTU

- *Tagamet®* (cimetidine)

- *Tapazole®* (methimazole)

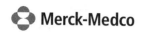

Beta blockers *may increase* the side effects of these medications:

- *DHE-45®* (dihydroergotamine)

- *Ergomar®* (ergotamine)

- *Migranal®* (dihydroergotamine)

These medications *may decrease* how well beta blockers work:

- Barbiturates such as *Butisol®* (butabarbital), *Luminal®* (phenobarbital), *Mebaral®* (mephobarbital), and others—see Glossary

- NSAIDs such as *Motrin®* (ibuprofen), *Aleve®* (naproxen), *Vioxx®* (rofecoxib), *Celebrex®* (celecoxib), and others—see Glossary

- *Rifadin®* (rifampin)

- Theophylline such as *Theo-Dur®*, *Uniphyl®*, and others—see Glossary

- Thyroid medications such as *Cytomel®* (liothyronine), *Levoxyl®* (levothyroxine), *Synthroid®* (levothyroxine), and others—see Glossary

---

Tell your doctor or other healthcare professional about all medications (both prescription and nonprescription [over-the-counter] medications) that you are taking.

Why Else Do People Take Beta Blockers?

Beta blockers may also help prevent a heart attack (myocardial infarction), heart rhythm problem (arrhythmia), cardiac chest pain (angina), migraine headaches, and shakiness (tremors). Some people also take beta blockers for congestive heart failure.

What Else Should I Know about Beta Blockers?

Medications cannot cure high blood pressure, but they can help control it and help reduce the chance of stroke, heart attack (myocardial infarction), congestive heart failure, kidney failure, and death. It is important to take your blood pressure medication daily as prescribed to reduce your risks. Keeping your weight down, eating a healthy diet that is low in salt (sodium), and exercising regularly will also help control your blood pressure. Ask your doctor or other healthcare professional for a diet and exercise plan.

Have your blood pressure checked regularly as directed by your doctor or other healthcare professional.

 # Warning!

To give you the best care, your doctor or other healthcare professional needs to know about the diseases and medical conditions you have had—your full medical history. Tell your doctor or other healthcare professional if you have or have ever had any of the following:

- Allergy or previous reaction to beta blockers
- Breathing problems (asthma and COPD, including emphysema and chronic bronchitis)
- Congestive heart failure
- Diabetes
- Poor circulation (peripheral vascular disease)
- Sadness, feeling blue or down, depressed mood (depression)

Beta blockers may worsen the symptoms of some lung problems, especially asthma and COPD, including emphysema and chronic bronchitis. Tell your doctor or other healthcare professional if you have trouble breathing or shortness of breath.

Taking beta blockers may hide the symptoms of low blood sugar (hypoglycemia). This may cause problems for people with diabetes. Ask your doctor or other healthcare professional whether you need to check your blood sugar to help prevent the dangers of hypoglycemia or other side effects.

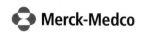

Beta blockers may worsen the symptoms of poor circulation (peripheral vascular disease). Tell your doctor or other healthcare professional if you develop symptoms of poor circulation such as pain, numbness, or coldness of your legs, feet, and hands.

Beta blockers may make you unsteady on your feet, causing you to fall and possibly break a bone. If you have fallen recently, tell your doctor or other healthcare professional about it. Taking a different medication or a lower dose may make you less likely to fall. You should not stop taking this medication without first talking to your doctor or other healthcare professional.

Under certain circumstances, your doctor or other healthcare professional may decide that you should stop taking this medication. If you have taken it for more than a couple of weeks, he or she may want you to decrease it gradually, lowering the dose over a few weeks or months. Stopping suddenly may cause unpleasant withdrawal symptoms or may worsen your medical problems. Pay careful attention to the instructions your doctor or other healthcare professional gives you about how much less to take and for how long.

Angiotensin-Converting Enzyme (ACE) Inhibitors

Angiotensin-converting enzyme (ACE) inhibitors relax blood vessels. These medications help to lower blood pressure and make it easier for the heart to pump blood.

Many blood pressure pills contain two different medications in one pill. Names of combination medications are not listed below. This section only contains information on ACE inhibitors. Check the Medication and Chapter Table to find out which other sections to review for more information on your second medication.

Brand Name	Generic Name
Accupril®	quinapril
Aceon®	perindopril
Altace®	ramipril
Capoten®	captopril
Lotensin®	benazepril
Mavik®	trandolapril
Monopril®	fosinopril
Prinivil®	lisinopril
Univasc®	moexipril
Vasotec®	enalapril
Zestril®	lisinopril

How Will I Take ACE Inhibitors?

ACE inhibitors are usually taken 1 to 3 times a day. *Capoten®* (captopril) and *Univasc®* (moexipril) should be taken on an empty stomach 1 hour before or 2 hours after meals. Other ACE inhibitors can be taken with or without food. Your doctor or other healthcare professional will tell you how many times a day to take your medication.

If you miss a dose of this medication, take the dose you missed as soon as possible. However, if it is almost time for your next dose, skip the missed dose and just take the next one. Do not double your dose. Take your medication exactly as directed by your doctor or other healthcare professional. Do not stop taking a prescription medication unless directed by your doctor or other healthcare professional.

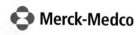

What Side Effects Can ACE Inhibitors Cause?

More Common

- Dizziness when standing up from a bed or a chair
- Dry cough that will not go away
- High potassium in your blood (hyperkalemia)
- Rash (skin redness, bumps, itching, or irritation)
- Tiredness or sluggishness (fatigue)

Less Common

- Change in taste
- Diarrhea
- Kidney problems
- Nausea
- Swelling of the face, lips, tongue, arms, and legs (angioedema)

Rare

- Easy bruising ("black-and-blue" marks on the skin)
- Erection problems (erectile dysfunction)
- Frequent fever, sore throat, or flu-like symptoms that may be a sign of low white blood cells

---

Tell your doctor or other healthcare professional if you have side effects that bother you, do not go away, make you worried about taking your medication, or make you want to stop taking your medication.

Do Other Medications Interact with ACE Inhibitors?

Many nonprescription (over-the-counter [OTC]) medications such as antacids, laxatives, pain, cough, cold, and allergy medications contain medications that *may increase* blood pressure. If you are taking blood pressure medication, you should talk to your doctor or other healthcare professional before taking any new OTC medications.

ACE inhibitors *may increase* the side effects of lithium such as *Eskalith®*, *Lithobid®*, and others—see Glossary.

ACE inhibitors *may increase* the side effects of other high blood pressure medications—see Glossary.

The following *may increase* potassium blood levels and *may increase* the side effects of ACE inhibitors:

- Potassium-sparing diuretics such as *Aldactazide®* (spironolactone/ hydrochlorothiazide), *Dyazide®* (triamterene/hydrochlorothiazide), *Moduretic®* (amiloride/hydrochlorothiazide), and others—see Glossary

- Potassium supplements such as *K-Dur®*, *Klor-Con®*, *Slow K®*, and others—see Glossary

- Salt substitutes

Nonsteroidal anti-inflammatory drugs (NSAIDs), such as *Motrin®* (ibuprofen), *Aleve®* (naproxen), *Vioxx®* (rofecoxib), *Celebrex®* (celecoxib), and others (see Glossary), *may decrease* how well an ACE inhibitor works.

Tell your doctor or other healthcare professional about all medications (both prescription and nonprescription [over-the-counter] medications) that you are taking.

Why Else Do People Take ACE Inhibitors?

ACE inhibitors may be used in congestive heart failure and to help prevent kidney problems in people with diabetes.

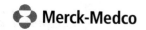

What Else Should I Know about ACE Inhibitors?

Cough may be a common side effect of ACE inhibitors. Talk to your doctor or other healthcare professional if you develop a cough. This should be checked because it may be a sign of another medical problem.

Medications cannot cure high blood pressure, but they can help control it and help reduce the chance of stroke, heart attack (myocardial infarction), congestive heart failure, kidney failure, and death. It is important to take your blood pressure medications daily as prescribed to reduce your risks. Keeping your weight down, eating a healthy diet that is low in salt (sodium), and exercising regularly will also help control your blood pressure. Ask your doctor or other healthcare professional for a diet and exercise plan.

Have your blood pressure checked regularly as directed by your doctor or other healthcare professional.

 # Warning!

To give you the best care, your doctor or other healthcare professional needs to know about the diseases and medical conditions you have had—your full medical history. Tell your doctor or other healthcare professional if you have or have ever had, or presently take, any of the following:

- Allergy or previous reaction to ACE inhibitors
- Congestive heart failure
- High potassium in your blood (hyperkalemia)
- Kidney problems
- Liver problems
- Low blood pressure (hypotension)
- Potassium-sparing diuretics such as *Aldactazide*® (spironolactone/hydrochlorothiazide), *Dyazide*® (triamterene/hydrochlorothiazide), *Moduretic*® (amiloride/hydrochlorothiazide), and others—see Glossary

- Potassium supplements such as *K-Dur*®, *Klor-Con*®, *Slow K*®, and others—see Glossary

- Swelling of the face, lips, tongue, arms, and legs (angioedema)

Kidney problems or diabetes may increase the amount of potassium in the blood. Your doctor or other healthcare professional may order blood tests to make sure your potassium blood levels do not get too high while taking ACE inhibitors.

ACE inhibitors may make you unsteady on your feet, causing you to fall and possibly break a bone. If you have fallen recently, tell your doctor or other healthcare professional about it. Taking a different medication or a lower dose may make you less likely to fall. You should not stop taking this medication without first talking to your doctor or other healthcare professional.

Ask your doctor or other healthcare professional before using salt substitutes because many contain potassium that could increase your potassium blood levels.

Angiotensin II (A-II) Blockers

Angiotensin II (A-II) blockers help to relax the blood vessels by blocking angiotensin II, a substance in the body that causes the blood vessels to tighten (constrict). This helps to lower blood pressure.

Many blood pressure pills contain two different medications in one pill. Names of combination medications are not listed below. This section only contains information on A-II blockers. Check the Medication and Chapter Table to find out which other sections to review for more information on your second medication.

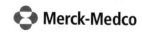
Brand Name	Generic Name
Atacand®	candesartan
Avapro®	irbesartan
Cozaar®	losartan
Diovan®	valsartan
Micardis®	telmisartan
Teveten®	eprosartan

How Will I Take A-II Blockers?

Angiotensin II blockers are usually taken 1 to 2 times a day. You may take them with or without food. Your doctor or other healthcare professional will tell you how many times a day to take your medication.

If you miss a dose of this medication, take the dose you missed as soon as possible. However, if it is almost time for your next dose, skip the missed dose and just take the next one. Do not double your dose. Take your medication exactly as directed by your doctor or other healthcare professional. Do not stop taking a prescription medication unless directed by your doctor or other healthcare professional.

What Side Effects Can A-II Blockers Cause?

More Common

- Dizziness

- Headache

- Nasal congestion, sinus infections, and head colds

- Tiredness or sluggishness (fatigue)

Less Common

- Back pain

- Diarrhea

- Difficulty falling asleep or staying asleep (insomnia)

- Dizziness when standing up from a bed or a chair

- High potassium in your blood (hyperkalemia)

- Muscle aches and pain

- Nausea

Rare

- Liver problems that may cause yellowing of the skin or eyes (jaundice)

Tell your doctor or other healthcare professional if you have side effects that bother you, do not go away, make you worried about taking your medication, or make you want to stop taking your medication.

Do Other Medications Interact with A-II Blockers?

Nonsteroidal anti-inflammatory drugs (NSAIDs), such as *Motrin*® (ibuprofen), *Aleve*® (naproxen), *Vioxx*® (rofecoxib), *Celebrex*® (celecoxib), and others (see Glossary), *may decrease* how well A-II blockers work.

These medications *may increase* the side effects of A-II blockers:

- *Diflucan*® (fluconazole)

- Diuretics (water pills) such as *HydroDIURIL*® (hydrochlorothiazide or HCTZ), *Lasix*® (furosemide), and others—see Glossary

- High blood pressure medications—see Glossary

- *Nizoral*® (ketoconazole)

- *Sporanox*®(itraconazole)

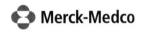

Micardis® (telmisartan) *may increase* the effects of *Lanoxin*® (digoxin).

Many nonprescription (over-the-counter [OTC]) medications such as antacids, laxatives, pain, cough, cold, and allergy medications contain medications that *may increase* blood pressure. If you are taking blood pressure medication, you should talk to your doctor or other healthcare professional before taking any new OTC medications.

Tell your doctor or other healthcare professional about all medications (both prescription and nonprescription [over-the-counter] medications) that you are taking.

What Else Should I Know about A-II Blockers?

Medications cannot cure high blood pressure, but they can help control it and help reduce the chance of stroke, heart attack (myocardial infarction), congestive heart failure, kidney failure, and death. It is important to take your blood pressure medications daily as prescribed to reduce your risks. Keeping your weight down, eating a healthy diet that is low in salt (sodium), and exercising regularly will also help control your blood pressure. Ask your doctor or other healthcare professional for a diet and exercise plan.

Have your blood pressure checked regularly as directed by your doctor or other healthcare professional.

 # Warning!

To give you the best care, your doctor or other healthcare professional needs to know about the diseases and medical conditions you have had—your full medical history. Tell your doctor or other healthcare professional if you have or have ever had any of the following:

- Allergy or previous reaction to A-II blockers

- Heart problems

- Kidney problems

- Liver problems

- Swelling of the face, lips, tongue, arms, and legs (angioedema)

A-II blockers may make you unsteady on your feet, causing you to fall and possibly break a bone. If you have fallen recently, tell your doctor or other healthcare professional about it. Taking a different medication or a lower dose may make you less likely to fall. You should not stop taking this medication without first talking to your doctor or other healthcare professional.

Calcium Channel Blockers

Calcium channel blockers help lower blood pressure by relaxing the blood vessels.

Many blood pressure pills contain two different medications in one pill. Names of combination medications are not listed below. This section only contains information on calcium channel blockers. Check the Medication and Chapter Table to find out which other sections to review for more information on your second medication.

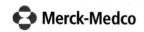
Brand Name	Generic Name
Adalat®	nifedipine
Calan®	verapamil
Cardene®	nicardipine
Cardizem®	diltiazem
Covera-HS®	verapamil
Dilacor®	diltiazem
DynaCirc®	isradipine
Isoptin®	verapamil
Norvasc®	amlodipine
Plendil®	felodipine
Procardia®	nifedipine
Sular®	nisoldipine
Tiamate®	diltiazem
Tiazac®	diltiazem
Vascor®	bepridil
Verelan®	verapamil

How Will I Take Calcium Channel Blockers?

Calcium channel blockers are generally taken 1 to 3 times a day. *Plendil®* (felodipine), *Cardene®* (nicardipine), nifedipine, and diltiazem should be taken on an empty stomach 1 hour before or 2 hours after meals. Verapamil should be taken with food or meals. *DynaCirc®* (isradipine) should be taken with food to help prevent an upset stomach. *Sular®* (nisoldipine) should not be taken with high-fat meals. Your doctor or other healthcare professional will tell you how many times a day to take your medication.

When a medication has initials after its name, such as XL, XR, SR, BID, DUR, and others, it usually means that the body absorbs the medication slowly over time, so you usually have to take it only once or twice a day. The body will absorb some medications of this type too fast if you crush or break them or dissolve them in liquid, and their effects will not last as long as they should. Check with your doctor or other healthcare professional before crushing or breaking your pills or dissolving your pills in liquid.

If you miss a dose of this medication, take the dose you missed as soon as possible. However, if it is almost time for your next dose, skip the missed dose and just take the next one. Do not double your dose. Take your medication exactly as directed by your doctor or other healthcare professional. Do not stop taking a prescription medication unless directed by your doctor or other healthcare professional.

What Side Effects Can Calcium Channel Blockers Cause?

More Common

- Constipation
- Dizziness when standing up from a bed or a chair
- Headache
- Reddening of the face (flushing)
- Swelling or puffiness of feet, ankles, or lower legs (edema)

Less Common

- Congestive heart failure
- Diarrhea
- Nausea
- Rash (skin redness, bumps, itching, or irritation)
- Slow, fast, or irregular heartbeat (palpitations)

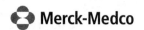

Tell your doctor or other healthcare professional if you have side effects that bother you, do not go away, make you worried about taking your medication, or make you want to stop taking your medication.

 ## Do Other Medications Interact with Calcium Channel Blockers?

Many nonprescription (over-the-counter [OTC]) medications such as antacids, laxatives, pain, cough, cold, and allergy medications contain medications that *may increase* blood pressure. If you are taking blood pressure medication, you should talk to your doctor or other healthcare professional before taking any new OTC medications.

Calcium channel blockers *may increase* the side effects of these medications:

- *BuSpar®* (buspirone)
- Heart rhythm problem (arrhythmia) medications—see Glossary
- High blood pressure (hypertension) medications and diuretics (water pills)—see Glossary
- *Lanoxin®* (digoxin)
- Lithium such as *Eskalith®*, *Lithobid®*, and others—see Glossary
- *Neoral®* (cyclosporine)
- Quinidine such as *Quinaglute®*, *Quinidex®*, and others—see Glossary
- *Sandimmune®* (cyclosporine)
- Statins such as *Lipitor®* (atorvastatin), *Pravachol®* (pravastatin), *Zocor®* (simvastatin), and others—see Glossary
- *Tegretol®* (carbamazepine)
- Theophylline such as *Theo-Dur®*, *Uniphyl®*, and others—see Glossary

These medications *may increase* the side effects of calcium channel blockers:

- *Tagamet®* (cimetidine)
- *Zantac®* (ranitidine)

Ethmozine® (moricizine) **may decrease** how well diltiazem works, and diltiazem **may increase** the side effects of *Ethmozine*® (moricizine).

These medications **may decrease** how well calcium channel blockers work:

- Barbiturates such as *Butisol*® (butabarbital), *Luminal*® (phenobarbital), *Mebaral*® (mephobarbital), and others—see Glossary

- *Rifadin*® (rifampin)

These medications **may increase** the side effects of *Adalat*® (nifedipine), *Cardene*® (nicardipine), *DynaCirc*® (isradipine), *Plendil*® (felodipine), *Procardia*® (nifedipine), and *Sular*® (nisoldipine):

- *Diflucan*® (fluconazole)

- *Nizoral*® (ketoconazole)

- *Sporanox*® (itraconazole)

Nonsteroidal anti-inflammatory drugs (NSAIDs) such as *Motrin*® (ibuprofen), *Aleve*® (naproxen), *Vioxx*® (rofecoxib), *Celebrex*® (celecoxib), and others (see Glossary) **may decrease** how well calcium channel blockers work.

Erythromycin, such as *Ery-Tab*®, *Erythrocin*®, and others (see Glossary), **may increase** the side effects of *Plendil*® (felodipine).

Norvir® (ritonavir) **may cause** serious or life-threatening side effects if taken by someone who is also taking *Vascor*® (bepridil).

Vascor® (bepridil) is generally not prescribed for anyone who is taking *Propulsid*® (cisapride [withdrawn from general distribution; available only by special arrangement with the manufacturer]), *Seldane*® (terfenadine [no longer commercially available]), or *Hismanal*® (astemizole [no longer commercially available]), because together they **may cause** serious, sometimes fatal, heart problems.

Grapefruit and grapefruit juice may increase the side effects of calcium channel blockers. This interaction can happen whether you eat the grapefruit or drink the grapefruit juice at the same time as you take your medication or if you take

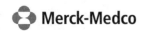

the medication separately from the grapefruit or grapefruit juice. Talk to your doctor or other healthcare professional before eating grapefruit or drinking grapefruit juice if you are taking this medication. Please also read the discussion on A Warning about Grapefruit and Grapefruit Juice on pages i-ii.

Tell your doctor or other healthcare professional about all medications (both prescription and nonprescription [over-the-counter] medications) that you are taking.

Why Else Do People Take Calcium Channel Blockers?

Calcium channel blockers may be helpful for cardiac chest pain (angina), heart rhythm problems (arrhythmia), and prevention of migraine headaches.

What Else Should I Know about Calcium Channel Blockers?

Medications cannot cure high blood pressure, but they can help control it and help reduce the chance of stroke, heart attack (myocardial infarction), congestive heart failure, kidney failure, and death. It is important to take your blood pressure medications daily as prescribed to reduce your risks. Keeping your weight down, eating a healthy diet that is low in salt (sodium), and exercising regularly will also help to control your blood pressure. Ask your doctor or other healthcare professional for a diet and exercise plan.

Have your blood pressure checked regularly as directed by your doctor or other healthcare professional.

 # Warning!

To give you the best care, your doctor or other healthcare professional needs to know about the diseases and medical conditions you have had—your full

medical history. Tell your doctor or other healthcare professional if you have or have ever had any of the following:

- Allergy or previous reaction to calcium channel blockers

- Congestive heart failure

- Heart rhythm problems (arrhythmia)

- Kidney problems

- Liver problems

- Low blood pressure (hypotension)

Sustained-released or long-acting types of calcium channel blockers (released into the body slowly over 12 to 24 hours) are usually recommended for high blood pressure because short-acting calcium channel blockers may cause more serious side effects than long-acting types. Long-acting medications usually have initials after their name such as CD, CR, CC, XL, XR, SR, HS, BID, or others. If you are not taking a medication with any of these initials after the name, talk to your doctor or other healthcare professional to see if this medication is right for you.

Calcium channel blockers may make you unsteady on your feet, causing you to fall and possibly break a bone. If you have fallen recently, tell your doctor or other healthcare professional about it. Taking a different medication or a lower dose may make you less likely to fall. You should not stop taking this medication without first talking to your doctor or other healthcare professional.

Under certain circumstances, your doctor or other healthcare professional may decide that you should stop taking this medication. If you have taken it for more than a couple of weeks, he or she may want you to decrease it gradually, lowering the dose over a few weeks or months. Stopping suddenly may cause unpleasant withdrawal symptoms or may worsen your medical problems. Pay careful attention to the instructions your doctor or other healthcare professional gives you about how much less to take and for how long.

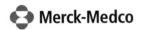

▲*Aldomet*® (methyldopa)

Aldomet® (methyldopa) helps to relax the blood vessels, which helps to lower blood pressure.

Many blood pressure pills contain two different medications in one pill. Names of combination medications are not listed below. This section only contains information on *Aldomet*® (methyldopa). Check the Medication and Chapter Table to find out which other sections to review for more information on your second medication.

▲ Indicates medications that are more likely to cause unpleasant or dangerous side effects. These medications are generally not recommended for people over 65. The side effects may not be very obvious and may be mistaken for "just a part of getting older" but may be serious. If you are taking one of these medications, you might want to talk to your doctor or other healthcare professional to see if this medication is best for you. Safer medications may be available and lower dosages may be required. You should not stop taking these medications without first talking to your doctor or other healthcare professional.

See the WARNING section on page 412 for the specific safety problems associated with this medication ▲.

 ## How Will I Take *Aldomet*® (methyldopa)?

Aldomet® (methyldopa) is usually taken 1 to 4 times a day. Your doctor or other healthcare professional will tell you how many times a day to take your medication.

If you miss a dose of this medication, take the dose you missed as soon as possible. However, if it is almost time for your next dose, skip the missed dose and just take the next one. Do not double your dose. Take your medication exactly as directed by your doctor or other healthcare professional. Do not stop taking a prescription medication unless directed by your doctor or other healthcare professional.

What Side Effects Can *Aldomet*® (methyldopa) Cause?

More Common

- Cardiac chest pain (angina)

- Congestive heart failure

- Dizziness when standing up from a bed or a chair

- Dry mouth

- Ejaculation and erection problems (erectile dysfunction)

- Headache

- Leg pain, warmth, redness, or swelling

- Loss of interest in sex (decreased libido)

- Swelling or puffiness of the feet, ankles, or lower legs (edema)

- Tiredness or sluggishness (fatigue)

Less Common

- Difficulty concentrating

- Fever

- Low red blood cells (anemia)

- Rash (skin redness, bumps, itching, or irritation)

- Red or brown (tea-colored) urine

- Sadness, feeling blue or down, depressed mood (depression)

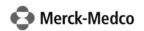

Rare

- Frequent fever, sore throat, or flu-like symptoms that may be a sign of low white blood cells

- Liver problems that may cause yellowing of the skin or eyes (jaundice)

- Skin rash with fever and joint pain or swelling that may be a sign of lupus

---

Tell your doctor or other healthcare professional if you have side effects that bother you, do not go away, make you worried about taking your medication, or make you want to stop taking your medication.

Do Other Medications Interact with *Aldomet*® (methyldopa)?

Many nonprescription (over-the-counter [OTC]) medications such as antacids, laxatives, pain, cough, cold, and allergy medications contain medications that ***may increase*** blood pressure. If you are taking blood pressure medication, you should talk to your doctor or other healthcare professional before taking any new OTC medications.

Aldomet® (methyldopa) ***may increase*** the side effects of lithium such as *Eskalith*®, *Lithobid*®, and others—see Glossary.

Nonsteroidal anti-inflammatory drugs (NSAIDs), such as *Motrin*® (ibuprofen), *Aleve*® (naproxen), *Vioxx*® (rofecoxib), *Celebrex*® (celecoxib), and others (see Glossary), ***may decrease*** how well *Aldomet*® (methyldopa) works.

Aldomet® (methyldopa) is generally not prescribed for anyone who is taking MAO inhibitors, such as *Marplan*® (isocarboxazid), *Nardil*® (phenelzine), or *Parnate*® (tranylcypromine), because together they ***may cause*** serious or even fatal reactions. If your doctor or other healthcare professional wants you to stop taking one medication and start taking the other, you should wait at least 2 weeks between stopping one and starting the other.

These medications *may increase* the side effects of *Aldomet®* (methyldopa):

- *Comtan®* (entacapone)
- *Tasmar®* (tolcapone)

Other blood pressure medications *may increase* the side effects of *Aldomet®* (methyldopa).

Aldomet® (methyldopa) *may increase* the side effects of *Sinemet®* (carbidopa/levodopa), and *Sinemet®* (carbidopa/levodopa) *may increase* the side effects of *Aldomet®* (methyldopa).

Aldomet® (methyldopa) *may increase* the side effects of other medications that cause drowsiness, including anticholinergic medications, antidepressants, antihistamines (allergy medications), antispasmodics, benzodiazepines (a type of tranquilizer), anxiety medications, narcotics (pain relievers), muscle relaxants, neuroleptic medications (a type of tranquilizer), seizure medications, or sleep medications. Avoid driving a car and other activities that need mental alertness, like using a knife or operating machinery, while taking these medications together.

Drinking alcoholic beverages (such as beer, wine, whiskey, and others) *may increase* the side effects of *Aldomet®* (methyldopa).

Tell your doctor or other healthcare professional about all medications (both prescription and nonprescription [over-the-counter] medications) that you are taking.

What Else Should I Know about *Aldomet®* (methyldopa)?

Medications cannot cure high blood pressure, but they can help control it and help reduce the chance of stroke, heart attack (myocardial infarction), congestive heart failure, kidney failure, and death. It is important to take your blood pressure medications daily as prescribed to help reduce your risks. Keeping your weight down, eating a healthy diet that is low in salt (sodium), and exercising regularly will also help control your blood pressure. Ask your doctor or other healthcare professional for a diet and exercise plan.

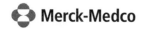

Have your blood pressure checked regularly as directed by your doctor or other healthcare professional.

 # Warning!

To give you the best care, your doctor or other healthcare professional needs to know about the diseases and medical conditions you have had—your full medical history. Tell your doctor or other healthcare professional if you have or have ever had or are presently taking any of the following:

- Allergy or previous reaction to *Aldomet*® (methyldopa)
- Congestive heart failure
- Liver problems
- Low blood pressure (hypotension)
- MAO inhibitors, such as *Marplan*® (isocarboxazid), *Nardil*® (phenelzine), or *Parnate*® (tranylcypromine)

Aldomet® (methyldopa) is generally not prescribed for people over 65 because it has side effects such as dizziness, drowsiness, sadness, feeling blue or down, depressed mood (depression), and erection and ejaculation problems (erectile dysfunction). If you are taking *Aldomet*® (methyldopa), ask your doctor or other healthcare professional if it is the right medication for you. Do not stop taking this medication without talking to your doctor or other healthcare professional.

Aldomet® (methyldopa) may make you unsteady on your feet, causing you to fall and possibly break a bone. If you have fallen recently, tell your doctor or other healthcare professional about it. Taking a different medication or a lower dose may make you less likely to fall. You should not stop taking this medication without first talking to your doctor or other healthcare professional.

Since *Aldomet*® (methyldopa) may cause damage to your liver, your doctor or other healthcare professional may order blood tests to find out early on if the medication is causing liver problems, before they become serious.

Aldomet® (methyldopa) may cause drowsiness. Avoid driving a car and other activities that need mental alertness, like using a knife or operating machinery, while taking this medication. Drinking alcoholic beverages (such as beer, wine, whiskey, and others) may increase the side effects.

Under certain circumstances, your doctor or other healthcare professional may decide that you should stop taking this medication. If you have taken it for more than a couple of weeks, he or she may want you to decrease it gradually, lowering the dose over a few weeks or months. Stopping suddenly may cause unpleasant withdrawal symptoms or may worsen your medical problems. Pay careful attention to the instructions your doctor or other healthcare professional gives you about how much less to take and for how long.

Catapres® (clonidine)

Catapres® (clonidine) helps to relax the blood vessels, which helps to reduce blood pressure.

Some blood pressure pills contain two different medications in one pill. Names of combination medications are not listed below. This section only contains information on *Catapres*® (clonidine). Check the Medication and Chapter Table to find out which other sections to review for more information on your second medication.

How Will I Take *Catapres*® (clonidine)?

Catapres® (clonidine) is usually taken 1 to 2 times a day. *Catapres*® (clonidine) may be taken with or without food. Your doctor or other healthcare professional will tell you how many times a day to take your medication.

Catapres® (clonidine) also comes as a patch, which is usually applied once a week like a *Band-Aid*®. If you use the patch, apply it to a clean, dry area of skin on your upper arm or chest. Avoid any part of your skin that has hair or a cut or is irritated. Keep the patch in place when you take a shower or bath or go

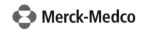

swimming. If the patch gets loose before it is time to change it, cover the loose part with adhesive tape. If it becomes too loose to fix or actually falls off, put a new patch on instead. Change the patch once a week. To keep the patch from irritating your skin, put the new patch in a different area of the skin from the previous one. When you take off an old patch, make sure you throw it away where children and pets cannot get it as it still will contain some medication that may be harmful to them.

If you miss a dose of this medication, take the dose you missed as soon as possible. However, if it is almost time for your next dose, skip the missed dose and just take the next one. Do not double your dose. Take your medication exactly as directed by your doctor or other healthcare professional. Do not stop taking a prescription medication unless directed by your doctor or other healthcare professional.

What Side Effects Can *Catapres*® (clonidine) Cause?

More Common

- Constipation
- Dizziness when standing up from a bed or a chair
- Drowsiness
- Dry mouth
- Headache
- Muscle aches and pains
- Tiredness or sluggishness (fatigue)

Less Common

- Erection problems (erectile dysfunction)
- Fast heartbeat (palpitations)
- Leg pain when walking
- Loss of interest in sex (decreased libido)

- Nausea

- Nervousness (anxiety)

- Rash (skin redness, bumps, itching, or irritation)

- Sadness, feeling blue or down, depressed mood (depression)

- Strange dreams and nightmares

Tell your doctor or other healthcare professional if you have side effects that bother you, do not go away, make you worried about taking your medication, or make you want to stop taking your medication.

Do Other Medications Interact with *Catapres*® (clonidine)?

Many nonprescription (over-the-counter [OTC]) medications such as antacids, laxatives, pain, cough, cold, and allergy medications contain medications that *may increase* blood pressure. If you are taking blood pressure medication, you should talk to your doctor or other healthcare professional before taking any new OTC medications.

Tricyclic antidepressants, such as *Elavil*® (amitriptyline), *Pamelor*® (nortriptyline), *Sinequan*® (doxepin), and others (see Glossary), *may decrease* how well *Catapres*® (clonidine) works.

Beta blockers, such as *Inderal*® (propranolol), *Tenormin*® (atenolol), *Toprol*® (metoprolol), and others (see Glossary), *may decrease* how well *Catapres*® (clonidine) works.

Nonsteroidal anti-inflammatory drugs (NSAIDs), such as *Motrin*® (ibuprofen), *Aleve*® (naproxen), *Vioxx*® (rofecoxib), *Celebrex*® (celecoxib), and others (see Glossary), *may decrease* how well *Catapres*® (clonidine) works.

Catapres® (clonidine) *may increase* the side effects of other medications that cause drowsiness, including anticholinergic medications, antidepressants, antihistamines (allergy medications), antispasmodics, benzodiazepines (a type of tranquilizer), anxiety medications, narcotics (pain relievers), muscle relaxants,

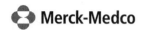
neuroleptic medications (a type of tranquilizer), seizure medications, or sleep medications. Avoid driving a car and other activities that need mental alertness, like using a knife or operating machinery, while taking these medications together.

Drinking alcoholic beverages (such as beer, wine, whiskey, and others) *may increase* the side effects of *Catapres®* (clonidine).

Tell your doctor or other healthcare professional about all medications (both prescription and nonprescription [over-the-counter] medications) that you are taking.

What Else Should I Know about *Catapres®* (clonidine)?

Medications cannot cure high blood pressure, but they can help control it and help reduce the chance of stroke, heart attack (myocardial infarction), congestive heart failure, kidney failure, and death. It is important to take your blood pressure medications daily as prescribed to help reduce your risks. Keeping your weight down, eating a healthy diet that is low in salt (sodium), and exercising regularly will also help control your blood pressure. Ask your doctor or other healthcare professional for a diet and exercise plan.

Have your blood pressure checked regularly as directed by your doctor or other healthcare professional.

 # Warning!

To give you the best care, your doctor or other healthcare professional needs to know about the diseases and medical conditions you have had—your full medical history. Tell your doctor or other healthcare professional if you have or have ever had any of the following:

- Allergy or previous reaction to adhesives or skin (transdermal) patches
- Allergy or previous reaction to *Catapres®* (clonidine)

- Heart attack (myocardial infarction)

- Heart problems

- Kidney problems

Catapres® (clonidine) may make you unsteady on your feet, causing you to fall and possibly break a bone. If you have fallen recently, tell your doctor or other healthcare professional about it. Taking a different medication or a lower dose may make you less likely to fall. You should not stop taking this medication without first talking to your doctor or other healthcare professional.

Catapres® (clonidine) may cause drowsiness. Avoid driving a car and other activities that need mental alertness, like using a knife or operating machinery, while taking this medication. Drinking alcoholic beverages (such as beer, wine, whiskey, and others) may increase the side effects.

Under certain circumstances, your doctor or other healthcare professional may decide that you should stop taking this medication. If you have taken it for more than a couple of weeks, he or she may want you to decrease it gradually, lowering the dose over a few weeks or months. Stopping suddenly may cause unpleasant withdrawal symptoms or may worsen your medical problems. Pay careful attention to the instructions your doctor or other healthcare professional gives you about how much less to take and for how long.

Alpha Blockers

Alpha blockers help to lower blood pressure by relaxing blood vessels so blood can flow through arteries more easily.

Some blood pressure pills contain two different medications in one pill. Names of combination medications are not listed below. This section only contains information on alpha blockers. Check the Medication and Chapter Table to find out which other sections to review for more information on your second medication.

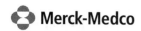

Merck-Medco   High Blood Pressure

Brand Name	Generic Name
Cardura®	doxazosin
Hytrin®	terazosin
Minipress®	prazosin

How Will I Take Alpha Blockers?

People take alpha blockers from 1 to 3 times a day. They may be taken with food to help prevent stomach upset. Your doctor or other healthcare professional will tell you how many times a day to take your medication.

If you miss a dose of this medication, take the dose you missed as soon as possible. However, if it is almost time for your next dose, skip the missed dose and just take the next one. Do not double your dose. Take your medication exactly as directed by your doctor or other healthcare professional. Do not stop taking a prescription medication unless directed by your doctor or other healthcare professional.

What Side Effects Can Alpha Blockers Cause?

More Common

- Dizziness when standing up from a bed or a chair, especially with the first dose
- Drowsiness
- Tiredness or sluggishness (fatigue)

Less Common

- Dry mouth
- Fast heartbeat (palpitations)

418

- Headache

- Loss of bladder control (urinary incontinence)

- Nervousness (anxiety)

- Swelling or puffiness of the feet, ankles, or lower legs (edema)

Tell your doctor or other healthcare professional if you have side effects that bother you, do not go away, make you worried about taking your medication, or make you want to stop taking your medication.

Do Other Medications Interact with Alpha Blockers?

These medications *may increase* the side effects of alpha blockers:

- Other high blood pressure medications—see Glossary

- Diuretics (water pills) such as *HydroDIURIL*® (hydrochlorothiazide or HCTZ), *Lasix*® (furosemide), and others—see Glossary

Alpha blockers *may increase* the side effects of other medications that cause drowsiness, including antidepressants, antihistamines (allergy medications), benzodiazepines (a type of tranquilizer), anxiety medications, narcotics (pain relievers), muscle relaxants, neuroleptic medications (a type of tranquilizer), seizure medications, or sleep medications. Avoid driving a car and other activities that need mental alertness, like using a knife or operating machinery, while taking this medication.

Drinking alcoholic beverages (such as beer, wine, whiskey, and others) *may increase* the side effects of alpha blockers.

Nonsteroidal anti-inflammatory drugs (NSAIDs), such as *Motrin*® (ibuprofen), *Aleve*® (naproxen), *Vioxx*® (rofecoxib), *Celebrex*® (celecoxib), and others (see Glossary), *may decrease* how well alpha blockers work.

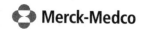

Many nonprescription (over-the-counter [OTC]) medications such as antacids, laxatives, pain, cough, cold, and allergy medications contain medications that **_may increase_** blood pressure. If you are taking blood pressure medication, you should talk to your doctor or other healthcare professional before taking any new OTC medications.

Tell your doctor or other healthcare professional about all medications (both prescription and nonprescription [over-the-counter] medications) that you are taking.

Why Else Do People Take Alpha Blockers?

Alpha blockers help relieve problems with urinating in men who have an enlarged prostate (benign prostatic hypertrophy).

What Else Should I Know about Alpha Blockers?

Medications cannot cure high blood pressure but they can help control it and help reduce the chance of stroke, heart attack (myocardial infarction), congestive heart failure, kidney failure, and death. It is important to take your blood pressure medications daily as prescribed to help reduce your risks. Keeping your weight down, eating a healthy diet that is low in salt (sodium), and exercising regularly will also help control your blood pressure. Ask your doctor or other healthcare professional for a diet and exercise plan.

Have your blood pressure checked regularly as directed by your doctor or other healthcare professional.

 # Warning!

To give you the best care, your doctor or other healthcare professional needs to know about the diseases and medical conditions you have had—your full

medical history. Tell your doctor or other healthcare professional if you have or have ever had any of the following:

- Allergy or previous reaction to alpha blockers

- Dizziness when standing up from a bed or a chair

- Prostate cancer or previous testing for prostate cancer

Be careful when taking your first dose. Some people have a fainting spell within the first hour and a half after taking the first dose of an alpha blocker. Ask a friend or family member to be with you when you take your first dose. If you feel dizzy, lie down so that you do not faint. Getting up slowly may reduce any dizziness or lightheadedness that you might feel after taking the first dose.

Alpha blockers may make you unsteady on your feet, causing you to fall and possibly break a bone. If you have fallen recently, tell your doctor or other healthcare professional about it. Taking a different medication or a lower dose may make you less likely to fall. You should not stop taking this medication without first talking to your doctor or other healthcare professional.

Alpha blockers may cause drowsiness. Avoid driving a car and other activities that need mental alertness, like using a knife or operating machinery, while taking this medication. Drinking alcoholic beverages (such as beer, wine, whiskey, and others) may increase the side effects.

Under certain circumstances, your doctor or other healthcare professional may decide that you should stop taking this medication. If you have taken it for more than a couple of weeks, he or she may want you to decrease it gradually, lowering the dose over a few weeks or months. Stopping suddenly may cause unpleasant withdrawal symptoms or may worsen your medical problems. Pay careful attention to the instructions your doctor or other healthcare professional gives you about how much less to take and for how long.

Apresoline® (hydralazine)

Apresoline® (hydralazine) is a vasodilator, which helps to lower blood pressure by relaxing blood vessels.

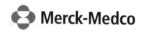

Some blood pressure pills contain two different medications in one pill. Names of combination medications are not listed below. This section only contains information on *Apresoline®* (hydralazine). Check the Medication and Chapter Table to find out which other sections to review for more information on your second medication.

How Will I Take *Apresoline®* (hydralazine)?

Apresoline® (hydralazine) is usually taken 2 to 4 times a day. It may be taken with or without food. However, the way you take it should be consistent. It should either always be taken with food or always be taken without food. Your doctor or other healthcare professional will tell you how many times a day to take your medication.

If you miss a dose of this medication, take the dose you missed as soon as possible. However, if it is almost time for your next dose, skip the missed dose and just take the next one. Do not double your dose. Take your medication exactly as directed by your doctor or other healthcare professional. Do not stop taking a prescription medication unless directed by your doctor or other healthcare professional.

What Side Effects Can *Apresoline®* (hydralazine) Cause?

More Common

- Diarrhea

- Fast heartbeat (palpitations)

- Headache

- Increased sensitivity to the sun (bad sunburn)

- Nausea

- Poor appetite

Less Common

- Cardiac chest pain (angina)

- Constipation

- Dizziness

- Increased tearing (watery eyes)

- Liver problems that may cause yellowing of the skin or eyes (jaundice)

- Reddening of the face (flushing)

- Skin rash with fever and joint pain or swelling that may be a sign of lupus

- Stuffy, runny nose (rhinitis)

- Swelling or puffiness of the of the feet, ankles, or lower legs (edema)

- Tingling, pain, or weakness in hands and feet

Tell your doctor or other healthcare professional if you have side effects that bother you, do not go away, make you worried about taking your medication, or make you want to stop taking your medication.

Do Other Medications Interact with *Apresoline*® (hydralazine)?

Apresoline® (hydralazine) ***may increase*** the side effects of other high blood pressure medications—see Glossary.

Apresoline® (hydralazine) ***may decrease*** how well diuretics (water pills) such as *HydroDIURIL*® (hydrochlorothiazide or HCTZ), *Lasix*® (furosemide), and others (see Glossary) work.

Many nonprescription (over-the-counter [OTC]) medications such as antacids, laxatives, pain, cough, cold, and allergy medications contain medications that ***may increase*** blood pressure. If you are taking blood pressure medication, you should talk to your doctor or other healthcare professional before taking any new OTC medications.

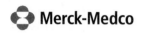
Nonsteroidal anti-inflammatory drugs (NSAIDs) such as *Motrin*® (ibuprofen), *Aleve*® (naproxen), *Vioxx*® (rofecoxib), *Celebrex*® (celecoxib), and others (see Glossary) ***may decrease*** how well *Apresoline*® (hydralazine) works.

Tell your doctor or other healthcare professional about all medications (both prescription and nonprescription [over-the-counter] medications) that you are taking.

Why Else Do People Take *Apresoline*® (hydralazine)?

Apresoline® (hydralazine) is sometimes used for congestive heart failure.

What Else Should I Know about *Apresoline*® (hydralazine)?

Medications cannot cure high blood pressure, but they can help control it and help reduce the chance of stroke, heart attack (myocardial infarction), congestive heart failure, kidney failure, and death. It is important to take your blood pressure medications daily as prescribed to help reduce your risks. Keeping your weight down, eating a healthy diet that is low in salt (sodium), and exercising regularly will also help control your blood pressure. Ask your doctor or other healthcare professional for a diet and exercise plan.

Have your blood pressure checked regularly as directed by your doctor or other healthcare professional.

 # Warning!

To give you the best care, your doctor or other healthcare professional needs to know about the diseases and medical conditions you have had—your full medical history. Tell your doctor or other healthcare professional if you have or have ever had any of the following:

- Allergy or previous reaction to *Apresoline*® (hydralazine)

- Cardiac chest pain (angina)

- Coronary artery disease

- Kidney problems

- Lupus

- Stroke

Call your doctor or other healthcare professional right away if you get a skin rash with pain or swelling in your joints (elbows, knees, and others) while taking *Apresoline*® (hydralazine).

If you are taking *Apresoline*® (hydralazine), stay out of the sun as much as you can to avoid a serious sunburn. When you do go out in the sun, use sunblock or sunscreen, and wear protective clothing, such as a wide-brimmed hat and a long-sleeved shirt.

Apresoline® (hydralazine) may cause fluid retention and swelling or puffiness of the feet, ankles, or lower legs (edema). This medication is sometimes prescribed with a diuretic (water pill) to help prevent swelling. Ask your doctor or other healthcare professional about diuretics if you have edema.

Apresoline® (hydralazine) may make you unsteady on your feet, causing you to fall and possibly break a bone. If you have fallen recently, tell your doctor or other healthcare professional about it. Taking a different medication or a lower dose may make you less likely to fall. You should not stop taking this medication without first talking to your doctor or other healthcare professional.

Under certain circumstances, your doctor or other healthcare professional may decide that you should stop taking this medication. If you have taken it for more than a couple of weeks, he or she may want you to decrease it gradually, lowering the dose over a few weeks or months. Stopping suddenly may cause unpleasant withdrawal symptoms or may worsen your medical problems. Pay careful attention to the instructions your doctor or other healthcare professional gives you about how much less to take and for how long.

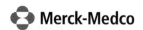

Loniten® (minoxidil)

Loniten® (minoxidil) helps to lower blood pressure by relaxing blood vessels.

How Will I Take *Loniten®* (minoxidil)?

Loniten® (minoxidil) is usually taken 1 to 2 times a day. It may be taken with food to help prevent stomach upset. Your doctor or other healthcare professional will tell you how many times a day to take your medication.

If you miss a dose of this medication, take the dose you missed as soon as possible. However, if it is almost time for your next dose, skip the missed dose and just take the next one. Do not double your dose. Take your medication exactly as directed by your doctor or other healthcare professional. Do not stop taking a prescription medication unless directed by your doctor or other healthcare professional.

What Side Effects Can *Loniten®* (minoxidil) Cause?

More Common

- Fast heartbeat (palpitations)
- Increased hair growth, usually on the face, arms, and back
- Swelling or puffiness of the feet, ankles, or lower legs (edema)
- Weight gain

Less Common

- Cardiac chest pain (angina)
- Rash (skin redness, bumps, itching, or irritation)
- Shortness of breath

Rare

- Breast tenderness

Tell your doctor or other healthcare professional if you have side effects that bother you, do not go away, make you worried about taking your medication, or make you want to stop taking your medication.

Do Other Medications Interact with *Loniten®* (minoxidil)?

Other high blood pressure medications (see Glossary) *may increase* the side effects of *Loniten®* (minoxidil).

Loniten® (minoxidil) *may decrease* how well diuretics (water pills) such as *HydroDIURIL®* (hydrochlorothiazide or HCTZ), *Lasix®* (furosemide), and others (see Glossary) work.

Nonsteroidal anti-inflammatory drugs (NSAIDs) such as *Motrin®* (ibuprofen), *Aleve®* (naproxen), *Vioxx®* (rofecoxib), *Celebrex®* (celecoxib), and others (see Glossary) *may decrease* how well *Loniten®* (minoxidil) works.

Many nonprescription (over-the-counter [OTC]) medications such as antacids, laxatives, pain, cough, cold, and allergy medications contain medications that *may increase* blood pressure. If you are taking blood pressure medication, you should talk to your doctor or other healthcare professional before taking any new OTC medications.

Tell your doctor or other healthcare professional about all medications (both prescription and nonprescription [over-the-counter] medications) that you are taking.

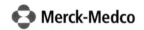
Why Else Do People Take *Loniten*® (minoxidil)?

Rogaine®, which is a liquid form of minoxidil, may help grow hair in men with baldness.

What Else Should I Know about *Loniten*® (minoxidil)?

Medications cannot cure high blood pressure, but they can help control it and help reduce the chance of stroke, heart attack (myocardial infarction), congestive heart failure, kidney failure, and death. It is important to take your blood pressure medications daily as prescribed to help reduce your risks. Keeping your weight down, eating a healthy diet that is low in salt (sodium), and exercising regularly will also help control your blood pressure. Ask your doctor or other healthcare professional for a diet and exercise plan.

Have your blood pressure checked regularly as directed by your doctor or other healthcare professional.

 # Warning!

To give you the best care, your doctor or other healthcare professional needs to know about the diseases and medical conditions you have had—your full medical history. Tell your doctor or other healthcare professional if you have or have ever had any of the following:

- Allergy or previous reaction to *Loniten*® (minoxidil)
- Cardiac chest pain (angina)
- Congestive heart failure
- Heart attack (myocardial infarction)
- Heart rhythm problems (arrhythmia)

Loniten® (minoxidil) may cause fluid retention and swelling or puffiness of the feet, ankles, or lower legs (edema). This medication is sometimes prescribed with a diuretic (water pill) to help prevent swelling. Ask your doctor or other healthcare professional about diuretics if you have edema.

Loniten® (minoxidil) may make you unsteady on your feet, causing you to fall and possibly break a bone. If you have fallen recently, tell your doctor or other healthcare professional about it. Taking a different medication or a lower dose may make you less likely to fall. You should not stop taking this medication without first talking to your doctor or other healthcare professional.

High Cholesterol

What Is Cholesterol?

Cholesterol is a fatty substance made by the body and found in the blood. Having the right amount of cholesterol is important to the healthy functioning of the body. People with too much cholesterol in the blood have a greater chance of developing heart disease.

Cholesterol comes from two sources. Your body itself makes some cholesterol and brings in some with the food you eat. Food from animal sources, such as meat, poultry, fish, seafood, and dairy products, contains cholesterol. Vegetables and other kinds of food that come from plants, such as wheat and other grains, do not contain cholesterol.

Although the oils and fats that come from vegetables and plants do not contain cholesterol, some may be as harmful as animal fat when they are eaten in large amounts. These are the saturated fats, such as coconut oil, palm oil, and cocoa butter. Other plant fats can be part of a healthy diet when eaten in recommended amounts. These include monounsaturated fats, such as canola oil and olive oil, and polyunsaturated fats, such as corn oil, sunflower oil, and soybean oil.

Cholesterol and other fats are carried through the bloodstream by lipoproteins, a type of protein. Two common types of lipoproteins are high-density lipoproteins (also called HDLs), which are sometimes called "good cholesterol" because they carry cholesterol to the liver to be removed from the body, and low-density lipoproteins (LDLs), which are sometimes called "bad cholesterol" because they deposit cholesterol in your arteries, causing buildup.

The body makes both kinds of cholesterol. Both are needed for several normal body functions. The foods you eat play only one part in how much of each kind of cholesterol is in your body. You also have an inborn cholesterol-making tendency that you inherited from past generations of your family. Some

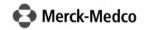

people's bodies make too much "bad cholesterol" even when they have very healthy diets and stay away from fatty foods that are high in cholesterol.

Having too much LDL (bad cholesterol) in your blood, especially when there is too little HDL (good cholesterol) at the same time, increases the risk that your arteries will become hard and clogged, a condition called atherosclerosis. Arteries are the blood vessels that carry blood through your heart and from your heart to other parts of your body. Arteries in the heart and brain are particularly prone to clogging and hardening. If an artery in your heart clogs, it can cause a heart attack. If an artery in your brain clogs, it can cause a stroke.

Your doctor or other healthcare professional needs to know about the balance between the amount of HDL and LDL in your blood. It is one important way to find out how likely you are to develop heart disease or have a stroke.

Another type of fat found in the blood is triglycerides. Triglycerides may not be a direct cause of heart disease, but very high amounts in a person's blood suggest that the person may not be eating as healthy a diet as he or she should. Eating an unhealthy diet can cause other problems that may lead to heart disease and/or stroke. People with diabetes must be especially careful to keep their triglyceride levels within the normal range.

How Is High Cholesterol Treated?

If you have high cholesterol, you can do a number of things to improve it. You can reduce the amount of fat that you eat, particularly saturated fat and hydrogenated fat, as are found especially in eggs, butter, and red meat. You can lose weight, which will be helped by eating less fat. You can exercise more with the approval of your doctor or other healthcare professional. If you smoke, you can stop. While stopping smoking may not directly lower your cholesterol level, it will help to reduce the risk of coronary artery disease.

If all these do not lower your cholesterol enough, or if your cholesterol count is already dangerously high, your doctor or other healthcare professional may prescribe medications that are designed to improve the amounts of different kinds of cholesterol in your blood—to reduce the "bad" ones and increase the "good" ones. But medications cannot do it all. Even after you start to take a medication for high cholesterol, you have to eat properly, exercise regularly, keep your weight down, and not smoke. Talk to your doctor or other healthcare professional before starting an exercise program.

Tips for Lowering High Cholesterol and Reducing Your Chance of Heart Disease

These are some ways you may be able to help lower your cholesterol if it is too high:

- **Watch your weight.** Losing weight and eating foods that are low in fat often lower cholesterol.

- **Exercise.** Regular exercise increases the amount of "good" cholesterol (HDL) in the blood and slightly lowers the amount of "bad" cholesterol (LDL). Talk to your doctor or other healthcare professional before you start an exercise program.

- **Do not smoke.** Smoking increases your chance of heart disease.

- **Eat well.** About two thirds of what you eat should be fruits, vegetables, and whole grains. Only one third should be meat and dairy products.

Medications for High Cholesterol

Several kinds of medications may be taken for high cholesterol. This chapter discusses these medications and/or categories of medications:

MEDICATIONS	See Page
Statins	434
Fibrates	438
Bile Acid Binders	442
Niacin	446

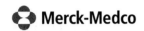

If you do not see the exact name of the medication that you take for high cholesterol listed above, check the Medication and Chapter Table to find out which category your medication falls under or check the Index.

Statins

Statins may help lower high LDL (bad cholesterol), even in people whose high cholesterol has already started to harden their arteries, and can help lower cholesterol in people without heart disease to help prevent heart disease. Some statins can also lower triglyceride levels and help to raise HDL (good cholesterol). Note that the generic name of each cholesterol medication in this list ends in "statin."

Brand Name	Generic Name
Baycol®	cerivastatin
Lescol®	fluvastatin
Lipitor®	atorvastatin
Mevacor®	lovastatin
Pravachol®	pravastatin
Zocor®	simvastatin

 ## How Will I Take Statins?

Statins come as pills and are usually taken once daily. *Baycol®* (cerivastatin) and *Zocor®* (simvastatin) are usually taken in the evening, with or without food. *Lescol®* (fluvastatin) is usually taken at bedtime with or without food. *Lipitor®* (atorvastatin) and *Pravachol®* (pravastatin) may be taken at any time, with or without food. *Mevacor®* (lovastatin) is usually taken with your evening meal. It may take up to 4 weeks to see changes in your cholesterol blood tests. Your doctor or other healthcare professional will tell you how often to take your medication.

If you miss a dose of this medication, take the dose you missed as soon as possible. However, if it is almost time for your next dose, skip the missed dose and just take the next one. Do not double your dose. Take your medication exactly as directed by your doctor or other healthcare professional. Do not stop taking a prescription medication unless directed by your doctor or other healthcare professional.

What Side Effects Can Statins Cause?

More Common

- Constipation
- Diarrhea
- Dizziness
- Gas
- Headache
- Nausea
- Rash (skin redness, bumps, itching, or irritation)
- Stomach pain

Less Common

- Erection problems (erectile dysfunction)
- Flu-like symptoms (fever, chills, runny nose)
- General aches and pains
- Heartburn
- Trouble falling asleep or staying asleep (insomnia)

Rare

- Liver problems that may cause yellowing of the skin or eyes (jaundice)
- Severe muscle cramps and weakness which can be very serious—see Warning on page 437

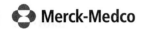

Tell your doctor or other healthcare professional if you have side effects that bother you, do not go away, make you worried about taking your medication, or make you want to stop taking your medication.

Do Other Medications Interact with Statins?

These medications *may increase* the side effects of statins:

- *Atromid-S*® (clofibrate)
- *Biaxin*® (clarithromycin)
- Calcium channel blockers such as *Cardizem*® (diltiazem), *Norvasc*® (amlodipine), *Procardia*® (nifedipine), and others—see Glossary
- *Diflucan*® (fluconazole)
- Erythromycin such as *Ery-Tab*®, *Erythrocin*®, and others—see Glossary
- *Lopid*® (gemfibrozil)
- *Neoral*® (cyclosporine)
- Niacin
- *Nizoral*® (ketoconazole)
- *Sandimmune*® (cyclosporine)
- *Serzone*® (nefazodone)
- *Sporanox*® (itraconazole)
- *Tricor*® (fenofibrate)

Statins *may increase* the side effects of *Coumadin*® (warfarin).

Bile acid binders such as *Questran*® (cholestyramine) or *Colestid*® (colestipol), or a bulk-forming laxative like *Metamucil*® (psyllium) *may decrease* the effects of statins by preventing them from being absorbed completely. To help make sure they are absorbed so they can work properly, take statins 1 hour before or 4 to 6 hours after taking a bile acid binder or a bulk-forming laxative.

Grapefruit and grapefruit juice *may increase* the side effects of statins. This interaction can happen whether you eat the grapefruit or drink the grapefruit juice at the same time as you take your medication or if you take the medication separately from the grapefruit or grapefruit juice. Talk to your doctor or other healthcare professional before eating grapefruit or drinking grapefruit juice if you are taking this medication. Please also read the discussion on A Warning about Grapefruit and Grapefruit Juice on pages i-ii.

Tell your doctor or other healthcare professional about all medications (both prescription and nonprescription [over-the-counter] medications) that you are taking.

What Else Should I Know about Statins?

If you are going to have any kind of surgery, tell your doctor or other healthcare professional about it. He or she may want you to stop taking your statin medication for a short time before the operation because you may have an increased risk of muscle breakdown during surgery, which can lead to kidney failure.

 # Warning!

To give you the best care, your doctor or other healthcare professional needs to know about the diseases and medical conditions you have had—your full medical history. Tell your doctor or other healthcare professional if you have or have ever had any of the following:

- Allergy or previous reaction to statins
- Any organ transplant
- High alcohol intake (drinking 3 or more alcoholic beverages, such as beer, wine, whiskey, and others, every day)
- Liver problems
- Low blood pressure (hypotension)

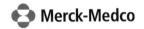

- Overactive thyroid (hyperthyroidism)
- Poorly controlled diabetes requiring frequent hospitalizations
- Recent (within the past month) major surgery or traumatic accident
- Underactive thyroid (hypothyroidism)

If you are having chest pain, pain in the left shoulder, down the inside of the left arm, or pain in the throat, jaw, teeth, back (between the shoulder blades), or abdomen (stomach), you may be having a heart attack. Other symptoms of a heart attack might include fullness, pressure, heaviness, discomfort, numbness, or tightness on your chest. If you take nitroglycerin and the dose that has been prescribed for you does not relieve your symptoms, or you do not have nitroglycerin, go to the emergency room of the nearest hospital where you will be evaluated and your doctor or other healthcare professional will be contacted.

If you have severe muscle cramps or weakness, contact your doctor or other healthcare professional immediately. This may be a sign of muscle breakdown, which may lead to kidney failure.

Since statins may cause damage to your liver, your doctor or other healthcare professional may order blood tests to find out early on if the medication is causing liver problems, before they become serious.

Fibrates

Fibrates, also called fibric acid derivatives, are medications that help lower triglyceride levels and LDL (bad cholesterol). They may also help raise HDL (good cholesterol).

Brand Name	Generic Name
Atromid-S®	clofibrate
Lopid®	gemfibrozil
Tricor®	fenofibrate

How Will I Take Fibrates?

Fibrates come as pills and are usually taken 1 to 4 times daily. *Lopid®* (gemfibrozil) is usually taken before meals. *Atromid-S®* (clofibrate) and *Tricor®* (fenofibrate) are usually taken during a meal. It may take up to 6 to 8 weeks to see changes in your cholesterol blood tests. Your doctor or other healthcare professional will tell you how many times a day to take your medication.

If you miss a dose of this medication, take the dose you missed as soon as possible. However, if it is almost time for your next dose, skip the missed dose and just take the next one. Do not double your dose. Take your medication exactly as directed by your doctor or other healthcare professional. Do not stop taking a prescription medication unless directed by your doctor or other healthcare professional.

What Side Effects Can Fibrates Cause?

More Common

- Diarrhea
- Gas or bloating
- Headache
- Heartburn
- Nausea
- Tiredness or sluggishness (fatigue)

Less Common

- Cardiac chest pain (angina)
- Constipation
- Fast heartbeat (palpitations)
- Flu-like symptoms (fever, chills, runny nose)
- Gallstones

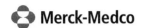

Rare

- Liver problems that may cause yellowing of the skin or eyes (jaundice)

- Low red blood cells (anemia)

- Pancreas problems (pancreatitis)

- Rash (skin redness, bumps, itching, or irritation)

- Severe muscle cramps and weakness which can be very serious—see Warning on page 441

- Swelling or puffiness of the feet, ankles, or lower legs (edema)

Tell your doctor or other healthcare professional if you have side effects that bother you, do not go away, make you worried about taking your medication, or make you want to stop taking your medication.

 ## Do Other Medications Interact with Fibrates?

Fibrates *may increase* the side effects of these medications:

- *Coumadin*® (warfarin)

- Statins such as *Lipitor*® (atorvastatin), *Pravachol*® (pravastatin), *Zocor*® (simvastatin), and others—see Glossary

Bile acid binders such as *Questran*® (cholestyramine) or *Colestid*® (colestipol), or a bulk-forming laxative like *Metamucil*® (psyllium) *may decrease* the effects of fibrates by preventing them from being absorbed completely. To help make sure they are absorbed so they can work properly, take fibrates 1 hour before or 4 to 6 hours after taking a bile acid binder or a bulk-forming laxative.

Tell your doctor or other healthcare professional about all medications (both prescription and nonprescription [over-the-counter] medications) that you are taking.

Warning!

To give you the best care, your doctor or other healthcare professional needs to know about the diseases and medical conditions you have had—your full medical history. Tell your doctor or other healthcare professional if you have or have ever had any of the following:

- Allergy or previous reaction to *Lopid*® (gemfibrozil), *Tricor*® (fenofibrate), or *Atromid-S*® (clofibrate)

- Cardiac chest pain (angina)

- Gallbladder problems

- Heart rhythm problems (arrhythmias)

- Kidney problems

- Liver problems

- Overactive thyroid (hyperthyroidism)

- Stomach problems (ulcers)

- Underactive thyroid (hypothyroidism)

If you are having chest pain, pain in the left shoulder, down the inside of the left arm, or pain in the throat, jaw, teeth, back (between the shoulder blades), or abdomen (stomach), you may be having a heart attack. Other symptoms of a heart attack might include fullness, pressure, heaviness, discomfort, numbness, or tightness on your chest. If you take nitroglycerin and the dose that has been prescribed for you does not relieve your symptoms, or you do not have nitroglycerin, go to the emergency room of the nearest hospital where you will be evaluated and your doctor or other healthcare professional will be contacted.

If you have severe muscle cramps or weakness, contact your doctor or other healthcare professional immediately. This may be a sign of muscle breakdown, which may lead to kidney failure.

Since fibrates may cause damage to your liver, your doctor or other healthcare professional may order blood tests to find out early on if the medication is causing liver problems, before they become serious.

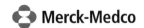

Bile Acid Binders

Bile acid binders lower LDL (bad cholesterol) levels by binding cholesterol and helping prevent its reabsorption into the body.

Brand Name	Generic Name
Colestid®	colestipol
LoCHOLEST®	cholestyramine
Prevalite®	cholestyramine
Questran®	cholestyramine

How Will I Take Bile Acid Binders?

Bile acid binders are usually taken twice a day. Mix your powdered bile acid binder with at least 8 ounces of water or juice, or mix it with milk, cereal, or soup. Bile acid binders are usually taken 1 hour after or 4 to 6 hours before other medications so that both will work as well as possible. It may take up to 1 to 2 months to see changes in your cholesterol blood tests. Your doctor or other healthcare professional will tell you how many times a day to take your medication.

If you miss a dose of this medication, take the dose you missed as soon as possible. However, if it is almost time for your next dose, skip the missed dose and just take the next one. Do not double your dose. Take your medication exactly as directed by your doctor or other healthcare professional. Do not stop taking a prescription medication unless directed by your doctor or other healthcare professional.

What Side Effects Can Bile Acid Binders Cause?

More Common

- Bloating
- Constipation
- Dizziness when standing up from a bed or a chair
- Gas
- Headache
- Heartburn
- Nausea
- Poor appetite
- Stomach pain
- Vomiting

Less Common

- Bleeding that does not stop easily (nose bleeds, bleeding while brushing your teeth, and cuts)
- Bowel movements that float or are unusually loose or smelly (fatty stools)
- Decreased absorption of certain foods and nutrients
- Easy bruising ("black-and-blue" marks on the skin)
- Gallstones
- Pancreas problems (pancreatitis)
- Vitamin deficiencies

Tell your doctor or other healthcare professional if you have side effects that bother you, do not go away, make you worried about taking your medication, or make you want to stop taking your medication.

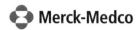

Do Other Medications Interact with Bile Acid Binders?

Many medications do not work well if they are taken at about the same time as a bile acid binder. The bile acid binder "binds" these medications just as it binds the bile acid, preventing the body from absorbing them properly. This is why you should not take your bile acid binder at the same time as other medications. Bile acid binders are usually taken 1 hour after or 4 to 6 hours before other medications so that both will work as well as possible. These are only some of the medications that should not be taken at the same time as bile acid binders:

- *Actigall*® (ursodiol)
- *Actonel*® (risedronate)
- Antibiotics
- *Atromid-S*® (clofibrate)
- Corticosteroids such as prednisone and others—see Glossary
- *Coumadin*® (warfarin)
- Diabetes medications such as *DiaBeta*® (glyburide), *Glucophage*® (metformin), *Glucotrol*® (glipizide), and others—see Glossary
- Diuretics (water pills) such as *HydroDIURIL*® (hydrochlorothiazide or HCTZ), *Lasix*® (furosemide), and others—see Glossary
- Estrogens such as *Estrace*®, *Premarin*®, *Prempro*™, and others—see Glossary
- *Fosamax*® (alendronate)
- High blood pressure (hypertension) medications—see Glossary
- *Lanoxin*® (digoxin)
- *Lopid*® (gemfibrozil)
- Multivitamins (especially those that contain folic acid and the fat-soluble vitamins A, D, E, and K)
- Nonsteroidal anti-inflammatory drugs (NSAIDs) such as *Motrin*® (ibuprofen), *Aleve*® (naproxen), *Vioxx*® (rofecoxib), *Celebrex*® (celecoxib), and others—see Glossary

- Seizure medications such as *Dilantin®* (phenytoin), *Depakote®* (valproic acid), *Neurontin®* (gabapentin), *Tegretol®* (carbamazepine), and others—see Glossary

- Statins such as *Lipitor®* (atorvastatin), *Pravachol®* (pravastatin), *Zocor®* (simvastatin), and others—see Glossary

- Thyroid medications such as *Cytomel®* (liothyronine), *Levoxyl®* (levothyroxine), *Synthroid®* (levothyroxine), and others—see Glossary

- *Tricor®* (fenofibrate)

- Tricyclic antidepressants such as *Elavil®* (amitriptyline), *Pamelor®* (nortriptyline), *Sinequan®* (doxepin), and others—see Glossary

Questran® (cholestyramine) ***may increase*** the side effects of *Comtan®* (entacapone).

Tell your doctor or other healthcare professional about all medications (both prescription and nonprescription [over-the-counter] medications) that you are taking.

 # Warning!

To give you the best care, your doctor or other healthcare professional needs to know about the diseases and medical conditions you have had—your full medical history. Tell your doctor or other healthcare professional if you have or have ever had any of the following:

- Allergy or previous reaction to bile acid binders

- Constipation

- Gallbladder problems

- Liver problems

- Underactive thyroid (hypothyroidism)

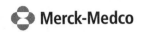

If you are having chest pain, pain in the left shoulder, down the inside of the left arm, or pain in the throat, jaw, teeth, back (between the shoulder blades), or abdomen (stomach), you may be having a heart attack. Other symptoms of a heart attack might include fullness, pressure, heaviness, discomfort, numbness, or tightness on your chest. If you take nitroglycerin and the dose that has been prescribed for you does not relieve your symptoms, or you do not have nitroglycerin, go to the emergency room of the nearest hospital where you will be evaluated and your doctor or other healthcare professional will be contacted.

If you become very constipated, have stomach or abdominal pain, or lose a lot of weight for no apparent reason over the course of a few weeks, tell your doctor or other healthcare professional about it.

Niacin

Niacin is a vitamin that lowers cholesterol by helping prevent the body from making cholesterol in the liver. It may lower LDL (bad cholesterol) and increase HDL (good cholesterol). Niacin is usually available as a nonprescription (over-the-counter) medication. Some forms of niacin are available only with a prescription.

How Will I Take Niacin?

Niacin is usually taken 1 to 3 times daily. Niacin may be taken with a meal, snack, or glass of milk to help prevent stomach upset. Your doctor or other healthcare professional will tell you how often to take your medication.

To help prevent side effects, your doctor or other healthcare professional may start by giving you a low dose of this medication and increase the amount slowly until it works well for you.

When a medication has initials after its name, such as XL, XR, SR, BID, DUR, and others, it usually means that the body absorbs the medication slowly over time, so you usually have to take it only once or twice a day. The body will absorb some medications of this type too fast if you crush or break them or dissolve them in liquid, and their effects will not last as long as they should.

Check with your doctor or other healthcare professional before crushing or breaking your pills or dissolving your pills in liquid.

If you miss a dose of this medication, take the dose you missed as soon as possible. However, if it is almost time for your next dose, skip the missed dose and just take the next one. Do not double your dose. Take your medication exactly as directed by your doctor or other healthcare professional. Do not stop taking a prescription medication unless directed by your doctor or other healthcare professional.

What Side Effects Can Niacin Cause?

More Common

- Headache
- Itching or tingling
- Nausea
- Reddening of the face (flushing)
- Stomach pain
- Vomiting

Less Common

- Diarrhea
- Dizziness when standing up from a bed or a chair
- Dry skin or eyes
- Fast heartbeat (palpitations)
- Gout (very painful, swollen joints)
- Increased blood sugar (hyperglycemia)

Rare

- Liver problems that may cause yellowing of the skin or eyes (jaundice)

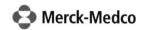

Tell your doctor or other healthcare professional if you have side effects that bother you, do not go away, make you worried about taking your medication, or make you want to stop taking your medication.

 ## Do Other Medications Interact with Niacin?

Niacin *may increase* the side effects of statins such as *Lipitor*® (atorvastatin), *Pravachol*® (pravastatin), *Zocor*® (simvastatin), and others—see Glossary.

Bile acid binders such as *Questran*® (cholestyramine) or *Colestid*® (colestipol), or a bulk-forming laxative like *Metamucil*® (psyllium) *may decrease* the effects of niacin by preventing it from being absorbed completely. To help make sure it is absorbed so it can work properly, take niacin 1 hour before or 4 to 6 hours after taking a bile acid binder or a bulk-forming laxative.

Tell your doctor or other healthcare professional about all medications (both prescription and nonprescription [over-the-counter] medications) that you are taking.

What Else Should I Know about Niacin?

When you first start to take niacin, you may have brief reddening (flushing) and a sensation of warmth, especially on your face and upper body. These symptoms usually go away after you have been taking niacin for 3 to 6 weeks. Drinking alcoholic beverages (such as beer, wine, whiskey, and others) or hot drinks when you take your niacin may make these symptoms worse. If these symptoms are bothersome, talk to your doctor or other healthcare professional about taking one 325-mg aspirin tablet (plain, uncoated tablet) or an NSAID 30 minutes before you take your niacin to help prevent this side effect from happening or help make it less bothersome.

Warning!

To give you the best care, your doctor or other healthcare professional needs to know about the diseases and medical conditions you have had—your full medical history. Tell your doctor or other healthcare professional if you have or have ever had any of the following:

- Allergy or previous reaction to niacin

- Bleeding problems

- Diabetes

- Easy bruising ("black and blue" marks on the skin)

- Gallbladder problems

- Glaucoma (an eye disease)

- Gout

- High alcohol intake (drinking 3 or more alcoholic beverages, such as beer, wine, whiskey and others, every day)

- Kidney problems

- Liver problems

- Low blood pressure (hypotension)

- Stomach problems (ulcer)

- Underactive thyroid (hypothyroidism)

If you are having chest pain, pain in the left shoulder, down the inside of the left arm, or pain in the throat, jaw, teeth, back (between the shoulder blades), or abdomen (stomach), you may be having a heart attack. Other symptoms of a heart attack might include fullness, pressure, heaviness, discomfort, numbness, or tightness on your chest. If you take nitroglycerin and the dose that has been prescribed for you does not relieve your symptoms, or you do not have nitroglycerin, go to the emergency room of the nearest hospital where you will be evaluated and your doctor or other healthcare professional will be contacted.

Niacin may make you unsteady on your feet, causing you to fall and possibly break a bone. If you have fallen recently, tell your doctor or other healthcare

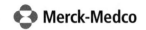

professional about it. Taking a different medication or a lower dose may make you less likely to fall. You should not stop taking this medication without first talking to your doctor or other healthcare professional.

Since niacin may cause damage to your liver, your doctor or other healthcare professional may order blood tests to find out early on if the medication is causing liver problems, before they become serious.

Chapter 14

Irregular or Abnormal Heartbeat

What Is an Irregular or Abnormal Heartbeat (Arrhythmia)?

An arrhythmia is a condition in which the heart beats abnormally. The heart can feel like it has skipped a beat or has had an extra beat. This feeling is sometimes described as a palpitation. It could also mean the heart is beating too slow or too fast. An arrhythmia may keep the heart from working as well as it should.

The heart consists of two upper chambers called the atria and two lower chambers called the ventricles. Arrhythmias may occur in any of these chambers. In some arrhythmias, like atrial fibrillation, the heart may not work well enough to pump out all of the blood. When the blood does not move through the heart normally, blood clots may form in the heart. These clots can then move out of the heart into the bloodstream.

A stroke is what happens when a clot blocks one of the blood vessels in the brain. The brain needs a constant supply of oxygen to function normally. When any part of the brain does not get enough oxygen, it may be permanently damaged.

Not all arrhythmias need treatment. But of those that do, some may be treated with medication, some may be treated with a pacemaker or other device, and, rarely, some need to be treated with surgery. Talk to your doctor or other healthcare professional to find out which treatment is right for you.

Many different types of heart rhythm problem (arrythmia) medications are used to help prevent or control abnormal heart rhythms or irregular heartbeat. There are different types of classes of heart rhythm problem (arrythmia) medications, and each has a different way of working to help prevent or control

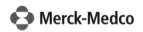
an irregular heartbeat. Heart rhythm medications work on specific substances in the heart that control the electrical signals and beating of the heart.

Medications for Arrhythmia

Several kinds of medications may be taken for arrhythmias. This chapter discusses these medications and/or categories of medications:

MEDICATIONS	See Page
Digoxin	453
Norpace® (disopyramide)	458
Procainamide	463
Quinidine	467
Rythmol® (propafenone)	473
Tambocor® (flecainide)	477
Tonocard® (tocainide)	481
Mexitil® (mexiletine)	485
Beta Blockers	489
Amiodarone	494
Betapace® (sotalol)	499
Diltiazem and Verapamil	504

If you do not see the exact name of the medication that you take for an irregular or abnormal heartbeat listed above, check the Medication and Chapter Table to find out which category your medication falls under or check the Index.

Digoxin

Digoxin treats an abnormally fast heartbeat that starts in the upper chambers (atria) of the heart. Atrial fibrillation and atrial flutter are examples of this type of irregular heartbeat. Taking digoxin slows the abnormally fast heartbeat and helps improve the symptoms of arrhythmia.

Brand Name	Generic Name
Lanoxicaps®	digoxin
Lanoxin®	digoxin

How Will I Take Digoxin?

Lanoxin® (digoxin) or *Lanoxicaps®* (digoxin) are usually taken as a pill or liquid once a day or possibly once every other day. Some people take different doses on different days to get the right amount of medication into the blood. Your doctor or other healthcare professional will tell you how often to take your medication.

If you miss a dose of this medication, take the dose you missed as soon as possible. However, if it is almost time for your next dose, skip the missed dose and just take the next one. Do not double your dose. Take your medication exactly as directed by your doctor or other healthcare professional. Do not stop taking a prescription medication unless directed by your doctor or other healthcare professional.

What Side Effects Can Digoxin Cause?

More Common
- Diarrhea
- Headache

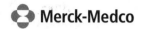

- Nausea

- Poor appetite

- Slow heartbeat (palpitations)*

- Vomiting

Less Common

- Blurred vision

- Confusion

- Dizziness

- Heart rhythm problems (arrhythmia)*

- Passing out or fainting

- Seeing "halos" around bright objects

- Tiredness or sluggishness (fatigue)

Rare

- Increased breast size in men

*Sometimes medications may actually cause or worsen the same symptoms they are being used to help relieve. Talk to your doctor or other healthcare professional if your symptoms get worse instead of better while taking this medication.

Tell your doctor or other healthcare professional if you have side effects that bother you, do not go away, make you worried about taking your medication, or make you want to stop taking your medication.

 Do Other Medications Interact with Digoxin?

These medications *may increase* the side effects of digoxin:

- Beta blockers such as *Inderal*® (propranolol), *Tenormin*® (atenolol), *Toprol*® (metoprolol), and others—see Glossary

- *Biaxin*® (clarithromycin)

- Calcium channel blockers such as *Cardizem*® (diltiazem), *Norvasc*® (amlodipine), *Procardia*® (nifedipine), and others—see Glossary

- Corticosteroids such as prednisone and others—see Glossary

- *Diflucan*® (fluconazole)

- Diuretics (water pills) such as *HydroDIURIL*® (hydrochlorothiazide or HCTZ), *Lasix*® (furosemide), and others—see Glossary

- Erythromycin such as *Ery-Tab*®, *Erythrocin*®, and others—see Glossary

- *Micardis*® (telmisartan)

- *Neoral*® (cyclosporine)

- *Nizoral*® (ketoconazole)

- Other heart rhythm problem (arrhythmia) medications—see Glossary

- *Plaquenil*® (hydroxychloroquine)

- Propylthiouracil or PTU

- Quinidine such as *Quinaglute*®, *Quinidex*®, and others—see Glossary

- *Sandimmune*® (cyclosporine)

- *Serzone*® (nefazodone)

- *Sporanox*® (itraconazole)

- *Tapazole*® (methimazole)

- Tetracycline antibiotics such as *Dynacin*® (minocycline), *Sumycin*® (tetracycline), *Vibramycin*® (doxycycline), and others—see Glossary

These medications ***may decrease*** how well digoxin works:

- *Azulfidine*® (sulfasalazine)

- *Neo-Tabs*™ (neomycin)

- *Precose*® (acarbose)

- *Reglan*® (metoclopramide)

- *Rheumatrex*® (methotrexate)

- Thyroid medications such as *Cytomel*® (liothyronine), *Levoxyl*® (levothyroxine), *Synthroid*® (levothyroxine), and others—see Glossary

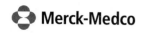

Antacids such as *Maalox®* or *Mylanta®* (aluminum hydroxide/magnesium hydroxide), *Rolaids®* or *Tums®* (calcium carbonate), or *Amphojel®* (aluminum hydroxide) ***may decrease*** the effects of digoxin when taken at the same time. If you are using antacids, take your digoxin dose 1 hour before or 2 hours after taking your antacid.

Bile acid binders such as *Questran®* (cholestyramine) or *Colestid®* (colestipol) or bulk-forming laxatives like *Metamucil®* (psyllium) ***may decrease*** the effects of digoxin by preventing it from being absorbed completely. To help make sure it is absorbed so it can work properly, take your digoxin dose 1 hour before or 4 to 6 hours after taking a bile acid binder or a bulk-forming laxative.

Many nonprescription (over-the-counter [OTC]) medications such as cough, cold, and allergy medications contain decongestants which ***may decrease*** how well heart rhythm medications work. If you are taking digoxin, you should talk to your doctor or other healthcare professional before taking any new OTC medications.

Tell your doctor or other healthcare professional about all medications (both prescription and nonprescription [over-the-counter] medications) that you are taking.

Why Else Do People Take Digoxin?

Lanoxin® (digoxin) and *Lanoxicaps®* (digoxin) are also taken for congestive heart failure.

 # Warning!

To give you the best care, your doctor or other healthcare professional needs to know about the diseases and medical conditions you have had—your full medical history. Tell your doctor or other healthcare professional if you have or have ever had any of the following:

- Allergy or previous reaction to *Lanoxin*® (digoxin) or *Lanoxicaps*® (digoxin)

- Heart attack (myocardial infarction)

- Kidney problems

- Low potassium in your blood (hypokalemia)

- Overactive thyroid (hyperthyroidism)

- Underactive thyroid (hypothyroidism)

Not having enough potassium in the blood (hypokalemia) may lead to increased side effects from digoxin and make the heart beat abnormally. If you are taking any of the medications listed below, they may lower potassium levels in your blood. Follow your doctor or other healthcare professional's instructions about what to eat or whether to take potassium supplements (pills, liquid, or powder) to help keep your potassium level normal, and have your blood tested as recommended. The following medications may lower potassium levels in your blood:

- Diuretics (water pills) such as *HydroDIURIL*® (hydrochlorothiazide or HCTZ), *Lasix*® (furosemide), and others—see Glossary

- Corticosteroids such as prednisone and others—see Glossary

Since digoxin may cause side effects if you get too much medication and may not work well if you do not get enough, your doctor or other healthcare professional may order blood tests to see if you are getting the right amount of this medication. Nausea, vomiting, diarrhea, dizziness, and blurred vision may be early signs that you are getting too much medication. Talk to your doctor or other healthcare professional if you have any of these symptoms, and be sure to get your blood tests as ordered. Do not change your dose or stop taking this medication unless directed by your doctor or other healthcare professional.

Digoxin may make you unsteady on your feet, causing you to fall and possibly break a bone. If you have fallen recently, tell your doctor or other healthcare professional about it. Taking a different medication or a lower dose may make you less likely to fall. You should not stop taking this medication without first talking to your doctor or other healthcare professional.

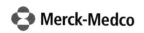

If you suddenly have leg or arm weakness, a change in or loss of vision, trouble speaking, or confusion, you may be having a stroke. This is serious and needs to be treated immediately. If you have these symptoms, go to the emergency room of the nearest hospital where you will be examined and your doctor or other healthcare professional will be contacted.

▲ *Norpace*® (disopyramide)

This medication works by changing the electrical impulses in the heart to help control abnormal heart rhythms and heartbeat.

▲ Indicates medications that are more likely to cause unpleasant or dangerous side effects. These medications are generally not recommended for people over 65. The side effects may not be very obvious and may be mistaken for "just a part of getting older" but may be serious. If you are taking one of these medications, you might want to talk to your doctor or other healthcare professional to see if this medication is best for you. Safer medications may be available and lower dosages may be required. You should not stop taking these medications without first talking to your doctor or other healthcare professional.

See the WARNING section on page 461 for the specific safety problems associated with this medication ▲.

 ## How Will I Take *Norpace*® (disopyramide)?

Norpace® (disopyramide) is usually taken 1 to 4 times a day. It may be taken with or without food. Your doctor or other healthcare professional will tell you how many times a day to take your medication.

When a medication has initials after its name, such as XL, XR, SR, BID, DUR, and others, it usually means that the body absorbs the medication slowly over time, so you usually have to take it only once or twice a day. The body will absorb some medications of this type too fast if you crush or break them or dissolve them in liquid, and their effects will not last as long as they should. Check with your doctor or other healthcare professional before crushing or breaking your pills or dissolving your pills in liquid.

If you miss a dose of this medication, take the dose you missed as soon as possible. However, if it is almost time for your next dose, skip the missed dose and just take the next one. Do not double your dose. Take your medication exactly as directed by your doctor or other healthcare professional. Do not stop taking a prescription medication unless directed by your doctor or other healthcare professional.

What Side Effects Can *Norpace*® (disopyramide) Cause?

More Common

- Blurred vision

- Constipation

- Dizziness

- Dry mouth, eyes, and nose

- Irregular heartbeat (palpitations)*

- Trouble urinating or emptying the bladder

Rare

- Decreased blood sugar (hypoglycemia)

- Liver problems that may cause yellowing of the skin or eyes (jaundice)

*Sometimes medications may actually cause or worsen the same symptoms they are being used to help relieve. Talk to your doctor or other healthcare professional if your symptoms get worse instead of better while taking this medication.

Tell your doctor or other healthcare professional if you have side effects that bother you, do not go away, make you worried about taking your medication, or make you want to stop taking your medication.

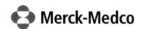 **Merck-Medco**

Do Other Medications Interact with *Norpace®* (disopyramide)?

These medications *may increase* the side effects of *Norpace®* (disopyramide):

- Beta blockers such as *Inderal®* (propranolol), *Tenormin®* (atenolol), *Toprol®* (metoprolol), and others—see Glossary

- *Biaxin®* (clarithromycin)

- Calcium channel blockers such as *Cardizem®* (diltiazem), *Norvasc®* (amlodipine), *Procardia®* (nifedipine), and others—see Glossary

- Erythromycin such as *Ery-Tab®*, *Erythrocin®*, and others—see Glossary

- Other heart rhythm problem (arrhythmia) medications—see Glossary

- *Zagam®* (sparfloxacin)

These medications *may decrease* how well *Norpace®* (disopyramide) works:

- Barbiturates such as *Butisol®* (butabarbital), *Luminal®* (phenobarbital), *Mebaral®* (mephobarbital), and others—see Glossary

- *Dilantin®* (phenytoin)

- *Rifadin®* (rifampin)

Norpace® (disopyramide) is generally not prescribed for anyone who is taking *Propulsid®* (cisapride [withdrawn from general distribution; available only by special arrangement with the manufacturer]), *Seldane®* (terfenadine [no longer commercially available]), or *Hismanal®* (astemizole [no longer commercially available]), because together they *may cause* serious, sometimes fatal, heart problems.

Norpace® (disopyramide) *may increase* the side effects of other medications that cause drowsiness, including antidepressants, antihistamines (allergy medications), benzodiazepines (a type of tranquilizer), anxiety medications, narcotics (pain relievers), muscle relaxants, neuroleptic medications (a type of tranquilizer), seizure medications, or sleep medications. Avoid driving a car and other activities that need mental alertness, like using a knife or operating machinery, while taking this medication.

Drinking alcoholic beverages (such as beer, wine, whiskey, and others) *may increase* the side effects of *Norpace*® (disopyramide).

Many nonprescription (over-the-counter [OTC]) medications such as cough, cold, and allergy medications contain decongestants which *may decrease* how well heart rhythm medications work. If you are taking *Norpace*® (disopyramide), you should talk to your doctor or other healthcare professional before taking any new OTC medications.

Tell your doctor or other healthcare professional about all medications (both prescription and nonprescription [over-the-counter] medications) that you are taking.

Warning!

To give you the best care, your doctor or other healthcare professional needs to know about the diseases and medical conditions you have had—your full medical history. Tell your doctor or other healthcare professional if you have or have ever had any of the following:

- Allergy or previous reaction to *Norpace*® (disopyramide)
- Congestive heart failure
- Diabetes
- Enlarged prostate (benign prostatic hypertrophy)
- Glaucoma (an eye disease)
- Kidney problems
- Liver problems
- Trouble urinating or emptying the bladder

Since *Norpace*® (disopyramide) may cause side effects if you get too much medication and may not work well if you do not get enough, your doctor or other healthcare professional may order blood tests to see if you are getting the right amount of this medication. Dizziness, constipation, and blurred vision

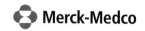

may be early signs that you are getting too much medication. Talk to your doctor or other healthcare professional if you have any of these symptoms, and be sure to get your blood tests as ordered. Do not change your dose or stop taking this medication unless directed by your doctor or other healthcare professional.

Norpace® (disopyramide) may cause side effects such as trouble urinating or urinary retention, dizziness, and constipation. This medication is generally not recommended for use in people over 65. If you are taking *Norpace®* (disopyramide), ask your doctor or other healthcare professional if it is the right medication for you. Do not stop taking the medication without talking to your doctor or other healthcare professional.

Norpace® (disopyramide) may cause drowsiness. Avoid driving a car and other activities that need mental alertness, like using a knife or operating machinery, while taking this medication. Drinking alcoholic beverages (such as beer, wine, whiskey, and others) may increase the side effects.

Norpace® (disopyramide) may make you unsteady on your feet, causing you to fall and possibly break a bone. If you have fallen recently, tell your doctor or other healthcare professional about it. Taking a different medication or a lower dose may make you less likely to fall. You should not stop taking this medication without first talking to your doctor or other healthcare professional.

If you suddenly have leg or arm weakness, a change in or loss of vision, trouble speaking, or confusion, you may be having a stroke. This is serious and needs to be treated immediately. If you have these symptoms, go to the emergency room of the nearest hospital where you will be examined and your doctor or other healthcare professional will be contacted.

Under certain circumstances, your doctor or other healthcare professional may decide that you should stop taking this medication. If you have taken it for more than a couple of weeks, he or she may want you to decrease it gradually, lowering the dose over a few weeks or months. Stopping suddenly may cause unpleasant withdrawal symptoms or may worsen your medical problems. Pay careful attention to the instructions your doctor or other healthcare professional gives you about how much less to take and for how long.

Procainamide

This medication works by changing the electrical impulses in the heart to help control abnormal heart rhythms and heartbeat.

How Will I Take Procainamide?

Procainamide is usually taken 2 to 6 times a day. It should be taken on an empty stomach 1 hour before meals or 2 hours after meals. Ask your doctor or other healthcare professional about taking it with food if it upsets your stomach. Your doctor or other healthcare professional will tell you how many times a day to take your medication.

When a medication has initials after its name, such as XL, XR, SR, BID, DUR, and others, it usually means that the body absorbs the medication slowly over time, so you usually have to take it only 2 to 4 times a day. The body will absorb some medications of this type too fast if you crush or break them or dissolve them in liquid, and their effects will not last as long as they should. Check with your doctor or other healthcare professional before crushing or breaking your pills or dissolving your pills in liquid.

If you miss a dose of this medication, take the dose you missed as soon as possible. However, if it is almost time for your next dose, skip the missed dose and just take the next one. Do not double your dose. Take your medication exactly as directed by your doctor or other healthcare professional. Do not stop taking a prescription medication unless directed by your doctor or other healthcare professional.

What Side Effects Can Procainamide Cause?

More Common

- Bitter taste
- Diarrhea

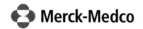

- Dizziness

- Nausea

- Poor appetite

- Vomiting

Less Common

- Allergic reactions such as rash (skin redness, bumps, itching, or irritation), swelling of the face and throat, or trouble breathing

- Easy bruising ("black-and-blue" marks on the skin)

- Frequent fever, sore throat, or flu-like symptoms that may be a sign of low white blood cells

- Heart rhythm problems (arrhythmia)*

- Skin rash with fever and joint pain and swelling that may be a sign of lupus

- Sadness, feeling blue or down, depressed mood (depression)

- Tingling, pain, or weakness in the hands and feet

- Tiredness or sluggishness (fatigue)

Rare

- Liver problems that may cause yellowing of the skin or eyes (jaundice)

*Sometimes medications may actually cause or worsen the same symptoms they are being used to help relieve. Talk to your doctor or other healthcare professional if your symptoms get worse instead of better while taking this medication.

Tell your doctor or other healthcare professional if you have side effects that bother you, do not go away, make you worried about taking your medication, or make you want to stop taking your medication.

Do Other Medications Interact with Procainamide?

These medications *may increase* the side effects of procainamide:

- Beta blockers such as *Inderal*® (propranolol), *Tenormin*® (atenolol), *Toprol*® (metoprolol), and others—see Glossary

- Calcium channel blockers such as *Cardizem*® (diltiazem), *Norvasc*® (amlodipine), *Procardia*® (nifedipine), and others—see Glossary

- *Floxin*® (ofloxacin)

- Other heart rhythm problem (arrhythmia) medications—see Glossary

- *Proloprim*® (trimethoprim)

- *Tagamet*® (cimetidine)

- *Trimpex*® (trimethoprim)

- *Zagam*® (sparfloxacin)

Procainamide *may increase* the side effects of *Glucophage*® (metformin).

Procainamide is generally not prescribed for anyone who is taking *Propulsid*® (cisapride [withdrawn from general distribution; available only by special arrangement with the manufacturer]), *Seldane*® (terfenadine [no longer commercially available]), or *Hismanal*® (astemizole [no longer commercially available]), because together they *may cause* serious, sometimes fatal, heart problems.

Many nonprescription (over-the-counter [OTC]) medications such as cough, cold, and allergy medications contain decongestants which *may decrease* how well heart rhythm medications work. If you are taking procainamide, you should talk to your doctor or other healthcare professional before taking any new OTC medications.

Tell your doctor or other healthcare professional about all medications (both prescription and nonprescription [over-the-counter] medications) that you are taking.

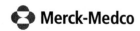

🛑 Warning!

To give you the best care, your doctor or other healthcare professional needs to know about the diseases and medical conditions you have had—your full medical history. Tell your doctor or other healthcare professional if you have or have ever had any of the following:

- Allergy or previous reaction to procainamide

- Blood problems

- Cardiac chest pain (angina)

- Congestive heart failure

- Kidney problems

- Liver problems

- Lupus

If you get a skin rash with pain or swelling in your joints (elbows, knees, and others), especially while taking procainamide, call your doctor or other healthcare professional.

Since procainamide may cause side effects if you get too much medication and may not work well if you do not get enough, your doctor or other healthcare professional may order blood tests to see if you are getting the right amount of this medication. Poor appetite, dizziness, and nausea may be early signs that you are getting too much medication. Talk to your doctor or other healthcare professional if you have any of these symptoms, and be sure to get your blood tests as ordered. Do not change your dose or stop taking this medication unless directed by your doctor or other healthcare professional.

If you suddenly have leg or arm weakness, a change in or loss of vision, trouble speaking, or confusion, you may be having a stroke. This is serious and needs to be treated immediately. If you have these symptoms, go to the emergency room of the nearest hospital where you will be examined and your doctor or other healthcare professional will be contacted.

Procainamide may make you unsteady on your feet, causing you to fall and possibly break a bone. If you have fallen recently, tell your doctor or other healthcare professional about it. Taking a different medication or a lower dose may make you less likely to fall. You should not stop taking this medication without first talking to your doctor or other healthcare professional.

Under certain circumstances, your doctor or other healthcare professional may decide that you should stop taking this medication. If you have taken it for more than a couple of weeks, he or she may want you to decrease it gradually, lowering the dose over a few weeks or months. Stopping suddenly may cause unpleasant withdrawal symptoms or may worsen your medical problems. Pay careful attention to the instructions your doctor or other healthcare professional gives you about how much less to take and for how long.

Quinidine

This medication works by changing the electrical impulses in the heart to help control abnormal heart rhythms.

 ## How Will I Take Quinidine?

Quinidine is usually taken 1 to 4 times a day. It should be taken on an empty stomach 1 hour before meals or 2 hours after meals. Ask your doctor or other healthcare professional about taking it with food if it upsets your stomach. Your doctor or other healthcare professional will tell you how many times a day to take your medication.

When a medication has initials after its name, such as XL, XR, SR, BID, DUR, and others, it usually means that the body absorbs the medication slowly over time, so you usually have to take it only once or twice a day. The body will absorb some medications of this type too fast if you crush or break them or dissolve them in liquid, and their effects will not last as long as they should. Check with your doctor or other healthcare professional before crushing or breaking your pills or dissolving your pills in liquid.

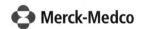

If you miss a dose of this medication, take the dose you missed as soon as possible. However, if it is almost time for your next dose, skip the missed dose and just take the next one. Do not double your dose. Take your medication exactly as directed by your doctor or other healthcare professional. Do not stop taking a prescription medication unless directed by your doctor or other healthcare professional.

 ## What Side Effects Can Quinidine Cause?

More Common
- Diarrhea
- Nausea
- Poor appetite
- Stomach pain
- Vomiting

Less Common
- Blurred vision
- Cardiac chest pain (angina)
- Confusion
- Dizziness
- Increased sensitivity to the sun (bad sunburn)
- Nervousness (anxiety)
- Passing out or fainting
- Sadness, feeling blue or down, depressed mood (depression)
- Seeing or hearing things that are not there (hallucinations)

Rare
- Allergic reactions such as rash (skin redness, bumps, itching, or irritation), swelling of the face and throat, or trouble breathing

- Easy bruising ("black-and-blue" marks on the skin)
- Frequent fever, sore throat, or flu-like symptoms that may be a sign of low white blood cells
- Headache
- Hearing problems
- Kidney problems
- Liver problems that may cause yellowing of the skin or eyes (jaundice)
- Reddening of the face (flushing)
- Ringing in the ears (tinnitus)

Tell your doctor or other healthcare professional if you have side effects that bother you, do not go away, make you worried about taking your medication, or make you want to stop taking your medication.

Do Other Medications Interact with Quinidine?

These medications *may increase* the side effects of quinidine:

- Antacids containing magnesium such as *Maalox®*, *Mylanta®*, *Phillips'® Milk of Magnesia*, and others—see Glossary
- Calcium channel blockers such as *Cardizem®* (diltiazem), *Norvasc®* (amlodipine), *Procardia®* (nifedipine), and others—see Glossary
- *Daranide®* (dichlorphenamide)
- *Diamox®* (acetazolamide)
- *Diflucan®* (fluconazole)
- Diuretics (water pills) such as *HydroDIURIL®* (hydrochlorothiazide or HCTZ), *Lasix®* (furosemide), and others—see Glossary
- *Neptazane®* (methazolamide)
- *Nizoral®* (ketoconazole)

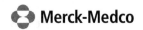

- *Norvir*® (ritonavir)
- *Sporanox*® (itraconazole)
- *Tagamet*® (cimetidine)
- *Zagam*® (sparfloxacin)

These medications *may decrease* how well quinidine works:
- Barbiturates such as *Butisol*® (butabarbital), *Luminal*® (phenobarbital), *Mebaral*® (mephobarbital), and others—see Glossary
- *Dilantin*® (phenytoin)
- *Mexitil*® (mexiletine)
- *Midamor*® (amiloride)
- *Rifadin*® (rifampin)

Quinidine *may increase* the side effects of these medications:
- *Coumadin*® (warfarin)
- *Lanoxin*® (digoxin) or *Lanoxicaps*® (digoxin)
- *Glucophage*® (metformin)
- Other heart rhythm problem (arrhythmia) medications—see Glossary
- Tricyclic antidepressants such as *Elavil*® (amitriptyline), *Pamelor*® (nortriptyline), *Sinequan*® (doxepin), and others—see Glossary

Quinidine *may decrease* how well codeine (various brand names) works.

Quinidine is generally not prescribed for anyone who is taking *Propulsid*® (cisapride [withdrawn from general distribution; available only by special arrangement with the manufacturer]), *Seldane*® (terfenadine [no longer commercially available]), or *Hismanal*® (astemizole [no longer commercially available]), because together they *may cause* serious, sometimes fatal, heart problems.

Grapefruit and grapefruit juice *may increase* the side effects of quinidine. This interaction can happen whether you eat the grapefruit or drink the grapefruit juice at the same time as you take your medication or if you take the medication separately from the grapefruit or grapefruit juice. Talk to your doctor or other healthcare professional before eating grapefruit or drinking grapefruit juice if you are taking this medication. Please also read the discussion on A Warning about Grapefruit and Grapefruit Juice on pages i-ii.

Many nonprescription (over-the-counter [OTC]) medications such as cough, cold, and allergy medications contain decongestants which *may decrease* how well heart rhythm medications work. If you are taking quinidine, you should talk to your doctor or other healthcare professional before taking any new OTC medications.

Tell your doctor or other healthcare professional about all medications (both prescription and nonprescription [over-the-counter] medications) that you are taking.

Warning!

To give you the best care, your doctor or other healthcare professional needs to know about the diseases and medical conditions you have had—your full medical history. Tell your doctor or other healthcare professional if you have or have ever had any of the following:

- Allergy or previous reaction to quinidine or quinine
- Congestive heart failure
- Kidney problems
- Liver problems
- Low blood pressure (hypotension)
- Lupus
- Myasthenia gravis

Since quinidine may cause side effects if you get too much medication and may not work well if you do not get enough, your doctor or other healthcare

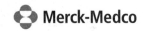

professional may order blood tests to see if you are getting the right amount of this medication. Nausea, vomiting, and poor appetite may be early signs that you are getting too much medication. Talk to your doctor or other healthcare professional if you have any of these symptoms, and be sure to get your blood tests as ordered. Do not change your dose or stop taking this medication unless directed by your doctor or other healthcare professional.

Quinidine may make you unsteady on your feet, causing you to fall and possibly break a bone. If you have fallen recently, tell your doctor or other healthcare professional about it. Taking a different medication or a lower dose may make you less likely to fall. You should not stop taking this medication without first talking to your doctor or other healthcare professional.

If you suddenly have leg or arm weakness, a change in or loss of vision, trouble speaking, or confusion, you may be having a stroke. This is serious and needs to be treated immediately. If you have these symptoms, go to the emergency room of the nearest hospital where you will be examined and your doctor or other healthcare professional will be contacted.

Since quinidine may cause damage to your liver, your doctor or other healthcare professional may order blood tests to find out early on if the medication is causing liver problems, before they become serious.

If you are taking quinidine, stay out of the sun as much as you can to avoid a serious sunburn. When you do go out in the sun, use sunblock or sunscreen, and wear protective clothing, such as a wide-brimmed hat and a long-sleeved shirt.

Under certain circumstances, your doctor or other healthcare professional may decide that you should stop taking this medication. If you have taken it for more than a couple of weeks, he or she may want you to decrease it gradually, lowering the dose over a few weeks or months. Stopping suddenly may cause unpleasant withdrawal symptoms or may worsen your medical problems. Pay careful attention to the instructions your doctor or other healthcare professional gives you about how much less to take and for how long.

Rythmol® (propafenone)

This medication works by changing the electrical impulses in the heart to help control abnormal heart rhythms.

How Will I Take *Rythmol*® (propafenone)?

This medication is usually taken 3 times daily. It may be taken with or without food. Your doctor or other healthcare professional will tell you how often to take your medication.

To help prevent side effects, your doctor or other healthcare professional may start by giving you a low dose of this medication, increasing the amount slowly until it works well for you.

If you miss a dose of this medication, take the dose you missed as soon as possible. However, if it is almost time for your next dose, skip the missed dose and just take the next one. Do not double your dose. Take your medication exactly as directed by your doctor or other healthcare professional. Do not stop taking a prescription medication unless directed by your doctor or other healthcare professional.

What Side Effects Can *Rythmol*® (propafenone) Cause?

More Common

- Constipation

- Dizziness

- Headache

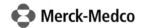

- Irregular heartbeat (palpitations)*

- Nausea

- Tiredness or sluggishness (fatigue)

- Vomiting

Less Common

- Blurred vision

- Diarrhea

- Drowsiness

- Poor coordination and unsteadiness when walking or standing

- Shakiness or tremors

- Trouble falling asleep or staying asleep (insomnia)

Rare

- Allergic reactions such as rash (skin redness, bumps, itching, or irritation), swelling of the face and throat, or trouble breathing

- Frequent fever, sore throat, or flu-like symptoms that may be a sign of low white blood cells

- Liver problems that may cause yellowing of the skin or eyes (jaundice)

*Sometimes medications may actually cause or worsen the same symptoms they are being used to help relieve. Talk to your doctor or other healthcare professional if your symptoms get worse instead of better while taking this medication.

Tell your doctor or other healthcare professional if you have side effects that bother you, do not go away, make you worried about taking your medication, or make you want to stop taking your medication.

Do Other Medications Interact with *Rythmol*® (propafenone)?

These medications *may increase* the side effects of *Rythmol*® (propafenone):

- *Norvir*® (ritonavir)
- Quinidine such as *Quinaglute*®, *Quinidex*®, and others—see Glossary
- *Tagamet*® (cimetidine)

Rifadin® (rifampin) *may decrease* how well *Rythmol*® (propafenone) works.

Rythmol® (propafenone) *may increase* the side effects of these medications:

- Beta blockers such as *Inderal*® (propranolol), *Tenormin*® (atenolol), *Toprol*® (metoprolol), and others—see Glossary
- Calcium channel blockers such as *Cardizem*® (diltiazem), *Norvasc*® (amlodipine), *Procardia*® (nifedipine), and others—see Glossary
- *Coumadin*® (warfarin)
- *Lanoxin*® (digoxin) or *Lanoxicaps*® (digoxin)
- *Neoral*® (cyclosporine)
- *Sandimmune*® (cyclosporine)
- Theophylline such as *Theo-Dur*®, *Uniphyl*®, and others—see Glossary
- Tricyclic antidepressants such as *Elavil*® (amitriptyline), *Pamelor*® (nortriptyline), *Sinequan*® (doxepin), and others—see Glossary

Rythmol® (propafenone) is generally not prescribed for anyone who is taking *Propulsid*® (cisapride [withdrawn from general distribution; available only by special arrangement with the manufacturer]), *Seldane*® (terfenadine [no longer commercially available]), or *Hismanal*® (astemizole [no longer commercially available]), because together they *may cause* serious, sometimes fatal, heart problems.

Many nonprescription (over-the-counter [OTC]) medications such as cough, cold, and allergy medications contain decongestants which *may decrease* how well heart rhythm medications work. If you are taking *Rythmol*® (propafenone), you should talk to your doctor or other healthcare professional before taking any new OTC medications.

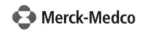

Tell your doctor or other healthcare professional about all medications (both prescription and nonprescription [over-the-counter] medications) that you are taking.

Warning!

To give you the best care, your doctor or other healthcare professional needs to know about the diseases and medical conditions you have had—your full medical history. Tell your doctor or other healthcare professional if you have or have ever had any of the following:

- Allergy or previous reaction to *Rythmol*® (propafenone)

- Blood problems

- Breathing problems (asthma and COPD, including emphysema or chronic bronchitis)

- Congestive heart failure

- Kidney problems

- Liver problems

- Low blood pressure (hypotension)

- Low potassium in your blood (hypokalemia)

If you suddenly have leg or arm weakness, a change in or loss of vision, trouble speaking, or confusion, you may be having a stroke. This is serious and needs to be treated immediately. If you have these symptoms, go to the emergency room of the nearest hospital where you will be examined and your doctor or other healthcare professional will be contacted.

Rythmol® (propafenone) may make you unsteady on your feet, causing you to fall and possibly break a bone. If you have fallen recently, tell your doctor or other healthcare professional about it. Taking a different medication or a lower dose may make you less likely to fall. You should not stop taking this medication without first talking to your doctor or other healthcare professional.

Under certain circumstances, your doctor or other healthcare professional may decide that you should stop taking this medication. If you have taken it for more than a couple of weeks, he or she may want you to decrease it gradually, lowering the dose over a few weeks or months. Stopping suddenly may cause unpleasant withdrawal symptoms or may worsen your medical problems. Pay careful attention to the instructions your doctor or other healthcare professional gives you about how much less to take and for how long.

Tambocor® (flecainide)

This medication works by changing the electrical impulses in the heart to help control abnormal heart rhythms and heartbeat.

 ### How Will I Take *Tambocor*® (flecainide)?

This medication is usually taken 2 times daily. It can be taken with or without food. Your doctor or other healthcare professional will tell you how often to take your medication.

To help prevent side effects, your doctor or other healthcare professional may start by giving you a low dose of this medication, increasing the amount slowly until it works well for you.

If you miss a dose of this medication, take the dose you missed as soon as possible. However, if it is almost time for your next dose, skip the missed dose and just take the next one. Do not double your dose. Take your medication exactly as directed by your doctor or other healthcare professional. Do not stop taking a prescription medication unless directed by your doctor or other healthcare professional.

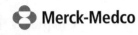

⚠ What Side Effects Can *Tambocor*® (flecainide) Cause?

More Common

- Cardiac chest pain (angina)
- Constipation
- Dizziness
- Headache
- Irregular heartbeat (palpitations)*
- Nausea
- Nervousness (anxiety)
- Tiredness or sluggishness (fatigue)
- Trouble breathing or shortness of breath
- Unusual or metallic taste
- Vomiting

Less Common

- Blurred vision
- Rash (skin redness, bumps, itching, or irritation)
- Shakiness or tremors
- Stomach pain

*Sometimes medications may actually cause or worsen the same symptoms they are being used to help relieve. Talk to your doctor or other healthcare professional if your symptoms get worse instead of better while taking this medication.

Tell your doctor or other healthcare professional if you have side effects that bother you, do not go away, make you worried about taking your medication, or make you want to stop taking your medication.

Do Other Medications Interact with *Tambocor*® (flecainide)?

These medications *may increase* the side effects of *Tambocor*® (flecainide):

- Beta blockers such as *Inderal*® (propranolol), *Tenormin*® (atenolol), *Toprol*® (metoprolol), and others—see Glossary

- Calcium channel blockers such as *Cardizem*® (diltiazem), *Norvasc*® (amlodipine), *Procardia*® (nifedipine), and others—see Glossary

- *Norvir*® (ritonavir)

- Other heart rhythm problem (arrhythmia) medications—see Glossary

- *Tagamet*® (cimetidine)

Tambocor® (flecainide) *may increase* the side effects of *Lanoxin*® (digoxin) or *Lanoxicaps*® (digoxin).

Tambocor® (flecainide) is generally not prescribed for anyone who is taking *Propulsid*® (cisapride [withdrawn from general distribution; available only by special arrangement with the manufacturer]), *Seldane*® (terfenadine [no longer commercially available]), or *Hismanal*® (astemizole [no longer commercially available]), because together they *may cause* serious, sometimes fatal, heart problems.

Many nonprescription (over-the-counter [OTC]) medications such as cough, cold, and allergy medications contain decongestants which *may decrease* how well heart rhythm medications work. If you are taking *Tambocor*® (flecainide), you should talk to your doctor or other healthcare professional before taking any new OTC medications.

Tell your doctor or other healthcare professional about all medications (both prescription and nonprescription [over-the-counter] medications) that you are taking.

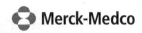

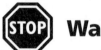 # Warning!

To give you the best care, your doctor or other healthcare professional needs to know about the diseases and medical conditions you have had—your full medical history. Tell your doctor or other healthcare professional if you have or have ever had any of the following:

- Allergy or previous reaction to *Tambocor*® (flecainide)

- Congestive heart failure

- Kidney problems

- Liver problems

- Low potassium in your blood (hypokalemia)

Tambocor® (flecainide) may make you unsteady on your feet, causing you to fall and possibly break a bone. If you have fallen recently, tell your doctor or other healthcare professional about it. Taking a different medication or a lower dose may make you less likely to fall. You should not stop taking this medication without first talking to your doctor or other healthcare professional.

If you suddenly have leg or arm weakness, a change in or loss of vision, trouble speaking, or confusion, you may be having a stroke. This is serious and needs to be treated immediately. If you have these symptoms, go to the emergency room of the nearest hospital where you will be examined and your doctor or other healthcare professional will be contacted.

Under certain circumstances, your doctor or other healthcare professional may decide that you should stop taking this medication. If you have taken it for more than a couple of weeks, he or she may want you to decrease it gradually, lowering the dose over a few weeks or months. Stopping suddenly may cause unpleasant withdrawal symptoms or may worsen your medical problems. Pay careful attention to the instructions your doctor or other healthcare professional gives you about how much less to take and for how long.

Tonocard® (tocainide)

This medication works by changing the electrical impulses in the heart to help control abnormal heart rhythms and heartbeat.

How Will I Take *Tonocard*® (tocainide)?

This medication is usually taken 3 times daily. It may be taken with or without food. Your doctor or other healthcare professional will tell you how often to take your medication.

To help prevent side effects, your doctor or other healthcare professional may start by giving you a low dose of this medication, increasing the amount slowly until it works well for you.

If you miss a dose of this medication, take the dose you missed as soon as possible. However, if it is almost time for your next dose, skip the missed dose and just take the next one. Do not double your dose. Take your medication exactly as directed by your doctor or other healthcare professional. Do not stop taking a prescription medication unless directed by your doctor or other healthcare professional.

What Side Effects Can *Tonocard*® (tocainide) Cause?

More Common

- Dizziness

- Headache

- Irregular heartbeat (palpitations)*

- Nausea

*Sometimes medications may actually cause or worsen the same symptoms they are being used to help relieve. Talk to your doctor or other healthcare professional if your symptoms get worse instead of better while taking this medication.

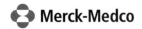

- Nervousness (anxiety)
- Poor coordination and unsteadiness when walking or standing
- Shakiness or tremors
- Tingling, numbness, or pain in hands and feet
- Trouble breathing or shortness of breath

Less Common

- Blurred vision
- Diarrhea
- Low blood pressure (hypotension)
- Poor appetite
- Rash (skin redness, bumps, itching, or irritation)
- Ringing in the ears (tinnitus)
- Stomach pain
- Vomiting

Rare

- Easy bruising ("black-and-blue" marks on the skin)
- Frequent fever, sore throat, or flu-like symptoms that may be a sign of low white blood cells
- Hair loss
- Low red blood cells (anemia)
- Skin rash with fever and joint pain and swelling that may be a sign of lupus

---

Tell your doctor or other healthcare professional if you have side effects that bother you, do not go away, make you worried about taking your medication, or make you want to stop taking your medication.

Do Other Medications Interact with *Tonocard*® (tocainide)?

These medications *may increase* the side effects of *Tonocard*® (tocainide):

- Beta blockers such as *Inderal*® (propranolol), *Tenormin*® (atenolol), *Toprol*® (metoprolol), and others—see Glossary

- Other heart rhythm problem (arrhythmia) medications—see Glossary

Tonocard® (tocainide) *may increase* the side effects of *Lanoxin*® (digoxin) or *Lanoxicaps*® (digoxin).

Rifadin® (rifampin) *may decrease* the side effects of *Tonocard*® (tocainide).

Tonocard® (tocainide) is generally not prescribed for anyone who is taking *Propulsid*® (cisapride [withdrawn from general distribution; available only by special arrangement with the manufacturer]), *Seldane*® (terfenadine [no longer commercially available]), or *Hismanal*® (astemizole [no longer commercially available]), because together they *may cause* serious, sometimes fatal, heart problems.

Many nonprescription (over-the-counter [OTC]) medications such as cough, cold, and allergy medications contain decongestants which *may decrease* how well heart rhythm medications work. If you are taking *Tonocard*® (tocainide), you should talk to your doctor or other healthcare professional before taking any new OTC medications.

Tell your doctor or other healthcare professional about all medications (both prescription and nonprescription [over-the-counter] medications) that you are taking.

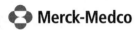

⬟ **STOP** Warning!

To give you the best care, your doctor or other healthcare professional needs to know about the diseases and medical conditions you have had—your full medical history. Tell your doctor or other healthcare professional if you have or have ever had any of the following:

- Allergy or previous reaction to *Tonocard*® (tocainide) or lidocaine

- Congestive heart failure

- Heart attack (myocardial infarction)

- Kidney problems

- Liver problems

- Low potassium in your blood (hypokalemia)

Tonocard® (tocainide) may make you unsteady on your feet, causing you to fall and possibly break a bone. If you have fallen recently, tell your doctor or other healthcare professional about it. Taking a different medication or a lower dose may make you less likely to fall. You should not stop taking this medication without first talking to your doctor or other healthcare professional.

Under certain circumstances, your doctor or other healthcare professional may decide that you should stop taking this medication. If you have taken it for more than a couple of weeks, he or she may want you to decrease it gradually, lowering the dose over a few weeks or months. Stopping suddenly may cause unpleasant withdrawal symptoms or may worsen your medical problems. Pay careful attention to the instructions your doctor or other healthcare professional gives you about how much less to take and for how long.

Mexitil® (mexiletine)

This medication works by changing the electrical impulses in the heart to help control abnormal heart rhythms and heartbeat.

How Will I Take *Mexitil*® (mexiletine)?

This medication is usually taken 3 to 4 times daily. It may be taken with or without food. It may be taken with food to help prevent stomach upset. Your doctor or other healthcare professional will tell you how often to take your medication.

If you miss a dose of this medication, take the dose you missed as soon as possible. However, if it is almost time for your next dose, skip the missed dose and just take the next one. Do not double your dose. Take your medication exactly as directed by your doctor or other healthcare professional. Do not stop taking a prescription medication unless directed by your doctor or other healthcare professional.

What Side Effects Can *Mexitil*® (mexiletine) Cause?

More Common

- Cardiac chest pain (angina)

- Confusion

- Diarrhea

- Dizziness

- Headache

- Irregular heartbeat (palpitations)*

*Sometimes medications may actually cause or worsen the same symptoms they are being used to help relieve. Talk to your doctor or other healthcare professional if your symptoms get worse instead of better while taking this medication.

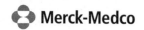

- Nausea

- Shakiness or tremors

- Tiredness or sluggishness (fatigue)

- Unpleasant taste

- Vomiting

Less Common

- Blurred vision

- Congestive heart failure

- Dry mouth

- Passing out or fainting

- Rash (skin redness, bumps, itching, or irritation)

- Ringing in the ears (tinnitus)

- Sadness, feeling blue or down, depressed mood (depression)

- Stomach pain

- Trouble breathing or shortness of breath

Rare

- Easy bruising ("black-and-blue" marks on the skin)

- Frequent fever, sore throat, or flu-like symptoms that may be a sign of low white blood cells

- Liver problems that may cause yellowing of the skin or eyes (jaundice)

- Seizures

- Skin rash with fever and joint pain and swelling that may be a sign of lupus

- Swelling or puffiness of the feet, ankles, or lower legs (edema)

- Ulcers in the stomach that may cause black, tarry-looking bowel movements

Tell your doctor or other healthcare professional if you have side effects that bother you, do not go away, make you worried about taking your medication, or make you want to stop taking your medication.

Do Other Medications Interact with *Mexitil*® (mexiletine)?

These medications *may increase* the side effects of *Mexitil*® (mexiletine):

- Beta blockers such as *Inderal*® (propranolol), *Tenormin*® (atenolol), *Toprol*® (metoprolol), and others—see Glossary

- Calcium channel blockers such as *Cardizem*® (diltiazem), *Norvasc*® (amlodipine), *Procardia*® (nifedipine), and others—see Glossary

- Other heart rhythm problem (arrhythmia) medications—see Glossary

Mexitil® (mexiletine) *may increase* the side effects of the following:

- Caffeine, such as in coffee, tea, colas, chocolate, and other foods

- Theophylline such as *Theo-Dur*®, *Uniphyl*®, and others—see Glossary

These medications *may decrease* the side effects of *Mexitil*® (mexiletine):

- *Dilantin*® (phenytoin)

- *Rifadin*® (rifampin)

Many nonprescription (over-the-counter [OTC]) medications such as cough, cold, and allergy medications contain decongestants which *may decrease* how well heart rhythm medications work. If you are taking *Mexitil*® (mexiletine), you should talk to your doctor or other healthcare professional before taking any new OTC medications.

Tell your doctor or other healthcare professional about all medications (both prescription and nonprescription [over-the-counter] medications) that you are taking.

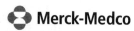

STOP **Warning!**

To give you the best care, your doctor or other healthcare professional needs to know about the diseases and medical conditions you have had—your full medical history. Tell your doctor or other healthcare professional if you have or have ever had any of the following:

- Allergy or previous reaction to *Mexitil®* (mexiletine)
- Blood problems
- Congestive heart failure
- Heart attack (myocardial infarction)
- Liver problems
- Low blood pressure (hypotension)
- Parkinson's disease
- Seizures (epilepsy)
- Stomach problems (ulcers)

Mexitil® (mexiletine) may make you unsteady on your feet, causing you to fall and possibly break a bone. If you have fallen recently, tell your doctor or other healthcare professional about it. Taking a different medication or a lower dose may make you less likely to fall. You should not stop taking this medication without first talking to your doctor or other healthcare professional.

Mexitil® (mexiletine) may cause stomach pain, which may be a sign of an ulcer. However, you may have an ulcer without feeling any pain at all. If ulcers are not treated, they may cause serious stomach or intestinal bleeding. Tell your doctor or other healthcare professional if you have severe stomach pain or stomach pain that keeps returning or if you have ever had peptic ulcer disease. Call your doctor or other healthcare professional right away if you have black, tarry-looking bowel movements (stools), if you vomit dark material that looks like coffee grounds, or if you notice any blood in your bowel movements. Any of these symptoms may be a sign of a bleeding ulcer.

Since *Mexitil®* (mexiletine) may cause damage to your liver, your doctor or other healthcare professional may order blood tests to find out early on if the medication is causing liver problems, before they become serious.

If you have had seizures in the past, tell your doctor or other healthcare professional because *Mexitil®* (mexiletine) may cause seizures. Stopping this medication suddenly may also cause seizures. If your doctor or other healthcare professional decides that you should stop taking *Mexitil®* (mexiletine), pay careful attention to the instructions he or she gives you about how much less to take and for how long.

Under certain circumstances, your doctor or other healthcare professional may decide that you should stop taking this medication. If you have taken it for more than a couple of weeks, he or she may want you to decrease it gradually, lowering the dose over a few weeks or months. Stopping suddenly may cause unpleasant withdrawal symptoms or may worsen your medical problems. Pay careful attention to the instructions your doctor or other healthcare professional gives you about how much less to take and for how long.

Beta Blockers

These medications work by slowing down the heartbeat to help control abnormal heart rhythms and heartbeat.

Brand Name	Generic Name
Blocadren®	timolol
Corgard®	nadolol
Inderal®	propranolol
Kerlone®	betaxolol
Lopressor®	metoprolol
Tenormin®	atenolol
Toprol®	metoprolol
Zebeta®	bisoprolol

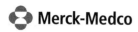

How Will I Take Beta Blockers?

Beta blockers are usually taken 1 to 3 times daily. They may be taken with or without food. However, the way you take most of them should be consistent. They should either always be taken with food or always be taken without food. Your doctor or other healthcare professional will tell you how often to take your medication.

When a medication has initials after its name, such as XL, XR, SR, BID, DUR, and others, it usually means that the body absorbs the medication slowly over time, so you usually have to take it only once or twice a day. The body will absorb some medications of this type too fast if you crush or break them or dissolve them in liquid, and their effects will not last as long as they should. Check with your doctor or other healthcare professional before crushing or breaking your pills or dissolving your pills in liquid.

If you miss a dose of this medication, take the dose you missed as soon as possible. However, if it is almost time for your next dose, skip the missed dose and just take the next one. Do not double your dose. Take your medication exactly as directed by your doctor or other healthcare professional. Do not stop taking a prescription medication unless directed by your doctor or other healthcare professional.

What Side Effects Can Beta Blockers Cause?

More Common

- Dizziness when standing up from a bed or a chair
- Erection problems (erectile dysfunction)
- Loss of interest in sex (decreased libido)
- Tiredness or sluggishness (fatigue)
- Weakness

Less Common

- Change in blood sugar

- Congestive heart failure

- Heartburn

- Leg pain when walking

- Rash (skin redness, bumps, itching, or irritation)

- Sadness, feeling blue or down, depressed mood (depression)

- Slow or irregular heartbeat (palpitations)*

- Strange dreams and nightmares

- Trouble breathing or shortness of breath with asthma and COPD, including emphysema or chronic bronchitis

*Sometimes medications may actually cause or worsen the same symptoms they are being used to help relieve. Talk to your doctor or other healthcare professional if your symptoms get worse instead of better while taking this medication.

Tell your doctor or other healthcare professional if you have side effects that bother you, do not go away, make you worried about taking your medication, or make you want to stop taking your medication.

 Do Other Medications Interact with Beta Blockers?

Beta blockers **may decrease** how well these medications work:

- Diabetes medications such as *DiaBeta*® (glyburide), *Glucophage*® (metformin), *Glucotrol*® (glipizide), and others—see Glossary

These medications **may increase** the side effects of beta blockers:

- High blood pressure (hypertension) medications and diuretics (water pills)—see Glossary

- *Lanoxin*® (digoxin) or *Lanoxicaps*® (digoxin)

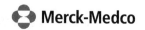

- Neuroleptic medications such as *Risperdal®* (risperidone), *Thorazine®* (chlorpromazine), *Zyprexa®* (olanzapine), and others—see Glossary

- Other heart rhythm problem (arrhythmia) medications—see Glossary

- Propylthiouracil or PTU

- *Tagamet®* (cimetidine)

- *Tapazole®* (methimazole)

Beta blockers *may increase* the side effects of these medications:

- *DHE-45®* (dihydroergotamine)

- *Ergomar®* (ergotamine)

- *Migranal®* (dihydroergotamine)

These medications *may decrease* how well beta blockers work:

- Barbiturates such as *Butisol®* (butabarbital), *Luminal®* (phenobarbital), *Mebaral®* (mephobarbital), and others—see Glossary

- Nonsteroidal anti-inflammatory drugs (NSAIDs) such as *Motrin®* (ibuprofen), *Aleve®* (naproxen), *Vioxx®* (rofecoxib), *Celebrex®* (celecoxib), and others—see Glossary

- *Rifadin®* (rifampin)

- Theophylline such as *Theo-Dur®*, *Uniphyl®*, and others—see Glossary

- Thyroid medications such as *Cytomel®* (liothyronine), *Levoxyl®* (levothyroxine), *Synthroid®* (levothyroxine), and others—see Glossary

Many nonprescription (over-the-counter [OTC]) medications such as cough, cold, and allergy medications contain decongestants which *may decrease* how well heart rhythm medications work. If you are taking beta blockers, you should talk to your doctor or other healthcare professional before taking any new OTC medications.

Tell your doctor or other healthcare professional about all medications (both prescription and nonprescription [over-the-counter] medications) that you are taking.

Why Else Do People Take Beta Blockers?

Beta blockers may also help prevent heart attacks (myocardial infarctions), cardiac chest pain (angina), migraine headaches, and shakiness or tremors. People also take beta blockers for high blood pressure and congestive heart failure.

 # Warning!

To give you the best care, your doctor or other healthcare professional needs to know about the diseases and conditions you have had—your full medical history. Tell your doctor or other healthcare professional if you have or have ever had any of the following:

- Allergy or previous reaction to beta blockers
- Breathing problems (asthma and COPD, including emphysema and chronic bronchitis)
- Congestive heart failure
- Diabetes
- Poor circulation (peripheral vascular disease)
- Sadness, feeling blue or down, depressed mood (depression)

Beta blockers may worsen the symptoms of some lung problems, especially asthma and COPD, including emphysema or chronic bronchitis. Tell your doctor or other healthcare professional if you have trouble breathing or shortness of breath.

Beta blockers may hide the symptoms of low blood sugar (hypoglycemia). This may cause problems for people with diabetes. Ask your doctor or other healthcare professional how often you should check your blood sugar.

Beta blockers may worsen the symptoms of poor circulation (peripheral vascular disease). Tell your doctor or other healthcare professional if you develop symptoms of poor circulation such as pain, numbness, or coldness of your legs, feet, and hands.

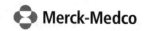

Beta blockers may make you unsteady on your feet, causing you to fall and possibly break a bone. If you have fallen recently, tell your doctor or other healthcare professional about it. Taking a different medication or a lower dose may make you less likely to fall. You should not stop taking this medication without first talking to your doctor or other healthcare professional.

If you suddenly have leg or arm weakness, a change in or loss of vision, trouble speaking, or confusion, you may be having a stroke. This is serious and needs to be treated immediately. If you have these symptoms, go to the emergency room of the nearest hospital where you will be examined and your doctor or other healthcare professional will be contacted.

Under certain circumstances, your doctor or other healthcare professional may decide that you should stop taking this medication. If you have taken it for more than a couple of weeks, he or she may want you to decrease it gradually, lowering the dose over a few weeks or months. Stopping suddenly may cause unpleasant withdrawal symptoms or may worsen your medical problems. Pay careful attention to the instructions your doctor or other healthcare professional gives you about how much less to take and for how long.

Amiodarone

This medication works by changing the electrical impulses in the heart and slowing the heartbeat to help control abnormal heart rhythms and heartbeat.

Brand Name	Generic Name
Cordarone®	amiodarone
Pacerone®	amiodarone

How Will I Take Amiodarone?

Amiodarone is usually taken 1 to 2 times daily. It may be taken with food to help prevent stomach upset. Your doctor or other healthcare professional will tell you how often to take your medication.

If you miss a dose of this medication, take the dose you missed as soon as possible. However, if it is almost time for your next dose, skip the missed dose and just take the next one. Do not double your dose. Take your medication exactly as directed by your doctor or other healthcare professional. Do not stop taking a prescription medication unless directed by your doctor or other healthcare professional.

What Side Effects Can Amiodarone Cause?

More Common

- Blurred vision

- Dizziness

- Increased sensitivity to the sun (bad sunburn)

- Nausea

- Poor coordination and unsteadiness when walking or standing

- Shakiness or tremors

- Slow heartbeat (palpitations)*

- Tingling, numbness, or pain of the hands and feet

- Tiredness or sluggishness (fatigue)

- Trouble breathing or shortness of breath

*Sometimes medications may actually cause or worsen the same symptoms they are being used to help relieve. Talk to your doctor or other healthcare professional if your symptoms get worse instead of better while taking this medication.

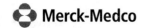

- Vomiting
- Yellow and brown spots in the eyes (these do not affect vision)

Less Common

- Blue-gray skin coloring
- Constipation
- Headache
- Irregular heartbeat (palpitations)*
- Liver problems that may cause yellowing of the skin or eyes (jaundice)
- Overactive thyroid (hyperthyroidism)
- Poor appetite
- Stomach pain
- Trouble falling asleep or staying asleep (insomnia)
- Underactive thyroid (hypothyroidism)

Rare

- Allergic reactions such as rash (skin redness, bumps, itching, or irritation), swelling of the face and throat, or trouble breathing
- Bleeding that does not stop easily (nose bleeds, bleeding while brushing your teeth, and cuts)

*Sometimes medications may actually cause or worsen the same symptoms they are being used to help relieve. Talk to your doctor or other healthcare professional if your symptoms get worse instead of better while taking this medication.

Tell your doctor or other healthcare professional if you have side effects that bother you, do not go away, make you worried about taking your medication, or make you want to stop taking your medication.

Do Other Medications Interact with Amiodarone?

These medications *may increase* the side effects of amiodarone:

- *Norvir*® (ritonavir)
- *Zagam*® (sparfloxacin)

Dilantin® (phenytoin) *may decrease* how well amiodarone works.

Amiodarone *may increase* the side effects of these medications:

- Beta blockers such as *Inderal*® (propranolol), *Tenormin*® (atenolol), *Toprol*® (metoprolol), and others—see Glossary
- Calcium channel blockers such as *Cardizem*® (diltiazem), *Norvasc*® (amlodipine), *Procardia*® (nifedipine), and others—see Glossary
- *Coumadin*® (warfarin)
- *Dilantin*® (phenytoin)
- *Lanoxin*® (digoxin) or *Lanoxicaps*® (digoxin)
- *Neoral*® (cyclosporine)
- Other heart rhythm problem (arrhythmia) medications—see Glossary
- *Sandimmune*® (cyclosporine)

Amiodarone is generally not prescribed for anyone who is taking *Propulsid*® (cisapride [withdrawn from general distribution; available only by special arrangement with the manufacturer]), *Seldane*® (terfenadine [no longer commercially available]), or *Hismanal*® (astemizole [no longer commercially available]), because together they *may cause* serious, sometimes fatal, heart problems.

Many nonprescription (over-the-counter [OTC]) medications such as cough, cold, and allergy medications contain decongestants which *may decrease* how well heart rhythm medications work. If you are taking amiodarone, you should talk to your doctor or other healthcare professional before taking any new OTC medications.

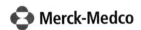
Tell your doctor or other healthcare professional about all medications (both prescription and nonprescription [over-the-counter] medications) that you are taking.

 # Warning!

To give you the best care, your doctor or other healthcare professional needs to know about the diseases and medical conditions you have had—your full medical history. Tell your doctor or other healthcare professional if you have or have ever had any of the following:

- Allergy or previous reaction to amiodarone
- Breathing problems
- Congestive heart failure
- Heart attack (myocardial infarction)
- Liver problems
- Low potassium in your blood (hypokalemia)
- Overactive thyroid (hyperthyroidism)
- Underactive thyroid (hypothyroidism)

Since amiodarone may cause damage to your liver, your doctor or other healthcare professional may order blood tests to find out early on if the medication is causing liver problems, before they become serious.

If you are taking amiodarone, stay out of the sun as much as you can to avoid a serious sunburn. When you do go out in the sun, use sunblock or sunscreen, and wear protective clothing, such as a wide-brimmed hat and a long-sleeved shirt.

Amiodarone may cause serious lung problems. In some patients these problems may be life threatening. Contact your doctor or other healthcare professional if you develop a cough or have trouble breathing while taking this medication.

Amiodarone may make you unsteady on your feet, causing you to fall and possibly break a bone. If you have fallen recently, tell your doctor or other healthcare professional about it. Taking a different medication or a lower dose may make you less likely to fall. You should not stop taking this medication without first talking to your doctor or other healthcare professional.

If you suddenly have leg or arm weakness, a change in or loss of vision, trouble speaking, or confusion, you may be having a stroke. This is serious and needs to be treated immediately. If you have these symptoms, go to the emergency room of the nearest hospital where you will be examined and your doctor or other healthcare professional will be contacted.

Betapace® (sotalol)

This medication works by changing the electrical impulses in the heart to help control abnormal heart rhythms and heartbeat.

 ## How Will I Take *Betapace*® (sotalol)?

Betapace® (sotalol) is usually taken 2 to 3 times daily. It should be taken on an empty stomach 1 hour before meals or 2 hours after meals. Your doctor or other healthcare professional will tell you how often to take your medication.

To help prevent side effects, your doctor or other healthcare professional may start by giving you a low dose of this medication, increasing the amount slowly until it works well for you.

If you miss a dose of this medication, take the dose you missed as soon as possible. However, if it is almost time for your next dose, skip the missed dose and just take the next one. Do not double your dose. Take your medication exactly as directed by your doctor or other healthcare professional. Do not stop taking a prescription medication unless directed by your doctor or other healthcare professional.

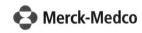

What Side Effects Can *Betapace*® (sotalol) Cause?

More Common

- Diarrhea

- Dizziness when standing up from a bed or a chair

- Headache

- Nausea

- Slow or irregular heartbeat (palpitations)*

- Tiredness or sluggishness (fatigue)

- Trouble breathing or shortness of breath with asthma and COPD, including emphysema or chronic bronchitis

- Vision problems

- Vomiting

- Weakness

Less Common

- Change in blood sugar

- Congestive heart failure

- Erection problems (erectile dysfunction)

- Gas or bloating

- Increased or excessive sweating (perspiration)

- Leg pain when walking

- Loss of interest in sex (decreased libido)

- Muscle pain

- Rash (skin redness, bumps, itching, or irritation)

*Sometimes medications may actually cause or worsen the same symptoms they are being used to help relieve. Talk to your doctor or other healthcare professional if your symptoms get worse instead of better while taking this medication.

- Sadness, feeling blue or down, depressed mood (depression)

- Strange dreams and nightmares

Tell your doctor or other healthcare professional if you have side effects that bother you, do not go away, make you worried about taking your medication, or make you want to stop taking your medication.

Do Other Medications Interact with *Betapace*® (sotalol)?

These medications *may increase* the side effects of *Betapace*® (sotalol):

- Beta blockers such as *Inderal*® (propranolol), *Tenormin*® (atenolol), *Toprol*® (metoprolol), and others—see Glossary

- Calcium channel blockers such as *Cardizem*® (diltiazem), *Norvasc*® (amlodipine), *Procardia*® (nifedipine), and others—see Glossary

- High blood pressure (hypertension) medications—see Glossary

- Neuroleptic medications such as *Risperdal*® (risperidone), *Thorazine*® (chlorpromazine), *Zyprexa*® (olanzapine), and others—see Glossary

- Other heart rhythm problem (arrhythmia) medications—see Glossary

- Tricyclic antidepressants such as *Elavil*® (amitriptyline), *Pamelor*® (nortriptyline), *Sinequan*® (doxepin), and others—see Glossary

- *Zagam*® (sparfloxacin)

Betapace® (sotalol) *may increase* the side effects of *Lanoxin*® (digoxin) or *Lanoxicaps*® (digoxin).

Betapace® (sotalol) is generally not prescribed for anyone who is taking *Propulsid*® (cisapride [withdrawn from general distribution; available only by special arrangement with the manufacturer]), *Seldane*® (terfenadine [no longer commercially available]), or *Hismanal*® (astemizole [no longer commercially available]), because together they *may cause* serious, sometimes fatal, heart problems.

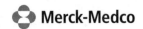

Betapace® (sotalol) ***may decrease*** how well beta-adrenergic bronchodilators such as *Proventil®* (albuterol), *Serevent®* (salmeterol), and others (see Glossary) work.

Many nonprescription (over-the-counter [OTC]) medications such as cough, cold, and allergy medications contain decongestants which ***may decrease*** how well heart rhythm medications work. If you are taking *Betapace®* (sotalol), you should talk to your doctor or other healthcare professional before taking any new OTC medications.

Antacids such as *Maalox®* or *Mylanta®* (aluminum hydroxide/magnesium hydroxide), *Rolaids®* or *Tums®* (calcium carbonate), or *Amphojel®* (aluminum hydroxide) ***may decrease*** the effects of *Betapace®* (sotalol) when taken at the same time. If you are using antacids, take the *Betapace®* (sotalol) 1 hour before or 2 hours after taking your antacid.

Tell your doctor or other healthcare professional about all medications (both prescription and nonprescription [over-the-counter] medications) that you are taking.

 # Warning!

To give you the best care, your doctor or other healthcare professional needs to know about the diseases and medical conditions you have had—your full medical history. Tell your doctor or other healthcare professional if you have or have ever had any of the following:

- Allergy or previous reaction to *Betapace®* (sotalol) or beta blockers such as *Inderal®* (propranolol), *Tenormin®* (atenolol), *Toprol®* (metoprolol), and others—see Glossary

- Breathing problems (asthma and COPD, including emphysema or chronic bronchitis)

- Congestive heart failure

- Diabetes

- Kidney problems

- Liver problems

- Low potassium in your blood (hypokalemia)

- Overactive thyroid (hyperthyroidism)

- Poor circulation (peripheral vascular disease)

- Sadness, feeling blue or down, depressed mood (depression)

Betapace® (sotalol) may worsen the symptoms of some lung problems, especially asthma and COPD, including emphysema or chronic bronchitis. Tell your doctor or other healthcare professional if you have trouble breathing or shortness of breath.

Betapace® (sotalol) may hide the symptoms of low blood sugar (hypoglycemia). This may cause problems for people with diabetes. Ask your doctor or other healthcare professional how often you should check your blood sugar.

Betapace® (sotalol) may worsen the symptoms of poor circulation (peripheral vascular disease). Tell your doctor or other healthcare professional if you develop symptoms of poor circulation such as pain, numbness, or coldness of your legs, feet, and hands.

Betapace® (sotalol) may make you unsteady on your feet, causing you to fall and possibly break a bone. If you have fallen recently, tell your doctor or other healthcare professional about it. Taking a different medication or a lower dose may make you less likely to fall. You should not stop taking this medication without first talking to your doctor or other healthcare professional.

If you suddenly have leg or arm weakness, a change in or loss of vision, trouble speaking, or confusion, you may be having a stroke. This is serious and needs to be treated immediately. If you have these symptoms, go to the emergency room of the nearest hospital where you will be examined and your doctor or other healthcare professional will be contacted.

Under certain circumstances, your doctor or other healthcare professional may decide that you should stop taking this medication. If you have taken it for more than a couple of weeks, he or she may want you to decrease it gradually, lowering the dose over a few weeks or months. Stopping suddenly may cause unpleasant withdrawal symptoms or may worsen your medical problems. Pay

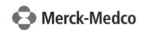

careful attention to the instructions your doctor or other healthcare professional gives you about how much less to take and for how long.

Diltiazem and Verapamil

These medications work by slowing down the heartbeat to help control abnormal heart rhythms and heartbeat.

Brand Name	Generic Name
Calan®	verapamil
Cardizem®	diltiazem
Covera®	verapamil
Dilacor®	diltiazem
Isoptin®	verapamil
Tiazac®	diltiazem
Verelan®	verapamil

How Will I Take Diltiazem and Verapamil?

Diltiazem and verapamil are usually taken 1 to 4 times a day. Diltiazem should be taken on an empty stomach 1 hour before or 2 hours after meals. Verapamil should be taken with meals. Your doctor or other healthcare professional will tell you how many times a day to take your medication.

When a medication has initials after its name, such as XL, XR, SR, BID, DUR, and others, it usually means that the body absorbs the medication slowly over time, so you usually have to take it only once or twice a day. The body will absorb some medications of this type too fast if you crush or break them or dissolve them in liquid, and their effects will not last as long as they should. Check with your doctor or other healthcare professional before crushing or breaking your pills or dissolving your pills in liquid.

If you miss a dose of this medication, take the dose you missed as soon as possible. However, if it is almost time for your next dose, skip the missed dose and just take the next one. Do not double your dose. Take your medication exactly as directed by your doctor or other healthcare professional. Do not stop taking a prescription medication unless directed by your doctor or other healthcare professional.

What Side Effects Can Diltiazem and Verapamil Cause?

More Common

- Constipation
- Dizziness when standing up from a bed or a chair
- Headache
- Reddening of the face (flushing)
- Swelling or puffiness of feet, ankles, or lower legs (edema)

Less Common

- Congestive heart failure
- Diarrhea
- Nausea
- Rash (skin redness, bumps, itching, or irritation)
- Slow, fast, or irregular heartbeat (palpitations)*

*Sometimes medications may actually cause or worsen the same symptoms they are being used to help relieve. Talk to your doctor or other healthcare professional if your symptoms get worse instead of better while taking this medication.

Tell your doctor or other healthcare professional if you have side effects that bother you, do not go away, make you worried about taking your medication, or make you want to stop taking your medication.

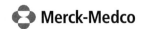

Do Other Medications Interact with Diltiazem and Verapamil?

Diltiazem and verapamil *may increase* the side effects of these medications:

- Benzodiazepines such as *Ativan*® (lorazepam), *Klonopin*® (clonazepam), *Xanax*® (alprazolam), and others—see Glossary

- *BuSpar*® (buspirone)

- High blood pressure (hypertension) medications and diuretics (water pills)—see Glossary

- *Lanoxin*® (digoxin) or *Lanoxicaps*® (digoxin)

- Lithium such as *Eskalith*®, *Lithobid*®, and others—see Glossary

- *Neoral*® (cyclosporine)

- Other heart rhythm problem (arrhythmia) medications—see Glossary

- Quinidine such as *Quinaglute*®, *Quinidex*®, and others—see Glossary

- *Sandimmune*® (cyclosporine)

- Statins such as *Lipitor*® (atorvastatin), *Pravachol*® (pravastatin), *Zocor*® (simvastatin), and others—see Glossary

- *Tegretol*® (carbamazepine)

- Theophylline such as *Theo-Dur*®, *Uniphyl*®, and others—see Glossary

These medications *may increase* the side effects of diltiazem and verapamil:

- *Tagamet*® (cimetidine)

- *Zantac*® (ranitidine)

Ethmozine® (moricizine) *may decrease* how well diltiazem works, and diltiazem *may increase* the side effects of *Ethmozine*® (moricizine).

These medications *may decrease* how well diltiazem and verapamil work:

- Barbiturates such as *Butisol*® (butabarbital), *Luminal*® (phenobarbital), *Mebaral*® (mephobarbital), and others—see Glossary

- *Rifadin*® (rifampin)

Many nonprescription (over-the-counter [OTC]) medications such as cough, cold, and allergy medications contain decongestants which *may decrease* how well heart rhythm medications work. If you are taking diltiazem or verapamil, you should talk to your doctor or other healthcare professional before taking any new OTC medications.

Grapefruit and grapefruit juice *may increase* the side effects of diltiazem and verapamil. This interaction can happen whether you eat the grapefruit or drink the grapefruit juice at the same time as you take your medication or if you take the medication separately from the grapefruit or grapefruit juice. Talk to your doctor or other healthcare professional before eating grapefruit or drinking grapefruit juice if you are taking this medication. Please also read the discussion on A Warning about Grapefruit and Grapefruit Juice on pages i-ii.

Tell your doctor or other healthcare professional about all medications (both prescription and nonprescription [over-the-counter] medications) that you are taking.

Why Else Do People Take Diltiazem and Verapamil?

Diltiazem and verapamil are helpful for high blood pressure (hypertension), cardiac chest pain (angina), and to help prevent migraine headaches.

 # Warning!

To give you the best care, your doctor or other healthcare professional needs to know about the diseases and medical conditions you have had—your full medical history. Tell your doctor or other healthcare professional if you have or have ever had any of the following:

- Allergy or previous reaction to diltiazem or verapamil
- Cardiac chest pain (angina)
- Congestive heart failure

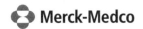

- Kidney problems
- Liver problems

If you suddenly have leg or arm weakness, a change in or loss of vision, trouble speaking, or confusion, you may be having a stroke. This is serious and needs to be treated immediately. If you have these symptoms, go to the emergency room of the nearest hospital where you will be examined and your doctor or other healthcare professional will be contacted.

Diltiazem and verapamil may make you unsteady on your feet, causing you to fall and possibly break a bone. If you have fallen recently, tell your doctor or other healthcare professional about it. Taking a different medication or a lower dose may make you less likely to fall. You should not stop taking this medication without first talking to your doctor or other healthcare professional.

Under certain circumstances, your doctor or other healthcare professional may decide that you should stop taking this medication. If you have taken it for more than a couple of weeks, he or she may want you to decrease it gradually, lowering the dose over a few weeks or months. Stopping suddenly may cause unpleasant withdrawal symptoms or may worsen your medical problems. Pay careful attention to the instructions your doctor or other healthcare professional gives you about how much less to take and for how long.

Chapter 15

Irritable Bowel Syndrome

What Is Irritable Bowel Syndrome?

Irritable bowel syndrome (IBS) affects the intestines and is sometimes called "spastic colon." With IBS the digestive system is often sensitive to stress, diet, and medications. Symptoms of IBS include constipation, diarrhea, or a change back and forth between constipation and diarrhea. People with IBS can also have bloating and cramping pain.

Treatment for IBS depends on whether the main problem is diarrhea or constipation. If a particular food can be identified as the cause, not eating it anymore should help to take care of the problem. If stress makes the symptoms of IBS worse, reducing the stress in your life should help improve the symptoms. If constipation is a problem, getting regular exercise and eating plenty of foods containing fiber, such as fresh fruits, vegetables, and whole grains, can help. Please read the chapter about constipation on pages 169-192 for advice on treating constipation. Your doctor or other healthcare professional may recommend taking bulk-forming laxatives, which are discussed in the chapter about constipation.

Medications for Irritable Bowel Syndrome

Several kinds of medications may be taken for the diarrhea and cramping pain caused by irritable bowel syndrome. This chapter discusses these medications and/or categories of medications:

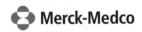
MEDICATIONS	See Page
Antispasmodic Medications	510
Loperamide	515

If you do not see the exact name of the medication that you take for irritable bowel syndrome listed above, check the Medication and Chapter Table to find out which category your medication falls under or check the Index.

Antispasmodic Medications

Antispasmodic medications are usually used for short periods of time to temporarily relieve the discomfort and diarrhea caused by irritable bowel syndrome.

▲ Indicates medications that are more likely to cause unpleasant or dangerous side effects. These medications are generally not recommended for people over 65. The side effects may not be very obvious and may be mistaken for "just a part of getting older" but may be serious. If you are taking one of these medications, you might want to talk to your doctor or other healthcare professional to see if this medication is best for you. Safer medications may be available and lower dosages may be required. You should not stop taking these medications without first talking to your doctor or other healthcare professional.

See the WARNING section on page 513 for the specific safety problems associated with these medications ▲.

Brand Name	Generic Name
▲Anaspaz®	hyoscyamine
▲Bentyl®	dicyclomine
▲Cystospaz®	hyoscyamine
▲Donnatal®	belladonna/phenobarbital
▲Levsin®	hyoscyamine
▲Librax®	clidinium/chlordiazepoxide
Lomotil®	diphenoxylate/atropine
Pamine®	methscopolamine
▲Pro-Banthine®	propantheline
▲Quarzan®	clidinium

How Will I Take Antispasmodic Medications?

An antispasmodic medication is taken as a tablet or liquid. Usually it is taken 1 to 4 times a day. Your doctor or other healthcare professional will tell you how many times a day to take your medication.

This medication is often used "as needed," so missing a dose should not be a problem. If you miss a dose and it is almost time for the next dose, you should skip the forgotten dose. Do not double the dose. Take your medication as directed by your doctor or other healthcare professional.

What Side Effects Can Antispasmodic Medications Cause?

More Common

- Blurred vision
- Constipation

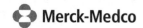
- Dizziness when standing up from a bed or a chair
- Drowsiness
- Dry mouth, eyes, and nose
- Eyes that are too sensitive to light
- Fast heartbeat (palpitations)
- Increased size of pupils in the eyes (dilated pupils)
- Trouble urinating or emptying the bladder

Less Common

- Confusion
- Nausea
- Nervousness (anxiety)
- Rash (skin redness, bumps, itching, or irritation)
- Reddening of the face (flushing)
- Seeing or hearing things that are not there (hallucinations)
- Trouble swallowing
- Vomiting

Tell your doctor or other healthcare professional if you have side effects that bother you, do not go away, make you worried about taking your medication, or make you want to stop taking your medication.

 ## Do Other Medications Interact with Antispasmodic Medications?

Antispasmodic medications *may increase* the side effects of other medications that cause drowsiness, including anticholinergic medications, antidepressants, antihistamines (allergy medications), other antispasmodics, benzodiazepines (a type of tranquilizer), anxiety medications, narcotics (pain relievers), muscle relaxants, neuroleptic medications (a type of tranquilizer), seizure medications, or sleep medications. Avoid driving a car and other activities that need mental alertness, like using a knife or operating machinery, while taking these medications together.

Drinking alcoholic beverages (such as beer, wine, whiskey, and others) *may increase* the side effects of antispasmodic medications.

Tell your doctor or other healthcare professional if you have side effects that bother you, do not go away, make you worried about taking your medication, or make you want to stop taking your medication.

Why Else Do People Take Antispasmodic Medications?

These medications are occasionally used for stomach ulcers or bladder control problems (urinary incontinence).

What Else Should I Know about Antispasmodic Medications?

Antispasmodic medications do not work for everyone. If your symptoms do not improve after a few weeks of taking an antispasmodic medication, discuss it with your doctor or other healthcare professional. You may be able to take something else that will work better for you.

 # Warning!

To give you the best care, your doctor or other healthcare professional needs to know about the diseases and medical conditions you have had—your full medical history. Tell your doctor or other healthcare professional if you have or have ever had any of the following:

- Allergy or previous reaction to antispasmodic medications
- Alzheimer's disease

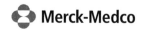

- Breathing problems (asthma and COPD, including emphysema or chronic bronchitis)

- Dizziness when standing up from a bed or a chair

- Enlarged prostate (benign prostatic hypertrophy)

- Glaucoma (an eye disease)

- Congestive heart failure

- Inflammatory bowel disease (ulcerative colitis or Crohn's disease)

- Kidney problems

- Liver problems

- Low blood pressure (hypotension)

- Trouble urinating

Antispasmodic medications are generally not recommended for people over 65 because they cause serious side effects, including dizziness, blurred vision, trouble urinating or emptying the bladder, confusion, and a fast heartbeat. If you are taking one of these medications, talk to your doctor or other healthcare professional to see if it is right for you. Do not stop taking this medication without first talking to your doctor or other healthcare professional.

Antispasmodic medications may make you unsteady on your feet, causing you to fall and possibly break a bone. If you have fallen recently, tell your doctor or other healthcare professional about it. Taking a different medication or a lower dose may make you less likely to fall. You should not stop taking this medication without first talking to your doctor or other healthcare professional.

Antispasmodic medications may cause drowsiness. Avoid driving a car and other activities that need mental alertness, like using a knife or operating machinery, while taking this medication. Drinking alcoholic beverages (such as beer, wine, whiskey, and others) may increase the side effects.

If your abdominal (stomach) pain becomes worse or if you have blood or mucus in your bowel movements, contact your doctor or other healthcare professional right away. These might be signs of a more serious problem.

Diarrhea may cause excessive fluid loss from your body. If you lose too much fluid from the diarrhea, it may cause a problem called dehydration. Tell your doctor or other healthcare professional if you have any of these symptoms:

- Confusion
- Dizziness
- Dry mouth
- Dry, wrinkled skin
- Increased thirst

It is important to drink plenty of clear, caffeine-free liquids while you have diarrhea to prevent dehydration. Talk to your doctor or other healthcare professional before increasing your fluids if you have heart or kidney problems.

You should talk to your doctor or other healthcare professional before taking antispasmodic medications if you are constipated. Antispasmodic medications will not help you if you are constipated; they may actually make the constipation worse.

Under certain circumstances your doctor or other healthcare professional may decide that you should stop taking this medication. If you have taken it for more than a couple of weeks, he or she may want you to decrease it gradually, lowering the dose over a few weeks or months. Stopping suddenly may cause unpleasant withdrawal symptoms or may worsen your medical problems. Pay careful attention to the instructions your doctor or other healthcare professional gives you about how much less to take and for how long.

Loperamide

Loperamide is a nonprescription (over-the-counter) medication that may be used to help treat diarrhea associated with irritable bowel syndrome. It helps stop diarrhea by slowing down the movements of the intestines. This allows the body to absorb more water from the intestines and make the bowel movements more solid, and decreases the urgency to go to the bathroom.

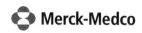
Brand Name	Generic Name
Diar-Aid®	loperamide
Imodium®	loperamide
Kaopectate® II	loperamide
Pepto Diarrhea Control®	loperamide

How Will I Take Loperamide?

Loperamide comes in pills and liquids. Loperamide is usually taken after each bowel movement 2 to 4 times a day. You should not take more than 16 mg in one day without talking to your doctor or other healthcare professional. It may be taken with or without food. Follow the instructions on the package or ask your doctor or other healthcare professional how often and when to take this medication.

This medication is often used "as needed," so missing a dose should not be a problem. If you miss a dose and it is almost time for the next dose, you should skip the forgotten dose. Do not double the dose. Take your medication as directed by your doctor or other healthcare professional.

What Side Effects Can Loperamide Cause?

Less Common

- Constipation
- Dizziness
- Drowsiness
- Dry mouth
- Nausea
- Poor appetite

- Stomach bloating

- Stomach pain

Rare

- Allergic reactions such as rash (skin redness, bumps, itching, or irritation), swelling of the face and throat, or trouble breathing

---

Tell your doctor or other healthcare professional if you have side effects that bother you, do not go away, make you worried about taking your medication, or make you want to stop taking your medication.

Do Other Medications Interact with Loperamide?

Loperamide *may increase* the side effects of other medications that cause drowsiness, including anticholinergic medications, antidepressants, antihistamines (allergy medications), antispasmodics, benzodiazepines (a type of tranquilizer), anxiety medications, narcotics (pain relievers), muscle relaxants, neuroleptic medications (a type of tranquilizer), seizure medications, or sleep medications. Avoid driving a car and other activities that need mental alertness, like using a knife or operating machinery, while taking these medications together.

Drinking alcoholic beverages (such as beer, wine, whiskey, and others) *may increase* the side effects of loperamide.

Tell your doctor or other healthcare professional about all medications (both prescription and nonprescription [over-the-counter] medications) that you are taking.

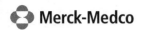

Why Else Do People Take Loperamide?

Loperamide may be used in inflammatory bowel disease, travelers' diarrhea, and to help reduce the amount of bowel movements in people who have had surgery for other intestinal problems.

 # Warning!

To give you the best care, your doctor or other healthcare professional needs to know about the diseases and medical conditions you have had—your full medical history. Tell your doctor or other healthcare professional if you have or have ever had any of the following:

- Allergy or previous reaction to loperamide
- Inflammatory bowel disease (ulcerative colitis or Crohn's disease)
- Liver problems

Loperamide may cause drowsiness. Avoid driving a car and other activities that need mental alertness, like using a knife or operating machinery, while taking this medication. Drinking alcoholic beverages (such as beer, wine, whiskey, and others) may increase the side effects.

If your abdominal (stomach) pain becomes worse or if you have blood or mucus in your bowel movements, contact your doctor or other healthcare professional right away. These might be signs of a more serious problem.

Diarrhea may cause excessive fluid loss from your body. If you lose too much fluid from the diarrhea, it may cause a problem called dehydration. Tell your doctor or other healthcare professional if you have any of these symptoms:

- Confusion
- Dizziness
- Dry mouth
- Dry, wrinkled skin
- Increased thirst

It is important to drink plenty of clear, caffeine-free liquids while you have diarrhea to prevent dehydration. Talk to your doctor or other healthcare professional before increasing your fluids if you have heart or kidney problems.

You should talk to your doctor or other healthcare professional before taking loperamide if you are constipated. Loperamide will not help you if you are constipated; it may actually make the constipation worse.

Osteoporosis

What Is Osteoporosis?

Osteoporosis is a disease in which bones become thin, weak, and brittle, so they break more easily. If osteoporosis is not treated, the bones thin and weaken gradually over the course of many years. People with osteoporosis usually have no symptoms when their bones are thinning. Pain occurs when a weakened bone breaks (fractures). Osteoporosis is a major cause of broken bones in older people, especially fractures in the spine, hip, and wrist.

Important causes of osteoporosis include changes in the amount of some hormones in the body as women age, an inherited tendency to develop osteoporosis (heredity), not eating enough food that contains calcium, not getting enough vitamin D, and not getting enough exercise.

Women are much more likely than men to develop osteoporosis, but many men also have osteoporosis. Women are more likely to develop osteoporosis if they are small-boned and thin and are of Caucasian or Asian ancestry, if others in their family have had osteoporosis, or if they stopped having menstrual periods before the age of 50. Men and women are also more likely to develop osteoporosis if they smoke or drink more than 3 alcoholic beverages (such as beer, wine, whiskey, and others) daily.

The following medications may increase the risk of developing osteoporosis:

- Barbiturates such as *Butisol*® (butabarbital), *Luminal*® (phenobarbital), *Mebaral*® (mephobarbital), and others—see Glossary

- Corticosteroids such as prednisone and others—see Glossary

- Seizure medications such as *Dilantin*® (phenytoin), *Depakote*® (valproic acid), *Neurontin*® (gabapentin), *Tegretol*® (carbamazepine), and others— see Glossary

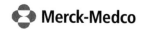

- Thyroid medications such as *Cytomel*® (liothyronine), *Levoxyl*® (levothyroxine), *Synthroid*® (levothyroxine), and others—see Glossary

Some of the ways to help prevent osteoporosis and help prevent osteoporosis from getting worse after it begins include:

- Eating more foods that contain calcium and vitamin D
- Doing weight-bearing exercises, such as walking or weight lifting, regularly
- Decreasing intake of caffeine (such as in coffee, tea, colas, chocolate, and others)
- Drinking fewer alcoholic beverages (such as beer, wine, whiskey, and others)
- Stopping smoking
- Taking medications that strengthen bones

Talk to your doctor or other healthcare professional about starting an exercise program, and taking calcium and vitamin supplements and other medications that may help prevent osteoporosis.

Some calcium-rich foods are listed on the next page.

Calcium-Rich Foods

Food	Serving Size	Average Amount of Calcium
DAIRY PRODUCTS (LOW-FAT TYPES ARE HEALTHIEST AND HAVE AS MUCH CALCIUM AS HIGH-FAT TYPES.)		
American cheese	1 ounce (slice)	165 to 200 mg
Cheddar cheese	1 ounce (slice)	About 200 mg
Cottage cheese	1 cup	125 to 155 mg
Milk (skim)	1 cup (8 ounces)	About 303 mg
Milk (whole)	1 cup (8 ounces)	About 288 mg
Swiss cheese	1 ounce (slice)	250 to 270 mg
Yogurt	1 cup	275 to 450 mg
FRUIT		
Figs	10, dried	About 270 mg
Orange	1	About 50 mg
SEAFOOD (CANNED, EATEN WITH BONES)		
Sardines packed in oil	8 medium	About 354 mg
Red salmon	1/2 cup	About 250 mg
VEGETABLES		
Broccoli	1 cup, cooked	About 70 mg
Cabbage	1 cup, cooked	About 50 mg
Cauliflower	1 cup, cooked	About 30 mg
Spinach	1 cup, cooked	250 to 275 mg
Turnip greens	1 cup, cooked	200 to 250 mg
OTHER		
Beans	1 cup, dried	About 90 mg
Tofu	1/2 cup	About 130 mg

Adapted from *Nutritive Value of Foods*, U.S. Department of Agriculture, 1999.

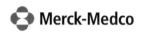

Medications for Osteoporosis

Several kinds of medications may be taken to help prevent or treat osteoporosis. This chapter discusses these medications and/or categories of medications:

MEDICATIONS	See Page
Estrogen*	524
Evista® (raloxifene)*	530
Calcium Supplements	532
Vitamin D	536
Bisphosphonates	539
Calcitonin	542

*For women only

If you do not see the exact name of the medication that you take to help prevent or treat osteoporosis listed above, check the Medication and Chapter Table to find out which category your medication falls under or check the Index.

Estrogen

Women may get the estrogen they need in two ways. First, the body makes it. But the amount the body makes becomes much less after menopause. Second, women can take estrogen in the form of pills they swallow or patches they apply to their skin.

Women begin to lose bone strength several years before they go through menopause (sometimes called "change of life" when women stop having menstrual periods), and that loss of bone strength is increased after menopause. If a woman can safely take estrogen, taking estrogen by mouth or by patches applied to the skin during and after menopause helps keep her bones strong and helps lower her chances of breaking bones when she gets older. In order to get benefits from estrogen, it should be taken for a number of years. Some women have medical conditions that make it unhealthy for them to take estrogen supplements. Talk to your doctor or other healthcare professional to see whether and for how long you should take estrogen.

Brand Name	Generic Name
Alora® Patch	estradiol
Cenestin® Pill	conjugated estrogens
Climara® Patch	estradiol
Combipatch™ Patch	estradiol/norethindrone
E$_2$III™ Patch	estradiol
Estrace® Pill	estradiol
Estraderm® Patch	estradiol
Estratab® Pill	esterified estrogens
FemPatch® Patch	estradiol
Menest® Pill	esterified estrogens
Ogen® Pill	estropipate
Ortho-Est® Pill	estropipate
Ortho-Prefest® Pill	estradiol
Premarin® Pill	conjugated estrogens
Premphase® Pill	conjugated estrogens every day plus medroxyprogesterone for 14 of every 28 days
Prempro™ Pill	conjugated estrogens and medroxyprogesterone taken every day
Vivelle® Patch	estradiol

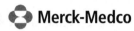 ## How Will I Take Estrogen?

Many women who take estrogen to help prevent osteoporosis take it as a pill. Another form of estrogen for osteoporosis is a patch (transdermal medication), which is applied to the skin like a *Band-Aid®*. Estrogen pills are usually taken once daily. Estrogen patches are usually applied once or twice a week. To help keep patches from irritating your skin, you should put each new patch in a different area from the old patch. Put on a new patch if the first one falls off. When you take a patch off, make sure you throw it away where children or pets cannot get it as it still contains medication that may be harmful to them. Your doctor or other healthcare professional will tell you how often to take your medication.

Some women take estrogen only while others take both estrogen and a medication called a progestin. Common brand names for oral progestins are *Provera®* (medroxyprogesterone) and *Prometrium®* (micronized progesterone). If you have had surgery to remove your uterus (hysterectomy), you do not need to take progestins. If your uterus has not been removed, a progestin is usually taken with estrogen to help prevent cancer of the lining of the uterus (endometrial cancer) from developing. For some women, the progestin is taken daily, and for others it is taken on certain days of the month. Your doctor or other healthcare professional will decide which is best for you.

Sometimes estrogen is combined with the progestin in pills or patches like *Prempro™*, *Premphase®*, or *Combipatch™*. With *Prempro™* and *Combipatch™*, you take both estrogen and progestins every day. If you are taking *Premphase®*, you take estrogen every day and progestins for only 14 days. The package is designed so you know when to take which pills.

If you miss a dose of this medication, take the dose you missed as soon as possible. However, if it is almost time for your next dose, skip the missed dose and just take the next one. Do not double your dose. Take your medication exactly as directed by your doctor or other healthcare professional. Do not stop taking a prescription medication unless directed by your doctor or other healthcare professional.

What Side Effects Can Estrogen Cause?

More Common

- Breast fullness, swelling, or tenderness

- Nausea

- Return of period-like bleeding (menstrual periods), if taking progestin with estrogen

- Swelling or puffiness of the feet, ankles, or lower legs (edema)

- Weight gain

Less Common

- Diarrhea

- Increased or decreased interest in sex

- Worsening of migraine headaches

Rare

- Chest pain with shortness of breath and/or coughing up blood

- Gallstones

- Heavy vaginal bleeding

- Increased risk of cancer of the lining of the uterus (endometrial cancer), if you are taking estrogen without progestins and you have not had a hysterectomy

- Increased risk of breast cancer. Most studies have not shown an increase, but some have reported up to twice the usual rate of breast cancer in women who used estrogens for more than 10 years.

- Leg pain, warmth, redness, or swelling

Tell your doctor or other healthcare professional if you have side effects that bother you, do not go away, make you worried about taking your medication, or make you want to stop taking your medication.

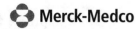

Do Other Medications Interact with Estrogen?

These medications *may decrease* how well estrogen works:

- Barbiturates such as *Butisol*® (butabarbital), *Luminal*® (phenobarbital), *Mebaral*® (mephobarbital), and others—see Glossary

- *Dilantin*® (phenytoin)

- *Rifadin*® (rifampin)

- *Topamax*® (topiramate)

Estrogen *may increase* the side effects of corticosteroids such as prednisone and others—see Glossary.

Estrogen *may decrease* how well *Coumadin*® (warfarin) works.

Tell your doctor or other healthcare professional about all medications (both prescription and nonprescription [over-the-counter] medications) that you are taking.

Why Else Do People Take Estrogen?

Estrogen also helps to relieve dryness, bleeding, or itching in the vagina. For this purpose, it may be used as a cream in the vagina. It can relieve some of the symptoms that are common after menopause, such as a sudden warm or hot feeling with sweating and reddening of the face and neck ("hot flashes") and leaking of urine and loss of bladder control (urinary incontinence). It may also be used to help reduce the risk of developing heart problems.

What Else Should I Know about Estrogen?

When estrogen is taken with a progestin such as in *Provera*®, *Prometrium*®, *Prempro*™, *Premphase*®, or *Combipatch*™, you may see a return of your menstrual (period-like) bleeding. You may have light spotting, or moderate-to-heavy bleeding, which may be normal. However, you should talk to your doctor or other healthcare professional if you have bleeding while taking these medications because it may be a sign of a more serious problem.

 # Warning!

To give you the best care, your doctor or other healthcare professional needs to know about the diseases and medical conditions you have had—your full medical history. Tell your doctor or other healthcare professional if you have or have ever had any of the following:

- Allergy or previous reaction to adhesives or skin (transdermal) patches
- Allergy or previous reaction to estrogen
- Blood clots (phlebitis or embolism)
- Breast cancer
- Cancer of the lining of the uterus (endometrial cancer)
- Endometriosis
- Fibroid (a type of noncancerous growth) in the uterus
- Gallbladder problems
- Liver problems

Women who have not had a hysterectomy increase their chance of developing cancer of the lining of the uterus (endometrial cancer) if they take estrogen without another medication called progestin. If you have not had a hysterectomy and estrogen is prescribed for you, you should discuss taking a progestin such as *Provera*® (medroxyprogesterone) or *Prometrium*® (micronized progesterone) with your doctor or other healthcare professional.

If you are having leg pain, warmth, redness, or swelling, you may have a blood clot (venous thrombosis). This is serious and needs to be treated. If you have these symptoms, go to the emergency room of the nearest hospital where you will be examined and your doctor or other healthcare professional will be contacted.

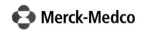

If you are having chest pain with shortness of breath and/or you are coughing up blood, you may have a blood clot in your lungs (pulmonary embolism). This is serious and needs to be treated immediately. If you have these symptoms, go to the emergency room of the nearest hospital where you will be examined and your doctor or other healthcare professional will be contacted.

Evista® (raloxifene)

Evista® (raloxifene) is a type of medication called a selective estrogen receptor modulator (SERM). *Evista*® acts like estrogen in some ways (helps protect the skeleton and heart) but is unlike estrogen in other ways (does not stimulate the breast and uterus). *Evista*® (raloxifene) is used to help prevent and treat postmenopausal osteoporosis.

Evista® (raloxifene) does not prevent hot flashes the way estrogen does and it can even make hot flashes worse during the first 6 months of use. *Evista*® (raloxifene) helps to keep bones strong and may make it less likely that women who take it will break bones in their spines.

 ## How Will I Take *Evista*® (raloxifene)

Evista® (raloxifene) is usually taken once a day with or without food. Your doctor or other healthcare professional will tell you how often to take this medication.

If you miss a dose of this medication, take the dose you missed as soon as possible. However, if it is almost time for your next dose, skip the missed dose and just take the next one. Do not double your dose. Take your medication exactly as directed by your doctor or other healthcare professional. Do not stop taking a prescription medication unless directed by your doctor or other healthcare professional.

What Side Effects Can *Evista*® (raloxifene) Cause?

More Common

- Hot flashes
- Leg cramps

Less Common

- Chest pain with shortness of breath and/or coughing up blood
- Leg pain, warmth, redness, or swelling

Tell your doctor or other healthcare professional if you have side effects that bother you, do not go away, make you worried about taking your medication, or make you want to stop taking your medication.

Do Other Medications Interact with *Evista*® (raloxifene)?

Bile acid binders such as *Questran*® (cholestyramine) or *Colestid*® (colestipol) or bulk-forming laxatives like *Metamucil*® (psyllium) **may decrease** the effects of *Evista*® (raloxifene) by preventing it from being absorbed completely. To help make sure it is absorbed so it can work properly, take *Evista*® (raloxifene) 1 hour before or 4 to 6 hours after taking a bile acid binder or a bulk-forming laxative.

Evista® (raloxifene) **may decrease** how well *Coumadin*® (warfarin) works.

Tell your doctor or other healthcare professional about all medications (both prescription and nonprescription [over-the-counter] medications) that you are taking.

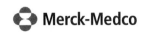

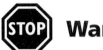 # Warning!

To give you the best care, your doctor or other healthcare professional needs to know about the diseases and medical conditions you have had—your full medical history. Tell your doctor or other healthcare professional if you have or have ever had any of the following:

- Allergy or previous reaction to *Evista*® (raloxifene)
- Blood clots (phlebitis or pulmonary embolism)
- Liver problems

If you are having leg pain, warmth, redness, or swelling, you may have a blood clot (venous thrombosis). This is serious and needs to be treated. If you have these symptoms, go to the emergency room of the nearest hospital where you will be examined and your doctor or other healthcare professional will be contacted.

If you are having chest pain with shortness of breath and/or you are coughing up blood, you may have a blood clot in your lungs (pulmonary embolism). This is serious and needs to be treated immediately. If you have these symptoms, go to the emergency room of the nearest hospital where you will be examined and your doctor or other healthcare professional will be contacted.

Calcium Supplements

Calcium is a mineral that is an important part of bones as well as other tissues and body functions. Almost all of the calcium in the body is stored in the bones. When the body does not have all the calcium it needs, it "steals" calcium from the bones, making them weaker and more likely to break. Eating enough calcium or taking supplements as directed by your doctor or other healthcare professional can help prevent this from happening. In older people, getting enough calcium helps to keep the bones from thinning too much and can help strengthen bones that have already been weakened by osteoporosis.

About half the people who live in the United States do not get enough calcium from the food they eat. If you do not get enough calcium from your food, calcium is available in a pill or a liquid form. There are many different calcium supplement products, including antacids containing calcium such as *Rolaids®* (calcium carbonate), *Tums®* (calcium carbonate), and others—see Glossary and the list below. Calcium carbonate and calcium citrate are the most commonly used calcium supplements. Some forms of calcium are combined with vitamin D, because vitamin D is also needed for strong bones (see next section on vitamin D). Calcium is available without a prescription. Ask your doctor or other healthcare professional if you are getting enough calcium from your diet or if you need a supplement. Do not take bone meal preparations unless directed by your doctor or other healthcare professional, as these preparations may contain impurities.

Brand Name	Generic Name
Alka-Mints®	calcium carbonate
Calcium Rich Rolaids®	calcium carbonate
Caltrate®	calcium carbonate
Citracal®	calcium citrate
Neo-Calglucon® (syrup)	calcium gluconate/calcium lactobionate
Os-Cal®	oyster shell powder
Posture®	tribasic calcium phosphate
Tums®	calcium carbonate
Viactiv®	calcium carbonate/vitamin D/ vitamin K

How Will I Take Calcium?

A person over 50 years of age should get about 1000 to 1500 mg of calcium every day from food and supplements. It is sometimes hard to get this much calcium in your diet. If, on a given day, you drank 1 glass of milk, ate 1 ounce of cheddar cheese, and had a cup of spinach for dinner, you would get about 750 mg of calcium in your diet and would still need to get 250–750 mg more calcium to meet the recommendations.

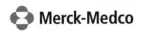

There are different kinds of calcium supplements. Calcium carbonate is absorbed best when taken with food or meals. Calcium citrate can be taken with or without food. Ask your doctor or other healthcare professional for advice about which kind of calcium supplements to take and how much to take.

To absorb calcium, the body needs vitamin D. The main ways to get vitamin D are by being out in the sun and by eating food that contains vitamin D. Some people do not get enough vitamin D. Ask your doctor or other healthcare professional whether you should be taking vitamin D. You can take it either in a pill that contains only vitamin D, a calcium supplement that contains vitamin D, or a multivitamin that contains many other vitamins and minerals as well.

If you miss a dose of this medication, take the dose you missed as soon as possible. However, if it is almost time for your next dose, skip the missed dose and just take the next one. Do not double your dose. Take your medication exactly as directed by your doctor or other healthcare professional.

 ## What Side Effects Can Calcium Cause?

More Common

- Constipation

- Gas

Rare

- Confusion

- Kidney stones

- Nausea

- Nervousness (anxiety)

- Stomach pain

- Thirst

- Vomiting

Tell your doctor or other healthcare professional if you have side effects that bother you, do not go away, make you worried about taking your medication, or make you want to stop taking your medication.

Do Other Medications Interact with Calcium?

Calcium *may decrease* how well these medications work, so these medications should be taken 1 hour before or 2 hours after taking calcium:

- *Aciphex*® (rabeprazole)

- *Axid*® (nizatidine)

- *Pepcid*® (famotidine)

- *Prevacid*® (lansoprazole)

- *Prilosec*® (omeprazole)

- Quinolone antibiotics such as *Cipro*® (ciprofloxacin), *Floxin*® (ofloxacin), and *Levaquin*® (levofloxacin)—see Glossary

- *Tagamet*® (cimetidine)

- Tetracycline antibiotics such as *Dynacin*® (minocycline), *Sumycin*® (tetracycline), *Vibramycin*® (doxycycline), and others—see Glossary

- *Zantac*® (ranitidine)

Viactiv® (calcium carbonate/vitamin D/vitamin K) contains vitamin K, which *may decrease* how well *Coumadin*® (warfarin) works.

Calcium or antacids that contain calcium can keep many other medications from being absorbed into the body. To get the most out of your medications, take calcium or an antacid 1 hour before or 2 hours after taking any other medication.

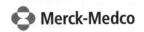
Tell your doctor or other healthcare professional about all medications (both prescription and nonprescription [over-the-counter] medications) that you are taking.

Warning!

To give you the best care, your doctor or other healthcare professional needs to know about the diseases and medical conditions you have had—your full medical history. Tell your doctor or other healthcare professional if you have or have ever had any of the following:

- Heart problems
- Kidney problems
- Kidney stones

Vitamin D

Vitamin D helps the body to absorb calcium. When you go out in the sun, your skin makes this important vitamin by itself. It is recommended that everyone get 400 to 800 international units (IU) of vitamin D every day. You can get your daily dose of vitamin D from a combination of sunlight, drinking milk and eating other dairy products, and taking vitamin or calcium supplements. Older people, especially those who live in northern climates or who stay inside all day, often do not get enough sunlight. Vitamin D is available without a prescription. If you do not already take a multiple vitamin with vitamin D, talk to your doctor or other healthcare professional to see if you should take a multiple vitamin or calcium supplement that contains vitamin D.

How Will I Take Vitamin D?

Vitamin D is usually taken once a day. It can be taken with or without food. Follow the instructions given on the package, or ask your doctor or other healthcare professional how often to use this medication.

If you miss a dose of this medication, take the dose you missed as soon as possible. However, if it is almost time for your next dose, skip the missed dose and just take the next one. Do not double your dose. Take your medication exactly as directed by your doctor or other healthcare professional.

What Side Effects Can Vitamin D Cause?

Less Common

Taking too much vitamin D may cause a person to absorb large amounts of calcium, creating a condition called hypercalcemia. These are the symptoms of hypercalcemia:

- Confusion
- Kidney stones
- Nausea
- Nervousness (anxiety)
- Severe constipation
- Stomach pain
- Thirst
- Vomiting
- Weakness

Tell your doctor or other healthcare professional if you have side effects that bother you, do not go away, make you worried about taking your medication, or make you want to stop taking your medication.

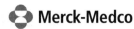

 ## Do Other Medications Interact with Vitamin D?

Mineral oil *may decrease* how well vitamin D works.

Bile acid binders such as *Questran*® (cholestyramine) or *Colestid*® (colestipol) or bulk-forming laxatives like *Metamucil*® (psyllium) *may decrease* the effects of vitamin D by preventing it from being absorbed completely. To help make sure it is absorbed so it can work properly, take vitamin D 1 hour before or 4 to 6 hours after taking a bile acid binder or a bulk-forming laxative.

Tell your doctor or other healthcare professional about all medications (both prescription and nonprescription [over-the-counter] medications) that you are taking.

Why Else Do People Take Vitamin D?

Vitamin D is also taken for rickets, a bone problem that is caused by having too little vitamin D in the diet (vitamin D deficiency).

 # Warning!

To give you the best care, your doctor or other healthcare professional needs to know about the diseases and medical conditions you have had—your full medical history. Tell your doctor or other healthcare professional if you have or have ever had high calcium in your blood (hypercalcemia) or kidney problems.

Bisphosphonates

Bisphosphonates help prevent bones from breaking down and becoming weaker. Bisphosphonates are used to help prevent and treat osteoporosis.

Brand Name	Generic Name
Actonel®	risedronate
Didronel®	etidronate
Fosamax®	alendronate

How Will I Take Bisphosphonates?

Didronel® (etidronate) is usually taken once a day for 2 weeks out of a 3-month period along with calcium taken every day. It should be taken 2 hours before or after meals and apart from other medications, calcium, and vitamins.

Fosamax® (alendronate) and *Actonel*® (risedronate) must be taken as described below to be absorbed and to help prevent side effects.

Fosamax® (alendronate) or *Actonel*® (risedronate) is usually taken once a day. It should be taken as soon as you wake up in the morning, at least 30 minutes before you have anything to eat or drink and before you take other medications. With your pill, drink a full 8-ounce glass of plain water (not juice, coffee, tea, milk, or any other beverages). Do not lie down for at least 30 minutes after taking *Fosamax*® (alendronate) or *Actonel*® (risedronate) to help prevent irritation of the tube that connects your mouth to your stomach (esophagus). You may sit or stand. If possible, wait 1 hour before eating so the medication can be absorbed better. These pills should be swallowed whole. Do not crush, chew, or break them. Your doctor or other healthcare professional will tell you how often to take your medication.

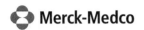
If you miss a dose of this medication, take the dose you missed as soon as possible. However, if it is almost time for your next dose, skip the missed dose and just take the next one. Do not double your dose. Take your medication exactly as directed by your doctor or other healthcare professional. Do not stop taking a prescription medication unless directed by your doctor or other healthcare professional.

What Side Effects Can Bisphosphonates Cause?

More Common

- Gas
- Headache
- Heartburn
- Stomach pain

Less Common

- Back pain
- Bone pain
- Burning in the tube that connects your mouth to your stomach (esophagus)
- Fever
- Pain when swallowing

Rare

- Rash (skin redness, bumps, itching, or irritation)
- Ulcers in the stomach that may cause black, tarry-looking bowel movements

Tell your doctor or other healthcare professional if you have side effects that bother you, do not go away, make you worried about taking your medication, or make you want to stop taking your medication.

Do Other Medications Interact with Bisphosphonates?

These medications *may increase* the side effects of *Fosamax*® (alendronate):

- Aspirin, medications that contain aspirin, and aspirin-like medications (salicylates)—see Glossary

- Nonsteroidal anti-inflammatory drugs (NSAIDs) such as *Motrin*® (ibuprofen), *Aleve*® (naproxen), *Vioxx*® (rofecoxib), *Celebrex*® (celecoxib), and others—see Glossary

Didronel® (etidronate) *may increase* the side effects of *Coumadin*® (warfarin).

Take bisphosphonates 1 hour before taking other medications to help prevent poor absorption of the bisphosphonates.

Tell your doctor or other healthcare professional about all medications (both prescription and nonprescription [over-the-counter] medications) that you are taking.

Why Else Do People Take Bisphosphonates?

Bisphosphonates are sometimes taken to help lower the amount of calcium in the blood when it is too high (hypercalcemia) or to help treat Paget's disease (a bone disease).

Warning!

To give you the best care, your doctor or other healthcare professional needs to know about the diseases and medical conditions you have had—your full medical history. Tell your doctor or other healthcare professional if you have or have ever had any of the following:

- Allergy or previous reaction to bisphosphonates

- Heartburn or gastroesophageal reflux disease (GERD)

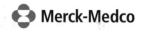

- Kidney problems

- Low calcium in your blood (hypocalcemia)

- Problems with the tube that connects your mouth with your stomach (esophagus) such as stricture

Bisphosphonates may cause stomach pain, which may be a sign of an ulcer. However, you may have an ulcer without feeling any pain at all. If ulcers are not treated, they may cause serious stomach or intestinal bleeding. Tell your doctor or other healthcare professional if you have severe stomach pain or stomach pain that keeps returning or if you have ever had peptic ulcer disease. Call your doctor or other healthcare professional right away if you have black, tarry-looking bowel movements (stools), if you vomit dark material that looks like coffee grounds, or if you notice any blood in your bowel movements. Any of these symptoms may be a sign of a bleeding ulcer.

Calcitonin

Calcitonin is a hormone that helps to treat osteoporosis by helping to prevent bones from releasing calcium.

Brand Name	Generic Name
Calcimar® Injection	salmon calcitonin
Miacalcin® Injection	salmon calcitonin
Miacalcin® Nasal Spray	salmon calcitonin

 ## How Will I Take Calcitonin?

If you use calcitonin as a nasal spray, you will usually spray it into your right nostril the first day and the left nostril the next day. Alternating nostrils helps keep your nose from getting sore. To get the spray ready for use, press down on the white side arms of the container about 6 times until a light spray comes out. You only have to do this the first time you use a new spray bottle of calcitonin.

If you take calcitonin as a shot (injection), you will usually take it once a day or once every other day. You can give yourself the injection or your caregiver can do it. Ask your doctor or other healthcare professional to show you how to give an injection. Do not use the medication if it looks lumpy or discolored or if you see specks floating in the liquid.

If you miss a dose of this medication, take the dose you missed as soon as possible. However, if it is almost time for your next dose, skip the missed dose and just take the next one. Do not double your dose. Take your medication exactly as directed by your doctor or other healthcare professional. Do not stop taking a prescription medication unless directed by your doctor or other healthcare professional.

What Side Effects Can Calcitonin Cause?

More Common

- Diarrhea

- Headache

- Loss of appetite

- Nausea

- Pain or irritation where shot (injection) was given

- Reddening of the face (flushing)

- Runny nose (when you use nasal spray)

Less Common

- Chest tightness or trouble breathing

- Constipation

- Itching or swelling

- Nose irritation or bleeding where nasal spray is used

- Rash (skin redness, bumps, itching, or irritation)

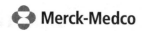

Tell your doctor or other healthcare professional if you have side effects that bother you, do not go away, make you worried about taking your medication, or make you want to stop taking your medication.

Why Else Do People Take Calcitonin?

Calcitonin injection is also used for Paget's disease (a bone disease) and for reducing very high levels of calcium in the blood (hypercalcemia).

What Else Should I Know about Calcitonin?

If using the nasal spray, keep each new package in the refrigerator at 36°F to 46°F (do not freeze) until you have opened it. Once it has been opened, you can keep it at room temperature (59°F to 86°F) for up to 1 month. Throw away any unused medication 1 month after opening the bottle.

If using the shots (injections), keep the bottle (vial) in the refrigerator at 36°F to 46°F (do not freeze).

 # Warning!

To give you the best care, your doctor or other healthcare professional needs to know about the diseases and medical conditions you have had—your full medical history. Tell your doctor or other healthcare professional if you have or have ever had an allergy or previous reaction to calcitonin or low calcium in your blood (hypocalcemia).

Your doctor or other healthcare professional may give you a skin test for allergy before prescribing calcitonin. The skin test will show whether you are allergic to calcitonin or to either of its main ingredients, salmon and gelatin. If so, this medication could give you a severe allergic reaction such as hives, swelling, or trouble breathing.

If you are using the nasal spray, your doctor or other healthcare professional may want to check your nasal passages for signs of irritation from the medication.

Chapter 17

Parkinson's Disease

What Is Parkinson's Disease?

Parkinson's disease is an illness that affects the part of the brain that controls body movement. The brain controls body movement by sending messages to the muscles. With Parkinson's disease there is a loss of dopamine (a chemical in the brain that controls movement) and an imbalance between dopamine and acetylcholine (another chemical in the brain that transmits messages to the muscles). The changes in dopamine and acetylcholine decrease the body's ability to control muscle movement.

Symptoms may not be noticed at first, but they get worse over time. A typical first indication that a person has Parkinson's disease is that his or her hands shake when they are not busy doing something, a condition called tremor. Other symptoms may occur later.

Early symptoms that frequently occur in Parkinson's disease include:
- A shuffling walk
- Difficulty making facial expressions
- Difficulty starting to walk
- Hand shaking (tremor) at rest
- Muscle stiffness
- Slower body movements

Later symptoms that frequently occur in Parkinson's disease include:
- Confusion
- Depression
- Drooling
- Memory loss

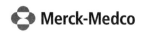

Medications may be used to help reduce the symptoms of Parkinson's disease. The kinds of medications taken for Parkinson's disease depend on which symptoms a person has and how severe the symptoms are. A person may have to take more than one kind of medication to help reduce symptoms. Surgery may be an option to help treat Parkinson's disease in some people.

Medications for Parkinson's Disease

Several kinds of medications may be taken for Parkinson's disease. This chapter discusses these medications and/or categories of medications:

MEDICATIONS	See Page
Anticholinergic Medications	548
Parlodel® (bromocriptine) and *Permax*® (pergolide)	553
Mirapex® (pramipexole) and *Requip*® (ropinirole)	557
Levodopa	562
Symmetrel® (amantadine)	567
Selegiline	570
Tasmar® (tolcapone)	573
Comtan® (entacapone)	577

If you do not see the exact name of the medication that you take for Parkinson's disease listed above, check the Medication and Chapter Table to find out which category your medication falls under or check the Index.

Anticholinergic Medications

Anticholinergic medications are most often used in early stages of Parkinson's disease to help reduce shakiness (tremors). They work by decreasing acetylcholine.

Brand Name	Generic Name
Akineton®	biperiden
Artane®	trihexyphenidyl
Cogentin®	benztropine
Kemadrin®	procyclidine

How Will I Take Anticholinergic Medications?

Anticholinergic medications usually are taken as pills 1 to 4 times a day. *Artane*® (trihexyphenidyl) is also available as a liquid. Taking these medications with food can help prevent stomach upset. Your doctor or other healthcare professional will tell you how many times a day to take your medication.

To help prevent side effects, your doctor or other healthcare professional may start by giving you a low dose of this medication, increasing the amount slowly until it works well for you.

When a medication has the word "sequel" after its name, it usually means that the body absorbs the medication slowly over time, so you usually have to take it only once or twice a day. The body will absorb some medications of this type too fast if you crush or break them or dissolve them in liquid, and their effects will not last as long as they should. Check with your doctor or other healthcare professional before crushing or breaking your pills or dissolving your pills in liquid.

If you miss a dose of this medication, take the dose you missed as soon as possible. However, if it is almost time for your next dose, skip the missed dose and just take the next one. Do not double your dose. Take your medication exactly as directed by your doctor or other healthcare professional. Do not stop taking a prescription medication unless directed by your doctor or other healthcare professional.

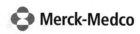

⚠️ What Side Effects Can Anticholinergic Medications Cause?

More Common

- Blurred vision
- Constipation
- Drowsiness
- Dry mouth, nose, throat, or eyes
- Fast heartbeat (palpitations)
- Increased sensitivity to light
- Trouble urinating or emptying the bladder
- Widening of the pupils in the eye (dilation)

Less Common

- Confusion
- Dizziness when standing up from a bed or a chair
- Nausea
- Nervousness (anxiety)
- Reddening of the face (flushing)
- Seeing or hearing things that are not there (hallucinations)
- Vomiting

Tell your doctor or other healthcare professional if you have side effects that bother you, do not go away, make you worried about taking your medication, or make you want to stop taking your medication.

Do Other Medications Interact with Anticholinergic Medications?

Anticholinergic medications **_may increase_** the side effects of other medications that cause drowsiness, including other anticholinergic medications, antidepressants, antihistamines (allergy medications), antispasmodics, benzodiazepines (a type of tranquilizer), anxiety medications, narcotics (pain relievers), muscle relaxants, neuroleptic medications (a type of tranquilizer), seizure medications, or sleep medications. Avoid driving a car and other activities that need mental alertness, like using a knife or operating machinery, while taking these medications together.

Drinking alcoholic beverages (such as beer, wine, whiskey, and others) *may increase* the side effects of anticholinergic medications.

These medications *may increase* the symptoms of Parkinson's disease:

- *Compazine*® (prochlorperazine)
- Neuroleptic medications such as *Risperdal*® (risperidone), *Thorazine*® (chlorpromazine), *Zyprexa*® (olanzapine), and others—see Glossary
- *Reglan*® (metoclopramide)

Tell your doctor or other healthcare professional about all medications (both prescription and nonprescription [over-the-counter] medications) that you are taking.

Why Else Do People Take Anticholinergic Medications?

Anticholinergic medications are sometimes used for shakiness (tremor) that is caused by neuroleptic medications such as *Risperdal*® (risperidone), *Thorazine*® (chlorpromazine), *Zyprexa*® (olanzapine), and others—see Glossary.

What Else Should I Know about Anticholinergic Medications?

Anticholinergic medications do not work for everyone. Talk to your doctor or other healthcare professional if you take one for Parkinson's disease and your symptoms do not improve. He or she may be able to prescribe another medication that will work better for you.

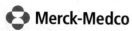

(STOP) **Warning!**

To give you the best care, your doctor or other healthcare professional needs to know about the diseases and medical conditions you have had—your full medical history. Tell your doctor or other healthcare professional if you have or have ever had any of the following:

- Allergy or previous reaction to anticholinergic medications
- Alzheimer's disease
- Congestive heart failure
- Enlarged prostate (benign prostatic hypertrophy)
- Glaucoma (an eye disease)
- Heart rhythm problems (arrhythmia)
- Inflammatory bowel disease (ulcerative colitis or Crohn's disease)
- Kidney problems
- Liver problems
- Severe constipation or bowel obstruction
- Trouble urinating

Anticholinergic medications may decrease the body's ability to perspire and may make it hard for your body to regulate its own temperature. Anticholinergic medications increase a person's chance of having heatstroke. Though not a true stroke, this rare but serious condition can cause high body temperature and sudden falling, fainting, or unconsciousness. Talk to your doctor or other healthcare professional about how you can avoid heatstroke.

Anticholinergic medications may cause drowsiness. Avoid driving a car and other activities that need mental alertness, like using a knife or operating machinery, while taking this medication. Drinking alcoholic beverages (such as beer, wine, whiskey, and others) may increase the side effects.

Anticholinergic medications may make you unsteady on your feet, causing you to fall and possibly break a bone. If you have fallen recently, tell your doctor or other healthcare professional about it. Taking a different medication or a lower dose may make you less likely to fall. You should not stop taking this medication without first talking to your doctor or other healthcare professional.

Anticholinergic medications sometimes cause many side effects in people over 65. Additionally, they may lose their effectiveness over time. Talk to your doctor or other healthcare professional if you have side effects, or have been taking an anticholinergic medication for a long time, to see if this medication is still right for you. Do not stop taking this medication without talking to your doctor or other healthcare professional.

Under certain circumstances your doctor or other healthcare professional may decide that you should stop taking this medication. If you have taken it for more than a couple of weeks, he or she may want you to decrease it gradually, lowering the dose over a few weeks or months. Stopping suddenly may cause unpleasant withdrawal symptoms or may worsen your medical problems. Pay careful attention to the instructions your doctor or other healthcare professional gives you about how much less to take and for how long.

Parlodel® (bromocriptine) and *Permax*® (pergolide)

Parlodel® (bromocriptine) and *Permax*® (pergolide) work like dopamine to help reduce the symptoms of Parkinson's disease.

 ### How Will I Take *Parlodel*® (bromocriptine) and *Permax*® (pergolide)?

Parlodel® (bromocriptine) and *Permax*® (pergolide) are usually taken 2 to 3 times a day. These medications are usually taken with food or meals to help prevent stomach upset. Talk to your doctor or other healthcare professional about how many times a day to take your medication.

To help prevent side effects, your doctor or other healthcare professional may start by giving you a low dose of this medication, increasing the amount slowly until it works well for you.

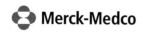

If you miss a dose of this medication, take the dose you missed as soon as possible. However, if it is almost time for your next dose, skip the missed dose and just take the next one. Do not double your dose. Take your medication exactly as directed by your doctor or other healthcare professional. Do not stop taking a prescription medication unless directed by your doctor or other healthcare professional.

What Side Effects Can *Parlodel*® (bromocriptine) and *Permax*® (pergolide) Cause?

More Common

- Blurred vision

- Confusion

- Constipation

- Dizziness when standing up from a bed or a chair

- Jerking motion, uncontrollable, repetitive movements of the face, neck, and arms

- Nasal congestion, runny nose

- Nausea

- Nervousness (anxiety)

- Seeing or hearing things that are not there (hallucinations)

- Tiredness or sluggishness (fatigue)

- Trouble falling asleep or staying asleep (insomnia)

Less Common

- Change in taste

- Double vision

- Increased urination

- Irregular heartbeat (palpitations)

- Memory problems
- Muscle aches and pains
- Swelling or puffiness of the feet, ankles, or lower legs (edema)
- Ulcers in the stomach that may cause black, tarry-looking bowel movements
- Vomiting

Rare

- Erection problems (erectile dysfunction)
- Frequent fever, sore throat, or flu-like symptoms that may be a sign of low white blood cells
- Low red blood cells (anemia)
- Seizures
- Stroke

Tell your doctor or other healthcare professional if you have side effects that bother you, do not go away, make you worried about taking your medication, or make you want to stop taking your medication.

Do Other Medications Interact with *Parlodel*® (bromocriptine) and *Permax*® (pergolide)?

Erythromycin such as *Ery-Tab*®, *Erythrocin*®, and others (see Glossary) *may increase* the side effects of *Parlodel*® (bromocriptine) and *Permax*® (pergolide).

Parlodel® (bromocriptine) and *Permax*® (pergolide) *may increase* the side effects of other medications that cause drowsiness, including anticholinergic medications, antidepressants, antihistamines (allergy medications), antispasmodics, benzodiazepines (a type of tranquilizer), anxiety medications, narcotics (pain relievers), muscle relaxants, neuroleptic medications (a type of tranquilizer), seizure medications, or sleep medications. Avoid driving a car and other

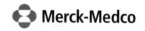

activities that need mental alertness, like using a knife or operating machinery, while taking these medications together.

Drinking alcoholic beverages (such as beer, wine, whiskey, and others) *may increase* the side effects of *Parlodel*® (bromocriptine) and *Permax*® (pergolide).

Parlodel® (bromocriptine) and *Permax*® (pergolide) *may increase* the side effects of these medications:

- *Neoral*® (cyclosporine)
- *Sandimmune*® (cyclosporine)

These medications *may increase* the symptoms of Parkinson's disease:

- *Compazine*® (prochlorperazine)
- Neuroleptic medications such as *Risperdal*® (risperidone), *Thorazine*® (chlorpromazine), *Zyprexa*® (olanzapine), and others—see Glossary
- *Reglan*® (metoclopramide)

Tell your doctor or other healthcare professional about all medications (both prescription and nonprescription [over-the-counter] medications) that you are taking.

 # Warning!

To give you the best care, your doctor or other healthcare professional needs to know about the diseases and medical conditions you have had—your full medical history. Tell your doctor or other healthcare professional if you have or have ever had any of the following:

- Allergy or previous reaction to *Parlodel*® (bromocriptine), *Permax*® (pergolide), or ergotamine (such as *Cafergot*® or *Ergostat*®)
- Dizziness when standing up from a bed or a chair
- Heart rhythm problems (arrhythmia)

- Seizures (epilepsy)

- Stomach problems (ulcers)

Parlodel® (bromocriptine) and *Permax*® (pergolide) may cause drowsiness. Avoid driving a car and other activities that need mental alertness, like using a knife or operating machinery, while taking this medication. Drinking alcoholic beverages (such as beer, wine, whiskey, and others) may increase the side effects.

Parlodel® (bromocriptine) and *Permax*® (pergolide) may make you unsteady on your feet, causing you to fall and possibly break a bone. If you have fallen recently, tell your doctor or other healthcare professional about it. Taking a different medication or a lower dose may make you less likely to fall. You should not stop taking this medication without first talking to your doctor or other healthcare professional.

If you have had seizures in the past, tell your doctor or other healthcare professional because *Parlodel*® (bromocriptine) and *Permax*® (pergolide) may cause seizures. Stopping this medication suddenly may also cause seizures. If your doctor or other healthcare professional decides that you should stop taking *Parlodel*® (bromocriptine) or *Permax*® (pergolide), pay careful attention to the instructions he or she gives you about how much less to take and for how long.

Under certain circumstances your doctor or other healthcare professional may decide that you should stop taking this medication. If you have taken it for more than a couple of weeks, he or she may want you to decrease it gradually, lowering the dose over a few weeks or months. Stopping suddenly may cause unpleasant withdrawal symptoms or may worsen your medical problems. Pay careful attention to the instructions your doctor or other healthcare professional gives you about how much less to take and for how long.

Mirapex® (pramipexole) and *Requip*® (ropinirole)

Mirapex® (pramipexole) and *Requip*® (ropinirole) work like dopamine to help reduce the symptoms of Parkinson's disease.

How Will I Take *Mirapex*® (pramipexole) and *Requip*® (ropinirole)?

Mirapex® (pramipexole) and *Requip*® (ropinirole) are usually taken 3 times a day. These medications are usually taken with food or meals to help prevent stomach upset. Talk to your doctor or other healthcare professional about how many times a day to take your medication.

To help prevent side effects, your doctor or other healthcare professional may start by giving you a low dose of this medication, increasing the amount slowly until it works well for you.

If you miss a dose of this medication, take the dose you missed as soon as possible. However, if it is almost time for your next dose, skip the missed dose and just take the next one. Do not double your dose. Take your medication exactly as directed by your doctor or other healthcare professional. Do not stop taking a prescription medication unless directed by your doctor or other healthcare professional.

What Side Effects Can *Mirapex*® (pramipexole) and *Requip*® (ropinirole) Cause?

More Common

- Blurred vision
- Confusion
- Constipation
- Dizziness when standing up from a bed or a chair
- Dry mouth
- Headache
- Jerking motion, uncontrollable, repetitive movements of the face, neck, and arms
- Nasal congestion, runny nose

- Nausea
- Seeing or hearing things that are not there (hallucinations)
- Tiredness or sluggishness (fatigue)
- Trouble falling asleep or staying asleep (insomnia)

Less Common

- Double vision
- Fast heartbeat (palpitations)
- Increased urination
- Memory problems
- Muscle aches and pains
- Nervousness (anxiety)
- Sleep attacks (sudden overwhelming sleepiness, without awareness of falling asleep)
- Swelling or puffiness of the feet, ankles, or lower legs (edema)
- Vomiting

Rare

- Erection problems (erectile dysfunction)
- Low red blood cells (anemia)

Tell your doctor or other healthcare professional if you have side effects that bother you, do not go away, make you worried about taking your medication, or make you want to stop taking your medication.

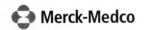

Do Other Medications Interact with *Mirapex*® (pramipexole) and *Requip*® (ropinirole)?

These medications *may increase* the side effects of *Mirapex*® (pramipexole) and *Requip*® (ropinirole):

- Erythromycin such as *Ery-Tab*®, *Erythrocin*®, and others—see Glossary

- Quinolone antibiotics such as *Cipro*® (ciprofloxacin), *Floxin*® (ofloxacin), and *Levaquin*® (levofloxacin)—see Glossary

- *Tagamet*® (cimetidine)

- *Zantac*® (ranitidine)

Mirapex® (pramipexole) and *Requip*® (ropinirole) *may increase* the side effects of other medications that cause drowsiness, including anticholinergic medications, antidepressants, antihistamines (allergy medications), antispasmodics, benzodiazepines (a type of tranquilizer), anxiety medications, narcotics (pain relievers), muscle relaxants, neuroleptic medications, (a type of tranquilizer), seizure medications, or sleep medications. Avoid driving a car and other activities that need mental alertness, like using a knife or operating machinery, while taking these medications together.

Drinking alcoholic beverages (such as beer, wine, whiskey, and others) *may increase* the side effects of *Mirapex*® (pramipexole) and *Requip*® (ropinirole).

These medications *may increase* the symptoms of Parkinson's disease:

- *Compazine*® (prochlorperazine)

- Neuroleptic medications such as *Risperdal*® (risperidone), *Thorazine*® (chlorpromazine), *Zyprexa*® (olanzapine), and others—see Glossary

- *Reglan*® (metoclopramide)

Tell your doctor or other healthcare professional about all medications (both prescription and nonprescription [over-the-counter] medications) that you are taking.

Warning!

To give you the best care, your doctor or other healthcare professional needs to know about the diseases and medical conditions you have had—your full medical history. Tell your doctor or other healthcare professional if you have or have ever had any of the following:

- Allergy or previous reaction to *Mirapex®* (pramipexole) or *Requip®* (ropinirole)

- Coronary artery disease

- Dementia or Alzheimer's disease

- Dizziness when standing up from a bed or a chair

- Heart attack (myocardial infarction)

- Kidney problems

- Schizophrenia (a mental illness that causes delusions and hallucinations)

Mirapex® (pramipexole) and *Requip®* (ropinirole) may cause drowsiness. Avoid driving a car and other activities that need mental alertness, like using a knife or operating machinery, while taking this medication. Drinking alcoholic beverages (such as beer, wine, whiskey, and others) may increase the side effects.

Mirapex® (pramipexole) and *Requip®* (ropinirole) may make you unsteady on your feet, causing you to fall and possibly break a bone. If you have fallen recently, tell your doctor or other healthcare professional about it. Taking a different medication or a lower dose may make you less likely to fall. You should not stop taking this medication without first talking to your doctor or other healthcare professional.

Under certain circumstances your doctor or other healthcare professional may decide that you should stop taking this medication. If you have taken it for more than a couple of weeks, he or she may want you to decrease it gradually, lowering the dose over a few weeks or months. Stopping suddenly may cause unpleasant withdrawal symptoms or may worsen your medical problems. Pay careful attention to the instructions your doctor or other healthcare professional gives you about how much less to take and for how long.

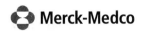
Levodopa

Levodopa is similar to a chemical called dopamine that is found in the brain that controls movement. Once levodopa reaches the brain it is changed into dopamine. Levodopa is often broken down in the bloodstream by enzymes before it can reach the brain. To help prevent the breakdown of levodopa before it reaches the brain, levodopa is often combined with carbidopa. Carbidopa helps prevent enzymes from breaking down levodopa in the bloodstream and helps more levodopa get into the brain. *Sinemet*® and *Atamet*® are a combination of levodopa and carbidopa. *Sinemet*® and *Atamet*® (carbidopa/levodopa) and *Larodopa*™ and *Dopar*® (levodopa only) help relieve the symptoms of Parkinson's disease.

Brand Name	Generic Name
Atamet®	carbidopa/levodopa
Dopar®	levodopa
Larodopa™	levodopa
Sinemet®	carbidopa/levodopa

 How Will I Take Levodopa?

Most people take levodopa 3 to 5 times a day. Levodopa should be taken on an empty stomach if possible. If stomach upset occurs, ask your doctor or other healthcare professional about taking it with food. Your doctor or other healthcare professional will tell you how many times a day to take your medication.

To help prevent side effects, your doctor or other healthcare professional may start by giving you a low dose of this medication, increasing the amount slowly until it works well for you.

When a medication has initials such as CR after its name, it usually means that the body absorbs the medication slowly over time, so you usually have to take it only once or twice a day. The body will absorb some medications of this type too fast if you crush or break them or dissolve them in liquid, and their effects will not last as long as they should. Check with your doctor or other healthcare professional before crushing or breaking your pills or dissolving your pills in liquid.

If you miss a dose of this medication, take the dose you missed as soon as possible. However, if it is almost time for your next dose, skip the missed dose and just take the next one. Do not double your dose. Take your medication exactly as directed by your doctor or other healthcare professional. Do not stop taking a prescription medication unless directed by your doctor or other healthcare professional.

What Side Effects Can Levodopa Cause?

More Common

- Blurred vision

- Confusion

- Constipation

- Dizziness when standing up from a bed or a chair

- Dry mouth

- Eyelid twitching

- Fast heartbeat (palpitations)

- Headache

- Nausea

Less Common

- High blood pressure (hypertension)

- Increased interest in sex

- Jerking motion, uncontrollable, repetitive movements of the face, neck, and arms

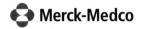

- Nervousness (anxiety)

- Nightmares

- Passing out or fainting

- Poor appetite

- Sadness, feeling blue or down, depressed mood (depression)

- Trouble breathing or shortness of breath

- Trouble falling asleep or staying asleep (insomnia)

- Trouble urinating or emptying the bladder

- Ulcers in the stomach that may cause black, tarry-looking bowel movements

- Urine that may appear darker or change color

- Vomiting

Tell your doctor or other healthcare professional if you have side effects that bother you, do not go away, make you worried about taking your medication, or make you want to stop taking your medication.

 Do Other Medications Interact with Levodopa?

These medications *may decrease* how well levodopa works:

- *Dilantin®* (phenytoin)

- Iron supplements (ferrous sulfate, ferrous gluconate, and ferrous fumarate)

- Isoniazid

- Vitamin B_6 (pyridoxine)

High blood pressure (hypertension) medications (see Glossary) *may increase* the side effects of levodopa.

Levodopa is generally not prescribed for anyone who is taking MAO inhibitors, such as *Marplan®* (isocarboxazid), *Nardil®* (phenelzine), or *Parnate®* (tranylcypromine), because together they **may cause** serious or even fatal reactions. If your doctor or other healthcare professional wants you to stop taking one medication and start taking the other, you should wait at least 2 weeks between stopping one and starting the other.

Antacids such as *Maalox®* or *Mylanta®* (aluminum hydroxide/magnesium hydroxide), *Rolaids®* or *Tums®* (calcium carbonate), or *Amphojel®* (aluminum hydroxide) **may decrease** the effects of levodopa when taken at the same time. If you are using antacids, take levodopa 1 hour before or 2 hours after taking your antacid.

These medications **may increase** the symptoms of Parkinson's disease:

- *Compazine®* (prochlorperazine)

- Neuroleptic medications such as *Risperdal®* (risperidone), *Thorazine®* (chlorpromazine), *Zyprexa®* (olanzapine), and others—see Glossary

- *Reglan®* (metoclopramide)

Tell your doctor or other healthcare professional about all medications (both prescription and nonprescription [over-the-counter] medications) that you are taking.

 # Warning!

To give you the best care, your doctor or other healthcare professional needs to know about the diseases and medical conditions you have had—your full medical history. Tell your doctor or other healthcare professional if you have or have ever had, or presently take, any of the following:

- Allergy or previous reaction to levodopa

- Asthma or nasal polyps (overgrowth of tissue in the nose)

- Glaucoma (an eye disease)

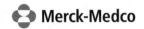

- Heart attack (myocardial infarction)

- Heart rhythm problems (arrhythmia)

- Kidney problems

- Liver problems

- MAO inhibitors such as *Marplan*® (isocarboxazid), *Nardil*® (phenelzine), or *Parnate*® (tranylcypromine)

- Melanoma (a form of skin cancer)

- Sadness, feeling blue or down, depressed mood (depression)

- Stomach problems (ulcers)

Protein changes in your diet may cause changes in how well your levodopa works. Divide the protein in your diet equally throughout the day instead of eating a lot of protein at one time and then little or none later in the day. Keeping a balance of protein in your diet will help levodopa keep working in your body at a steady rate. Major sources of protein include meat, fish and seafood, poultry, eggs, milk and other dairy products, nuts, and legumes (such as peas and beans).

Vitamin B_6 (pyridoxine) may decrease how well levodopa works. Avoid taking vitamin B_6 or eating large amounts of liver, fish, whole-grain cereals, and legumes (such as peas and beans). Talk to your doctor or other healthcare professional before taking a multivitamin.

Levodopa may make you unsteady on your feet, causing you to fall and possibly break a bone. If you have fallen recently, tell your doctor or other healthcare professional about it. Taking a different medication or a lower dose may make you less likely to fall. You should not stop taking this medication without first talking to your doctor or other healthcare professional.

Under certain circumstances your doctor or other healthcare professional may decide that you should stop taking this medication. If you have taken it for more than a couple of weeks, he or she may want you to decrease it gradually, lowering the dose over a few weeks or months. Stopping suddenly may cause unpleasant withdrawal symptoms or may worsen your medical problems. Pay careful attention to the instructions your doctor or other healthcare professional gives you about how much less to take and for how long.

Symmetrel® (amantadine)

Symmetrel® (amantadine) increases dopamine activity to help reduce the symptoms of Parkinson's disease.

How Will I Take *Symmetrel*® (amantadine)?

Symmetrel® (amantadine) comes as a pill or syrup that is usually taken 1 to 2 times a day. It may be taken with or without food. Your doctor or other healthcare professional will tell you how many times a day to take your medication.

If you miss a dose of this medication, take the dose you missed as soon as possible. However, if it is almost time for your next dose, skip the missed dose and just take the next one. Do not double your dose. Take your medication exactly as directed by your doctor or other healthcare professional. Do not stop taking a prescription medication unless directed by your doctor or other healthcare professional.

What Side Effects Can *Symmetrel*® (amantadine) Cause?

More Common

- Confusion
- Constipation
- Dizziness
- Dry mouth
- Headache
- Nausea
- Nervousness (anxiety)
- Swelling or puffiness of the feet, ankles, or lower legs (edema)

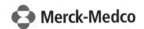

- Trouble breathing or shortness of breath
- Trouble falling asleep or staying asleep (insomnia)

Less Common

- Dizziness when standing up from a bed or a chair
- Nightmares
- Poor appetite
- Rash (skin redness, bumps, itching, or irritation)
- Sadness, feeling blue or down, depressed mood (depression)
- Seeing or hearing things that are not there (hallucinations)
- Seizures

Rare

- Frequent fever, sore throat, or flu-like symptoms that may be a sign of low white blood cells

---

Tell your doctor or other healthcare professional if you have side effects that bother you, do not go away, make you worried about taking your medication, or make you want to stop taking your medication.

 Do Other Medications Interact with *Symmetrel*® (amantadine)?

These medications **may increase** the side effects of *Symmetrel*® (amantadine):

- Sulfa medications such as *Bactrim*™, *Septra*®, and others—see Glossary
- *Trimpex*® (trimethoprim)

These medications **may increase** the symptoms of Parkinson's disease:

- *Compazine*® (prochlorperazine)

- Neuroleptic medications such as *Risperdal*® (risperidone), *Thorazine*® (chlorpromazine), *Zyprexa*® (olanzapine), and others—see Glossary

- *Reglan*® (metoclopramide)

Tell your doctor or other healthcare professional about all medications (both prescription and nonprescription [over-the-counter] medications) that you are taking.

Why Else Do People Take *Symmetrel*® (amantadine)?

Symmetrel® (amantadine) is sometimes used to help prevent or treat the flu (influenza).

 # Warning!

To give you the best care, your doctor or other healthcare professional needs to know about the diseases and medical conditions you have had—your full medical history. Tell your doctor or other healthcare professional if you have or have ever had any of the following:

- Allergy or previous reaction to *Symmetrel*® (amantadine) or *Flumadine*® (rimantadine)

- Dizziness when standing up from a bed or a chair

- Kidney problems

- Liver problems

- Seizures (epilepsy)

If you have had seizures in the past, tell your doctor or other healthcare professional because *Symmetrel*® (amantadine) may cause seizures. Stopping this medication suddenly may also cause seizures. If your doctor or other healthcare professional decides that you should stop taking *Symmetrel*® (amantadine), pay careful attention to the instructions he or she gives you about how much less to take and for how long.

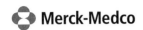

Selegiline

Selegiline is a type of monoamine oxidase (MAO) inhibitor, called an MAO-B inhibitor, which helps reduce the symptoms of Parkinson's disease.

Brand Name	Generic Name
Ataryl®	selegiline
Carbex®	selegiline
Eldepryl®	selegiline

How Will I Take Selegiline?

Selegiline is usually taken 1 to 2 times a day. If you take selegiline 2 times a day, it is usually taken at breakfast and lunch. If you take it later in the day, you might have trouble falling asleep. Your doctor or other healthcare professional will tell you how often to take this medication.

If you miss a dose of this medication, take the dose you missed as soon as possible. However, if it is almost time for your next dose, skip the missed dose and just take the next one. Do not double your dose. Take your medication exactly as directed by your doctor or other healthcare professional. Do not stop taking a prescription medication unless directed by your doctor or other healthcare professional.

What Side Effects Can Selegiline Cause?

More Common

- Difficulty starting to walk
- Dizziness
- Nausea

- Nervousness (anxiety)
- Slower body movements, difficulty walking
- Trouble falling asleep or staying asleep (insomnia)

Less Common

- Blurred vision
- Confusion
- Dizziness when standing up from a bed or a chair
- Dry mouth, eyes, and nose
- Fast heartbeat (palpitations)
- Passing out or fainting
- Trouble breathing or shortness of breath

Tell your doctor or other healthcare professional if you have side effects that bother you, do not go away, make you worried about taking your medication, or make you want to stop taking your medication.

Do Other Medications Interact with Selegiline?

Selegiline is generally not prescribed for anyone who is taking an SSRI, such as *Celexa*™ (citalopram), *Luvox*® (fluvoxamine), *Paxil*® (paroxetine), *Prozac*® (fluoxetine), or *Zoloft*® (sertraline), because together they *may cause* serious reactions, even a coma. If your doctor or other healthcare professional wants you to stop taking one medication and start taking the other, you should wait at least 2 to 6 weeks between stopping one and starting the other, depending on which medication you are taking.

Selegiline is generally not prescribed for anyone who is taking *Demerol*® (meperidine), because together they *may cause* serious reactions, even a coma. If your doctor or other healthcare professional wants you to stop taking one medication and start taking the other, you should wait at least 2 weeks between stopping one and starting the other, depending on which medication you are taking.

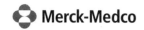

Selegiline *may cause* serious side effects when the dose is higher than 10 mg daily. If your doctor or other healthcare professional prescribes more than 10 mg daily, you may have to follow a special diet. Additionally, medication interactions may be more common or more serious. Ask your doctor or other healthcare professional about foods and medications to avoid if you are taking more than 10 mg daily.

These medications *may increase* the symptoms of Parkinson's disease:

- *Compazine*® (prochlorperazine)
- Neuroleptic medications such as *Risperdal*® (risperidone), *Thorazine*® (chlorpromazine), *Zyprexa*® (olanzapine), and others—see Glossary
- *Reglan*® (metoclopramide)

Tell your doctor or other healthcare professional about all medications (both prescription and nonprescription [over-the-counter] medications) that you are taking.

Why Else Do People Take Selegiline?

Selegiline is sometimes taken for Alzheimer's disease.

 # Warning!

To give you the best care, your doctor or other healthcare professional needs to know about the diseases and medical conditions you have had—your full medical history. Tell your doctor or other healthcare professional if you have or have ever had, or presently take, any of the following:

- Allergy or previous reaction to selegiline
- *Demerol*® (meperidine)
- Dizziness when standing up from a bed or a chair

- Liver problems

- Seizures (epilepsy)

- SSRIs such as *Celexa*™ (citalopram), *Luvox*® (fluvoxamine), *Paxil*® (paroxetine), *Prozac*® (fluoxetine), and *Zoloft*® (sertraline)

Selegiline may make you unsteady on your feet, causing you to fall and possibly break a bone. If you have fallen recently, tell your doctor or other healthcare professional about it. Taking a different medication or a lower dose may make you less likely to fall. You should not stop taking this medication without first talking to your doctor or other healthcare professional.

Selegiline may cause serious side effects when the dose is higher than 10 mg daily. If your doctor or other healthcare professional prescribes more than 10 mg daily, you may have to follow a special diet. Additionally, medication interactions may be more common or more serious. Ask your doctor or other healthcare professional about foods and medications to avoid if you are taking more than 10 mg daily.

Tasmar® (tolcapone)

Tasmar® (tolcapone) is usually given with levodopa because it helps decrease the breakdown of levodopa in the bloodstream and helps levodopa reach the brain, where it is changed to dopamine. This helps to improve the symptoms of Parkinson's disease.

 ## How Will I Take *Tasmar*® (tolcapone)?

Tasmar® (tolcapone) is usually taken 3 times a day at the same time you take *Sinemet*® or *Atamet*® (carbidopa/levodopa). It can be taken with or without food. It can be taken with food to help prevent stomach upset. Your doctor or other healthcare professional will tell you how many times a day to take your medication.

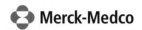

If you miss a dose of this medication, take the dose you missed as soon as possible. However, if it is almost time for your next dose, skip the missed dose and just take the next one. Do not double your dose. Take your medication exactly as directed by your doctor or other healthcare professional. Do not stop taking a prescription medication unless directed by your doctor or other healthcare professional.

 ## What Side Effects Can *Tasmar*® (tolcapone) Cause?

More Common

- Diarrhea
- Drowsiness
- Dry mouth
- Increased or excessive sweating (perspiration)
- Jerking motion, uncontrollable, repetitive movements of the face, neck, and arms
- Muscle contractions or abnormal posture
- Muscle cramps
- Nausea
- Poor appetite
- Seeing or hearing things that are not there (hallucinations)

Less Common

- Confusion
- Constipation
- Dizziness when standing up from a bed or a chair
- Frequent dreams
- Headache
- Nausea

- Trouble falling asleep or staying asleep (insomnia)

- Urine that may appear darker or change color

Rare

- Easy bruising ("black-and-blue" marks on the skin)

- Liver problems that may cause yellowing of the skin or eyes (jaundice)

Tell your doctor or other healthcare professional if you have side effects that bother you, do not go away, make you worried about taking your medication, or make you want to stop taking your medication.

Do Other Medications Interact with *Tasmar*® (tolcapone)?

Tasmar® (tolcapone) *may increase* the side effects of *Aldomet*® (methyldopa).

Tasmar® (tolcapone) is generally not prescribed for anyone who is taking MAO inhibitors, such as *Marplan*® (isocarboxazid), *Nardil*® (phenelzine), or *Parnate*® (tranylcypromine), because together they *may cause* serious or even fatal reactions. If your doctor or other healthcare professional wants you to stop taking one medication and start taking the other, you should wait at least 2 weeks between stopping one and starting the other.

Tasmar® (tolcapone) *may increase* the side effects of other medications that cause drowsiness, including antidepressants, antihistamines (allergy medications), benzodiazepines (a type of tranquilizer), anxiety medications, narcotics (pain relievers), muscle relaxants, neuroleptic medications (a type of tranquilizer), seizure medications, or sleep medications. Avoid driving a car and other activities that need mental alertness, like using a knife or operating machinery, while taking this medication.

Drinking alcoholic beverages (such as beer, wine, whiskey, and others) *may increase* the side effects of *Tasmar*® (tolcapone).

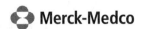

These medications may increase the symptoms of Parkinson's disease:

- *Compazine®* (prochlorperazine)

- Neuroleptic medications such as *Risperdal®* (risperidone), *Thorazine®* (chlorpromazine), *Zyprexa®* (olanzapine), and others—see Glossary

- *Reglan®* (metoclopramide)

Tell your doctor or other healthcare professional about all medications (both prescription and nonprescription [over-the-counter] medications) that you are taking.

 # Warning!

To give you the best care, your doctor or other healthcare professional needs to know about the diseases and medical conditions you have had—your full medical history. Tell your doctor or other healthcare professional if you have or have ever had, or presently take, any of the following:

- Allergy or previous reaction to *Tasmar®* (tolcapone)

- Dizziness when standing up from a bed or a chair

- Kidney problems

- Liver problems

- MAO inhibitors such as *Marplan®* (isocarboxazid), *Nardil®* (phenelzine), or *Parnate®* (tranylcypromine)

Since *Tasmar®* (tolcapone) may cause damage to your liver, your doctor or other healthcare professional may order blood tests to find out early on if the medication is causing liver problems, before they become serious.

Tasmar® (tolcapone) may make you unsteady on your feet, causing you to fall and possibly break a bone. If you have fallen recently, tell your doctor or other healthcare professional about it. Taking a different medication or a lower dose may make you less likely to fall. You should not stop taking this medication without first talking to your doctor or other healthcare professional.

Tasmar® (tolcapone) may cause drowsiness. Avoid driving a car and other activities that need mental alertness, like using a knife or operating machinery, while taking this medication. Drinking alcoholic beverages (such as beer, wine, whiskey, and others) may increase the side effects.

Under certain circumstances, your doctor or other healthcare professional may decide that you should stop taking this medication. If you have taken it for more than a couple of weeks, he or she may want you to decrease it gradually, lowering the dose over a few weeks or months. Stopping suddenly may cause unpleasant withdrawal symptoms or may worsen your medical problems. Pay careful attention to the instructions your doctor or other healthcare professional gives you about how much less to take and for how long.

Comtan® (entacapone)

Comtan® (entacapone) is usually given with levodopa because it helps decrease the breakdown of levodopa in the bloodstream and helps levodopa reach the brain where it is changed to dopamine. This helps to improve the symptoms of Parkinson's disease.

 ## How Will I Take *Comtan*® (entacapone)?

Comtan® (entacapone) is usually taken 3 times a day with *Sinemet*® or *Atamet*® (carbidopa/levodopa). It may be taken with or without food. Your doctor or other healthcare professional will tell you how many times a day to take your medication.

If you miss a dose of this medication, take the dose you missed as soon as possible. However, if it is almost time for your next dose, skip the missed dose and just take the next one. Do not double your dose. Take your medication exactly as directed by your doctor or other healthcare professional. Do not stop taking a prescription medication unless directed by your doctor or other healthcare professional.

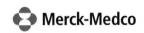

What Side Effects Can *Comtan*® (entacapone) Cause?

More Common

- Brownish-orange or dark yellow urine
- Confusion
- Diarrhea
- Dizziness
- Drowsiness
- Jerking motion, uncontrollable, repetitive movements of the face, neck, and arms
- Nausea
- Seeing or hearing things that are not there (hallucinations)
- Tiredness or sluggishness (fatigue)

Less Common

- Back pain
- Bloating and gas
- Constipation
- Dizziness when standing up from a bed or a chair
- Dry mouth
- Increased or excessive sweating (perspiration)
- Taste changes
- Trouble breathing or shortness of breath

Rare

- Easy bruising ("black-and-blue" marks on the skin)
- Severe muscle cramps and weakness

Tell your doctor or other healthcare professional if you have side effects that bother you, do not go away, make you worried about taking your medication, or make you want to stop taking your medication.

Do Other Medications Interact with *Comtan*® (entacapone)?

Comtan® (entacapone) *may increase* the side effects of these medications:

- *Aldomet*® (methyldopa)
- Epinephrine eyedrops such as *Epifrin*®, *E-Pilo*®, and *Glaucon*®
- *EpiPen*® (epinephrine)
- *Isuprel*® (isoproterenol)
- *Medihaler*® (isoproterenol)
- *Primatene*® (epinephrine)
- *Tornalate*® (bitolterol)

These medications *may increase* the side effects of *Comtan*® (entacapone):

- Ampicillin (various)
- *Benemid*® (probenecid)
- *Chloromycetin*® (chloramphenicol)
- Erythromycin such as *Ery-Tab*®, *Erythrocin*®, and others—see Glossary
- *Questran*® (cholestyramine)
- *Rifadin*® (rifampin)

These medications *may increase* the symptoms of Parkinson's disease:

- *Compazine*® (prochlorperazine)
- Neuroleptic medications such as *Risperdal*® (risperidone), *Thorazine*® (chlorpromazine), *Zyprexa*® (olanzapine), and others—see Glossary
- *Reglan*® (metoclopramide)

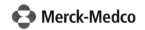

Comtan® (entacapone) is generally not prescribed for anyone who is taking MAO inhibitors, such as *Marplan*® (isocarboxazid), *Nardil*® (phenelzine), or *Parnate*® (tranylcypromine), because together they ***may cause*** serious or even fatal reactions. If your doctor or other healthcare professional wants you to stop taking one medication and start taking the other, you should wait at least 2 weeks between stopping one and starting the other.

Comtan® (entacapone) ***may increase*** the side effects of other medications that cause drowsiness, including antidepressants, antihistamines (allergy medications), benzodiazepines (a type of tranquilizer), anxiety medications, narcotics (pain relievers), muscle relaxants, neuroleptic medications (a type of tranquilizer), seizure medications, or sleep medications. Avoid driving a car and other activities that need mental alertness, like using a knife or operating machinery, while taking this medication.

Drinking alcoholic beverages (such as beer, wine, whiskey, and others) ***may increase*** the side effects of *Comtan*® (entacapone).

Tell your doctor or other healthcare professional about all medications (both prescription and nonprescription [over-the-counter] medications) that you are taking.

 # Warning!

To give you the best care, your doctor or other healthcare professional needs to know about the diseases and medical conditions you have had—your full medical history. Tell your doctor or other healthcare professional if you have or have ever had, or presently take, any of the following:

- Allergy or previous reaction to *Comtan*® (entacapone)

- Liver problems

- MAO inhibitors such as *Marplan*® (isocarboxazid), *Nardil*® (phenelzine), or *Parnate*® (tranylcypromine)

Comtan® (entacapone) may make you unsteady on your feet, causing you to fall and possibly break a bone. If you have fallen recently, tell your doctor or other healthcare professional about it. Taking a different medication or a lower dose may make you less likely to fall. You should not stop taking this medication without first talking to your doctor or other healthcare professional.

Comtan® (entacapone) may cause drowsiness. Avoid driving a car and other activities that need mental alertness, like using a knife or operating machinery, while taking this medication. Drinking alcoholic beverages (such as beer, wine, whiskey, and others) may increase the side effects.

Under certain circumstances your doctor or other healthcare professional may decide that you should stop taking this medication. If you have taken it for more than a couple of weeks, he or she may want you to decrease it gradually, lowering the dose over a few weeks or months. Stopping suddenly may cause unpleasant withdrawal symptoms or may worsen your medical problems. Pay careful attention to the instructions your doctor or other healthcare professional gives you about how much less to take and for how long.

Chapter 18

Sleeping Difficulty (Insomnia)

What Is Insomnia?

Insomnia is difficulty in falling asleep or staying asleep. Insomnia causes daytime drowsiness, irritability, and problems concentrating. A person with insomnia usually takes more than 30 to 45 minutes to fall asleep, wakes up many times at night, or wakes up too early without a feeling of restfulness.

Insomnia may be caused by medical problems, such as heart or lung conditions, heartburn, enlarged prostate (benign prostatic hypertrophy), incontinence (problems with bladder control), congestive heart failure, anxiety (nervousness), depression, pain, thyroid problems, and others. Talk to your doctor or other healthcare professional if you have insomnia. He or she may be able to treat your medical problems to help you sleep better.

Insomnia may also be caused by medications such as:

- Beta-adrenergic bronchodilators such as *Proventil®* (albuterol), *Serevent®* (salmeterol), and others—see Glossary

- Caffeine contained in some over-the-counter (nonprescription) medications

- Cough, cold, and allergy medications

- Diuretics (water pills) such as *HydroDIURIL®* (hydrochlorothiazide or HCTZ), *Lasix®* (furosemide), and others—see Glossary

- *Eldepryl®* (selegiline)

- *Prozac®* (fluoxetine)

- *Ritalin®* (methylphenidate)

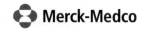

- *Symmetrel*® (amantadine)
- Theophylline such as *Theo-Dur*®, *Uniphyl*®, and others—see Glossary

Talk to your doctor or other healthcare professional if you have trouble sleeping and are taking any of these medications. He or she may be able to try a different medication or lower your dose to help reduce your insomnia. Do not stop taking the medications unless directed by your doctor or other healthcare professional.

Insomnia may be worsened by other factors such as your sleeping and eating habits. Some recommendations to help improve your sleeping include:

- Avoid drinking alcoholic beverages (such as beer, wine, whiskey, and others).

- Create a routine in which you go to sleep at the same time every night and wake up at the same time every morning.

- Do not eat or drink anything that contains caffeine (such as colas, coffee, and chocolate) in the afternoon and evening.

- Avoid heavy meals and snacks in the evening.

- Get a moderate amount of exercise every day. If you exercise in the evening, finish at least 2 to 4 hours before bedtime.

- Keep your bedroom dark and quiet, and keep it at a temperature that is not too warm or too cold.

- Try to limit your bedroom to a place for sleep. Avoid watching television, reading, eating, paying bills, and other activities associated with being awake.

- Avoid daytime naps.

- Avoid going to bed early.

- Relax before bedtime with a warm bath or by reading.

Medications for Insomnia

Several kinds of medications may be taken to help people sleep better.
This chapter discusses these medications and/or categories of medications:

MEDICATIONS	See Page
Benzodiazepines	585
Ambien® (zolpidem)	592
Sonata® (zaleplon)	594
Chloral Hydrate	597
Desyrel® (trazodone)	600
Tricyclic Antidepressants	604
Antihistamines	609
Meprobamate	614
Barbiturates	618

If you do not see the exact name of the medication that you take for insomnia
listed above, check the Medication and Chapter Table to find out which
category your medication falls under or check the Index.

Benzodiazepines

Benzodiazepines cause drowsiness and may help to relieve insomnia.

▲ Indicates medications that are more likely to cause unpleasant or dangerous
side effects. These medications are generally not recommended for people
over 65. The side effects may not be very obvious and may be mistaken for
"just a part of getting older" but may be serious. If you are taking one of
these medications, you might want to talk to your doctor or other healthcare
professional to see if this medication is best for you. Safer medications may
be available and lower dosages may be required. You should not stop taking
these medications without first talking to your doctor or other healthcare
professional.

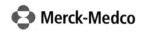
See the WARNING section on page 590 for the specific safety problems associated with these medications ▲.

Brand Name	Generic Name
Ativan®	lorazepam
▲Dalmane®	flurazepam
▲Doral®	quazepam
Halcion®	triazolam
▲Klonopin®	clonazepam
▲Libritabs®	chlordiazepoxide
▲Librium®	chlordiazepoxide
▲Paxipam®	halazepam
ProSom™	estazolam
Restoril®	temazepam
Serax®	oxazepam
▲Tranxene®	clorazepate
▲Valium®	diazepam
Xanax®	alprazolam

 ## How Will I Take Benzodiazepines?

Benzodiazepines that are prescribed for sleeping problems are usually taken, as pills or liquids, before bedtime as needed for sleep. Benzodiazepines do not work right away for sleep. In most cases they do not work for at least 30 minutes to 1 hour after being taken. They may take as long as 2 hours to work. Your doctor or other healthcare professional will tell you when to take your medication.

What Side Effects Can Benzodiazepines Cause?

More Common

- Confusion
- Dizziness when standing up from a bed or a chair
- Drowsiness
- Falling
- Increased sensitivity to the sun (bad sunburn)
- Poor coordination or balance when walking
- Tiredness or sluggishness (fatigue)

Less Common

- Bitter taste
- Blurred or double vision
- Constipation
- Fast heartbeat (palpitations)
- Headache
- Increased chance of breaking a hip
- Long-term memory problems (amnesia)
- Low blood pressure (hypotension)
- Nausea
- Nervousness (anxiety)
- Rash (skin redness, bumps, itching, or irritation)
- Sadness, feeling blue or down, depressed mood (depression)
- Seeing or hearing things that are not there (hallucinations)
- Shakiness or tremors
- Slowed breathing
- Slurred speech
- Trouble urinating or emptying the bladder

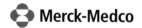

Rare

- Frequent fever, sore throat, or flu-like symptoms that may be a sign of low white blood cells

- Increased breast size in men

- Liver problems that may cause yellowing of the skin or eyes (jaundice)

- Ringing in the ears (tinnitus)

Tell your doctor or other healthcare professional if you have side effects that bother you, do not go away, make you worried about taking your medication, or make you want to stop taking your medication.

 ## Do Other Medications Interact with Benzodiazepines?

These medications *may increase* the side effects of *Halcion*® (triazolam):

- *Diflucan*® (fluconazole)

- *Nizoral*® (ketoconazole)

- *Serzone*® (nefazodone)

- *Sporanox*® (itraconazole)

Benzodiazepines *may increase* the side effects of other medications that cause drowsiness, including anticholinergic medications, antidepressants, antihistamines (allergy medications), antispasmodics, anxiety medications, narcotics (pain relievers), muscle relaxants, neuroleptic medications (a type of tranquilizer), seizure medications, or other sleep medications. Avoid driving a car and other activities that need mental alertness, like using a knife or operating machinery, while taking these medications together.

Drinking alcoholic beverages (such as beer, wine, whiskey, and others) *may increase* the side effects of benzodiazepines.

These medications ***may increase*** the side effects of benzodiazepines:

- *Antabuse*® (disulfiram)
- *Biaxin*® (clarithromycin)
- *Crixivan*® (indinavir)
- Erythromycin such as *Ery-Tab*®, *Erythrocin*®, and others—see Glossary
- *Norvir*® (ritonavir)
- *Prilosec*® (omeprazole)
- *Sporanox*® (itraconazole)
- *Tagamet*® (cimetidine)
- *Zantac*® (ranitidine)

These medications ***may decrease*** how well benzodiazepines work:

- *Cerebyx*® (fosphenytoin)
- *Dilantin*® (phenytoin)
- *Rifadin*® (rifampin)
- *Tegretol*® (carbamazepine)

Grapefruit and grapefruit juice ***may increase*** the side effects of benzodiazepines. This interaction can happen whether you eat the grapefruit or drink the grapefruit juice at the same time as you take your medication or if you take the medication separately from the grapefruit or grapefruit juice. Talk to your doctor or other healthcare professional before eating grapefruit or drinking grapefruit juice if you are taking one of these medications. Please also read the discussion on A Warning about Grapefruit and Grapefruit Juice on pages i-ii.

Tell your doctor or other healthcare professional about all medications (both prescription and nonprescription [over-the-counter] medications) that you are taking.

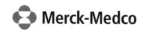

Why Else Do People Take Benzodiazepines?

Some benzodiazepines may also be used to help reduce seizures, muscle spasms, and restless leg syndrome. Benzodiazepines are also used to help treat nervousness (anxiety).

 # Warning!

To give you the best care, your doctor or other healthcare professional needs to know about the diseases and medical conditions you have had—your full medical history. Tell your doctor or other healthcare professional if you have or have ever had any of the following:

- Allergy or previous reaction to benzodiazepines

- Breathing problems (asthma and COPD, including emphysema and chronic bronchitis)

- Glaucoma (an eye disease)

- High alcohol intake (drinking 3 or more alcoholic beverages, such as beer, wine, whiskey, and others, every day)

- Kidney problems

- Liver problems

- Sadness, feeling blue or down, depressed mood (depression)

Dalmane® (flurazepam), *Doral*® (quazepam), *Klonopin*® (clonazepam), *Libritabs*® (chlordiazepoxide), *Librium*® (chlordiazepoxide), *Paxipam*® (halazepam), *Tranxene*® (clorazepate), and *Valium*® (diazepam) are generally not recommended for use in people over the age of 65 because they are long-acting, and long-acting benzodiazepines have been associated with a higher risk of broken hips and car accidents than other, shorter-acting benzodiazepines. If you are taking any of these medications, ask your doctor or other healthcare professional if this medication is right for you. Do not stop taking this medication without talking to your doctor or other healthcare professional.

Benzodiazepines cause more side effects in older adults than in younger adults. Whenever possible, their use should be avoided. If a benzodiazepine is necessary, *Restoril®* (temazepam) or *ProSom™* (estazolam) are generally recommended for older people who have problems falling asleep or staying asleep.

After taking a benzodiazepine regularly, people may develop a strong need for it (dependence). To help prevent this from happening, do not take benzodiazepines more often than prescribed by your doctor or other healthcare professional.

Benzodiazepines may cause drowsiness. Avoid driving a car and other activities that need mental alertness, like using a knife or operating machinery, while taking this medication. Drinking alcoholic beverages (such as beer, wine, whiskey, and others) may increase the side effects.

Benzodiazepines may make you unsteady on your feet, causing you to fall and possibly break a bone. If you have fallen recently, tell your doctor or other healthcare professional about it. Taking a different medication or a lower dose may make you less likely to fall. You should not stop taking this medication without first talking to your doctor or other healthcare professional.

If you are taking a benzodiazepine, stay out of the sun as much as you can to avoid a serious sunburn. When you do go out in the sun, use sunblock or sunscreen, and wear protective clothing, such as a wide-brimmed hat and a long-sleeved shirt.

Klonopin® (clonazepam) is sometimes confused with clonidine, which is taken for high blood pressure (hypertension). The names of the medications sound similar, but the medications themselves are very different. Talk to your doctor or other healthcare professional to make sure you are taking the right medication.

Sleep medications are only recommended for short-term use. Many have side effects that can be dangerous in people over the age of 65. Talk to your doctor or other healthcare professional if you have been taking these medications regularly for more than 3 weeks. Do not stop taking them without talking to your doctor or other healthcare professional.

Under certain circumstances your doctor or other healthcare professional may decide that you should stop taking this medication. If you have taken it for more than a couple of weeks, he or she may want you to decrease it gradually,

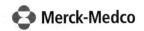

lowering the dose over a few weeks or months. Stopping suddenly may cause unpleasant withdrawal symptoms or may worsen your medical problems. Pay careful attention to the instructions your doctor or other healthcare professional gives you about how much less to take and for how long.

Ambien® (zolpidem)

Ambien® (zolpidem) causes drowsiness and may help to relieve insomnia.

How Will I Take *Ambien*® (zolpidem)?

Ambien® (zolpidem) is usually taken before bedtime, as needed for sleep. It works in up to 30 minutes. Your doctor or other healthcare professional will tell you how to take your medication.

What Side Effects Can *Ambien*® (zolpidem) Cause?

More Common

- Diarrhea
- Dizziness
- Drowsiness

Less Common

- Tiredness or sluggishness (fatigue) during the day

Tell your doctor or other healthcare professional if you have side effects that bother you, do not go away, make you worried about taking your medication, or make you want to stop taking your medication.

Do Other Medications Interact with *Ambien*® (zolpidem)?

Ambien® (zolpidem) **may increase** the side effects of other medications that cause drowsiness, including anticholinergic medications, antidepressants, antihistamines (allergy medications), antispasmodics, benzodiazepines (a type of tranquilizer), anxiety medications, narcotics (pain relievers), muscle relaxants, neuroleptic medications (a type of tranquilizer), seizure medications, or other sleep medications. Avoid driving a car and other activities that need mental alertness, like using a knife or operating machinery, while taking these medications together.

Drinking alcoholic beverages (such as beer, wine, whiskey, and others) **may increase** the side effects of *Ambien*® (zolpidem).

Rifadin® (rifampin) **may decrease** how well *Ambien*® (zolpidem) works.

Tell your doctor or other healthcare professional about all medications (both prescription and nonprescription [over-the-counter] medications) that you are taking.

Warning!

To give you the best care, your doctor or other healthcare professional needs to know about the diseases and medical conditions you have had—your full medical history. Tell your doctor or other healthcare professional if you have or have ever had an allergy or previous reaction to *Ambien*® (zolpidem) and/or liver problems.

Ambien® (zolpidem) may make you unsteady on your feet, causing you to fall and possibly break a bone. If you have fallen recently, tell your doctor or other healthcare professional about it. Taking a different medication or a lower dose may make you less likely to fall. You should not stop taking this medication without first talking to your doctor or other healthcare professional.

Ambien® (zolpidem) may cause drowsiness. Avoid driving a car and other activities that need mental alertness, like using a knife or operating machinery,

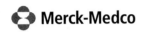
while taking this medication. Drinking alcoholic beverages (such as beer, wine, whiskey, and others) may increase the side effects.

After taking *Ambien*® (zolpidem) regularly, people may develop a strong need for it (dependence). To help prevent this from happening, do not take *Ambien*® (zolpidem) more often than prescribed by your doctor or other healthcare professional.

Sleep medications are only recommended for short-term use. Many have side effects that can be dangerous in people over the age of 65. Talk to your doctor or other healthcare professional if you have been taking this medication regularly for more than 3 weeks. Do not stop taking it without talking to your doctor or other healthcare professional.

Under certain circumstances your doctor or other healthcare professional may decide that you should stop taking this medication. If you have taken it for more than a couple of weeks, he or she may want you to decrease it gradually, lowering the dose over a few weeks or months. Stopping suddenly may cause unpleasant withdrawal symptoms or may worsen your medical problems. Pay careful attention to the instructions your doctor or other healthcare professional gives you about how much less to take and for how long.

Sonata® (zaleplon)

Sonata® (zaleplon) causes drowsiness and may help to relieve insomnia.

 ## How Will I Take *Sonata*® (zaleplon)?

Sonata® (zaleplon) should be taken before bedtime, as needed for sleep. *Sonata*® (zaleplon) usually works in up to 30 minutes. *Sonata*® (zaleplon) should not be taken with or immediately after eating a heavy or fatty meal because this may cause *Sonata*® (zaleplon) to work more slowly than usual. Your doctor or other healthcare professional will tell you how often to take this medication.

What Side Effects Can *Sonata*® (zaleplon) Cause?

More Common

- Confusion

- Dizziness

- Drowsiness

- Headache

- Muscle aches

- Nausea

Less Common

- Blurred vision

- Constipation

- Dry mouth

- Memory loss

- Nervousness (anxiety)

Tell your doctor or other healthcare professional if you have side effects that bother you, do not go away, make you worried about taking your medication, or make you want to stop taking your medication.

Do Other Medications Interact with *Sonata*® (zaleplon)?

Sonata® (zaleplon) ***may increase*** the side effects of other medications that cause drowsiness, including anticholinergic medications, antidepressants, antihistamines (allergy medications), antispasmodics, benzodiazepines (a type of tranquilizer), anxiety medications, narcotics (pain relievers), muscle relaxants, neuroleptic medications (a type of tranquilizer), seizure medications, or other sleep medications. Avoid driving a car and other activities that need mental alertness, like using a knife or operating machinery, while taking these medications together.

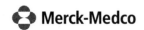

Drinking alcoholic beverages (such as beer, wine, whiskey, and others) *may increase* the side effects of *Sonata*® (zaleplon).

Tagamet® (cimetidine) *may increase* the side effects of *Sonata*® (zaleplon).

Rifadin® (rifampin) *may decrease* how well *Sonata*® (zaleplon) works.

Tell your doctor or other healthcare professional about all medications (both prescription and nonprescription [over-the-counter] medications) that you are taking.

 # Warning!

To give you the best care, your doctor or other healthcare professional needs to know about the diseases and medical conditions you have had—your full medical history. Tell your doctor or other healthcare professional if you have or have ever had any of the following:

- Allergy or previous reaction to *Sonata*® (zaleplon)
- Breathing problems (asthma and COPD, including emphysema and chronic bronchitis)
- Liver problems
- Sadness, feeling blue or down, depressed mood (depression)

Sonata® (zaleplon) may make you unsteady on your feet, causing you to fall and possibly break a bone. If you have fallen recently, tell your doctor or other healthcare professional about it. Taking a different medication or a lower dose may make you less likely to fall. You should not stop taking this medication without first talking to your doctor or other healthcare professional.

Sonata® (zaleplon) may cause drowsiness. Avoid driving a car and other activities that need mental alertness, like using a knife or operating machinery, while taking this medication. Drinking alcoholic beverages (such as beer, wine, whiskey, and others) may increase the side effects.

After taking *Sonata*® (zaleplon) regularly, people may develop a strong need for it (dependence). To help prevent this from happening, do not take *Sonata*® (zaleplon) more often than prescribed by your doctor or other healthcare professional.

Sleep medications are only recommended for short-term use. Many have side effects that can be dangerous in people over the age of 65. Talk to your doctor or other healthcare professional if you have been taking this medication regularly for more than 3 weeks. Do not stop taking it without talking to your doctor or other healthcare professional.

Under certain circumstances your doctor or other healthcare professional may decide that you should stop taking this medication. If you have taken it for more than a couple of weeks, he or she may want you to decrease it gradually, lowering the dose over a few weeks or months. Stopping suddenly may cause unpleasant withdrawal symptoms or may worsen your medical problems. Pay careful attention to the instructions your doctor or other healthcare professional gives you about how much less to take and for how long.

Chloral Hydrate

Chloral hydrate causes drowsiness and may help to relieve insomnia.

 ## How Will I Take Chloral Hydrate?

Chloral hydrate is usually taken at bedtime, as needed for sleep. It usually takes 30 to 60 minutes to start working. Chloral hydrate is available as capsules, syrups, or suppositories to be inserted in the rectum. Your doctor or other healthcare professional will tell you how often to take your medication.

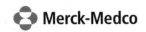

What Side Effects Can Chloral Hydrate Cause?

More Common

- Bad breath
- Dizziness
- Drowsiness
- Stomach cramps

Less Common

- Excitement
- Nausea
- Vomiting
- Ulcers in the stomach that may cause black, tarry-looking bowel movements

---

Tell your doctor or other healthcare professional if you have side effects that bother you, do not go away, make you worried about taking your medication, or make you want to stop taking your medication.

Do Other Medications Interact with Chloral Hydrate?

Chloral hydrate *may increase* the side effects of *Coumadin*® (warfarin).

Chloral hydrate *may increase* the side effects of other medications that cause drowsiness, including anticholinergic medications, antidepressants, antihistamines (allergy medications), antispasmodics, benzodiazepines (a type of tranquilizer), anxiety medications, narcotics (pain relievers), muscle relaxants, neuroleptic medications (a type of tranquilizer), seizure medications, or other sleep medications. Avoid driving a car and other activities that need mental alertness, like using a knife or operating machinery, while taking these medications together.

Drinking alcoholic beverages (such as beer, wine, whiskey, and others) *may increase* the side effects of chloral hydrate.

Tell your doctor or other healthcare professional about all medications (both prescription and nonprescription [over-the-counter] medications) that you are taking.

 # Warning!

To give you the best care, your doctor or other healthcare professional needs to know about the diseases and medical conditions you have had—your full medical history. Tell your doctor or other healthcare professional if you have or have ever had any of the following:

- Allergy or previous reaction to chloral hydrate
- Heart problems
- Kidney problems
- Liver problems

Chloral hydrate may cause stomach pain, which may be a sign of an ulcer. However, you may have an ulcer without feeling any pain at all. If ulcers are not treated, they may cause serious stomach or intestinal bleeding. Tell your doctor or other healthcare professional if you have severe stomach pain or stomach pain that keeps returning or if you have ever had peptic ulcer disease. Call your doctor or other healthcare professional right away if you have black, tarry-looking bowel movements (stools), if you vomit dark material that looks like coffee grounds, or if you notice any blood in your bowel movements. Any of these symptoms may be a sign of a bleeding ulcer.

Chloral hydrate may make you unsteady on your feet, causing you to fall and possibly break a bone. If you have fallen recently, tell your doctor or other healthcare professional about it. Taking a different medication or a lower dose may make you less likely to fall. You should not stop taking this medication without first talking to your doctor or other healthcare professional.

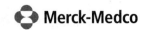

Chloral hydrate may cause drowsiness. Avoid driving a car and other activities that need mental alertness, like using a knife or operating machinery, while taking this medication. Drinking alcoholic beverages (such as beer, wine, whiskey, and others) may increase the side effects.

After taking chloral hydrate regularly, people may develop a strong need for it (dependence). To help prevent this from happening, do not take chloral hydrate more often than prescribed by your doctor or other healthcare professional.

Sleep medications are only recommended for short-term use. Many have side effects that can be dangerous in people over the age of 65. Talk to your doctor or other healthcare professional if you have been taking this medication regularly for more than 3 weeks. Do not stop taking it without talking to your doctor or other healthcare professional.

Under certain circumstances your doctor or other healthcare professional may decide that you should stop taking this medication. If you have taken it for more than a couple of weeks, he or she may want you to decrease it gradually, lowering the dose over a few weeks or months. Stopping suddenly may cause unpleasant withdrawal symptoms or may worsen your medical problems. Pay careful attention to the instructions your doctor or other healthcare professional gives you about how much less to take and for how long.

Desyrel® (trazodone)

Desyrel® (trazodone) causes drowsiness and is sometimes used to help relieve insomnia.

 ## How Will I Take *Desyrel*® (trazodone)?

Desyrel® (trazodone) is usually taken before bedtime, as needed for sleep. *Desyrel*® (trazodone) usually takes 30 to 60 minutes to start working. Your doctor or other healthcare professional will tell you how to take your medication.

What Side Effects Can *Desyrel*® (trazodone) Cause?

More Common

- Drowsiness
- Dry mouth
- Headache
- Nausea
- Nervousness (anxiety)

Less Common

- Constipation
- Dizziness when standing up from a bed or a chair
- Trouble falling asleep or staying asleep (insomnia)*
- Trouble urinating or emptying the bladder

Rare

- Lasting, painful erection (priapism)
- Seizures

*Sometimes medications may actually cause or worsen the same symptoms they are being used to help relieve. Talk to your doctor or other healthcare professional if your symptoms get worse instead of better while taking this medication.

Tell your doctor or other healthcare professional if you have side effects that bother you, do not go away, make you worried about taking your medication, or make you want to stop taking your medication.

Do Other Medications Interact with *Desyrel*® (trazodone)?

Desyrel® (trazodone) is generally not prescribed for anyone who is taking MAO inhibitors, such as *Marplan*® (isocarboxazid), *Nardil*® (phenelzine), or *Parnate*®

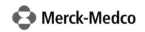

(tranylcypromine), because together they *may cause* serious or even fatal reactions. If your doctor or other healthcare professional wants you to stop taking one medication and start taking the other, you should wait at least 2 weeks between stopping one and starting the other.

Desyrel® (trazodone) is generally not prescribed for anyone who is taking triptans (migraine medications) such as *Imitrex*® (sumatriptan), *Maxalt*® (rizatriptan), and others (see Glossary) or *Meridia*® (sibutramine) and other appetite suppressants because together they *may cause* serious or even fatal reactions. Taken together, they *may cause* nervousness (anxiety), muscle weakness, confusion, and seizures.

Desyrel® (trazodone) *may increase* the side effects of other medications that cause drowsiness, including anticholinergic medications, antidepressants, antihistamines (allergy medications), antispasmodics, benzodiazepines (a type of tranquilizer), anxiety medications, narcotics (pain relievers), muscle relaxants, neuroleptic medications (a type of tranquilizer), seizure medications, or other sleep medications. Avoid driving a car and other activities that need mental alertness, like using a knife or operating machinery, while taking these medications together.

Drinking alcoholic beverages (such as beer, wine, whiskey, and others) *may increase* the side effects of *Desyrel*® (trazodone).

Tell your doctor or other healthcare professional about all medications (both prescription and nonprescription [over-the-counter] medications) that you are taking.

Why Else Do People Take *Desyrel*® (trazodone)?

Desyrel® (trazodone) may also be used to help treat depression.

Warning!

To give you the best care, your doctor or other healthcare professional needs to know about the diseases and medical conditions you have had—your full medical history. Tell your doctor or other healthcare professional if you have or have ever had, or presently take, any of the following:

- Allergy or previous reaction to *Desyrel®* (trazodone)

- Heart problems

- Liver problems

- Manic depression

- MAO inhibitors such as *Marplan®* (isocarboxazid), *Nardil®* (phenelzine), or *Parnate®* (tranylcypromine)

- Seizures (epilepsy)

Desyrel® (trazodone) may make you unsteady on your feet, causing you to fall and possibly break a bone. If you have fallen recently, tell your doctor or other healthcare professional about it. Taking a different medication or a lower dose may make you less likely to fall. You should not stop taking this medication without first talking to your doctor or other healthcare professional.

Desyrel® (trazodone) may cause drowsiness. Avoid driving a car and other activities that need mental alertness, like using a knife or operating machinery, while taking this medication. Drinking alcoholic beverages (such as beer, wine, whiskey, and others) may increase the side effects.

Sleep medications are only recommended for short-term use. Many have side effects that can be dangerous in people over the age of 65. Talk to your doctor or other healthcare professional if you have been taking these medications regularly for more than 3 weeks. Do not stop taking them without talking to your doctor or other healthcare professional.

Note for men: Call your doctor or other healthcare professional immediately if you develop an erection that hurts and will not go away.

Under certain circumstances your doctor or other healthcare professional may decide that you should stop taking *Desyrel®* (trazodone). If you have taken it for

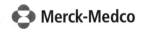

more than a couple of weeks, he or she may want you to decrease it gradually, lowering the dose over a few weeks or months. Stopping suddenly may cause unpleasant withdrawal symptoms or may worsen your medical problems. Pay careful attention to the instructions your doctor or other healthcare professional gives you about how much less to take and for how long.

Tricyclic Antidepressants

Tricyclic antidepressants cause drowsiness and are sometimes used to help relieve insomnia.

▲ Indicates medications that are more likely to cause unpleasant or dangerous side effects. These medications are generally not recommended for people over 65. The side effects may not be very obvious and may be mistaken for "just a part of getting older" but may be serious. If you are taking one of these medications, you might want to talk to your doctor or other healthcare professional to see if this medication is best for you. Safer medications may be available and lower dosages may be required. You should not stop taking these medications without first talking to your doctor or other healthcare professional.

See the WARNING section on page 607 for the specific safety problems associated with these medications ▲.

Brand Name	Generic Name
▲*Asendin*®	amoxapine
▲*Elavil*®	amitriptyline
Norpramin®	desipramine
Pamelor®	nortriptyline
▲*Sinequan*®	doxepin
▲*Surmontil*®	trimipramine
▲*Tofranil*®	imipramine

How Will I Take Tricyclic Antidepressants?

Tricyclic antidepressants taken for insomnia are usually taken before bedtime, as needed for sleep. Tricyclic antidepressants usually take 30 minutes to 2 hours to start working. Your doctor or other healthcare professional will tell you how to take your medication.

What Side Effects Can Tricyclic Antidepressants Cause?

More Common

- Constipation
- Dizziness when standing up from a bed or a chair
- Drowsiness
- Dry mouth, eyes, and nose
- Trouble urinating or emptying the bladder

Less Common

- Confusion
- Fast, slow, or irregular heartbeat (palpitations)
- Increased or decreased interest in sex
- Rash (skin redness, bumps, itching, or irritation)
- Worsening of glaucoma (an eye disease)

Rare

- Breast enlargement and tenderness (in both men and women)
- Hair loss
- Seizures
- Shakiness or tremors

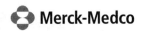 **Merck-Medco**

Tell your doctor or other healthcare professional if you have side effects that bother you, do not go away, make you worried about taking your medication, or make you want to stop taking your medication.

 ## Do Other Medications Interact with Tricyclic Antidepressants?

These medications *may increase* the side effects of tricyclic antidepressants:

- Quinidine such as *Quinaglute®*, *Quinidex®*, and others—see Glossary
- *Ritalin®* (methylphenidate)
- *Rythmol®* (propafenone)
- *Tagamet®* (cimetidine)

These medications *may decrease* how well tricyclic antidepressants work:

- Barbiturates such as *Butisol®* (butabarbital), *Luminal®* (phenobarbital), *Mebaral®* (mephobarbital), and others—see Glossary
- *Rifadin®* (rifampin)
- *Tegretol®* (carbamazepine)

Tricyclic antidepressants *may increase* the side effects of other medications that cause drowsiness, including anticholinergic medications, antidepressants, antihistamines (allergy medications), antispasmodics, benzodiazepines (a type of tranquilizer), anxiety medications, narcotics (pain relievers), muscle relaxants, neuroleptic medications (a type of tranquilizer), seizure medications, or other sleep medications. Avoid driving a car and other activities that need mental alertness, like using a knife or operating machinery, while taking these medications together.

Drinking alcoholic beverages (such as beer, wine, whiskey, and others) *may increase* the side effects of tricyclic antidepressants.

Taking a tricyclic antidepressant if you are also taking *Catapres®* (clonidine) or *Ismelin®* (guanethidine) *may raise* your blood pressure to dangerously high levels.

Tricyclic antidepressants are generally not prescribed for anyone who is taking MAO inhibitors, such as *Marplan®* (isocarboxazid), *Nardil®* (phenelzine), or *Parnate®* (tranylcypromine), because together they ***may cause*** serious or even fatal reactions. If your doctor or other healthcare professional wants you to stop taking one medication and start taking the other, you should wait at least 2 weeks between stopping one and starting the other.

Tricyclic antidepressants are generally not prescribed for anyone who is taking *Propulsid®* (cisapride [withdrawn from general distribution; available only by special arrangement with the manufacturer]), *Seldane®* (terfenadine [no longer commercially available]), or *Hismanal®* (astemizole [no longer commercially available]), because together they ***may cause*** serious, sometimes fatal, heart problems.

Tell your doctor or other healthcare professional about all medications (both prescription and nonprescription [over-the-counter] medications) that you are taking.

Why Else Do People Take Tricyclic Antidepressants?

Tricyclic antidepressants may help relieve depression, long-term pain, abnormal fears (phobias), panic attacks, inability to hold urine in (urinary incontinence), obsessive-compulsive disorders, headaches, and eating disorders such as anorexia and bulimia, and may help prevent migraine headaches.

 # Warning!

To give you the best care, your doctor or other healthcare professional needs to know about the diseases and medical conditions you have had—your full medical history. Tell your doctor or other healthcare professional if you have or have ever had, or presently take, any of the following:

- Allergy or previous reaction to tricyclic antidepressants, *Tegretol®* (carbamazepine), or *Trileptal®* (oxcarbazepine)

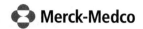

- Enlarged prostate (benign prostatic hypertrophy)

- Glaucoma (an eye disease)

- Liver problems

- Manic depression

- MAO inhibitors such as *Marplan*® (isocarboxazid), *Nardil*® (phenelzine), or *Parnate*® (tranylcypromine)

- Overactive thyroid (hyperthyroidism)

- Schizophrenia

- Seizures (epilepsy)

- Trouble urinating or emptying the bladder

Asendin® (amoxapine), *Elavil*® (amitriptyline), *Sinequan*® (doxepin), *Surmontil*® (trimipramine), and *Tofranil*® (imipramine) are generally not recommended for use in people over the age of 65 because these types of tricyclic antidepressants have been associated with a higher risk of broken hips and car accidents than other tricyclic antidepressants. If you are taking any of these medications, ask your doctor or other healthcare professional if this medication is right for you. Do not stop taking this medication without talking to your doctor or other healthcare professional.

Tricyclic antidepressants may make you unsteady on your feet, causing you to fall and possibly break a bone. If you have fallen recently, tell your doctor or other healthcare professional about it. Taking a different medication or a lower dose may make you less likely to fall. You should not stop taking this medication without first talking to your doctor or other healthcare professional.

Tricyclic antidepressants may cause drowsiness. Avoid driving a car and other activities that need mental alertness, like using a knife or operating machinery, while taking this medication. Drinking alcoholic beverages (such as beer, wine, whiskey, and others) may increase the side effects.

If you have had seizures in the past, tell your doctor or other healthcare professional because tricyclic antidepressants may cause seizures. Stopping this medication suddenly may also cause seizures. If your doctor or other healthcare professional decides that you should stop taking tricyclic antidepressants, pay careful attention to the instructions he or she gives you about how much less to take and for how long.

If you are taking a tricyclic antidepressant, stay out of the sun as much as you can to avoid a serious sunburn. When you do go out in the sun, use sunblock or sunscreen, and wear protective clothing, such as a wide-brimmed hat and a long-sleeved shirt.

Sleep medications are only recommended for short-term use. Many have side effects that can be dangerous in people over the age of 65. Talk to your doctor or other healthcare professional if you have been taking these medications regularly for more than 3 weeks. Do not stop taking them without talking to your doctor or other healthcare professional.

Under certain circumstances your doctor or other healthcare professional may decide that you should stop taking this medication. If you have taken it for more than a couple of weeks, he or she may want you to decrease it gradually, lowering the dose over a few weeks or months. Stopping suddenly may cause unpleasant withdrawal symptoms or may worsen your medical problems. Pay careful attention to the instructions your doctor or other healthcare professional gives you about how much less to take and for how long.

Antihistamines

Antihistamines were developed to relieve allergy symptoms such as sneezing, runny nose, and itchy eyes. Because they also make people sleepy, they are sometimes used for insomnia. Many nonprescription (over-the-counter [OTC]) sleeping pills and cold remedies contain antihistamines.

▲ Indicates medications that are more likely to cause unpleasant or dangerous side effects. These medications are generally not recommended for people over 65. The side effects may not be very obvious and may be mistaken for "just a part of getting older" but may be serious . If you are taking one of these medications, you might want to talk to your doctor or other healthcare professional to see if this medication is best for you. Safer medications may

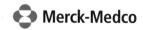

be available and lower dosages may be required. You should not stop taking these medications without first talking to your doctor or other healthcare professional.

See the WARNING section on page 612 for the specific safety problems associated with these medications ▲.

Brand Name	Generic Name
▲Benadryl®	diphenhydramine
▲Excedrin P.M.®	diphenhydramine/ acetaminophen
▲Nytol®	diphenhydramine
▲Sleep-Eze 3®	diphenhydramine
▲Sominex®	diphenhydramine
▲Tylenol PM®	diphenhydramine/ acetaminophen
▲Unisom®	doxylamine

How Will I Take Antihistamines?

Antihistamines are usually taken before bedtime, as needed for sleep. They do not work right away for sleep. Antihistamines usually take at least 30 minutes to start working. Follow the instructions given on the package, or ask your doctor or other healthcare professional how to take this medication.

What Side Effects Can Antihistamines Cause?

More Common

- Blurred vision

- Constipation

- Diarrhea
- Dizziness when standing up from a bed or a chair
- Double vision
- Drowsiness
- Dry mouth, eyes, and nose
- Poor coordination and trouble walking
- Trouble urinating or emptying the bladder

Less Common

- Confusion
- Fainting
- Fast heartbeat (palpitations)
- Memory problems
- Nausea
- Nervousness (anxiety)
- Poor appetite
- Reddening of the face (flushing)
- Shakiness or tremors
- Trouble breathing or shortness of breath
- Trouble falling asleep or staying asleep (insomnia)*
- Vomiting

*Sometimes medications may actually cause or worsen the same symptoms they are being used to help relieve. Talk to your doctor or other healthcare professional if your symptoms get worse instead of better while taking this medication.

Tell your doctor or other healthcare professional if you have side effects that bother you, do not go away, make you worried about taking your medication, or make you want to stop taking your medication.

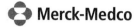

Do Other Medications Interact with Antihistamines?

Antihistamines *may increase* the side effects of other medications that cause drowsiness, including anticholinergic medications, antidepressants, other antihistamines (allergy medications), antispasmodics, benzodiazepines (a type of tranquilizer), anxiety medications, narcotics (pain relievers), muscle relaxants, neuroleptic medications (a type of tranquilizer), seizure medications, or other sleep medications. Avoid driving a car and other activities that need mental alertness, like using a knife or operating machinery, while taking these medications together.

Drinking alcoholic beverages (such as beer, wine, whiskey, and others) *may increase* the side effects of antihistamines.

Many nonprescription (over-the-counter [OTC]) medications such as pain, cough, cold, allergy, and sleep medications, contain antihistamines. If you are taking antihistamines regularly, you should talk to your doctor or other healthcare professional before taking any new OTC medications.

Tell your doctor or other healthcare professional about all medications (both prescription and nonprescription [over-the-counter] medications) that you are taking.

Why Else Do People Take Antihistamines?

Antihistamines may be taken for skin allergies, cold, flu, hay fever, and other allergic conditions. Some antihistamines may also be taken to help treat nervousness (anxiety).

 # Warning!

To give you the best care, your doctor or other healthcare professional needs to know about the diseases and medical conditions you have had—your full

medical history. Tell your doctor or other healthcare professional if you have or have ever had any of the following:

- Allergy or previous reaction to antihistamines
- Breathing problems (asthma and COPD, including emphysema and chronic bronchitis)
- Enlarged prostate (benign prostatic hypertrophy)
- Glaucoma (an eye disease)

Antihistamines that cause drowsiness are generally not recommended for people over the age of 65 for insomnia because they cause serious side effects, including dizziness, blurred vision, constipation, trouble urinating or emptying the bladder, confusion, and a fast heartbeat. If you are taking one of these medications, talk to your doctor or other healthcare professional to see if it is right for you. Do not stop taking this medication without first talking to your doctor or other healthcare professional.

Antihistamines may cause drowsiness. Avoid driving a car and other activities that need mental alertness, like using a knife or operating machinery, while taking this medication. Drinking alcoholic beverages (such as beer, wine, whiskey, and others) may increase the side effects.

Antihistamines may make you unsteady on your feet, causing you to fall and possibly break a bone. If you have fallen recently, tell your doctor or other healthcare professional about it. Taking a different medication or a lower dose may make you less likely to fall. You should not stop taking this medication without first talking to your doctor or other healthcare professional.

Sleep medications are only recommended for short-term use. Many have side effects that can be dangerous in people over the age of 65. Talk to your doctor or other healthcare professional if you have been taking these medications regularly for more than 3 weeks. Do not stop taking them without talking to your doctor or other healthcare professional.

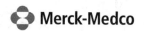

Meprobamate

Meprobamate causes drowsiness and is sometimes used to help relieve insomnia.

▲ Indicates medications that are more likely to cause unpleasant or dangerous side effects. These medications are generally not recommended for people over 65. The side effects may not be very obvious and may be mistaken for "just a part of getting older" but may be serious. If you are taking one of these medications, you might want to talk to your doctor or other healthcare professional to see if this medication is best for you. Safer medications may be available and lower dosages may be required. You should not stop taking these medications without first talking to your doctor or other healthcare professional.

See the WARNING section on page 616 for the specific safety problems associated with these medications ▲.

Brand Name	Generic Name
▲Equanil™	meprobamate
▲Miltown®	meprobamate

 ## How Will I Take Meprobamate?

Meprobamate is usually taken before bedtime, as needed for sleep. Meprobamate may take up to 2 hours to start working. Your doctor or other healthcare professional will tell you how to take this medication.

 ## What Side Effects Can Meprobamate Cause?

More Common

- Diarrhea

- Dizziness

- Drowsiness

- Nausea

- Vomiting

Less Common

- Excitement

- Headache

- Weakness

Rare

- Allergic reaction such as rash (skin redness, bumps, itching, or irritation), swelling of the face and throat, or trouble breathing

- Bleeding that does not stop easily (nose bleeds, bleeding while brushing your teeth, and cuts)

- Blurred vision

- Easy bruising ("black-and-blue" marks on the skin)

- Frequent fever, sore throat, or flu-like symptoms that may be a sign of low white blood cells

- Irregular heartbeat (palpitations)

- Seizures

- Slurred speech

Tell your doctor or other healthcare professional if you have side effects that bother you, do not go away, make you worried about taking your medication, or make you want to stop taking your medication.

 ## Do Other Medications Interact with Meprobamate?

Meprobamate *may increase* the side effects of other medications that cause drowsiness, including anticholinergic medications, antidepressants, antihistamines (allergy medications), antispasmodics, benzodiazepines (a type of

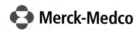
tranquilizer), anxiety medications, narcotics (pain relievers), muscle relaxants, neuroleptic medications (a type of tranquilizer), seizure medications, or other sleep medications. Avoid driving a car and other activities that need mental alertness, like using a knife or operating machinery, while taking these medications together.

Drinking alcoholic beverages (such as beer, wine, whiskey, and others) *may increase* the side effects of meprobamate.

Tell your doctor or other healthcare professional about all medications (both prescription and nonprescription [over-the-counter] medications) that you are taking.

Why Else Do People Take Meprobamate?

Meprobamate is sometimes used to help treat nervousness (anxiety).

 # Warning!

To give you the best care, your doctor or other healthcare professional needs to know about the diseases and medical conditions you have had—your full medical history. Tell your doctor or other healthcare professional if you have or have ever had any of the following:

- Allergy or previous reaction to meprobamate
- Kidney problems
- Liver problems
- Seizures (epilepsy)

Meprobamate is generally not recommended for people over the age of 65 for insomnia because it may cause a strong need for the medication (dependence) and serious side effects, including dizziness and blurred vision. If you are taking this medication, talk to your doctor or other healthcare professional to see if it is right for you. Do not stop taking this medication without first talking to your doctor or other healthcare professional.

Meprobamate may cause drowsiness. Avoid driving a car and other activities that need mental alertness, like using a knife or operating machinery, while taking this medication. Drinking alcoholic beverages (such as beer, wine, whiskey, and others) may increase the side effects.

Meprobamate may make you unsteady on your feet, causing you to fall and possibly break a bone. If you have fallen recently, tell your doctor or other healthcare professional about it. Taking a different medication or a lower dose may make you less likely to fall. You should not stop taking this medication without first talking to your doctor or other healthcare professional.

If you have had seizures in the past, tell your doctor or other healthcare professional because meprobamate may cause seizures. Stopping this medication suddenly may also cause seizures. If your doctor or other healthcare professional decides that you should stop taking meprobamate, pay careful attention to the instructions he or she gives you about how much less to take and for how long.

After taking meprobamate regularly, people may develop a strong need for it (dependence). To help prevent this from happening, do not take meprobamate more often than prescribed by your doctor or other healthcare professional.

Sleep medications are only recommended for short-term use. Many have side effects that can be dangerous in people over the age of 65. Talk to your doctor or other healthcare professional if you have been taking this medication regularly for more than 3 weeks. Do not stop taking it without talking to your doctor or other healthcare professional.

Under certain circumstances your doctor or other healthcare professional may decide that you should stop taking this medication. If you have taken it for more than a couple of weeks, he or she may want you to decrease it gradually, lowering the dose over a few weeks or months. Stopping suddenly may cause unpleasant withdrawal symptoms or may worsen your medical problems. Pay careful attention to the instructions your doctor or other healthcare professional gives you about how much less to take and for how long.

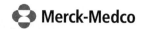

Barbiturates

Barbiturates cause drowsiness and are sometimes used to help relieve insomnia.

▲ Indicates medications that are more likely to cause unpleasant or dangerous side effects. These medications are generally not recommended for people over 65. The side effects may not be very obvious and may be mistaken for "just a part of getting older" but may be serious. If you are taking one of these medications, you might want to talk to your doctor or other healthcare professional to see if this medication is best for you. Safer medications may be available and lower dosages may be required. You should not stop taking these medications without first talking to your doctor or other healthcare professional.

See the WARNING section on page 621 for the specific safety problems associated with these medications ▲.

Brand Name	Generic Name
▲*Alurate®*	aprobarbital
▲*Butisol®*	butabarbital
▲*Mebaral®*	mephobarbital
▲*Nembutal®*	pentobarbital
▲*Seconal®*	secobarbital

 How Will I Take Barbiturates?

Barbiturates used to treat insomnia are taken before bedtime, as needed for sleep. Barbiturates generally take 1 to 2 hours to start working. Your doctor or other healthcare professional will tell you how to take your medication.

What Side Effects Can Barbiturates Cause?

More Common

- Drowsiness

Less Common

- Confusion

- Constipation

- Dizziness

- Nausea

- Nervousness (anxiety)

- Seeing or hearing things that are not there (hallucinations)

- Slow heartbeat

- Trouble breathing or shortness of breath

- Trouble falling asleep or staying asleep (insomnia)*

- Vomiting

Rare

- Allergic reactions such as rash (skin redness, bumps, itching, or irritation), swelling of the face and throat, or trouble breathing

- Fever

- Liver problems that may cause yellowing of the skin or eyes (jaundice)

- Low red blood cells (anemia)

*Sometimes medications may actually cause or worsen the same symptoms they are being used to help relieve. Talk to your doctor or other healthcare professional if your symptoms get worse instead of better while taking this medication.

Tell your doctor or other healthcare professional if you have side effects that bother you, do not go away, make you worried about taking your medication, or make you want to stop taking your medication.

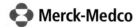 **Merck-Medco**

Do Other Medications Interact with Barbiturates?

Barbiturates *may decrease* how well these medications work:

- Beta blockers such as *Inderal*® (propranolol), *Tenormin*® (atenolol), *Toprol*® (metoprolol), and others—see Glossary

- Calcium channel blockers such as *Cardizem*® (diltiazem), *Norvasc*® (amlodipine), *Procardia*® (nifedipine), and others—see Glossary

- Corticosteroids such as prednisone and others—see Glossary

- *Coumadin*® (warfarin)

- Estrogens such as *Estrace*®, *Premarin*®, *Prempro*™, and others—see Glossary

- *Flagyl*® (metronidazole)

- *Gris-PEG*® (griseofulvin)

- *Norpace*® (disopyramide)

- *Prandin*® (repaglinide)

- Quinidine such as *Quinaglute*®, *Quinidex*®, and others—see Glossary

- *Tegretol*® (carbamazepine)

- Tetracycline antibiotics such as *Dynacin*® (minocycline), *Sumycin*® (tetracycline), *Vibramycin*® (doxycycline), and others—see Glossary

- Theophylline such as *Theo-Dur*®, *Uniphyl*®, and others—see Glossary

- Tricyclic antidepressants such as *Elavil*® (amitriptyline), *Pamelor*® (nortriptyline), *Sinequan*® (doxepin), and others—see Glossary

Barbiturates *may increase* the side effects of other medications that cause drowsiness, including anticholinergic medications, antidepressants, antihistamines (allergy medications), antispasmodics, benzodiazepines (a type of tranquilizer), anxiety medications, narcotics (pain relievers), muscle relaxants, neuroleptic medications (a type of tranquilizer), seizure medications, or other sleep medications. Avoid driving a car and other activities that need mental alertness, like using a knife or operating machinery, while taking these medications together.

Drinking alcoholic beverages (such as beer, wine, whiskey, and others) *may increase* the side effects of barbiturates.

Tell your doctor or other healthcare professional about all medications (both prescription and nonprescription [over-the-counter] medications) that you are taking.

Why Else Do People Take Barbiturates?

Barbiturates are sometimes used for seizures and anxiety (nervousness).

 # Warning!

To give you the best care, your doctor or other healthcare professional needs to know about the diseases and medical conditions you have had—your full medical history. Tell your doctor or other healthcare professional if you have or have ever had any of the following:

- Allergy or previous reaction to barbiturates
- Breathing problems (asthma and COPD, including emphysema and chronic bronchitis)
- Diabetes
- Liver problems
- Overactive thyroid (hyperthyroidism)
- Sadness, feeling blue or down, depressed mood (depression)

Barbiturates are generally not recommended for people over the age of 65 for insomnia because they may cause a strong need for the medication (dependence) and serious side effects, including dizziness and blurred vision. If you are taking this medication, talk to your doctor or other healthcare professional to see if it is right for you. Do not stop taking this medication without first talking to your doctor or other healthcare professional.

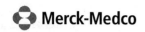

Barbiturates may make you unsteady on your feet, causing you to fall and possibly break a bone. If you have fallen recently, tell your doctor or other healthcare professional about it. Taking a different medication or a lower dose may make you less likely to fall. You should not stop taking this medication without first talking to your doctor or other healthcare professional.

Barbiturates may cause drowsiness. Avoid driving a car and other activities that need mental alertness, like using a knife or operating machinery, while taking this medication. Drinking alcoholic beverages (such as beer, wine, whiskey, and others) may increase the side effects.

Since barbiturates may cause damage to your liver, your doctor or other healthcare professional may order blood tests to find out early on if the medication is causing liver problems, before they become serious.

After taking barbiturates regularly, people may develop a strong need for it (dependence). To help prevent this from happening, do not take barbiturates more often than prescribed by your doctor or other healthcare professional.

Sleep medications are only recommended for short-term use. Many have side effects that can be dangerous in people over the age of 65. Talk to your doctor or other healthcare professional if you have been taking this medication regularly for more than 3 weeks. Do not stop taking it without talking to your doctor or other healthcare professional.

Under certain circumstances your doctor or other healthcare professional may decide that you should stop taking this medication. If you have taken it for more than a couple of weeks, he or she may want you to decrease it gradually, lowering the dose over a few weeks or months. Stopping suddenly may cause unpleasant withdrawal symptoms or may worsen your medical problems. Pay careful attention to the instructions your doctor or other healthcare professional gives you about how much less to take and for how long.

Stroke, Heart Attack, and Blood Clot Prevention

What Are Blood Clots?

Blood clotting is the way the body naturally stops bleeding, whether after a minor cut or major surgery. When blood vessels are damaged, proteins in the blood are triggered to attach to each other and to platelets (tiny cells in the blood) to form a clot or plug.

Sometimes a clot forms abnormally in a vein or artery; this is called a thrombus. A clot that forms in the veins may block the normal flow of blood and cause redness, pain, and swelling (phlebitis). A clot in the vein of a leg (venous thrombosis) may form after surgery or after long periods of bed rest or inactivity. Inactivity slows the flow of blood and lets it pool in the legs, increasing the chances that a clot will form. If a clot breaks off from the inner wall of a blood vessel, the blood can carry it to the lungs. The result can be a life-threatening disorder called pulmonary embolism (clot in the lung).

A clot in one of the arteries that carries blood to the heart may lead to a heart attack (myocardial infarction). A heart attack is what happens when a blood clot blocks one of the arteries that carry the oxygen-rich blood to the heart that it needs in order to function as it should. When this happens, a part of the heart may be permanently damaged.

A stroke is what happens when a clot blocks one of the blood vessels going to the brain. The brain needs a constant supply of oxygen to function as it should. When any part of the brain does not get enough oxygen, that part may become permanently damaged.

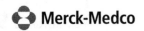
Several kinds of medications may be taken for the treatment or prevention of blood clots. This chapter discusses these medications and/or categories of medications:

MEDICATIONS	See Page
Coumadin® (warfarin)	624
Heparin and *Lovenox*® (enoxaparin)	632
Aspirin	637
Plavix® (clopidogrel) and *Ticlid*® (ticlopidine)	643
Dipyridamole *(Persantine*® and *Aggrenox*®)	648

If you do not see the exact name of the medication that you take for the treatment or prevention of blood clots listed above, check the Medication and Chapter Table to find out which category your medication falls under or check the Index.

Coumadin® (warfarin)

Coumadin® (warfarin) is an anticoagulant, sometimes called a "blood thinner." Anticoagulants cannot dissolve clots that have already formed and do not actually "thin" the blood. Their role is to stop new clots from forming and to stop existing clots from getting bigger. Anticoagulants are sometimes prescribed for people who have a heart rhythm problem (arrhythmia) like atrial fibrillation, for people who have had blood clots before, or for people who have had heart valve replacements.

Anticoagulants (blood thinners) cause the body to produce less of the proteins that are needed for clotting. When a person takes *Coumadin*® (warfarin), clots take longer to form, and clots that are already formed take longer to grow. A person who takes an anticoagulant is given a blood test to measure how long his or her blood takes to clot. Your doctor or other healthcare professional uses this information to adjust the dose of anticoagulants that you are taking.

How Will I Take *Coumadin*® (warfarin)?

Coumadin® (warfarin) is usually taken once daily. Sometimes a different dose is prescribed for different days of the week. Your doctor or other healthcare professional will tell you how much medication to take and how often to take it.

To help prevent side effects, your doctor or other healthcare professional may start by giving you a low dose of this medication, increasing the amount slowly until it works well for you.

If you miss a dose of this medication, take the dose you missed as soon as possible. However, if it is almost time for your next dose, skip the missed dose and just take the next one. Do not double your dose. Take your medication exactly as directed by your doctor or other healthcare professional. Do not stop taking a prescription medication unless directed by your doctor or other healthcare professional.

What Side Effects Can *Coumadin*® (warfarin) Cause?

More Common

- Bleeding that does not stop easily (nose bleeds, bleeding while brushing your teeth, and cuts)
- Easy bruising ("black-and-blue" marks on the skin)

Less Common

- Coughing up blood
- Diarrhea
- Low red blood cells (anemia)
- Nausea
- Red- or brown-colored urine
- Severe bleeding (hemorrhage)
- Severe headache

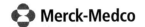

- Stomach pain
- Ulcers in the stomach that may cause black, tarry-looking bowel movements
- Vomiting

Rare

- Hair loss
- Liver problems that may cause yellowing of the skin or eyes (jaundice)
- Rash (skin redness, bumps, itching, or irritation)
- Severe peeling of skin

Tell your doctor or other healthcare professional if you have side effects that bother you, do not go away, make you worried about taking your medication, or make you want to stop taking your medication.

Do Other Medications Interact with *Coumadin*® (warfarin)?

It can be dangerous to take other medications with *Coumadin*® (warfarin). To help prevent side effects from a combination of medications (interactions), your doctor or other healthcare professional may have to change the amount or kind of medication you are taking. Do not start or stop taking any medication unless you have talked about it with your doctor or other healthcare professional first.

Many nonprescription (over-the-counter [OTC]) medications such as pain, cough, cold, allergy, and sleep medications contain aspirin or NSAIDs that *may increase* the side effects of *Coumadin*® (warfarin). If you are taking *Coumadin*® (warfarin), you should talk to your doctor or other healthcare professional before taking any new OTC medications.

Many antibiotics interact with *Coumadin*® (warfarin). Some antibiotics that interact with *Coumadin*® (warfarin) are listed on the next page. Check with your doctor or other healthcare professional before starting any new antibiotics if you are taking *Coumadin*® (warfarin).

These medications *may increase* the side effects of *Coumadin*® (warfarin):

- *Accolate*® (zafirlukast)
- *Aggrenox*® (dipyridamole/aspirin)
- Amiodarone such as *Cordarone*® or *Pacerone*®
- *Antabuse*® (disulfiram)
- *Anturane*® (sulfinpyrazone)
- Aspirin, medications that contain aspirin, and aspirin-like medications (salicylates)—see Glossary
- *Atromid-S*® (clofibrate)
- *Biaxin*® (clarithromycin)
- Chloral hydrate
- *Danocrine*® (danazol)
- *Didronel*® (etidronate)
- *Diflucan*® (fluconazole)
- *Dilantin*® (phenytoin)
- *Ergamisol*® (levamisole)
- Erythromycin such as *Ery-Tab*®, *Erythrocin*®, and others—see Glossary
- Glucagon
- *Halotestin*® (fluoxymesterone)
- Heparin
- *Lovenox*® (enoxaparin)
- *Metandren*® (methyltestosterone)
- *Nizoral*® (ketoconazole)
- Nonsteroidal anti-inflammatory drugs (NSAIDs) such as *Motrin*® (ibuprofen), *Aleve*® (naproxen), *Vioxx*® (rofecoxib), *Celebrex*® (celecoxib), and others—see Glossary
- *Persantine*® (dipyridamole)

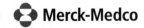

- Quinidine such as *Quinaglute*®, *Quinidex*®, and others—see Glossary

- Quinine

- *Rythmol*® (propafenone)

- *Sporanox*® (itraconazole)

- Statins such as *Lipitor*® (atorvastatin), *Pravachol*® (pravastatin), *Zocor*® (simvastatin), and others—see Glossary

- Sulfa medications such as *Bactrim*™ (sulfamethoxazole/trimethoprim) or *Septra*® (sulfamethoxazole/trimethoprim)

- *Tagamet*® (cimetidine)

- Thyroid medications such as *Cytomel*® (liothyronine), *Levoxyl*® (levothyroxine), *Synthroid*® (levothyroxine), and others—see Glossary

- *Tylenol*® (acetaminophen)

- Vitamin E

- *Zyflo*® (zileuton)

These medications *may decrease* how well *Coumadin*® (warfarin) works:

- Barbiturates such as *Butisol*® (butabarbital), *Luminal*® (phenobarbital), *Mebaral*® (mephobarbital), and others—see Glossary

- *Cytadren*® (aminoglutethimide)

- *Evista*® (raloxifene)

- *Grisactin*® (griseofulvin)

- Propylthiouracil (PTU)

- *Rifadin*® (rifampin)

- *Tapazole*® (methimazole)

- *Tegretol*® (carbamazepine)

- *Viactiv*® (calcium, vitamins D and K)

- Vitamin K

Drinking alcoholic beverages (such as beer, wine, whiskey, and others) *may increase* the side effects of *Coumadin®* (warfarin).

Bile acid binders such as *Questran®* (cholestyramine) or *Colestid®* (colestipol) or bulk-forming laxatives like *Metamucil®* (psyllium) *may decrease* the effects of *Coumadin®* (warfarin) by preventing it from being absorbed completely. To help make sure it is absorbed so it can work properly, take *Coumadin®* (warfarin) 1 hour before or 4 to 6 hours after taking a bile acid binder or a bulk-forming laxative.

Tell your doctor or other healthcare professional about all medications (both prescription and nonprescription [over-the-counter] medications) that you are taking.

What Else Should I Know about *Coumadin®* (warfarin)?

If you are taking an anticoagulant, it is important that you eat the same amount of fruits and vegetables every day. This is especially important when eating foods that contain a lot of vitamin K, which is found in fish, liver, green tea, and green, leafy vegetables. Do not take any medications or multivitamins that contain vitamin K unless your doctor or other healthcare professional has told you to do so. Do not make major changes in what you eat without first talking with your doctor or other healthcare professional.

 # Warning!

To give you the best care, your doctor or other healthcare professional needs to know about the diseases and medical conditions you have had—your full medical history. Tell your doctor or other healthcare professional if you have or have ever had any of the following:

- Allergy or previous reaction to *Coumadin®* (warfarin)
- Bleeding problems

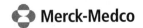

- Liver problems
- Overactive thyroid (hyperthyroidism)
- Recent surgery
- Stomach problems (ulcers)
- Underactive thyroid (hypothyroidism)

Coumadin® (warfarin) may cause side effects if you get too much medication and may not work well if you do not get enough. Your doctor or other healthcare professional may order a blood test that checks your clotting time, called an INR or a PT, to see if you are getting the right amount of this medication. Easy bruising ("black-and-blue" marks on the skin) or bleeding that does not stop easily (nose bleeds, bleeding while brushing your teeth, and cuts) may be early signs that you are getting too much medication. Talk to your doctor or other healthcare professional if you have any of these symptoms, and be sure to get your blood tests as ordered. Do not change your dose or stop taking this medication unless directed by your doctor or other healthcare professional.

Coumadin® (warfarin) may increase your risk of a bleeding ulcer. Stomach pain may be a sign of an ulcer. However, you may have an ulcer without feeling any pain at all. If ulcers are not treated, they may cause serious stomach or intestinal bleeding. Tell your doctor or other healthcare professional if you have severe stomach pain or stomach pain that keeps returning, or if you have ever had peptic ulcer disease. Call your doctor or other healthcare professional right away if you have black, tarry-looking bowel movements (stools), if you vomit dark material that looks like coffee grounds, or if you notice any blood in your bowel movements. Any of these symptoms may be a sign of a bleeding ulcer.

Because *Coumadin*® (warfarin) prevents blood from clotting as well as usual, you should talk to your doctor or other healthcare professional about whether you should stop taking this medication before surgery or dental procedures. Your doctor or other healthcare professional may need to lower your dosage or temporarily stop *Coumadin*® (warfarin) for a while in order to help prevent excessive bleeding during surgery or dental work.

As long as you are taking an anticoagulant, talk to your doctor or other healthcare professional before doing any strenuous physical activity (such as skiing or any other sport that could result in an injury). If you have an injury that results in bleeding, your medication could prevent the formation of clots that would be needed to stop the bleeding.

If you are injured in any way that causes you to bleed or bruise excessively, contact your doctor or other healthcare professional.

If you are having leg pain, redness, or swelling, you may have a blood clot (venous thrombosis). This is serious and needs to be treated. If you have these symptoms, go to the emergency room of the nearest hospital where you will be examined and your doctor or other healthcare professional will be contacted.

If you are having chest pain with shortness of breath and/or you are coughing up blood, you may have a blood clot in your lungs (pulmonary embolism). This is serious and needs to be treated immediately. If you have these symptoms, go to the emergency room of the nearest hospital where you will be examined and your doctor or other healthcare professional will be contacted.

If you are having chest pain, pain in the left shoulder, down the inside of the left arm, or pain in the throat, jaw, teeth, back (between the shoulder blades), or abdomen (stomach), you may be having a heart attack. Other symptoms of a heart attack might include fullness, pressure, heaviness, discomfort, numbness, or tightness on your chest. If you take nitroglycerin and the dose that has been prescribed for you does not relieve your symptoms, or you do not have nitroglycerin, go to the emergency room of the nearest hospital where you will be evaluated and your doctor or other healthcare professional will be contacted.

If you suddenly have leg or arm weakness, a change in or loss of vision, trouble speaking, or confusion, you may be having a stroke. This is serious and needs to be treated immediately. If you have these symptoms, go to the emergency room of the nearest hospital where you will be examined and your doctor or other healthcare professional will be contacted.

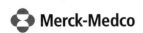

Heparin and *Lovenox*® (enoxaparin)

Heparin is an anticoagulant, sometimes called a "blood thinner." Anticoagulants (blood thinners) cannot dissolve clots that have already formed and do not actually "thin" the blood. *Lovenox*® (enoxaparin) is a type of heparin. The role of heparin is to stop new clots from forming and to stop existing clots from getting bigger. Anticoagulants are sometimes prescribed for people who have a heart rhythm problem (arrhythmia) like atrial fibrillation, for people who have had blood clots before, or for people who have had heart valve replacements. Heparin and *Lovenox*® (enoxaparin) are not absorbed when taken orally. They are injected either just under the skin or into a vein. They are usually used when it is important to prevent the formation of blood clots. They may be given before and after surgery to help prevent blood clots in the legs (venous thrombosis) and in the lungs (pulmonary embolism).

Anticoagulants (blood thinners) cause the body to produce less of the proteins that are needed for clotting. When a person uses heparin, clots take longer to form, and clots that are already formed take longer to grow. A person who takes an anticoagulant may be given a blood test to measure how long his or her blood takes to clot. Your doctor or other healthcare professional uses this information to adjust the dose of anticoagulants that you are taking.

Brand Name	Generic Name
Lovenox®	enoxaparin
Various	heparin

How Will I Take Heparin and *Lovenox*® (enoxaparin)?

When used at home, heparin and *Lovenox*® (enoxaparin) are usually given twice a day by a shot (injection) under the skin on the side of the stomach area. Ask your doctor or other healthcare professional to show you how to inject yourself. Do not use the medication if the liquid in the bottle (vial) looks lumpy or cloudy, or if you see specks floating in the liquid. Keep your medication bottles (vials) at room temperature (59°F to 86°F), and protect them from light. Your doctor or other healthcare professional will tell you how often to use this medication.

If you miss a dose of this medication, take the dose you missed as soon as possible. However, if it is almost time for your next dose, skip the missed dose and just take the next one. Do not double your dose. Take your medication exactly as directed by your doctor or other healthcare professional. Do not stop taking a prescription medication unless directed by your doctor or other healthcare professional.

What Side Effects Can Heparin and *Lovenox*® (enoxaparin) Cause?

More Common

- Bleeding that does not stop easily (nose bleeds, bleeding while brushing your teeth, and cuts)
- Easy bruising ("black-and-blue" marks on the skin)
- Rash (skin redness, bumps, itching, or irritation)

Less Common

- Coughing up blood
- Itching and burning of the feet
- Low red blood cells (anemia)
- Nausea
- Red- or brown-colored urine
- Severe bleeding (hemorrhage)
- Severe headache
- Skin irritation where the injection (shot) was given
- Ulcers in the stomach that may cause black, tarry-looking bowel movements

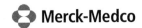

Rare

- Flu-like symptoms (fever, chills, runny nose)
- Headache
- Trouble breathing or shortness of breath
- Vomiting

Tell your doctor or other healthcare professional if you have side effects that bother you, do not go away, make you worried about taking your medication, or make you want to stop taking your medication.

Do Other Medications Interact with Heparin and *Lovenox*® (enoxaparin)?

Many nonprescription (over-the-counter [OTC]) medications such as pain, cough, cold, allergy, and sleep medications contain aspirin or NSAIDs that ***may increase*** the side effects of heparin and *Lovenox*® (enoxaparin). If you are taking heparin or *Lovenox*® (enoxaparin), you should talk to your doctor or other healthcare professional before taking any new OTC medications.

These medications ***may increase*** the side effects of heparin and *Lovenox*® (enoxaparin):

- *Aggrenox*® (dipyridamole/aspirin)
- Aspirin, medications that contain aspirin, and aspirin-like medications (salicylates)—see Glossary
- *Coumadin*® (warfarin)
- Nonsteroidal anti-inflammatory drugs (NSAIDs) such as *Motrin*® (ibuprofen), *Aleve*® (naproxen), *Vioxx*® (rofecoxib), *Celebrex*® (celecoxib), and others—see Glossary
- *Persantine*® (dipyridamole)
- *Plavix*® (clopidogrel)
- *Ticlid*® (ticlopidine)

Tell your doctor or other healthcare professional about all medications (both prescription and nonprescription [over-the-counter] medications) that you are taking.

 # Warning!

To give you the best care, your doctor or other healthcare professional needs to know about the diseases and medical conditions you have had—your full medical history. Tell your doctor or other healthcare professional if you have or have ever had any of the following:

- Allergy or previous reaction to heparin, *Lovenox®* (enoxaparin), or pork
- Bleeding problems
- Catheter in the bladder (only important if you have one now)
- Diabetes
- High alcohol intake (drinking 3 or more alcoholic beverages, such as beer, wine, whiskey, and others, every day)
- Kidney problems
- Liver problems
- Recent surgery
- Stomach problems (ulcers)

Since heparin and *Lovenox®* (enoxaparin) may cause side effects if you get too much medication and may not work well if you do not get enough, your doctor or other healthcare professional may order blood tests to see if you are getting the right amount of this medication. Easy bruising ("black-and-blue" marks on the skin) or bleeding that does not stop easily (nose bleeds, bleeding while brushing your teeth, and cuts) may be early signs that you are getting too much medication. Talk to your doctor or other healthcare professional if you have any of these symptoms and be sure to get your blood tests as ordered. Do not change your dose or stop taking this medication unless directed by your doctor or other healthcare professional.

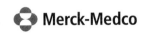

Heparin and *Lovenox*® (enoxaparin) may increase your risk of a bleeding ulcer. Stomach pain may be a sign of an ulcer. However, you may have an ulcer without feeling any pain at all. If ulcers are not treated, they may cause serious stomach or intestinal bleeding. Tell your doctor or other healthcare professional if you have severe stomach pain or stomach pain that keeps returning or if you have ever had peptic ulcer disease. Call your doctor or other healthcare professional right away if you have black, tarry-looking bowel movements (stools), if you vomit dark material that looks like coffee grounds, or if you notice any blood in your bowel movements. Any of these symptoms may be a sign of a bleeding ulcer.

Because heparin and *Lovenox*® (enoxaparin) prevent blood from clotting as well as usual, you should talk to your doctor or other healthcare professional about whether you should stop taking this medication before surgery or dental procedures. Your doctor or other healthcare professional may need you to temporarily stop your medication for a while in order to help prevent excessive bleeding during surgery or dental work.

As long as you are taking heparin and *Lovenox*® (enoxaparin), talk to your doctor or other healthcare professional before doing any strenuous physical activity (such as skiing or any other sport that could result in an injury). If you have an injury that results in bleeding, your medication could prevent the formation of clots that would be needed to stop the bleeding.

If you are injured in any way that causes you to bleed or bruise excessively, contact your doctor or other healthcare professional.

If you are having leg pain, redness, or swelling, you may have a blood clot (venous thrombosis). This is serious and needs to be treated. If you have these symptoms, go to the emergency room of the nearest hospital where you will be examined and your doctor or other healthcare professional will be contacted.

If you are having chest pain with shortness of breath and/or you are coughing up blood, you may have a blood clot in your lungs (pulmonary embolism). This is serious and needs to be treated immediately. If you have these symptoms, go to the emergency room of the nearest hospital where you will be examined and your doctor or other healthcare professional will be contacted.

If you are having chest pain, pain in the left shoulder, down the inside of the left arm, or pain in the throat, jaw, teeth, back (between the shoulder blades), or abdomen (stomach), you may be having a heart attack. Other symptoms of a heart attack might include fullness, pressure, heaviness, discomfort, numbness, or tightness on your chest. If you take nitroglycerin and the dose that has been prescribed for you does not relieve your symptoms, or you do not have nitroglycerin, go to the emergency room of the nearest hospital where you will be evaluated and your doctor or other healthcare professional will be contacted.

If you suddenly have leg or arm weakness, a change in or loss of vision, trouble speaking, or confusion, you may be having a stroke. This is serious and needs to be treated immediately. If you have these symptoms, go to the emergency room of the nearest hospital where you will be examined and your doctor or other healthcare professional will be contacted.

Aspirin

Aspirin is called an antiplatelet medication because it helps prevent strokes and heart attacks by preventing platelets (tiny cells in the blood) from clumping together and forming clots.

Because aspirin makes the blood clot more slowly, it may be used to help prevent the onset of a heart attack, and sometimes is used when people are having a heart attack. It is also used to help prevent some kinds of strokes. Taking aspirin to help prevent a heart attack or stroke is not recommended for everyone. Talk to your doctor or other healthcare professional before taking aspirin to help prevent a heart attack or stroke.

Brand Name	Generic Name
Bayer® Aspirin	aspirin
Bayer® Enteric-Coated	coated aspirin
Ecotrin®	coated aspirin
Halprin®	aspirin

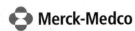

How Will I Take Aspirin?

When aspirin is used to help prevent heart attacks and strokes, it is used in smaller doses and less often than when it is used for pain. Sometimes only one children's aspirin pill is needed. Many people only have to take adult or children's aspirin once a day. Some only have to take aspirin a few days a week. Ask your doctor or other healthcare professional if and how often you should take aspirin.

Take aspirin with a full 8-ounce glass of water to keep pills from sticking in your throat, which may cause irritation. Aspirin may be taken with food to help reduce stomach upset. Some medications that contain aspirin are coated or have added ingredients called buffers to make the medication less irritating to the stomach. Buffers may reduce some side effects but not all. Do not crush or chew these pills unless directed by your doctor or other healthcare professional.

If you miss a dose of this medication, take the dose you missed as soon as possible. However, if it is almost time for your next dose, skip the missed dose and just take the next one. Do not double your dose. Take your medication exactly as directed by your doctor or other healthcare professional. Do not stop taking a prescribed medication unless directed by your doctor or other healthcare professional.

What Side Effects Can Aspirin Cause?

More Common

- Heartburn
- Nausea
- Vomiting

Less Common

- Bleeding that does not stop easily (nose bleeds, bleeding while brushing your teeth, and cuts)
- Easy bruising ("black-and-blue" marks on the skin)

- Hearing loss

- Low red blood cells (anemia)

- Ringing in the ears (tinnitus)

- Ulcers in the stomach that may cause black, tarry-looking bowel movements

Rare

- A combination of dizziness, diarrhea, confusion, headache, sweating, and fast, troubled breathing (hyperventilation) called salicylism

- Allergic reactions such as rash (skin redness, bumps, itching, or irritation), swelling of the face and throat, and trouble breathing

- Kidney problems

- Liver problems that may cause yellowing of the skin or eyes (jaundice)

- Severe bleeding

Tell your doctor or other healthcare professional if you have side effects that bother you, do not go away, make you worried about taking your medication, or make you want to stop taking your medication.

 Do Other Medications Interact with Aspirin?

Many nonprescription (over-the-counter [OTC]) medications such as pain, cough, cold, allergy, and sleep medications contain aspirin or NSAIDs. If you are taking aspirin, you should talk to your doctor or other healthcare professional before taking any new OTC medications.

Aspirin *may increase* the side effects of these medications:

- *Aggrenox®* (dipyridamole/aspirin)

- Aspirin-like medications (salicylates)—see Glossary

- Corticosteroids such as prednisone—see Glossary

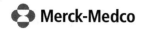
- *Coumadin*® (warfarin)
- *Depakene*® (valproic acid)
- *Depakote*® (divalproex)
- Diabetes medications such as *DiaBeta*® (glyburide), *Glucophage*® (metformin), *Glucotrol*® (glipizide), and others—see Glossary
- Heparin
- Insulin
- *Lovenox*® (enoxaparin)
- Nonsteroidal anti-inflammatory drugs (NSAIDs) such as *Motrin*® (ibuprofen), *Aleve*® (naproxen), *Vioxx*® (rofecoxib), *Celebrex*® (celecoxib), and others—see Glossary
- *Pepto-Bismol*® (bismuth subsalicylate)
- *Persantine*® (dipyridamole)
- *Plavix*® (clopidogrel)
- *Rheumatrex*® (methotrexate)
- *Ticlid*® (ticlopidine)

These medications ***may decrease*** how well aspirin works:

- *Anturane*® (sulfinpyrazone)
- *Benemid*® (probenecid)

Drinking alcoholic beverages (such as beer, wine, whiskey, and others) ***may increase*** the side effects of aspirin.

Tell your doctor or other healthcare professional about all medications (both prescription and nonprescription [over-the-counter] medications) that you are taking.

Why Else Do People Take Aspirin?

Aspirin is used to help relieve pain, arthritis, and fever.

 # Warning!

To give you the best care, your doctor or other healthcare professional needs to know about the diseases and medical conditions you have had—your full medical history. Tell your doctor or other healthcare professional if you have or have ever had any of the following:

- Allergy or previous reaction to aspirin, aspirin-like medications (salicylates), or NSAIDs
- Asthma or nasal polyps (overgrowth of tissue in the nose)
- Bleeding problems
- High alcohol intake (drinking 3 or more alcoholic beverages, such as beer, wine, whiskey, and others, every day)
- Liver problems
- Stomach problems (ulcers)

Aspirin may cause stomach pain, which may be a sign of an ulcer. However, you may have an ulcer without feeling any pain at all. If ulcers are not treated, they may cause serious stomach or intestinal bleeding. Tell your doctor or other healthcare professional if you have severe stomach pain or stomach pain that keeps returning or if you have ever had peptic ulcer disease. Call your doctor or other healthcare professional right away if you have black, tarry-looking bowel movements (stools), if you vomit dark material that looks like coffee grounds, or if you notice any blood in your bowel movements. Any of these symptoms may be a sign of a bleeding ulcer.

If you have asthma or a history of polyps in the nose, ask your doctor or other healthcare professional whether you can take aspirin safely.

If you are having leg pain, redness, or swelling, you may have a blood clot (venous thrombosis). This is serious and needs to be treated. If you have these

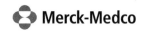

symptoms, go to the emergency room of the nearest hospital where you will be examined and your doctor or other healthcare professional will be contacted.

If you are having chest pain with shortness of breath and/or you are coughing up blood, you may have a blood clot in your lungs (pulmonary embolism). This is serious and needs to be treated immediately. If you have these symptoms, go to the emergency room of the nearest hospital where you will be examined and your doctor or other healthcare professional will be contacted.

If you are having chest pain, pain in the left shoulder, down the inside of the left arm, or pain in the throat, jaw, teeth, back (between the shoulder blades), or abdomen (stomach), you may be having a heart attack. Other symptoms of a heart attack might include fullness, pressure, heaviness, discomfort, numbness, or tightness on your chest. If you take nitroglycerin and the dose that has been prescribed for you does not relieve your symptoms, or you do not have nitroglycerin, go to the emergency room of the nearest hospital where you will be evaluated and your doctor or other healthcare professional will be contacted.

If you suddenly have leg or arm weakness, a change in or loss of vision, trouble speaking, or confusion, you may be having a stroke. This is serious and needs to be treated immediately. If you have any of these symptoms, go to the emergency room of the nearest hospital where you will be examined and your doctor or other healthcare professional will be contacted.

Because aspirin may prevent blood from clotting as well as usual, you should talk to your doctor or other healthcare professional about whether you should stop taking this medication before surgery or dental procedures. Your doctor or other healthcare professional may ask you to stop taking aspirin for a few days or a week before surgery or dental procedures.

Aspirin may cause a serious, even fatal, illness called Reye's syndrome when given to children with flu-like symptoms. Do not give aspirin to children without first talking to a doctor or other healthcare professional.

Plavix® (clopidogrel) and *Ticlid*® (ticlopidine)

Plavix® (clopidogrel) and *Ticlid*® (ticlopidine) are antiplatelet medications that decrease the stickiness of platelets and help prevent some kinds of strokes by helping to prevent blood clots from forming. These antiplatelet medications are available only by prescription.

How Will I Take *Plavix*® (clopidogrel) and *Ticlid*® (ticlopidine)?

Plavix® (clopidogrel) is usually taken once a day. It may be taken with or without food. *Ticlid*® (ticlopidine) is usually taken twice a day with food to help prevent stomach upset. Your doctor or other healthcare professional will tell you how often to take your medication.

If you miss a dose of this medication, take the dose you missed as soon as possible. However, if it is almost time for your next dose, skip the missed dose and just take the next one. Do not double your dose. Take your medication exactly as directed by your doctor or other healthcare professional. Do not stop taking a prescription medication unless directed by your doctor or other healthcare professional.

What Side Effects Can *Plavix*® (clopidogrel) and *Ticlid*® (ticlopidine) Cause?

More Common

- Diarrhea
- Easy bruising ("black-and-blue" marks on the skin)
- Gas or bloating
- Heartburn

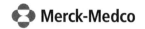

- Nausea

- Rash (skin redness, bumps, itching, or irritation)

Less Common

- Bleeding that does not stop easily (nose bleeds, bleeding while brushing your teeth, and cuts)

- Ulcers in the stomach that may cause black, tarry-looking bowel movements

Rare

With *Ticlid*® (ticlopidine) only:

- Frequent fever, sore throat, or flu-like symptoms that may be a sign of low white blood cells

- Hives

- Liver problems that may cause yellowing of the skin or eyes (jaundice)

- Ringing in the ears (tinnitus)

- Tingling, pain, or weakness in hands and feet

Tell your doctor or other healthcare professional if you have side effects that bother you, do not go away, make you worried about taking your medication, or make you want to stop taking your medication.

 Do Other Medications Interact with *Plavix*® (clopidogrel) and *Ticlid*® (ticlopidine)?

Many nonprescription (over-the-counter [OTC]) medications such as pain, cough, cold, allergy, and sleep medications contain aspirin or NSAIDs that *may increase* the side effects of antiplatelet medications. If you are taking *Plavix*® (clopidogrel) or *Ticlid*® (ticlopidine), you should talk to your doctor or other healthcare professional before taking any new OTC medications.

These medications *may increase* the side effects of *Plavix*® (clopidogrel) and *Ticlid*® (ticlopidine):

- *Aggrenox*® (dipyridamole/aspirin)

- Aspirin, medications that contain aspirin, and aspirin-like medications (salicylates)—see Glossary

- *Coumadin*® (warfarin)

- *Dilantin*® (phenytoin)

- Heparin

- *Lovenox*® (enoxaparin)

- Nonsteroidal anti-inflammatory drugs (NSAIDs) such as *Motrin*® (ibuprofen), *Aleve*® (naproxen), *Vioxx*® (rofecoxib), *Celebrex*® (celecoxib), and others—see Glossary

- *Persantine*® (dipyridamole)

Tagamet® (cimetidine) *may increase* the side effects of *Ticlid*® (ticlopidine).

Ticlid® (ticlopidine) *may increase* the side effects of theophylline such as *Theo-Dur*®, *Uniphyl*®, and others—see Glossary.

Plavix® (clopidogrel) *may increase* the side effects of *Nolvadex*® (tamoxifen).

Antacids such as *Maalox*® or *Mylanta*® (aluminum hydroxide/magnesium hydroxide), *Rolaids*® or *Tums*® (calcium carbonate), or *Amphojel*® (aluminum hydroxide) *may decrease* the effects of *Ticlid*® (ticlopidine) when taken at the same time. If you are using antacids, take *Ticlid*® (ticlopidine) 1 hour before or 2 hours after taking your antacid.

Tell your doctor or other healthcare professional about all medications (both prescription and nonprescription [over-the-counter] medications) that you are taking.

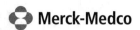

Warning!

To give you the best care, your doctor or other healthcare professional needs to know about the diseases and medical conditions you have had—your full medical history. Tell your doctor or other healthcare professional if you have or have ever had any of the following:

- Allergy or previous reaction to *Plavix*® (clopidogrel) or *Ticlid*® (ticlopidine)

- High cholesterol in your blood (hypercholesterolemia)

- Kidney problems

- Liver problems

- Low red blood cells (anemia)

- Stomach problems (ulcer)

Since *Ticlid*® (ticlopidine) may cause damage to your liver, your doctor or other healthcare professional may order blood tests to find out early on if the medication is causing liver problems, before they become serious.

If you are having leg pain, redness, or swelling, you may have a blood clot (venous thrombosis). This is serious and needs to be treated. If you have these symptoms, go to the emergency room of the nearest hospital where you will be examined and your doctor or other healthcare professional will be contacted.

If you are having chest pain with shortness of breath and/or you are coughing up blood, you may have a blood clot in your lungs (pulmonary embolism). This is serious and needs to be treated immediately. If you have these symptoms, go to the emergency room of the nearest hospital where you will be examined and your doctor or other healthcare professional will be contacted.

If you are having chest pain, pain in the left shoulder, down the inside of the left arm, or pain in the throat, jaw, teeth, back (between the shoulder blades), or abdomen (stomach), you may be having a heart attack. Other symptoms of a heart attack might include fullness, pressure, heaviness, discomfort, numbness, or tightness on your chest. If you take nitroglycerin and the dose that has been prescribed for you does not relieve your symptoms, or you do not have nitroglycerin, go to the emergency room of the nearest hospital where you will be evaluated and your doctor or other healthcare professional will be contacted.

If you suddenly have leg or arm weakness, a change in or loss of vision, trouble speaking, or confusion, you may be having a stroke. This is serious and needs to be treated immediately. If you have these symptoms, go to the emergency room of the nearest hospital where you will be examined and your doctor or other healthcare professional will be contacted.

Plavix® (clopidogrel) or *Ticlid*® (ticlopidine) may increase your risk of a bleeding ulcer. Stomach pain may be a sign of an ulcer. However, you may have an ulcer without feeling any pain at all. If ulcers are not treated, they may cause serious stomach or intestinal bleeding. Tell your doctor or other healthcare professional if you have severe stomach pain or stomach pain that keeps returning or if you have ever had peptic ulcer disease. Call your doctor or other healthcare professional right away if you have black, tarry-looking bowel movements (stools), if you vomit dark material that looks like coffee grounds, or if you notice any blood in your bowel movements. Any of these symptoms may be a sign of a bleeding ulcer.

Because antiplatelet medications may prevent blood from clotting as well as usual, you should talk to your doctor or other healthcare professional about whether you should stop taking your medication before surgery or dental procedures. Your doctor or other healthcare professional may ask you to stop taking your antiplatelet medication for 1 to 2 weeks before surgery or dental procedures.

As long as you are taking an antiplatelet medication, do not do any strenuous physical activity (such as skiing or any other sport that could result in an injury) without first talking with your doctor or other healthcare professional. If you have an injury that results in bleeding, your medication could prevent the formation of clots that would be needed to stop the bleeding.

If you are injured in any way that causes you to bleed or bruise excessively, contact your doctor or other healthcare professional immediately.

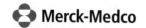

Dipyridamole

Persantine® (dipyridamole) and *Aggrenox®* (dipyridamole/aspirin) are antiplatelet medications that decrease the stickiness of platelets and help prevent heart attacks and some kinds of strokes by helping to prevent blood clots from forming. These medications are available only by prescription. Please see the previous section on aspirin on pages 637–642 for further information on interactions, side effects, and warnings if you are taking *Aggrenox®* because it contains aspirin.

Brand Name	Generic Name
Aggrenox®	dipyridamole/aspirin
Persantine®	dipyridamole

How Will I Take Dipyridamole?

Dipyridamole is usually taken 2 to 4 times a day. It is usually taken on an empty stomach 1 hour before or 2 hours after meals. If stomach upset occurs, it may be taken with food to help prevent stomach upset. *Aggrenox®* is usually taken twice daily. Your doctor or other healthcare professional will tell you how often to take your medication.

If you miss a dose of this medication, take the dose you missed as soon as possible. However, if it is almost time for your next dose, skip the missed dose and just take the next one. Do not double your dose. Take your medication exactly as directed by your doctor or other healthcare professional. Do not stop taking a prescription medication unless directed by your doctor or other healthcare professional.

What Side Effects Can Dipyridamole Cause?

More Common

- Dizziness

- Easy bruising ("black-and-blue" marks on the skin)

- Heartburn

- Nausea

Less Common

- Cardiac chest pain (angina)

- Rash (skin redness, bumps, itching, or irritation)

- Reddening of the face (flushing)

- Ulcers in the stomach that may cause black, tarry-looking bowel movements

Rare

- Bleeding that does not stop easily (nose bleeds, bleeding while brushing your teeth, and cuts)

- Liver problems that may cause yellowing of the skin or eyes (jaundice)

Tell your doctor or other healthcare professional if you have side effects that bother you, do not go away, make you worried about taking your medication, or make you want to stop taking your medication.

Do Other Medications Interact with Dipyridamole?

Many nonprescription (over-the-counter [OTC]) medications such as pain, cough, cold, allergy, and sleep medications contain aspirin or NSAIDs that *may increase* the side effects of dipyridamole. If you are taking dipyridamole, you should talk to your doctor or other healthcare professional before taking any new OTC medications.

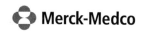

These medications *may increase* the side effects of dipyridamole:

- Aspirin and aspirin-like medications (salicylates)—see Glossary

- *Coumadin®* (warfarin)

- Heparin

- *Lovenox®* (enoxaparin)

- Nonsteroidal anti-inflammatory drugs (NSAIDs) such as *Motrin®* (ibuprofen), *Aleve®* (naproxen), *Vioxx®* (rofecoxib), and *Celebrex®* (celecoxib)—see Glossary

- *Plavix®* (clopidogrel)

- *Ticlid®* (ticlopidine)

Tell your doctor or other healthcare professional about all medications (both prescription and nonprescription [over-the-counter] medications) that you are taking.

 # Warning!

To give you the best care, your doctor or other healthcare professional needs to know about the diseases and medical conditions you have had—your full medical history. Tell your doctor or other healthcare professional if you have or have ever had any of the following:

- Allergy or previous reaction to *Persantine®* (dipyridamole), *Aggrenox®* (dipyridamole/aspirin), aspirin or aspirin-like medications (salicylates), or nonsteroidal anti-inflammatory drugs (NSAIDs) such as *Motrin®* (ibuprofen), *Aleve®* (naproxen), *Vioxx®* (rofecoxib), and *Celebrex®* (celecoxib)—see Glossary

- Cardiac chest pain (angina)

- Liver problems

- Low blood pressure (hypotension)

- Low red blood cells (anemia)

- Stomach problems (ulcer)

Since dipyridamole may cause damage to your liver, your doctor or other healthcare professional may order blood tests to find out early on if the medication is causing liver problems, before they become serious.

If you are having leg pain, redness, or swelling, you may have a blood clot (venous thrombosis). This is serious and needs to be treated. If you have these symptoms, go to the emergency room of the nearest hospital where you will be evaluated and your doctor or other healthcare professional will be contacted.

If you are having chest pain with shortness of breath and/or you are coughing up blood, you may have a blood clot in your lungs (pulmonary embolism). This is serious and needs to be treated immediately. If you have these symptoms, go to the emergency room of the nearest hospital where you will be examined and your doctor or other healthcare professional will be contacted.

If you are having chest pain, pain in the left shoulder, down the inside of the left arm, or pain in the throat, jaw, teeth, back (between the shoulder blades), or abdomen (stomach), you may be having a heart attack. Other symptoms of a heart attack might include fullness, pressure, heaviness, discomfort, numbness, or tightness on your chest. If you take nitroglycerin and the dose that has been prescribed for you does not relieve your symptoms, or you do not have nitroglycerin, go to the emergency room of the nearest hospital where you will be examined and your doctor or other healthcare professional will be contacted.

If you suddenly have leg or arm weakness, a change in or loss of vision, trouble speaking, or confusion, you may be having a stroke. This is serious and needs to be treated immediately. If you have these symptoms, go to the emergency room of the nearest hospital where you will be examined and your doctor or other healthcare professional will be contacted.

Dipyridamole may increase your risk of a bleeding ulcer. Stomach pain may be a sign of an ulcer. However, you may have an ulcer without feeling any pain at all. If ulcers are not treated, they may cause serious stomach or intestinal bleeding. Tell your doctor or other healthcare professional if you have severe

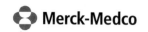

stomach pain or stomach pain that keeps returning or if you have ever had peptic ulcer disease. Call your doctor or other healthcare professional right away if you have black, tarry-looking bowel movements (stools), if you vomit dark material that looks like coffee grounds, or if you notice any blood in your bowel movements. Any of these symptoms may be a sign of a bleeding ulcer.

Because dipyridamole may prevent blood from clotting as well as usual, you should talk to your doctor or other healthcare professional about whether you should stop taking your medication before surgery or dental procedures. Your doctor or other healthcare professional may ask you to stop taking your dipyridamole for 1 to 2 weeks before surgery or dental procedures.

As long as you are taking dipyridamole, do not do any strenuous physical activity (such as skiing or any other sport that could result in an injury) without talking with your doctor or other healthcare professional. If you have an injury that results in bleeding, your medication could prevent the formation of clots that would be needed to stop the bleeding.

If you are injured in any way that causes you to bleed or bruise excessively, contact your doctor or other healthcare professional immediately.

Chapter 20

Thyroid Problems

What Are Thyroid Problems?

The thyroid is a small gland located in the front of the neck that produces natural chemicals (hormones) and releases them into the bloodstream. These hormones control many functions in your body. How fast your heart beats, your cholesterol level, the texture of your skin and hair, your energy level, your ability to think clearly and remember things, your intestinal function (constipation or diarrhea), and whether you feel hot or cold are but a few of the many functions thyroid hormones control. If a person's thyroid is underactive and does not produce enough thyroid hormone, that person is said to have a condition called hypothyroidism. If a person's thyroid is overactive and produces too much thyroid hormone, that person is said to have a condition called hyperthyroidism.

Underactive Thyroid (Hypothyroidism)

What Is Underactive Thyroid?

Underactive thyroid (hypothyroidism) is an abnormal condition in which the thyroid gland does not produce enough thyroid hormone. It is more common among women than men. It becomes more common as people get older. Not everyone with hypothyroidism will have symptoms. If you have hypothyroidism, you may have one or more of the following symptoms:

- Coarse hair

- Confusion

- Constipation

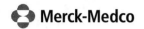

- Dry skin

- Hair loss

- High cholesterol blood level

- Hoarse voice

- Increased sensitivity to cold

- Memory problems

- Sadness, feeling blue or down, depressed mood (depression)

- Slowed speech

- Slow heartbeat (palpitations)

- Swelling or puffiness of the feet, ankles, or lower legs (edema)

- Tiredness or sluggishness (fatigue)

- Weight gain

Medications for Underactive Thyroid

Thyroid Medications

Thyroid medications are used to treat an underactive thyroid when your body's thyroid gland does not make enough thyroid hormone.

Brand Name	Generic Name
Armour® Thyroid	thyroid hormone
Cytomel®	liothyronine
Eltroxin®	levothyroxine
Levo-T®	levothyroxine
Levothroid®	levothyroxine
Levoxyl®	levothyroxine
Synthroid®	levothyroxine
Thyrolar®	levothyroxine/liothyronine

How Will I Take Thyroid Medications?

Thyroid hormone and levothyroxine are usually taken once a day at the same time each day. *Cytomel®* (liothyronine) is generally taken 2 to 3 times a day. Thyroid medications should be taken on an empty stomach 1 hour before or 2 hours after meals. Your doctor or other healthcare professional will tell you how often to take thyroid medications.

To help prevent side effects, your doctor or other healthcare professional may start by giving you a low dose of this medication, increasing the amount slowly until it works well for you.

Levothyroxine usually takes 6 to 8 weeks to have its maximum effects. Most people start to feel better in the first month after they start taking thyroid medication.

If you miss a dose of this medication, take the dose you missed as soon as possible. However, if it is almost time for your next dose, skip the missed dose and just take the next one. Do not double your dose. Take your medication exactly as directed by your doctor or other healthcare professional. Do not stop taking a prescription medication unless directed by your doctor or other healthcare professional.

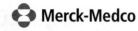

What Side Effects Can Thyroid Medications Cause?

Since thyroid hormone medications are identical to the hormones that the body makes naturally, side effects are usually uncommon. Most people who have side effects are taking too much medication, which may cause symptoms of an overactive thyroid. Your doctor or other healthcare professional may reduce the dose of your medication if side effects occur. Do not change your dose unless directed by your doctor or other healthcare professional.

More Common

- Headache
- Nervousness (anxiety)
- Trouble falling asleep or staying asleep (insomnia)

Less Common

- Cardiac chest pain (angina)
- Confusion
- Diarrhea
- Fast heartbeat (palpitations)
- Fine hair
- Increased appetite
- Increased or excessive sweating (perspiration)
- Increased sensitivity to heat
- Reddening of the face (flushing)
- Shakiness or tremors
- Weight loss

Tell your doctor or other healthcare professional if you have side effects that bother you, do not go away, make you worried about taking your medication, or make you want to stop taking your medication.

Do Other Medications Interact with Thyroid Medications?

Thyroid medications *may increase* the side effects of *Coumadin®* (warfarin).

Bile acid binders such as *Questran®* (cholestyramine) or *Colestid®* (colestipol) or bulk-forming laxatives like *Metamucil®* (psyllium) *may decrease* the effects of these thyroid medications by preventing them from being absorbed completely. To help make sure they are absorbed so they can work properly, take your thyroid medications 1 hour before or 4 to 6 hours after taking a bile acid binder or a bulk-forming laxative.

Antacids such as *Maalox®* or *Mylanta®* (aluminum hydroxide/magnesium hydroxide), *Rolaids®* or *Tums®* (calcium carbonate), or *Amphojel®* (aluminum hydroxide) *may decrease* the effects of these thyroid medications when taken at the same time. If you are using antacids, take your thyroid medication 1 hour before or 2 hours after taking your antacid.

Thyroid medications *may decrease* how well these medications work:

- Diabetes medications such as *DiaBeta®* (glyburide), *Glucophage®* (metformin), *Glucotrol®* (glipizide), and others—see Glossary

- Insulin

- *Lanoxicaps®* or *Lanoxin®* (digoxin)

- Theophylline such as *Theo-Dur®*, *Uniphyl®*, and others—see Glossary

---

Tell your doctor or other healthcare professional about all medications (both prescription and nonprescription [over-the-counter] medications) that you are taking.

Warning!

To give you the best care, your doctor or other healthcare professional needs to know about the diseases and medical conditions you have had—your full

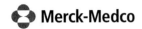

medical history. Tell your doctor or other healthcare professional if you have or have ever had any of the following:

- Adrenal gland problems (Addison's disease)
- Allergy or previous reaction to thyroid medications
- Diabetes
- Heart problems

Thyroid medications may affect the health of your bones. Taking too much thyroid medication may make you more likely to develop thinning bones (osteoporosis). Talk with your doctor or other healthcare professional about osteoporosis and ways to help prevent it.

Since thyroid medications may cause side effects if you get too much medication and may not work well if you do not get enough, your doctor or other healthcare professional may order blood tests to see if you are getting the right amount of medication. Headache, nervousness (anxiety), and trouble falling asleep or staying asleep (insomnia) may be early signs that you are getting too much medication. Talk to your doctor or other healthcare professional if you have any of these symptoms, and be sure to get your blood tests as ordered. Do not change your dose or stop taking this medication unless directed by your doctor or other healthcare professional.

If your symptoms do not improve after 6 to 8 weeks, it may mean that you are not getting enough of the medication. Talk to your doctor or other healthcare professional to see if you need more blood tests or a change in medication.

Overactive Thyroid (Hyperthyroidism)

What Is Overactive Thyroid?

Overactive thyroid (hyperthyroidism) is an abnormal condition in which the thyroid gland produces too much thyroid hormone. It is more common among women than men. It is most commonly seen in people with Grave's disease.

Not everyone with an overactive thyroid (hyperthyroidism) has symptoms. If you have hyperthyroidism, you may have one or more of the following symptoms:

- Cardiac chest pain (angina)

- Diarrhea

- Eye changes (bigger or bulging)

- Fast heartbeat (palpitations)

- Fine hair

- Increased appetite

- Increased or excessive sweating (perspiration)

- Increased sensitivity to heat

- Muscle weakness

- Nervousness (anxiety)

- Reddening of the face (flushing)

- Shakiness or tremors

- Trouble falling asleep or staying asleep (insomnia)

- Weight loss

Medications for Overactive Thyroid

Propylthiouracil (PTU) and *Tapazole*® (methimazole)

Propylthiouracil (PTU) and *Tapazole*® (methimazole) are used when your body's thyroid is overactive and produces too much thyroid hormone. These medications help bring your body's thyroid hormone down to a normal level.

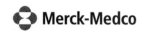

How Will I Take Propylthiouracil (PTU) and *Tapazole®* (methimazole)?

Tapazole® (methimazole) is generally taken once a day with a meal. Propylthiouracil (PTU) is generally taken 3 times a day. Your doctor or other healthcare professional will tell you how often to take your medication.

If you miss a dose of this medication, take the dose you missed as soon as possible. However, if it is almost time for your next dose, skip the missed dose and just take the next one. Do not double your dose. Take your medication exactly as directed by your doctor or other healthcare professional. Do not stop taking a prescription medication unless directed by your doctor or other healthcare professional.

What Side Effects Can Propylthiouracil (PTU) and *Tapazole®* (methimazole) Cause?

Many of the side effects from propylthiouracil (PTU) and *Tapazole®* (methimazole), such as developing symptoms of an underactive thyroid, may result from taking too much medication. Your doctor or other healthcare professional may reduce the dose of your medication if side effects occur. Do not change your dose unless directed by your doctor or other healthcare professional.

More Common

- Fever
- Rash (skin redness, bumps, itching, or irritation)

Less Common

- Coarse hair
- Confusion
- Constipation
- Dry skin
- Hair loss

- Hoarse voice

- Increased sensitivity to cold

- Memory problems

- Sadness, feeling blue or down, depressed mood (depression)

- Slowed speech

- Slow heartbeat (palpitations)

- Swelling or puffiness of the feet, ankles, or lower legs (edema)

- Tiredness or sluggishness (fatigue)

- Weight gain

Rare

- Frequent fevers, sore throats, or flu-like symptoms that may be a sign of low white blood cells.

Tell your doctor or other healthcare professional if you have side effects that bother you, do not go away, make you worried about taking your medication, or make you want to stop taking your medication.

Do Other Medications Interact with Propylthiouracil (PTU) and *Tapazole*® (methimazole)?

Propylthiouracil (PTU) and *Tapazole*® (methimazole) ***may increase*** the side effects of these medications:

- Beta blockers such as *Inderal*® (propranolol), *Tenormin*® (atenolol), *Toprol*® (metoprolol), and others—see Glossary

- *Lanoxicaps*® or *Lanoxin*® (digoxin)

- Theophylline such as *Theo-Dur*®, *Uniphyl*®, and others—see Glossary

Propylthiouracil (PTU) and *Tapazole*® (methimazole) ***may decrease*** how well *Coumadin*® (warfarin) works.

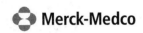

Tell your doctor or other healthcare professional about all medications (both prescription and nonprescription [over-the-counter] medications) that you are taking.

 # Warning!

To give you the best care, your doctor or other healthcare professional needs to know about the diseases and medical conditions you have had—your full medical history. Tell your doctor or other healthcare professional if you have or have ever had any of the following:

- Allergy or previous reaction to propylthiouracil (PTU) or *Tapazole®* (methimazole)

- Cardiac chest pain (angina)

- Liver problems

Since propylthiouracil (PTU) and *Tapazole®* (methimazole) may cause side effects if you get too much medication and may not work well if you do not get enough, your doctor or other healthcare professional may order blood tests to see if you are getting the right amount of this medication. Tiredness or sluggishness may be an early sign that you are getting too much medication. Talk to your doctor or other healthcare professional if you have these symptoms, and be sure to get your blood tests as ordered. Do not change your dose or stop taking this medication unless directed by your doctor or other healthcare professional.

These medications may cause a decrease in the number of white blood cells in your body needed to fight infections. If you have frequent fever, sore throat, or other flu-like symptoms, contact your doctor or other healthcare professional as soon as possible. Your doctor or other healthcare professional may order blood tests to see if the medication you take is causing these problems. Blood tests may help find these problems before they become serious.

Chapter 21

Urinary Problems

What Are Urinary Problems?

There are several common types of urinary problems. This chapter is devoted to two of them—loss of bladder control (urinary incontinence) and difficulty urinating due to an enlarged prostate (benign prostatic hypertrophy).

Loss of Bladder Control

Some older people find that they cannot hold their urine very well. Loss of bladder control (urinary incontinence) may occur with increasing frequency with advancing age. Sudden loss of bladder control may also be caused by illness or by some medications. For example, loss of bladder control may be the only sign that a person has a bladder infection. Bladder control usually returns after the infection has healed.

Each of the four main types of incontinence has a different cause. The four types are stress incontinence, urge incontinence, overflow incontinence, and functional incontinence. You may have more than one type of incontinence at the same time.

- **Stress incontinence** is loss of bladder control caused by pressure on the muscles that keep urine in the bladder. Small amounts of urine leak out when a person exercises, coughs, laughs, or sneezes. Many women who have previously given birth develop stress incontinence because delivering a baby weakens the muscles that keep urine in the bladder.

- **Urge incontinence** is the sudden feeling that you have to urinate. When this happens, you may not be able to hold in the urine long enough to reach a toilet. With this type of incontinence, the bladder squeezes inward (contracts) more often than it should (a condition called "overactive bladder") without giving the usual warning that it is time to urinate.

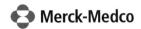

- **Overflow incontinence** leaves the bladder full almost all the time because the bladder cannot squeeze hard enough to empty very well. Small amounts of urine may leak out throughout the day.

- **Functional incontinence** is a problem that results from an inconvenient or unsuitable living situation. There is nothing wrong with the bladder itself, but a physical problem makes it hard for the person to get to a bathroom in time to urinate. For example, a person who has difficulty walking but has to climb a flight of stairs to reach the bathroom may need several minutes to get there—and may not make it in time.

Many people who lose some control over their bladders never see a doctor or other healthcare professional about the problem. Some assume that the situation is a normal part of aging. Others are too embarrassed to tell anyone about it. Yet, a lot can be done to help people control their urination again.

One way for people to regain bladder control is by changing their behavior in specific ways. For example, they may go to the bathroom every 2 hours. They may learn exercises that strengthen the muscles around the tube that carries urine from the bladder to the outside of the body (the urethra). Surgery and other devices can help some kinds of bladder control problems.

The kind of treatment for loss of bladder control that this chapter discusses is medication. The type of medication needed depends on the specific type (or types) of incontinence that a person has.

Medications Used for Loss of Bladder Control

Several kinds of medications may be taken for bladder control. This chapter discusses these medications and/or categories of medications:

MEDICATIONS	See Page
Anticholinergic Medications	665
Tricyclic Antidepressants	670
Sudafed® (pseudoephedrine)	676
Estrogen (for women only)	679

The second section of this chapter discusses urinary problems in men caused by an enlarged prostate (benign prostatic hypertrophy) and covers the following medications and/or categories of medications:

MEDICATIONS	See Page
Alpha Blockers	686
Proscar® (finasteride [for men only])	690

If you do not see the exact name of the medication that you take for bladder control or an enlarged prostate listed above, check the Medication and Chapter Table to find out which category your medication falls under or check the Index.

Anticholinergic Medications

Anticholinergic medications often help people who have urge incontinence. These medications help to relax the bladder and help prevent it from contracting so often.

▲ Indicates medications that are more likely to cause unpleasant or dangerous side effects. These medications are generally not recommended for people over 65. The side effects may not be very obvious and may be mistaken for "just a part of getting older" but may be serious. If you are taking one of these medications, you might want to talk to your doctor or other healthcare professional to see if this medication is best for you. Safer medications may be available and lower dosages may be required. You should not stop taking these medications without first talking to your doctor or other healthcare professional.

See the WARNING section on page 669 for the specific safety problems associated with these medications ▲.

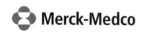
Brand Name	Generic Name
▲Cystospaz®	hyoscyamine
Detrol®	tolterodine
Ditropan®	oxybutynin
▲Levsin®	hyoscyamine
▲Levsinex®	hyoscyamine
▲Pro-Banthine®	propantheline
▲Urispas®	flavoxate

How Will I Take Anticholinergic Medications?

Most people take anticholinergic medications 2 to 4 times a day to help prevent accidental urine loss. Your doctor or other healthcare professional will tell you how many times a day to take your medication.

When a medication has initials after its name, such as XL, XR, SR, BID, DUR, and others, it usually means that the body absorbs the medication slowly over time, so you usually have to take it only once or twice a day. The body will absorb some medications of this type too fast if you crush or break them or dissolve them in liquid, and their effects will not last as long as they should. Check with your doctor or other healthcare professional before crushing or breaking your pills or dissolving your pills in liquid.

If you miss a dose of this medication, take the dose you missed as soon as possible. However, if it is almost time for your next dose, skip the missed dose and just take the next one. Do not double your dose. Take your medication exactly as directed by your doctor or other healthcare professional. Do not stop taking a prescription medication unless directed by your doctor or other healthcare professional.

What Side Effects Can Anticholinergic Medications Cause?

More Common
- Blurred vision
- Constipation
- Drowsiness
- Dry mouth, nose, throat, or eyes
- Eyes that are too sensitive to light
- Fast heartbeat (palpitations)
- Trouble urinating or emptying the bladder

Less Common
- Confusion
- Dizziness when standing up from a bed or a chair
- Fever
- Nausea
- Nervousness (anxiety)
- Rash (skin redness, bumps, itching, or irritation)
- Reddening of the face (flushing)
- Seeing or hearing things that are not there (hallucinations)
- Trouble swallowing
- Vomiting

Tell your doctor or other healthcare professional if you have side effects that bother you, do not go away, make you worried about taking your medication, or make you want to stop taking your medication.

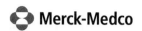

Do Other Medications Interact with Anticholinergic Medications?

Anticholinergic medications *may increase* the side effects of other medications that cause drowsiness, including other anticholinergic medications, antidepressants, antihistamines (allergy medications), antispasmodics, benzodiazepines (a type of tranquilizer), anxiety medications, narcotics (pain relievers), muscle relaxants, neuroleptic medications (a type of tranquilizer), seizure medications, or sleep medications. Avoid driving a car and other activities that need mental alertness, like using a knife or operating machinery, while taking these medications together.

Drinking alcoholic beverages (such as beer, wine, whiskey, and others) *may increase* the side effects of anticholinergic medications.

These medications *may increase* the side effects of *Detrol*® (tolterodine):

- *Biaxin*® (clarithromycin)
- *Diflucan*® (fluconazole)
- Erythromycin such as *Ery-Tab*®, *Erythrocin*®, and others—see Glossary
- *Nizoral*® (ketoconazole)
- *Sporanox*® (itraconazole)

Tell your doctor or other healthcare professional about all medications (both prescription and nonprescription [over-the-counter] medications) that you are taking.

Why Else Do People Take Anticholinergic Medications?

Bentyl® (dicyclomine), *Levsinex*® (hyoscyamine), and *Pro-Banthine*® (propantheline) may be prescribed for indigestion and irritable bowel syndrome.

What Else Should I Know about Anticholinergic Medications?

Anticholinergic medications do not work for everyone. If your symptoms do not improve within a few weeks after you start to take the medication, discuss this problem with your doctor or other healthcare professional. You may be able to take something else that will work better for you.

 # Warning!

To give you the best care, your doctor or other healthcare professional needs to know about the diseases and medical conditions you have had—your full medical history. Tell your doctor or other healthcare professional if you have or have ever had any of the following:

- Allergy or previous reaction to anticholinergic medications
- Breathing problems (asthma and COPD, including emphysema and chronic bronchitis)
- Congestive heart failure
- Dementia or Alzheimer's disease
- Dizziness when standing up from a bed or a chair
- Enlarged prostate (benign prostatic hypertrophy)
- Glaucoma (an eye disease)
- Inflammatory bowel disease (ulcerative colitis or Crohn's disease)
- Kidney problems
- Liver problems
- Low blood pressure (hypotension)
- Trouble urinating or emptying the bladder

Urispas® (flavoxate), *Cystospaz®* (hyoscyamine), *Levsin®* (hyoscyamine), *Levsinex®* (hyoscyamine) and *Pro-Banthine®* (propantheline) are generally not recommended for people over 65 because they cause serious side effects that include dizziness, blurred vision, constipation, confusion, and a fast heartbeat.

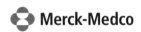

If you are taking one of these medications, talk to your doctor or other healthcare professional to see if it is right for you. Do not stop taking this medication without first talking to your doctor or other healthcare professional.

Anticholinergic medications may cause drowsiness. Avoid driving a car and other activities that need mental alertness, like using a knife or operating machinery, while taking this medication. Drinking alcoholic beverages (such as beer, wine, whiskey, and others) may increase the side effects.

Anticholinergic medications may make you unsteady on your feet, causing you to fall and possibly break a bone. If you have fallen recently, tell your doctor or other healthcare professional about it. Taking a different medication or a lower dose may make you less likely to fall. You should not stop taking this medication without first talking to your doctor or other healthcare professional.

Tricyclic Antidepressants

Tricyclic antidepressants may be taken for urge incontinence. These medications help keep the bladder from squeezing as often.

▲ Indicates medications that are more likely to cause unpleasant or dangerous side effects. These medications are generally not recommended for people over 65. The side effects may not be very obvious and may be mistaken for "just a part of getting older" but may be serious. If you are taking one of these medications, you might want to talk to your doctor or other healthcare professional to see if this medication is best for you. Safer medications may be available and lower dosages may be required. You should not stop taking these medications without first talking to your doctor or other healthcare professional.

See the WARNING section on page 674 for the specific safety problems associated with these medications ▲.

Brand Name	Generic Name
▲*Elavil*®	amitriptyline
Norpramin®	desipramine
Pamelor®	nortriptyline
▲*Sinequan*®	doxepin
▲*Surmontil*®	trimipramine
▲*Tofranil*®	imipramine

How Will I Take Tricyclic Antidepressants?

Tricyclic antidepressants are usually taken as pills 1 to 3 times a day. If taken only once a day, they are usually taken at bedtime to decrease the chance of daytime side effects. Your doctor or other healthcare professional will tell you how often to take your medication.

To help prevent side effects, your doctor or other healthcare professional may start by giving you a low dose of this medication, increasing the amount slowly until it works well for you.

If you miss a dose of this medication, take the dose you missed as soon as possible. However, if it is almost time for your next dose, skip the missed dose and just take the next one. Do not double your dose. Take your medication exactly as directed by your doctor or other healthcare professional. Do not stop taking a prescription medication unless directed by your doctor or other healthcare professional.

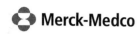

What Side Effects Can Tricyclic Antidepressants Cause?

More Common

- Constipation
- Dizziness when standing up from a bed or a chair
- Drowsiness
- Dry mouth, eyes, and nose
- Trouble urinating or emptying the bladder

Less Common

- Confusion
- Fast, slow, or irregular heartbeat (palpitations)
- Increased or decreased interest in sex
- Rash (skin redness, bumps, itching, or irritation)
- Worsening of glaucoma (an eye disease)

Rare

- Breast enlargement and tenderness (in both men and women)
- Hair loss
- Seizures
- Shakiness or tremors

Tell your doctor or other healthcare professional if you have side effects that bother you, do not go away, make you worried about taking your medication, or make you want to stop taking your medication.

Do Other Medications Interact with Tricyclic Antidepressants?

These medications *may increase* the side effects of tricyclic antidepressants:

- Quinidine such as *Quinaglute*®, *Quinidex*®, and others—see Glossary

- *Ritalin*® (methylphenidate)

- *Rythmol*® (propafenone)

- *Tagamet*® (cimetidine)

Tricyclic antidepressants *may increase* the side effects of other medications that cause drowsiness, including anticholinergic medications, antidepressants, antihistamines (allergy medications), antispasmodics, benzodiazepines (a type of tranquilizer), anxiety medications, narcotics (pain relievers), muscle relaxants, neuroleptic medications (a type of tranquilizer), seizure medications, or sleep medications. Avoid driving a car and other activities that need mental alertness, like using a knife or operating machinery, while taking these medications together.

Drinking alcoholic beverages (such as beer, wine, whiskey, and others) *may increase* the side effects of tricyclic antidepressants.

These medications *may decrease* how well tricyclic antidepressants work:

- Barbiturates such as *Butisol*® (butabarbital), *Luminal*® (phenobarbital), *Mebaral*® (mephobarbital), and others—see Glossary

- *Rifadin*® (rifampin)

- *Tegretol*® (carbamazepine)

Taking a tricyclic antidepressant and *Catapres*® (clonidine) or *Ismelin*® (guanethidine) *may raise* a person's blood pressure to dangerously high levels.

Tricyclic antidepressants are generally not prescribed for anyone who is taking MAO inhibitors, such as *Marplan*® (isocarboxazid), *Nardil*® (phenelzine), or *Parnate*® (tranylcypromine), because together they *may cause* serious or even fatal reactions. If your doctor or other healthcare professional wants you to stop

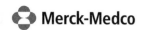

taking one medication and start taking the other, you should wait at least 2 weeks between stopping one and starting the other.

Tricyclic antidepressants are generally not used with *Propulsid*® (cisapride [withdrawn from general distribution; available only by special arrangement with the manufacturer]), *Seldane*® (terfenadine [no longer commercially available]), or *Hismanal*® (astemizole [no longer commercially available]), because together they ***may cause*** serious, sometimes fatal, heart problems.

Tell your doctor or other healthcare professional about all medications (both prescription and nonprescription [over-the-counter] medications) that you are taking.

Why Else Do People Take Tricyclic Antidepressants?

Tricyclic antidepressants can help to relieve depression, long-term pain, abnormal fears (phobias), panic attacks, obsessive-compulsive disorders, and eating disorders such as anorexia and bulimia.

 # Warning!

To give you the best care, your doctor or other healthcare professional needs to know about the diseases and medical conditions you have had—your full medical history. Tell your doctor or other healthcare professional if you have or have ever had, or presently take, any of the following:

- Allergy or previous reaction to tricyclic antidepressants, *Tegretol*® (carbamazepine), or *Trileptal*® (oxcarbazepine)

- Enlarged prostate (benign prostatic hypertrophy)

- Glaucoma (an eye disease)

- Liver problems

- Manic depression

- MAO inhibitors such as *Marplan*® (isocarboxazid), *Nardil*® (phenelzine), or *Parnate*® (tranylcypromine)

- Overactive thyroid (hyperthyroidism)

- Schizophrenia

- Seizures (epilepsy)

- Trouble urinating or emptying the bladder

Elavil® (amitriptyline), *Sinequan*® (doxepin), *Surmontil*® (trimipramine), and *Tofranil*® (imipramine) are generally not recommended for use in people over the age of 65 because these types of tricyclic antidepressants have been associated with a higher risk of broken hips than other tricyclic antidepressants. If you are taking any of these medications, ask your doctor or other healthcare professional if this medication is right for you. Do not stop taking this medication without talking to your doctor or other healthcare professional.

Tricyclic antidepressants may make you unsteady on your feet, causing you to fall and possibly break a bone. If you have fallen recently, tell your doctor or other healthcare professional about it. Taking a different medication or a lower dose may make you less likely to fall. You should not stop taking this medication without first talking to your doctor or other healthcare professional.

Tricyclic antidepressants may cause drowsiness. Avoid driving a car and other activities that need mental alertness, like using a knife or operating machinery, while taking this medication. Drinking alcoholic beverages (such as beer, wine, whiskey, and others) may increase the side effects.

If you are taking a tricyclic antidepressant, stay out of the sun as much as you can to avoid a serious sunburn. When you do go out in the sun, use sunblock or sunscreen, and wear protective clothing such as a wide-brimmed hat and a long-sleeved shirt.

Under certain circumstances, your doctor or other healthcare professional may decide that you should stop taking this medication. If you have taken it for more than a couple of weeks, he or she may want you to decrease it gradually, lowering the dose over a few weeks or months. Stopping suddenly may cause unpleasant withdrawal symptoms or may worsen your medical problems. Pay

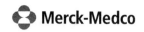

careful attention to the instructions your doctor or other healthcare professional gives you about how much less to take and for how long.

Sudafed® (pseudoephedrine)

Sudafed® (pseudoephedrine) may be taken for stress incontinence. *Sudafed®* (pseudoephedrine) helps tighten the muscles of the tube that carries urine from the bladder to the outside of the body (the urethra). Tightening those muscles, which may have been loosened during childbirth, can help to prevent urine from leaking out when a woman coughs, laughs, sneezes, or exercises, or during other activities. *Sudafed®* (pseudoephedrine) is available over-the-counter without a prescription.

How Will I Take *Sudafed®* (pseudoephedrine)?

Sudafed® (pseudoephedrine) is usually taken 2 or 3 times a day. Follow the instructions on the package or ask your doctor or other healthcare professional how many times a day to take your medication.

When a medication has 12-hour or 24-hour after its name, it usually means that the body absorbs the medication slowly over time, so you usually have to take it only once or twice a day. The body will absorb some medications of this type too fast if you crush or break them or dissolve them in liquid, and their effects will not last as long as they should. Check with your doctor or other healthcare professional before crushing or breaking your pills or dissolving your pills in liquid.

If you miss a dose of this medication, take the dose you missed as soon as possible. However, if it is almost time for your next dose, skip the missed dose and just take the next one. Do not double your dose. Take your medication exactly as directed by your doctor or other healthcare professional. Do not stop taking a prescription medication unless directed by your doctor or other healthcare professional.

What Side Effects Can *Sudafed*® (pseudoephedrine) Cause?

More Common

- Dizziness

- Nausea

- Nervousness (anxiety)

- Problems falling asleep or staying asleep (insomnia)

- Sweating

Less Common

- Difficulty breathing

- Fast heartbeat (palpitations)

- High blood pressure (hypertension)

Tell your doctor or other healthcare professional if you have side effects that bother you, do not go away, make you worried about taking your medication, or make you want to stop taking your medication.

Do Other Medications Interact with *Sudafed*® (pseudoephedrine)?

Sudafed® (pseudoephedrine) is generally not prescribed for someone who is taking MAO inhibitors, such as *Marplan*® (isocarboxazid), *Nardil*® (phenelzine), or *Parnate*® (tranylcypromine), because together they ***may cause*** serious or even fatal reactions. If your doctor or other healthcare professional wants you to stop taking one medication and start taking the other, you should wait at least 2 weeks between stopping one and starting the other.

These medications ***may increase*** the side effects of *Sudafed*® (pseudoephedrine):

- *Aldomet*® (methyldopa)

- *Celexa*™ (citalopram)

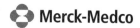

- *Furoxone*® (furazolidone)

- *Ismelin*® (guanethidine)

- *Luvox*® (fluvoxamine)

- *Paxil*® (paroxetine)

- *Prozac*® (fluoxetine)

- *Zoloft*® (sertraline)

Sudafed® (pseudoephedrine) ***may decrease*** how well high blood pressure (hypertension) medication works—see Glossary.

Many nonprescription (over-the-counter [OTC]) medications such as cough, cold, and allergy medications contain pseudoephedrine. You should talk to your doctor or other healthcare professional before taking any OTC medications.

Tell your doctor or other healthcare professional about all medications (both prescription and nonprescription [over-the-counter] medications) that you are taking.

Why Else Do People Take *Sudafed*® (pseudoephedrine)?

Sudafed® (pseudoephedrine) may also be used for colds, sinus problems, and allergies.

 # Warning!

To give you the best care, your doctor or other healthcare professional needs to know about the diseases and medical conditions you have had—your full medical history. Tell your doctor or other healthcare professional if you have or have ever had, or presently take, any of the following:

- Allergy or previous reaction to *Sudafed*® (pseudoephedrine)

- Diabetes
- Enlarged prostate (benign prostatic hypertrophy)
- Heart problems
- High blood pressure (hypertension)
- MAO inhibitors such as *Marplan*® (isocarboxazid), *Nardil*® (phenelzine), or *Parnate*® (tranylcypromine)
- Overactive thyroid (hyperthyroidism)

Estrogen

Before menopause, when a woman is still having menstrual periods, her body makes estrogen, the female hormone. After menopause, her body produces much less estrogen, triggering many physical changes as a direct result of her lower estrogen levels. In the urinary tract, the tube that carries urine from the bladder to the outside of the body (the urethra) may narrow, and the bladder muscles may weaken, causing bladder control problems. One reason why women take estrogen after menopause is to help strengthen the bladder muscles and restore control.

Brand Name	Generic Name
Alora® (patch)	estradiol
Cenestin® (pill)	synthetic conjugated estrogens
Climara® (patch)	estradiol
Combipatch™ (patch)	estradiol/norethindrone
E_2III™ (patch)	estradiol
Estrace® (pill or vaginal cream)	estradiol
Estraderm® (patch)	estradiol
Estratab® (pill)	esterified estrogens
Estring® (vaginal ring)	estradiol
FemPatch® (patch)	estradiol
Menest® (pill)	esterified estrogens

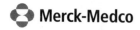
Brand Name	Generic Name
Ogen® (pill or vaginal cream)	estropipate
Ortho-Est® (pill)	estropipate
Ortho-Prefest® (pill)	estradiol
Premarin® (pill or vaginal cream)	conjugated estrogens
Premphase® (pill)	conjugated estrogens every day plus medroxyprogesterone for 14 of every 28 days
Prempro™ (pill)	conjugated estrogens and medroxyprogesterone taken every day
Vagifem® (vaginal tablet)	estradiol
Vivelle® (patch)	estradiol

How Will I Take Estrogen?

For urinary incontinence, a woman may use estrogen as a pill, as a vaginal ring, as a cream that is applied directly to the vagina, or as a patch, which is applied to the skin like a *Band-Aid®*. If taken as a pill, estrogen is usually taken once a day. A patch is usually applied once or twice a week. If used as a cream, the estrogen cream is usually applied inside the vagina at bedtime every day for 14 consecutive days. After that, the cream is usually applied inside the vagina 2 to 3 times a week. Estrogen may also be prescribed in a vaginal ring. A doctor or other healthcare professional inserts the ring high in the vagina once every 90 days. The ring slowly releases estrogen into the tissues around it. Your doctor or other healthcare professional will tell you how often to take your medication.

Some women take estrogen only, while others take both estrogen and a medication called a progestin. Common brand names for oral progestins are *Provera®* (medroxyprogesterone) and *Prometrium®* (micronized progesterone). If you have had surgery to remove your uterus (hysterectomy), you do not need to take a progestin. If your uterus has not been removed, a progestin is usually taken with estrogen to help prevent developing cancer of the lining of the uterus (endometrial cancer). For some women, the progestin is taken daily; for others it is taken on certain days of the month. Your doctor or other healthcare professional will decide which is best for you.

Sometimes estrogen is combined with the progestin in pills or patches like *Prempro*™, *Premphase*®, or *Combipatch*™. If you are taking *Premphase*®, you will take estrogen every day and progestins for only 14 days. The package is designed so you will know when to take which pills.

To help keep patches from irritating your skin, you should put each patch in a different area. Put on a new patch if the first one falls off. When you take a patch off, make sure you throw it away where children or pets cannot get it as it still will contain medication that may be harmful to them. Your doctor or other healthcare professional will tell you how often to take your medication.

If you miss a dose of this medication, take the dose you missed as soon as possible. However, if it is almost time for your next dose, skip the missed dose and just take the next one. Do not double your dose. Take your medication exactly as directed by your doctor or other healthcare professional. Do not stop taking a prescription medication unless directed by your doctor or other healthcare professional.

What Side Effects Can Estrogen Cause?

More Common

- Breast fullness, swelling, or tenderness

- Nausea

- Return of period-like bleeding (menstrual bleeding) if taking progestins

- Swelling or puffiness of the feet, ankles, or lower legs (edema)

- Weight gain

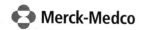

Less Common

- Diarrhea

- Increased or decreased interest in sex

- Worsening of migraine headaches

Rare

- Chest pain with shortness of breath and/or coughing up blood

- Gallstones

- Heavy vaginal bleeding

- Increased risk of breast cancer—Most studies have not shown an increase, but some have reported up to twice the usual rate of breast cancer in women who used estrogens for more than 10 years

- Increased risk of cancer of the lining of the uterus (endometrial cancer), if you are taking estrogen without progestins and you have not had a hysterectomy

- Leg pain, redness, or swelling

Tell your doctor or other healthcare professional if you have side effects that bother you, do not go away, make you worried about taking your medication, or make you want to stop taking your medication.

Do Other Medications Interact with Estrogen?

These medications **_may decrease_** how well estrogen works:

- Barbiturates such as _Butisol_® (butabarbital), _Luminal_® (phenobarbital), _Mebaral_® (mephobarbital), and others—see Glossary

- _Dilantin_® (phenytoin)

- _Rifadin_® (rifampin)

- _Topamax_® (topiramate)

Estrogen *may increase* the side effects of corticosteroids such as prednisone and others—see Glossary.

Estrogen *may decrease* how well *Coumadin*® (warfarin) works.

Tell your doctor or other healthcare professional about all medications (both prescription and nonprescription [over-the-counter] medications) that you are taking.

Why Else Do People Take Estrogen?

Estrogen also helps relieve dryness, bleeding, or itching in the vagina. For these purposes, it may be used as a cream in the vagina. It helps relieve some of the symptoms that are common after menopause (when women stop having menstrual periods altogether), such as a sudden warm or hot feeling with sweating and reddening of the face and neck ("hot flashes"). Estrogen is often used to help prevent or treat osteoporosis because it helps to slow bone loss after menopause. It may also be used to help reduce the risk of developing heart problems.

What Else Should I Know about Estrogen?

When estrogen is taken with a progestin such as *Provera*®, *Prometrium*®, *Prempro*™, *Premphase*®, or *Combipatch*™, there may be a return of menstrual (period-like) bleeding. It may be light spotting or moderate-to-heavy bleeding, which may be normal. However, you should talk to your doctor or other healthcare professional if you have bleeding while taking these medications because it may be a sign of a more serious problem.

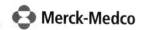

 # Warning!

To give you the best care, your doctor or other healthcare professional needs to know about the diseases and medical conditions you have had—your full medical history. Tell your doctor or other healthcare professional if you have or have ever had (or if any close blood relative has ever had) any of the following:

- Allergy or previous reaction to adhesives or skin (transdermal) patches

- Allergy or previous reaction to estrogen

- Blood clots (phlebitis or embolism)

- Breast cancer

- Cancer of the lining of the uterus (endometrial cancer)

- Endometriosis

- Fibroid (a type of noncancerous growth) in the uterus

- Gallbladder problems

- Liver problems

Women who have not had a hysterectomy may increase their chance of developing cancer of the lining of the uterus (endometrial cancer) if they take estrogen without another medication called progestin. If you have not had a hysterectomy and estrogen is prescribed for you, you should discuss taking a progestin such as *Provera*® (medroxyprogesterone) or *Prometrium*® (micronized progesterone) with your doctor or other healthcare professional.

If you are having leg pain, redness, or swelling, you may have a blood clot (venous thrombosis). This is serious and needs to be treated. If you have these symptoms, go to the emergency room of the nearest hospital where you will be examined and your doctor or other healthcare professional will be contacted.

If you are having chest pain with shortness of breath and/or you are coughing up blood, you may have a blood clot in your lungs (pulmonary embolism). This is serious and needs to be treated immediately. If you have these symptoms, go to the emergency room of the nearest hospital where you will be examined and your doctor or other healthcare professional will be contacted.

Enlarged Prostate (Benign Prostatic Hypertrophy)

Only men have a prostate gland (often called simply "the prostate"). It lies between the bladder and the rectum. As men grow older, it is common for the prostate gland to get larger. The medical term for an enlarged prostate that is otherwise healthy is benign (noncancerous) prostatic hyperplasia. This is sometimes called benign prostatic hypertrophy (BPH). After age 60, more than half of men have enlarged prostates.

As the prostate grows, it presses against the tube that carries urine from the bladder to the outside of the body (the urethra). Since the urethra is very narrow to begin with, even a little squeezing may block the flow of urine, like a kink in a tiny hose. Eventually, the bladder fills with more than the usual amount of urine, creating a condition that resembles overflow incontinence (described on page 664).

Men with an enlarged prostate may have some of the following symptoms:

- Awakening more than once at night to urinate
- Difficulty urinating or having a weak urine flow or one that stops and starts
- Fairly constant pain in the lower back, upper thighs, or pelvis
- Feeling that they cannot totally empty their bladders while urinating
- Having to urinate more often than they used to
- Leaking urine (incontinence)
- Need to push or strain to begin urination
- Pain while urinating

An enlarged prostate does not have to be treated unless it is causing problems. If the problems interfere with a man's usual activities, he may take medication or have surgery. Having an enlarged prostate gland does not cause prostate cancer.

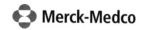

The following medications *may cause* or *worsen* symptoms of BPH:

- Anticholinergic medications such as *Artane*® (trihexyphenidyl), *Cogentin*® (benztropine), and others—see Glossary

- Antihistamines such as *Benadryl*® (diphenhydramine), *Chlor-trimeton*® (chlorpheniramine), and others—see Glossary

- Muscle relaxants such as *Flexeril*® (cyclobenzaprine), *Soma*® (carisoprodol), and others—see Glossary

- Neuroleptic medications such as *Risperdal*® (risperidone), *Thorazine*® (chlorpromazine), *Zyprexa*® (olanzapine), and others—see Glossary

- Some prescription and nonprescription cough, cold, and allergy medications

- Tricyclic antidepressants such as *Elavil*® (amitriptyline), *Pamelor*® (nortriptyline), *Sinequan*® (doxepin), and others—see Glossary

Talk to your doctor or other healthcare professional if you have BPH and are taking any of these medications. Do not stop taking these medications without talking to your doctor or other healthcare professional first.

Medications for Enlarged Prostate (Benign Prostatic Hypertrophy)

Alpha Blockers

Alpha blockers relax the muscle around the prostate. Relaxing that muscle may help relieve the uncomfortable symptoms of an enlarged prostate.

Brand Name	Generic Name
Cardura®	doxazosin
Flomax®	tamsulosin
Hytrin®	terazosin
Minipress®	prazosin

How Will I Take Alpha Blockers?

Alpha blockers are taken 1 to 3 times a day. They may be taken with food to help prevent stomach upset. Your doctor or other healthcare professional will tell you how many times a day to take your medication.

If you miss a dose of this medication, take the dose you missed as soon as possible. However, if it is almost time for your next dose, skip the missed dose and just take the next one. Do not double your dose. Take your medication exactly as directed by your doctor or other healthcare professional. Do not stop taking a prescription medication unless directed by your doctor or other healthcare professional.

What Side Effects Can Alpha Blockers Cause?

More Common

- Dizziness when standing up from a bed or a chair

- Drowsiness

- Tiredness or sluggishness (fatigue)

Less Common

- Dry mouth

- Fast heartbeat (palpitations)

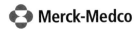
- Headache

- Nervousness (anxiety)

- Swelling or puffiness of the feet, ankles, or lower legs (edema)

Tell your doctor or other healthcare professional if you have side effects that bother you, do not go away, make you worried about taking your medication, or make you want to stop taking your medication.

Do Other Medications Interact with Alpha Blockers?

These medications *may increase* the side effects of alpha blockers:

- Diuretics (water pills) such as *HydroDIURIL®* (hydrochlorothiazide or HCTZ), *Lasix®* (furosemide), and others—see Glossary

- High blood pressure (hypertension) medications—see Glossary

Tagamet® (cimetidine) *may increase* the side effects of *Flomax®* (tamsulosin).

Alpha blockers *may increase* the side effects of other medications that cause drowsiness, including antidepressants, antihistamines (allergy medications), benzodiazepines (a type of tranquilizer), anxiety medications, narcotics (pain relievers), muscle relaxants, neuroleptic medications (a type of tranquilizer), seizure medications, or sleep medications. Avoid driving a car and other activities that need mental alertness, like using a knife or operating machinery, while taking this medication.

Drinking alcoholic beverages (such as beer, wine, whiskey, and others) *may increase* the side effects of alpha blockers.

Many nonprescription (over-the-counter [OTC]) medications such as cough, cold, allergy, and sleep medications contain medications that can worsen symptoms of an enlarged prostate. If you have an enlarged prostate, you should talk to your doctor or other healthcare professional before taking any new OTC medications.

Tell your doctor or other healthcare professional about all medications (both prescription and nonprescription [over-the-counter] medications) that you are taking.

Why Else Do People Take Alpha Blockers?

Alpha blockers can be used for high blood pressure (hypertension).

Warning!

To give you the best care, your doctor or other healthcare professional needs to know about the diseases and medical conditions you have had—your full medical history. Tell your doctor or other healthcare professional if you have or have ever had any of the following:

- Allergy or previous reaction to alpha blockers

- Dizziness when standing up from a bed or a chair

- Prostate cancer or previous testing for prostate cancer

Be careful when taking your first dose. Some people have a fainting spell within the first hour and a half. Ask a friend or family member to be with you when you take your first dose. If you feel dizzy, lie down so that you do not faint. Getting up slowly may reduce any dizziness or lightheadedness that you might feel after taking the first dose.

Alpha blockers may make you unsteady on your feet, causing you to fall and possibly break a bone. If you have fallen recently, tell your doctor or other healthcare professional about it. Taking a different medication or a lower dose may make you less likely to fall. You should not stop taking this medication without first talking to your doctor or other healthcare professional.

Alpha blockers may cause drowsiness. Avoid driving a car and other activities that need mental alertness, like using a knife or operating machinery, while taking this medication. Drinking alcoholic beverages (such as beer, wine, whiskey, and others) may increase the side effects.

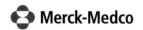

Proscar® (finasteride)

Proscar® (finasteride) shrinks the prostate by decreasing the amount of a hormone in the body that causes the prostate to grow. As the prostate gets smaller, the symptoms of enlarged prostate improve.

How Will I Take *Proscar*® (finasteride)?

Proscar® (finasteride) is usually taken as a pill every morning. *Proscar*® (finasteride) may take 3 to 6 months to work. It may be taken with or without food. Your doctor or other healthcare professional will tell you how many times a day to take your medication.

If you miss a dose of this medication, take the dose you missed as soon as possible. However, if it is almost time for your next dose, skip the missed dose and just take the next one. Do not double your dose. Take your medication exactly as directed by your doctor or other healthcare professional. Do not stop taking a prescription medication unless directed by your doctor or other healthcare professional.

What Side Effects Can *Proscar*® (finasteride) Cause?

Less Common

- Ejaculation and erection problems (erectile dysfunction)
- Loss of interest in sex (decreased libido)

Tell your doctor or other healthcare professional if you have side effects that bother you, do not go away, make you worried about taking your medication, or make you want to stop taking your medication.

Do Other Medications Interact with *Proscar*® (finasteride)?

Many nonprescription (over-the-counter [OTC]) medications such as cough, cold, allergy, and sleep medications contain medications that may worsen symptoms of an enlarged prostate. If you have an enlarged prostate, you should talk to your doctor or other healthcare professional before taking any new OTC medications.

Tell your doctor or other healthcare professional about all medications (both prescription and nonprescription [over-the-counter] medications) that you are taking.

Warning!

To give you the best care, your doctor or other healthcare professional needs to know about the diseases and medical conditions you have had—your full medical history. Tell your doctor or other healthcare professional if you have or have ever had any of the following:

- Allergy or previous reaction to *Proscar*® (finasteride)
- Liver problems
- Prostate cancer or previous testing for prostate cancer

Women who are pregnant or trying to become pregnant should not touch *Proscar*® (finasteride), especially when it has been crushed. This medication can cause birth defects in the babies of women who are exposed to it. Women who are pregnant or trying to become pregnant should not have any contact with the semen of a man who is taking *Proscar*® (finasteride). If a couple is planning pregnancy and the man is taking *Proscar*® (finasteride), he should stop taking it before they stop using birth control and contact his doctor or other healthcare professional.

Medication and Chapter Table

Name of Medication	Chapters	Medication Category
Accolate® (zafirlukast)	Asthma, Emphysema, & Chronic Bronchitis	Leukotriene modifiers
Accupril® (quinapril)	Congestive Heart Failure; High Blood Pressure	ACE inhibitors
Accuretic™ (hydrochlorothiazide/quinapril)	High Blood Pressure	Diuretics, thiazide; ACE inhibitors
Acebutolol	High Blood Pressure	Beta blockers
Aceon® (perindopril)	Congestive Heart Failure; High Blood Pressure	ACE inhibitors
Acetaminophen	Arthritis & Pain	Acetaminophen
Acetaminophen with codeine	Arthritis & Pain	Acetaminophen; Narcotics
Acetazolamide	Glaucoma	Carbonic anhydrase inhibitors
Acetohexamide	Diabetes	Sulfonylureas
Achromycin® (tetracycline)	Heartburn, Ulcers, & Indigestion	Tetracycline
AcipHex® (rabeprazole)	Heartburn, Ulcers, & Indigestion	Proton pump inhibitors
Actonel® (risedronate)	Osteoporosis	Bisphosphonates
Actos® (pioglitazone)	Diabetes	*Actos*® (pioglitazone) & *Avandia*® (rosiglitazone)
Acuprin 81® (aspirin)	Stroke, Heart Attack, & Blood Clot Prevention	Aspirin
Adalat® (nifedipine)	Coronary Artery Disease; High Blood Pressure	Calcium channel blockers
Adsorbocarpine™ (pilocarpine)	Glaucoma	Miotic medications
Advil® (ibuprofen)	Arthritis & Pain	Nonsteroidal anti-inflammatory drugs (NSAIDs)
AeroBid® (flunisolide)	Asthma, Emphysema, & Chronic Bronchitis	Corticosteroids
Aggrenox® (dipyridamole/aspirin)	Stroke, Heart Attack, & Blood Clot Prevention	Dipyridamole (*Persantine*®/*Aggrenox*®); Aspirin
Agoral® (senna)	Constipation	Laxatives, stimulant
Akineton® (biperiden)	Parkinson's Disease	Anticholinergic medications
Alamag® (aluminum hydroxide/ magnesium hydroxide)	Heartburn, Ulcers, & Indigestion	Antacids

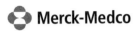
Name of Medication	Chapters	Medication Category
Albuterol	Asthma, Emphysema, & Chronic Bronchitis	Beta-adrenergic bronchodilators
Aldactazide® (spironolactone/ hydrochlorothiazide)	High Blood Pressure	Diuretics, potassium-sparing; Diuretics, thiazide
Aldactone® (spironolactone)	Congestive Heart Failure; High Blood Pressure	Diuretics, potassium-sparing
Aldoclor® (methyldopa/ chlorothiazide)	High Blood Pressure	*Aldomet®* (methyldopa); Diuretics, thiazide
Aldomet® (methyldopa)	High Blood Pressure	*Aldomet®* (methyldopa)
Aldoril® (methyldopa/ hydrochlorothiazide)	High Blood Pressure	*Aldomet®* (methyldopa); Diuretics, thiazide
Aleve® (naproxen)	Arthritis & Pain	Nonsteroidal anti-inflammatory drugs (NSAIDs)
Alka-Mints® (calcium carbonate)	Heartburn, Ulcers, & Indigestion; Osteoporosis	Antacids; Calcium supplements
Alkets® (calcium carbonate)	Heartburn, Ulcers, & Indigestion; Osteoporosis	Antacids; Calcium supplements
Alora® (estradiol)	Osteoporosis; Urinary Problems	Estrogen
Alphagan® (brimonidine)	Glaucoma	*Alphagan®* (brimonidine)
Alprazolam	Anxiety; Sleeping Difficulty	Benzodiazepines
Altace® (ramipril)	Congestive Heart Failure; High Blood Pressure	ACE inhibitors
AlternaGEL® (aluminum hydroxide)	Heartburn, Ulcers, & Indigestion	Antacids
Aluminum carbonate	Heartburn, Ulcers, & Indigestion	Antacids
Aluminum hydroxide/ magnesium hydroxide	Heartburn, Ulcers, & Indigestion	Antacids
Aluminum hydroxide/magnesium hydroxide/simethicone	Heartburn, Ulcers, & Indigestion	Antacids
Alupent® (metaproterenol)	Asthma, Emphysema, & Chronic Bronchitis	Beta-adrenergic bronchodilators
Alurate® (aprobarbital)	Sleeping Difficulty	Barbiturates
Amantadine	Parkinson's Disease	*Symmetrel®* (amantadine)
Amaryl® (glimepiride)	Diabetes	Sulfonylureas
Ambien® (zolpidem)	Sleeping Difficulty	*Ambien®* (zolpidem)
Amiodarone	Irregular Heartbeat	Amiodarone
Amitone® (calcium carbonate)	Heartburn, Ulcers, & Indigestion; Osteoporosis	Antacids; Calcium supplements
Amitriptyline	Arthritis & Pain; Depression; Sleeping Difficulty; Urinary Problems	Tricyclic antidepressants
Amoxapine	Arthritis & Pain; Depression; Sleeping Difficulty	Tricyclic antidepressants
Amoxicillin	Heartburn, Ulcers, & Indigestion	Amoxicillin

Name of Medication	Chapters	Medication Category
Amoxil® (amoxicillin)	Heartburn, Ulcers, & Indigestion	Amoxicillin
Amphojel® (aluminum hydroxide)	Heartburn, Ulcers, & Indigestion	Antacids
Anacin® (aspirin/caffeine)	Arthritis & Pain	Aspirin & aspirin-like medications (salicylates)
Anacin3® (acetaminophen)	Arthritis & Pain	Acetaminophen
Anafranil® (clomipramine)	Arthritis & Pain; Depression	Tricyclic antidepressants
Anaprox® (naproxen)	Arthritis & Pain	Nonsteroidal anti-inflammatory drugs (NSAIDs)
Anaspaz® (hyoscyamine)	Irritable Bowel Syndrome; Urinary Problems	Antispasmodic medications; Anticholinergic medications
Ansaid® (flurbiprofen)	Arthritis & Pain	Nonsteroidal anti-inflammatory drugs (NSAIDs)
Apresazide® (hydrochlorothiazide/hydralazine)	High Blood Pressure	Diuretics, thiazide; *Apresoline®* (hydralazine)
Apresoline® (hydralazine)	Congestive Heart Failure; High Blood Pressure	*Apresoline®* (hydralazine)
Aquachloral® (chloral hydrate)	Sleeping Difficulty	Chloral hydrate
Aquatensen® (methyclothiazide)	High Blood Pressure	Diuretics, thiazide
Aricept® (donepezil)	Alzheimer's Disease	Cholinesterase inhibitors
Aristocort® (triamcinolone)	Arthritis & Pain; Asthma, Emphysema, & Chronic Bronchitis	Corticosteroids
Armour® Thyroid (thyroid USP)	Thyroid Problems (Hypothyroidism)	Thyroid medications
Artane® (trihexyphenidyl)	Parkinson's Disease	Anticholinergic medications
Arthritis Pain Formula™ (aspirin)	Arthritis & Pain	Aspirin & aspirin-like medications (salicylates)
Arthrotec® (diclofenac/misoprostol)	Arthritis & Pain; Heartburn, Ulcers, & Indigestion	NSAIDs (nonsteroidal anti-inflammatory drugs); *Cytotec®* (misoprostol)
Ascriptin® (aspirin)	Arthritis & Pain; Stroke, Heart Attack, & Blood Clot Prevention	Aspirin & aspirin-like medications (salicylates)
Asendin® (amoxapine)	Arthritis & Pain; Depression; Sleeping Difficulty	Tricyclic antidepressants
Aspirin	Arthritis & Pain; Stroke, Heart Attack, & Blood Clot Prevention	Aspirin & aspirin-like medications (salicylates)
Aspirin Free Excedrin® (acetaminophen/caffeine)	Arthritis & Pain	Acetaminophen
AsthmaNefrin® (epinephrine)	Asthma, Emphysema, & Chronic Bronchitis	Beta-adrenergic bronchodilators
Atacand® (candesartan)	High Blood Pressure	A-II blockers
Atamet® (carbidopa/levodopa)	Parkinson's Disease	Levodopa
Atapryl™ (selegiline)	Parkinson's Disease	Selegiline
Atarax® (hydroxyzine)	Anxiety	Antihistamines

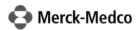 Medications

Name of Medication	Chapters	Medication Category
Atenolol	Congestive Heart Failure; Coronary Artery Disease; High Blood Pressure; Irregular Heartbeat	Beta blockers
Ativan® (lorazepam)	Anxiety; Sleeping Difficulty	Benzodiazepines
Atromid-S® (clofibrate)	High Cholesterol	Fibrates
Atrovent® (ipratropium)	Asthma, Emphysema, & Chronic Bronchitis	*Atrovent®* (ipratropium)
Avalide® (hydrochlorothiazide/irbesartan)	High Blood Pressure	Diuretics, thiazide; A-II blockers
Avandia® (rosiglitazone)	Diabetes	*Actos®* (pioglitazone) & *Avandia®* (rosiglitazone)
Avapro® (irbesartan)	High Blood Pressure	A-II blockers
Axid® (nizatidine)	Heartburn, Ulcers, & Indigestion	H₂ blockers
Azmacort® (triamcinolone)	Asthma, Emphysema, & Chronic Bronchitis	Corticosteroids
Azopt® (brinzolamide)	Glaucoma	Carbonic anhydrase inhibitors
Basaljel® (aluminum carbonate)	Heartburn, Ulcers, & Indigestion	Antacids
Baycol® (cerivastatin)	High Cholesterol	Statins
Bayer® (aspirin)	Arthritis & Pain; Stroke, Heart Attack, & Blood Clot Prevention	Aspirin & aspirin-like medications (salicylates)
Beclovent® (beclomethasone)	Asthma, Emphysema, & Chronic Bronchitis	Corticosteroids
Bell/ans™ (sodium bicarbonate)	Heartburn, Ulcers, & Indigestion	Antacids
Belladonna	Irritable Bowel Syndrome	Antispasmodic medications
Benadryl® (diphenhydramine)	Sleeping Difficulty	Antihistamines
Bentyl® (dicyclomine)	Irritable Bowel Syndrome	Antispasmodic medications
Benztropine	Parkinson's Disease	Anticholinergic medications
Betagan® (levobunolol)	Glaucoma	Beta blocker eyedrops
Betamethasone	Arthritis & Pain; Asthma, Emphysema, & Chronic Bronchitis	Corticosteroids
Betapace® (sotalol)	Irregular Heartbeat	Beta blockers
Betoptic® (betaxolol)	Glaucoma	Beta blocker eyedrops
Biaxin® (clarithromycin)	Heartburn, Ulcers, & Indigestion	*Biaxin®* (clarithromycin)
Bisacodyl	Constipation	Laxatives, stimulant
Bismuth subsalicylate	Heartburn, Ulcers, & Indigestion	*Pepto-Bismol®* (bismuth subsalicylate)
Blocadren® (timolol)	Congestive Heart Failure; Coronary Artery Disease; High Blood Pressure; Irregular Heartbeat	Beta blockers
Brethaire® (terbutaline)	Asthma, Emphysema, & Chronic Bronchitis	Beta-adrenergic bronchodilators
Brethine® (terbutaline)	Asthma, Emphysema, & Chronic Bronchitis	Beta-adrenergic bronchodilators

Name of Medication	Chapters	Medication Category
Bricanyl® (terbutaline)	Asthma, Emphysema, & Chronic Bronchitis	Beta-adrenergic bronchodilators
Bromo-Seltzer® (sodium bicarbonate)	Heartburn, Ulcers, & Indigestion	Antacids
Bufferin® (aspirin)	Arthritis & Pain; Stroke, Heart Attack, & Blood Clot Prevention	Aspirin & aspirin-like medications (salicylates)
Bumetanide	Congestive Heart Failure; High Blood Pressure	Diuretics, loop
Bumex® (bumetanide)	Congestive Heart Failure; High Blood Pressure	Diuretics, loop
Bupropion	Depression	*Wellbutrin®* (bupropion)
BuSpar® (buspirone)	Anxiety	*BuSpar®* (buspirone)
Butisol® (butabarbital)	Sleeping Difficulty	Barbiturates
Calan® (verapamil)	Coronary Artery Disease; High Blood Pressure; Irregular Heartbeat	Calcium channel blockers
Calcet Plus® (calcium carbonate/vitamin D)	Osteoporosis	Calcium supplements; Vitamin D
Calcimar® (salmon calcitonin)	Osteoporosis	Calcitonin
Calcitonin	Osteoporosis	Calcitonin
Calcium carbonate	Heartburn, Ulcers, & Indigestion; Osteoporosis	Antacids; Calcium Supplements
Calcium citrate	Osteoporosis	Calcium Supplements
Calcium gluconate	Osteoporosis	Calcium Supplements
Caltrate® (calcium carbonate)	Osteoporosis	Calcium Supplements
Cantil® (mepenzolate)	Irritable Bowel Syndrome	Antispasmodic medications
Capoten® (captopril)	Congestive Heart Failure; High Blood Pressure	ACE inhibitors
Capozide® (captopril/ hydrochlorothiazide)	High Blood Pressure	ACE inhibitors; Diuretics, thiazide
Capsaicin	Arthritis & Pain	Capsaicin
Capsin® (capsaicin)	Arthritis & Pain	Capsaicin
Captopril	Congestive Heart Failure; High Blood Pressure	ACE inhibitors
Carafate® (sucralfate)	Heartburn, Ulcers, & Indigestion	*Carafate®* (sucralfate)
Carbachol	Glaucoma	Miotic medications
Carbamazepine	Arthritis & Pain	*Tegretol®* (carbamazepine) & *Trileptal®* (oxcarbazepine)
Carbatrol® (carbamazepine)	Arthritis & Pain	*Tegretol®* (carbamazepine) & *Trileptal®* (oxcarbazepine)
Carbex® (selegiline)	Parkinson's Disease	Selegiline
Carboptic® (carbachol)	Glaucoma	Miotic medications
Cardene® (nicardipine)	Coronary Artery Disease; High Blood Pressure	Calcium channel blockers

Name of Medication	Chapters	Medication Category
Cardioquin® (quinidine)	Irregular Heartbeat	Quinidine
Cardizem® (diltiazem)	Coronary Artery Disease; High Blood Pressure; Irregular Heartbeat	Calcium channel blockers
Cardura® (doxazosin)	High Blood Pressure; Urinary Problems	Alpha blockers
Carteolol eyedrops	Glaucoma	Beta blocker eyedrops
Cartrol® (carteolol)	High Blood Pressure	Beta blockers
Cascara	Constipation	Laxatives, stimulant
Cataflam® (diclofenac)	Arthritis & Pain	Nonsteroidal anti-inflammatory drugs (NSAIDs)
Catapres® (clonidine)	High Blood Pressure	*Catapres®* (clonidine)
Celebrex® (celecoxib)	Arthritis & Pain	Cox-2 inhibitors
Celestone® (betamethasone)	Arthritis & Pain; Asthma, Emphysema, & Chronic Bronchitis	Corticosteroids
Celexa™ (citalopram)	Depression	Selective serotonin reuptake inhibitors (SSRIs)
Cenestin® (synthetic conjugated estrogens)	Osteoporosis; Urinary Problems	Estrogen
Cephulac® (lactulose)	Constipation	Lactulose
Chloral hydrate	Sleeping Difficulty	Chloral hydrate
Chlordiazepoxide	Anxiety; Sleeping Difficulty	Benzodiazepines
Chlordiazepoxide & clidinium	Anxiety; Irritable Bowel Syndrome	Benzodiazepines; Antispasmodic medications
Chlorpromazine	Alzheimer's Disease	Neuroleptic medications
Chlorpropamide	Diabetes	Sulfonylureas
Chlorthalidone	High Blood Pressure	Diuretics, thiazide
Cholestyramine	High Cholesterol	Bile acid binders
Choline magnesium trisalicylate	Arthritis & Pain	Aspirin & aspirin-like medications (salicylates)
Chooz® (calcium carbonate)	Heartburn, Ulcers, & Indigestion	Antacids
Chronulac® (lactulose)	Constipation	Lactulose
Cimetidine	Heartburn, Ulcers, & Indigestion	H$_2$ blockers
Citracal® (calcium citrate)	Osteoporosis	Calcium supplements
Citrocarbonate® (sodium bicarbonate/sodium citrate)	Heartburn, Ulcers, & Indigestion	Antacids
Citrucel® (methylcellulose)	Constipation	Laxatives, bulk-forming
Climara® (estradiol)	Osteoporosis; Urinary Problems	Estrogen
Clinoril® (sulindac)	Arthritis & Pain	Nonsteroidal anti-inflammatory drugs (NSAIDs)
Clomipramine	Arthritis & Pain; Depression	Tricyclic antidepressants
Clonazepam	Anxiety; Sleeping Difficulty	Benzodiazepines
Clonidine	High Blood Pressure	*Catapres®* (clonidine)

Name of Medication	Chapters	Medication Category
Clorazepate	Anxiety; Sleeping Difficulty	Benzodiazepines
Clorpres® (clonidine/ chlorthalidone)	High Blood Pressure	*Catapres®* (clonidine); Diuretics, thiazide
Clozapine	Alzheimer's Disease	Neuroleptic medications
Clozaril® (clozapine)	Alzheimer's Disease	Neuroleptic medications
Codeine	Arthritis & Pain	Narcotics
Cogentin® (benzotropine)	Parkinson's Disease	Anticholinergic medications
Cognex® (tacrine)	Alzheimer's Disease	Cholinesterase inhibitors
Colace® (docusate sodium)	Constipation	Stool softeners
Colestid® (colestipol)	High Cholesterol	Bile acid binders
CombiPatch® (estradiol/ norethindrone)	Osteoporosis; Urinary Problems	Estrogen
Combipres® (clonidine/ chlorthalidone)	High Blood Pressure	*Catapres®* (clonidine); Diuretics, thiazide
Combivent® (ipratropium/ albuterol)	Asthma, Emphysema, & Chronic Bronchitis	*Atrovent®* (ipratropium); Beta-adrenergic bronchodilators
Comtan® (entacapone)	Parkinson's Disease	*Comtan®* (entacapone)
Cordarone® (amiodarone)	Irregular Heartbeat	Amiodarone
Coreg® (carvedilol)	Congestive Heart Failure; High Blood Pressure	Beta blockers
Corgard® (nadolol)	Congestive Heart Failure; Coronary Artery Disease; High Blood Pressure; Irregular Heartbeat	Beta blockers
Correctol® (bisacodyl)	Constipation	Laxatives, stimulant
Cortef® (hydrocortisone)	Arthritis & Pain; Asthma, Emphysema, & Chronic Bronchitis	Corticosteroids
Cortisone	Arthritis & Pain; Asthma, Emphysema, & Chronic Bronchitis	Corticosteroids
Cortone® (cortisone)	Arthritis & Pain; Asthma, Emphysema, & Chronic Bronchitis	Corticosteroids
Corzide® (bendroflumethiazide/ nadolol)	High Blood Pressure	Diuretics, thiazide; Beta blockers
Cosopt® (dorzolamide/timolol)	Glaucoma	Carbonic anhydrase inhibitors; Beta blocker eyedrops
Coumadin® (warfarin)	Stroke, Heart Attack, & Blood Clot Prevention	*Coumadin®* (warfarin)
Covera® (verapamil)	Coronary Artery Disease; High Blood Pressure; Irregular Heartbeat	Calcium channel blockers
Cozaar® (losartan)	High Blood Pressure	A-II blockers
Cromolyn	Asthma, Emphysema, & Chronic Bronchitis	*Intal®* (cromolyn) & *Tilade®* (nedocromil)
Cystospaz® (hyoscyamine)	Irritable Bowel Syndrome; Urinary Problems	Antispasmodic medications; Anticholinergic medications
Cytomel® (liothyronine)	Thyroid Problems	Thyroid medications

Name of Medication	Chapters	Medication Category
Cytotec® (misoprostol)	Heartburn, Ulcers, & Indigestion	*Cytotec*® (misoprostol)
Dalmane® (flurazepam)	Sleeping Difficulty	Benzodiazepines
Daranide® (dichlorphenamide)	Glaucoma	Carbonic anhydrase inhibitors
Darvocet-N® (propoxyphene/ acetaminophen)	Arthritis & Pain	Narcotics; Acetaminophen
Darvon® (propoxyphene)	Arthritis & Pain	Narcotics
Darvon® Compound -65 (propoxyphene/aspirin/caffeine)	Arthritis & Pain	Narcotics; Aspirin & aspirin-like medications (salicylates)
Daypro® (oxaprozin)	Arthritis & Pain	Nonsteroidal anti-inflammatory drugs (NSAIDs)
Decadron® (dexamethasone)	Arthritis & Pain; Asthma, Emphysema, & Chronic Bronchitis	Corticosteroids
Delta-Cortef® (prednisolone)	Arthritis & Pain; Asthma, Emphysema, & Chronic Bronchitis	Corticosteroids
Demadex® (torsemide)	Congestive Heart Failure; High Blood Pressure	Diuretics, loop
Demerol® (meperidine)	Arthritis & Pain	Narcotics
Deponit® (nitroglycerin)	Congestive Heart Failure; Coronary artery disease	Nitrates
Desipramine	Arthritis & Pain; Depression; Sleeping Difficulty; Urinary Problems	Tricyclic antidepressants
Desyrel® (trazodone)	Depression; Sleeping Difficulty	*Desyrel*® (trazodone) & *Serzone*® (nefazodone)
Detrol® (tolterodine)	Urinary Problems	Anticholinergic medications
Dexamethasone	Arthritis & Pain; Asthma, Emphysema, & Chronic Bronchitis	Corticosteroids
DiaBeta® (glyburide)	Diabetes	Sulfonylureas
Diabinese® (chlorpropamide)	Diabetes	Sulfonylureas
Diamox® (acetazolamide)	Glaucoma	Carbonic anhydrase inhibitors
Diar-aid® (loperamide)	Irritable Bowel Syndrome	Loperamide
Diazepam	Anxiety; Sleeping Difficulty	Benzodiazepines
Dicarbosil® (calcium carbonate)	Heartburn, Ulcers, & Indigestion	Antacids
Diclofenac	Arthritis & Pain	Nonsteroidal anti-inflammatory drugs (NSAIDs)
Dicyclomine	Irritable Bowel Syndrome	Antispasmodic medications
Didronel® (etidronate)	Osteoporosis	Bisphosphonates
Diflunisal	Arthritis & Pain	Nonsteroidal anti-inflammatory drugs (NSAIDs)
Di-Gel® (aluminum/magnesium/ simethicone)	Heartburn, Ulcers, & Indigestion	Antacids
Digoxin	Congestive Heart Failure; Irregular Heartbeat	Digoxin

Name of Medication	Chapters	Medication Category
Dilacor® (diltiazem)	Coronary Artery Disease; High Blood Pressure; Irregular Heartbeat	Calcium channel blockers
Dilatrate® (isosorbide dinitrate)	Congestive Heart Failure; Coronary Artery Disease	Nitrates
Dilaudid® (hydromorphone)	Arthritis & Pain	Narcotics
Diltia® (diltiazem)	Coronary Artery Disease; High Blood Pressure; Irregular Heartbeat	Calcium channel blockers
Diltiazem	Coronary Artery Disease; High Blood Pressure; Irregular Heartbeat	Calcium channel blockers
Diocto-K® (docusate potassium)	Constipation	Stool softeners
Diovan® (valsartan)	High Blood Pressure	A-II blockers
Diovan HCT® (hydrochlorothiazide/valsartan)	High Blood Pressure	Diuretics, thiazide; A-II blockers
Diphenhydramine	Sleeping Difficulty	Antihistamines
Diphenoxylate & atropine	Irritable Bowel Syndrome	Antispasmodic medications
Dipivefrin	Glaucoma	Epinephrine & *Propine®* (dipivefrin)
Dipyridamole	Stroke, Heart Attack, & Blood Clot Prevention	Dipyridamole (*Persantine®* & *Aggrenox®*)
Disalcid® (salsalate)	Arthritis & Pain	Aspirin & aspirin-like medications (salicylates)
Disopyramide	Irregular Heartbeat	*Norpace®* (disopyramide)
Ditropan® (oxybutynin)	Urinary Problems	Anticholinergic medications
Diucardin® (hydroflumethiazide)	High Blood Pressure	Diuretics, thiazide
Diurese™ (trichlormethiazide)	High Blood Pressure	Diuretics, thiazide
Diuril® (chlorothiazide)	High Blood Pressure	Diuretics, thiazide
Doan's® Pills (magnesium salicylate)	Arthritis & Pain	Aspirin & aspirin-like medications (salicylates)
Docusate sodium	Constipation	Stool softeners
Dolobid® (diflunisal)	Arthritis & Pain	Aspirin & aspirin-like medications (salicylates)
Donnatal® (scopolamine/atropine/hyoscyamine/phenobarbital)	Irritable Bowel Syndrome	Antispasmodic medications
Dopar® (levodopa)	Parkinson's Disease	Levodopa
Doral® (quazepam)	Sleeping Difficulty	Benzodiazepines
Doxazosin	High Blood Pressure; Urinary Problems	Alpha blockers
Doxepin	Arthritis & Pain; Depression; Sleeping Difficulty; Urinary Problems	Tricyclic antidepressants
Doxidan® (docusate/phenolphthalein)	Constipation	Stool softeners; Laxatives, stimulant

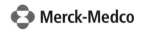

Name of Medication	Chapters	Medication Category
Dulcolax® (bisacodyl)	Constipation	Laxatives, stimulant
Duphalac® (lactulose)	Constipation	Lactulose
Duragesic® (fentanyl)	Arthritis & Pain	Narcotics
Dyazide® (triamterene/ hydrochlorothiazide)	High Blood Pressure	Diuretics, potassium-sparing; Diuretics, thiazide
Dymelor® (acetohexamide)	Diabetes	Sulfonylureas
DynaCirc® (isradipine)	Coronary Artery Disease; High Blood Pressure	Calcium channel blockers
Dyrenium® (triamterene)	High Blood Pressure	Diuretics, potassium-sparing
Ecotrin® (aspirin)	Arthritis & Pain; Stroke, Heart Attack, & Blood Clot Prevention	Aspirin & aspirin-like medications (salicylates)
Edecrin® (ethacrynic acid)	Congestive Heart Failure; High Blood Pressure	Diuretics, loop
Effexor® (venlafaxine)	Anxiety; Depression	*Effexor®* (venlafaxine)
Elavil® (amitriptyline)	Arthritis & Pain; Depression; Sleeping Difficulty; Urinary Problems	Tricyclic antidepressants
ELDEPRYL® (selegiline)	Parkinson's Disease	Selegiline
Eltroxin™ (levothyroxine)	Thyroid Problems	Thyroid medications
Empirin® (aspirin)	Arthritis & Pain; Stroke, Heart Attack, & Blood Clot Prevention	Aspirin & aspirin-like medications (salicylates)
Enalapril	Congestive Heart Failure; High Blood Pressure	ACE inhibitors
Enduron® (methyclothiazide)	High Blood Pressure	Diuretics, thiazide
Epifrin® (epinephrine)	Glaucoma	Epinephrine & *Propine®* (dipivefrin)
E-Pilo® (epinephrine/pilocarpine)	Glaucoma	Epinephrine & *Propine®* (dipivefrin); Miotic medications
Epinephrine	Asthma, Emphysema, & Chronic Bronchitis	Beta-adrenergic bronchodilators
Epinephrine eyedrops	Glaucoma	Epinephrine & *Propine®* (dipivefrin)
Equanil® (meprobamate)	Anxiety; Sleeping Difficulty	Meprobamate
Equilet® (calcium carbonate)	Heartburn, Ulcers, & Indigestion	Antacids
Esidrix® (hydrochlorothiazide)	High Blood Pressure	Diuretics, thiazide
Estazolam	Sleeping Difficulty	Benzodiazepines
Estrace® (estradiol)	Osteoporosis; Urinary Problems	Estrogen
Estraderm® (estradiol)	Osteoporosis; Urinary Problems	Estrogen
Estradiol	Osteoporosis; Urinary Problems	Estrogen
Estratab® (esterified estrogens)	Osteoporosis; Urinary Problems	Estrogen
Estratest® (esterified estrogens/ methyltestosterone)	Osteoporosis; Urinary Problems	Estrogen
Estring® (estradiol)	Urinary Problems	Estrogen

Name of Medication	Chapters	Medication Category
Estrogen	Osteoporosis; Urinary Problems	Estrogen
Estropipate	Osteoporosis; Urinary Problems	Estrogen
Ethacrynic acid	Congestive Heart Failure; High Blood Pressure	Diuretics, loop
Etodolac	Arthritis & Pain	Nonsteroidal anti-inflammatory drugs (NSAIDs)
Etrafon® (perphenazine/ amitriptyline)	Alzheimer's Disease; Depression	Neuroleptic medications; Tricyclic antidepressants
Evista® (raloxifene)	Osteoporosis	*Evista®* (raloxifene)
Excedrin® Migraine (acetaminophen/aspirin/caffeine)	Arthritis & Pain	Acetaminophen; Aspirin & aspirin-like medications (salicylates)
Excedrin P.M.® (acetaminophen/ diphenhydramine)	Arthritis & Pain; Sleeping Difficulty	Acetaminophen; Antihistamines
Exelon® (rivastigmine)	Alzheimer's Disease	Cholinesterase inhibitors
Ex-Lax® (senna)	Constipation	Laxatives, stimulant
Exna® (benzthiazide)	High Blood Pressure	Diuretics, thiazide
Extra Strength Excedrin® (acetaminophen/aspirin/caffeine)	Arthritis & Pain	Acetaminophen; Aspirin & aspirin-like medications (salicylates)
Famotidine	Heartburn, Ulcers, & Indigestion	H_2 blockers
Feldene® (piroxicam)	Arthritis & Pain	Nonsteroidal anti-inflammatory drugs (NSAIDs)
FemPatch® (estradiol)	Osteoporosis; Urinary Problems	Estrogen
Fenoprofen	Arthritis & Pain	Nonsteroidal anti-inflammatory drugs (NSAIDs)
Fiberall® (polycarbophil)	Constipation	Laxatives, bulk-forming
FiberCon® (polycarbophil)	Constipation	Laxatives, bulk-forming
Fioricet® (butalbital/ acetaminophen/caffeine)	Arthritis & Pain; Sleeping Difficulty	Barbiturates; Acetaminophen
Fioricet® with Codeine (acetaminophen/butalbital/ caffeine/codeine)	Arthritis & Pain; Sleeping Difficulty	Acetaminophen; Barbiturates; Narcotics
Fiorinal® (butalbital/aspirin/ caffeine)	Arthritis & Pain; Sleeping Difficulty	Barbiturates; Aspirin & aspirin-like medications (salicylates)
Fiorinal® with Codeine (aspirin/ caffeine/codeine/butalbital)	Arthritis & Pain; Sleeping Difficulty	Aspirin & aspirin-like medications (salicylates); Narcotics; Barbiturates
Flagyl® (metronidazole)	Heartburn, Ulcers, & Indigestion	*Flagyl®* (metronidazole)
Flavoxate	Urinary Problems	Anticholinergic medications
Fleet® (sodium phosphate/sodium biphosphate)	Constipation	Enemas
Fleet® Bisacodyl (bisacodyl)	Constipation	Enemas

Name of Medication	Chapters	Medication Category
Fleet® Phospho-soda (sodium phosphate/sodium biphosphate)	Constipation	Laxatives, saline
Flomax® (tamsulosin)	Urinary Problems	Alpha blockers
Flovent® (fluticasone)	Asthma, Emphysema, & Chronic Bronchitis	Corticosteroids
Fluphenazine	Alzheimer's Disease	Neuroleptic medications
Flurazepam	Sleeping Difficulty	Benzodiazepines
Flurbiprofen	Arthritis & Pain	Nonsteroidal anti-inflammatory drugs (NSAIDs)
Fosamax® (alendronate)	Osteoporosis	Bisphosphonates
Furosemide	Congestive Heart Failure; High Blood Pressure	Diuretics, loop
Gaviscon® (aluminum hydroxide/ alginic acid/sodium bicarbonate)	Heartburn, Ulcers, & Indigestion	Antacids
Gelusil® (aluminum hydroxide/ magnesium hydroxide/simethicone)	Heartburn, Ulcers, & Indigestion	Antacids
Gemfibrozil	High Cholesterol	Fibrates
Genapap™ (acetaminophen)	Arthritis & Pain	Acetaminophen
Glaucon® (epinephrine)	Glaucoma	Epinephrine & *Propine*® (dipivefrin)
Glipizide	Diabetes	Sulfonylureas
Glucophage® (metformin)	Diabetes	*Glucophage*® (metformin)
Glucotrol® (glipizide)	Diabetes	Sulfonylureas
Glyburide	Diabetes	Sulfonylureas
Glycerin Suppositories	Constipation	Glycerin Suppositories
Glynase® (glyburide)	Diabetes	Sulfonylureas
Glyset® (miglitol)	Diabetes	*Glyset*® (miglitol)
Halcion® (triazolam)	Sleeping Difficulty	Benzodiazepines
Haldol® (haloperidol)	Alzheimer's Disease	Neuroleptic medications
Halfprin® (aspirin)	Stroke, Heart Attack, & Blood Clot Prevention	Aspirin
Haloperidol	Alzheimer's Disease	Neuroleptic medications
Heparin	Stroke, Heart Attack, & Blood Clot Prevention	Heparin & *Lovenox*® (enoxaparin)
Hexadrol® (dexamethasone)	Arthritis & Pain; Asthma, Emphysema, & Chronic Bronchitis	Corticosteroids
Humalog® (insulin)	Diabetes	Insulin
Humorsol® (demecarium)	Glaucoma	Miotic medications
Hycodan® (hydrocodone/ homatropine)	Arthritis & Pain	Narcotics
Hydralazine	Congestive Heart Failure; High Blood Pressure	*Apresoline*® (hydralazine)
Hydrocet® (hydrocodone/ acetaminophen)	Arthritis & Pain	Narcotics; Acetaminophen

Name of Medication	Chapters	Medication Category
Hydrochlorothiazide (HCTZ)	High Blood Pressure	Diuretics, thiazide
Hydrocodone	Arthritis & Pain	Narcotics
Hydrocortisone	Arthritis & Pain; Asthma, Emphysema, & Chronic Bronchitis	Corticosteroids
Hydrocortone® (hydrocortisone)	Arthritis & Pain; Asthma, Emphysema, & Chronic Bronchitis	Corticosteroids
HydroDIURIL® (hydrochlorothiazide)	High Blood Pressure	Diuretics, thiazide
Hydroflumethiazide	High Blood Pressure	Diuretics, thiazide
Hydromorphone	Arthritis & Pain	Narcotics
Hydromox® (quinethazone)	High Blood Pressure	Diuretics, thiazide
Hydroxyzine	Anxiety	Antihistamines
Hygroton® (chlorthalidone)	High blood pressure	Diuretics, thiazide
Hyoscyamine	Irritable Bowel Syndrome; Urinary Problems	Antispasmodic medications; Anticholinergic medications
Hytrin® (terazosin)	High Blood Pressure; Urinary Problems	Alpha blockers
Hyzaar® (losartan/ hydrochlorothiazide)	High Blood Pressure	A-II blockers; Diuretics, thiazide
Ibuprofen	Arthritis & Pain	Nonsteroidal anti-inflammatory drugs (NSAIDs)
Imdur® (isosorbide mononitrate)	Congestive Heart Failure; Coronary Artery Disease	Nitrates
Imipramine	Arthritis & Pain; Depression; Sleeping Difficulty; Urinary Problems	Tricyclic antidepressants
Imodium® (loperamide)	Irritable Bowel Syndrome	Loperamide
Indapamide	Congestive Heart Failure; High Blood Pressure	Diuretics, thiazide
Inderal® (propranolol)	Congestive Heart Failure; Coronary Artery Disease; High Blood Pressure; Irregular Heartbeat	Beta blockers
Inderide® (propranolol/ hydrochlorothiazide)	High Blood Pressure	Beta blockers; Diuretics, thiazide
Indocin® (indomethacin)	Arthritis & Pain	Nonsteroidal anti-inflammatory drugs (NSAIDs)
Indomethacin	Arthritis & Pain	Nonsteroidal anti-inflammatory drugs (NSAIDs)
Insulin	Diabetes	Insulin
Intal® (cromolyn)	Asthma, Emphysema, & Chronic Bronchitis	*Intal*® (cromolyn) & *Tilade*® (nedocromil)
Iopidine® (apraclonidine)	Glaucoma	*Iopidine*® (apraclonidine)
Ipratropium	Asthma, Emphysema, & Chronic Bronchitis	*Atrovent*® (ipratropium)

Name of Medication	Chapters	Medication Category
ISMO® (isosorbide mononitrate)	Congestive Heart Failure; Coronary Artery Disease	Nitrates
Isoproterenol	Asthma, Emphysema, & Chronic Bronchitis	Beta-adrenergic bronchodilators
Isoptin® (verapamil)	Coronary Artery Disease; High Blood Pressure; Irregular Heartbeat	Calcium channel blockers
Isopto® Carbachol (carbachol)	Glaucoma	Miotic medications
Isopto® Carpine (pilocarpine)	Glaucoma	Miotic medications
Isordil® (isosorbide dinitrate)	Congestive Heart Failure; Coronary Artery Disease	Nitrates
Isosorbide dinitrate	Congestive Heart Failure; Coronary Artery Disease	Nitrates
Isosorbide mononitrate	Congestive Heart Failure; Coronary Artery Disease	Nitrates
Isuprel® (isoproterenol)	Asthma, Emphysema, & Chronic Bronchitis	Beta-adrenergic bronchodilators
KADIAN® (morphine)	Arthritis & Pain	Narcotics
Kaopectate® II (loperamide)	Irritable Bowel Syndrome	Loperamide
Kemadrin® (procyclidine)	Parkinson's Disease	Anticholinergic medications
Kerlone® (betaxolol)	Congestive Heart Failure; Coronary Artery Disease; High Blood Pressure; Irregular Heartbeat	Beta blockers
Ketoprofen	Arthritis & Pain	Nonsteroidal anti-inflammatory drugs (NSAIDs)
Ketorolac	Arthritis & Pain	Nonsteroidal anti-inflammatory drugs (NSAIDs)
Klonopin® (clonazepam)	Anxiety; Sleeping Difficulty	Benzodiazepines
Konsyl® (psyllium)	Constipation	Laxatives, bulk-forming
Kudrox® (aluminum hydroxide/ magnesium hydroxide/ simethicone)	Heartburn, Ulcers, & Indigestion	Antacids
Labetalol	Congestive Heart Failure; Coronary Artery Disease; High Blood Pressure	Beta blockers
Lactulose	Constipation	Lactulose
Lanoxicaps® (digoxin)	Congestive Heart Failure; Irregular Heartbeat	Digoxin
Lanoxin® (digoxin)	Congestive Heart Failure; Irregular Heartbeat	Digoxin
Larodopa® (levodopa)	Parkinson's Disease	Levodopa
Lasix® (furosemide)	Congestive Heart Failure; High Blood Pressure	Diuretics, loop
Lente insulin	Diabetes	Insulin
Lescol® (fluvastatin)	High Cholesterol	Statins

Name of Medication	Chapters	Medication Category
Levalbuterol	Asthma, Emphysema, & Chronic Bronchitis	Beta-adrenergic bronchodilators
Levatol® (penbutolol)	High Blood Pressure	Beta blockers
Levbid® (hyoscyamine)	Irritable Bowel Syndrome	Antispasmodic medications
Levobunolol eyedrops	Glaucoma	Beta blocker eyedrops
Levodopa	Parkinson's Disease	Levodopa
Levo-Dromoran® (levorphanol)	Arthritis & Pain	Narcotics
Levorphanol	Arthritis & Pain	Narcotics
Levo-T® (levothyroxine)	Thyroid Problems	Thyroid medications
Levothroid® (levothyroxine)	Thyroid Problems	Thyroid medications
Levothyroxine	Thyroid Problems	Thyroid medications
Levoxyl® (levothyroxine)	Thyroid Problems	Thyroid medications
Levsin® (hyoscyamine)	Irritable Bowel Syndrome; Urinary Problems	Antispasmodic medications; Anticholinergic medications
Levsinex® (hyoscyamine)	Irritable Bowel Syndrome; Urinary Problems	Antispasmodic medications; Anticholinergic medications
Lexxel® (enalapril/felodipine)	High Blood Pressure	ACE inhibitors; Calcium channel blockers
Librax® (chlordiazepoxide/clidinium)	Anxiety; Irritable Bowel Syndrome	Benzodiazepines; Antispasmodic medications
Libritabs® (chlordiazepoxide)	Anxiety; Sleeping Difficulty	Benzodiazepines
Librium® (chlordiazepoxide)	Anxiety; Sleeping Difficulty	Benzodiazepines
Limbitrol® (chlordiazepoxide/amitriptyline)	Anxiety; Depression; Sleeping Difficulty	Benzodiazepines; Tricyclic antidepressants
Liothyronine	Thyroid Problems (Hypothyroidism)	Thyroid medications
Lipitor® (atorvastatin)	High Cholesterol	Statins
Lisinopril	Congestive Heart Failure; High Blood Pressure	ACE inhibitors
LoCHOLEST® (cholestyramine)	High Cholesterol	Bile acid binders
Lodine® (etodolac)	Arthritis & Pain	Nonsteroidal anti-inflammatory drugs (NSAIDs)
Lomotil® (diphenoxylate/atropine)	Irritable Bowel Syndrome	Antispasmodic medications
Loniten® (minoxidil)	High Blood Pressure	*Loniten*® (minoxidil)
Loperamide	Irritable Bowel Syndrome	Loperamide
Lopid® (gemfibrozil)	High Cholesterol	Fibrates
Lopressor® (metoprolol)	Congestive Heart Failure; Coronary Artery Disease; High Blood Pressure; Irregular Heartbeat	Beta blockers
Lopressor HCT® (hydrochlorothiazide/metoprolol)	High Blood Pressure	Diuretics, thiazide; Beta blockers
Lorazepam	Anxiety; Sleeping Difficulty	Benzodiazepines
Lorcet® (hydrocodone/acetaminophen)	Arthritis & Pain	Narcotics; Acetaminophen

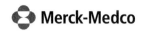

Name of Medication	Chapters	Medication Category
Lortab® (hydrocodone/acetaminophen)	Arthritis & Pain	Narcotics; Acetaminophen
Lotensin® (benazepril)	Congestive Heart Failure; High Blood Pressure	ACE inhibitors
Lotensin HCT® (benazepril/hydrochlorothiazide)	High Blood Pressure	ACE inhibitors; Diuretics, thiazide
Lotrel® (amlodipine/benazepril)	High Blood Pressure	Calcium channel blockers; ACE inhibitors
Lovenox® (enoxaparin)	Stroke, Heart Attack, & Blood Clot Prevention	Heparin & *Lovenox®* (enoxaparin)
Loxapine	Alzheimer's Disease	Neuroleptic medications
Loxitane® (loxapine)	Alzheimer's Disease	Neuroleptic medications
Lozol® (indapamide)	Congestive Heart Failure; High Blood Pressure	Diuretics, loop
Ludiomil® (maprotiline)	Arthritis & Pain; Depression	Tricyclic antidepressants
Luminal® (phenobarbital)	Sleeping Difficulty	Barbiturates
Luvox® (fluvoxamine)	Depression	Selective serotonin reuptake inhibitors (SSRIs)
Maalox® (aluminum hydroxide/magnesium hydroxide)	Heartburn, Ulcers, & Indigestion	Antacids
Magan® (magnesium salicylate)	Arthritis & Pain	Aspirin & aspirin-like medications (salicylates)
Magnalox (aluminum hydroxide/magnesium hydroxide)	Heartburn, Ulcers, & Indigestion	Antacids
Magnesium citrate	Constipation	Laxatives, saline
Magnesium hydroxide	Constipation; Heartburn, Ulcers, & Indigestion	Laxatives, saline; Antacids
Magnesium salicylate	Arthritis & Pain	Aspirin & aspirin-like medications (salicylates)
Magnesium sulfate	Constipation	Laxatives, saline
Mallamint® (calcium carbonate)	Heartburn, Ulcers, & Indigestion	Antacids
Maltsupex® (barley malt extract)	Constipation	Laxatives, bulk-forming
Maprotiline	Arthritis & Pain; Depression	Tricyclic antidepressants
Marblen™ (calcium carbonate/magnesium carbonate)	Heartburn, Ulcers, & Indigestion	Antacids
Marplan® (isocarboxazid)	Depression	MAO inhibitors
Mavik® (trandolapril)	Congestive Heart Failure; High Blood Pressure	ACE inhibitors
Maxair® (pirbuterol)	Asthma, Emphysema, & Chronic Bronchitis	Beta-adrenergic bronchodilators
Maxzide® (triamterene/hydrochlorothiazide)	High Blood Pressure	Diuretics, potassium-sparing; Diuretics, thiazide
Mebaral® (mephobarbital)	Sleeping Difficulty	Barbiturates

Name of Medication	Chapters	Medication Category
Meclofenamate	Arthritis & Pain	Nonsteroidal anti-inflammatory drugs (NSAIDs)
Medihaler-Iso® (isoproterenol)	Asthma, Emphysema, & Chronic Bronchitis	Beta-adrenergic bronchodilators
Medrol® (methylprednisolone)	Arthritis & Pain; Asthma, Emphysema, & Chronic Bronchitis	Corticosteroids
Mellaril® (thioridazine)	Alzheimer's Disease	Neuroleptic medications
Menest® (esterified estrogens)	Osteoporosis; Urinary Problems	Estrogen
Meperidine	Arthritis & Pain	Narcotics
Meprobamate	Anxiety; Sleeping Difficulty	Meprobamate
Metamucil® (psyllium)	Constipation	Laxatives, bulk-forming
Metaprel® (metaproterenol)	Asthma, Emphysema, & Chronic Bronchitis	Beta-adrenergic bronchodilators
Metaproterenol	Asthma, Emphysema, & Chronic Bronchitis	Beta-adrenergic bronchodilators
Methazolamide	Glaucoma	Carbonic anhydrase inhibitors
Methscopolamine	Irritable Bowel Syndrome	Antispasmodic medications
Methyclothiazide	High Blood Pressure	Diuretics, thiazide
Methyldopa	High Blood Pressure	*Aldomet*® (methyldopa)
Methylin® (methylphenidate)	Depression	*Ritalin*® (methylphenidate)
Methylphenidate	Depression	*Ritalin*® (methylphenidate)
Methylprednisolone	Arthritis & Pain; Asthma, Emphysema, & Chronic Bronchitis	Corticosteroids
Meticorten® (prednisone)	Arthritis & Pain; Asthma, Emphysema, & Chronic Bronchitis	Corticosteroids
Metoclopramide	Heartburn, Ulcers, & Indigestion	*Reglan*® (metoclopramide)
Metolazone	Congestive Heart Failure; High Blood Pressure	Diuretics, thiazide
Metoprolol	Congestive Heart Failure; Coronary Artery Disease; High Blood Pressure; Irregular Heartbeat	Beta blockers
Metronidazole	Heartburn, Ulcers, & Indigestion	*Flagyl*® (metronidazole)
Mevacor® (lovastatin)	High Cholesterol	Statins
Mexitil® (mexiletine)	Irregular Heartbeat	*Mexitil*® (mexiletine)
Miacalcin® (calcitonin salmon)	Osteoporosis	Calcitonin
Micardis® (telmisartan)	High Blood Pressure	A-II blockers
Micronase® (glyburide)	Diabetes	Sulfonylureas
Microzide® (hydrochlorothiazide)	High Blood Pressure	Diuretics, thiazide
Midamor® (amiloride)	High Blood Pressure	Diuretics, potassium-sparing
Miltown® (meprobamate)	Anxiety; Sleeping Difficulty	Meprobamate
Mineral oil	Constipation	Mineral oil
Minipress® (prazosin)	High Blood Pressure; Urinary Problems	Alpha blockers

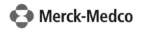 **Merck-Medco**

Name of Medication	Chapters	Medication Category
Minitran® (nitroglycerin)	Congestive Heart Failure; Coronary Artery Disease	Nitrates
Minizide® (polythiazide/prazosin)	High Blood Pressure	Diuretics, thiazide; Alpha blockers
Minoxidil	High Blood Pressure	*Loniten®* (minoxidil)
Mirapex® (pramipexole)	Parkinson's Disease	*Mirapex®* (pramipexole) & *Requip®* (ropinirole)
Mitrolan® (polycarbophil)	Constipation	Laxatives, bulk-forming
Moban® (molindone)	Alzheimer's Disease	Neuroleptic medications
Mobic® (meloxicam)	Arthritis & Pain	Nonsteroidal anti-inflammatory drugs (NSAIDs)
Mobidin® (magnesium salicylate)	Arthritis & Pain	Aspirin & aspirin-like medications (salicylates)
Moduretic® (amiloride/hydrochlorothiazide)	High Blood Pressure	Diuretics, potassium-sparing; Diuretics, thiazide
Monoket® (isosorbide mononitrate)	Congestive Heart Failure; Coronary Artery Disease	Nitrates
Monopril® (fosinopril)	Congestive Heart Failure; High Blood Pressure	ACE inhibitors
Morphine	Arthritis & Pain	Narcotics
Motrin® (ibuprofen)	Arthritis & Pain	Nonsteroidal anti-inflammatory drugs (NSAIDs)
MS Contin® (morphine)	Arthritis & Pain	Narcotics
MSIR® (morphine)	Arthritis & Pain	Narcotics
Mylanta® (aluminum hydroxide/magnesium hydroxide/simethicone)	Heartburn, Ulcers, & Indigestion	Antacids
Nabumetone	Arthritis & Pain	Nonsteroidal anti-inflammatory drugs (NSAIDs)
Nadolol	Congestive Heart Failure; Coronary Artery Disease; High Blood Pressure; Irregular Heartbeat	Beta blockers
Nalfon® (fenoprofen)	Arthritis & Pain	Nonsteroidal anti-inflammatory drugs (NSAIDs)
Naprelan® (naproxen)	Arthritis & Pain	Nonsteroidal anti-inflammatory drugs (NSAIDs)
Naprosyn® (naproxen)	Arthritis & Pain	Nonsteroidal anti-inflammatory drugs (NSAIDs)
Naproxen	Arthritis & Pain	Nonsteroidal anti-inflammatory drugs (NSAIDs)
Naqua® (trichlormethiazide)	High Blood Pressure	Diuretics, thiazide
Nardil® (phenelzine)	Depression	MAO inhibitors
Nature's Remedy® (cascara/aloe)	Constipation	Laxatives, stimulant
Naturetin® (bendroflumethiazide)	High Blood Pressure	Diuretics, thiazide
Navane® (thiothixene)	Alzheimer's Disease	Neuroleptic medications
Nembutal® (pentobarbital)	Sleeping Difficulty	Barbiturates

Name of Medication	Chapters	Medication Category
Neo-Calglucon® (calcium glubionate)	Osteoporosis	Calcium supplements
Neoloid® (castor oil)	Constipation	Laxatives, stimulant
Neptazane® (methazolamide)	Glaucoma	Carbonic anhydrase inhibitors
Neurontin® (gabapentin)	Arthritis & Pain	*Neurontin*® (gabapentin)
Niacin	High Cholesterol	Niacin
Niaspan® (niacin)	High Cholesterol	Niacin
Nicardipine	Coronary Artery Disease; High Blood Pressure	Calcium channel blockers
Nifedipine	Coronary Artery Disease; High Blood Pressure	Calcium channel blockers
Nitrek® (nitroglycerin)	Congestive Heart Failure; Coronary Artery Disease	Nitrates
Nitro-Bid® (nitroglycerin)	Congestive Heart Failure; Coronary Artery Disease	Nitrates
Nitrodisc® (nitroglycerin)	Congestive Heart Failure; Coronary Artery Disease	Nitrates
Nitro-Dur® (nitroglycerin)	Congestive Heart Failure; Coronary Artery Disease	Nitrates
Nitrogard® (nitroglycerin)	Coronary Artery Disease	Nitrates
Nitroglycerin	Congestive Heart Failure; Coronary Artery Disease	Nitrates
Nitroglyn® (nitroglycerin)	Congestive Heart Failure; Coronary Artery Disease	Nitrates
Nitrol® (nitroglycerin)	Congestive Heart Failure; Coronary Artery Disease	Nitrates
Nitrolingual® (nitroglycerin)	Coronary Artery Disease	Nitrates
Nitrong® (nitroglycerin)	Congestive Heart Failure; Coronary Artery Disease	Nitrates
NitroQuick® (nitroglycerin)	Coronary Artery Disease	Nitrates
Nitrostat® (nitroglycerin)	Coronary Artery Disease	Nitrates
Nitro-Time® (nitroglycerin)	Congestive Heart Failure; Coronary Artery Disease	Nitrates
Norco™ (hydrocodone/ acetaminophen)	Arthritis & Pain	Narcotics; Acetaminophen
Normodyne® (labetalol)	Congestive Heart Failure; Coronary Artery Disease; High Blood Pressure	Beta blockers
Norpace® (disopyramide)	Irregular Heartbeat	*Norpace*® (disopyramide)
Norpramin® (desipramine)	Arthritis & Pain; Depression; Sleeping Difficulty; Urinary Problems	Tricyclic antidepressants
Nortriptyline	Arthritis & Pain; Depression; Sleeping Difficulty; Urinary Problems	Tricyclic antidepressants

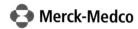
Name of Medication	Chapters	Medication Category
Norvasc® (amlodipine)	Coronary Artery Disease; High Blood Pressure	Calcium channel blockers
Novolin Prefilled™ (insulin)	Diabetes	Insulin
NovoPen® 3 (insulin)	Diabetes	Insulin
NPH Insulin	Diabetes	Insulin
Nytol® (diphenhydramine)	Sleeping Difficulty	Antihistamines
Ocupress® (carteolol)	Glaucoma	Beta blocker eyedrops
Ocusert® (pilocarpine)	Glaucoma	Miotic medications
Ogen® (estropipate)	Osteoporosis; Urinary Problems	Estrogen
OptiPranolol® (metipranolol)	Glaucoma	Beta blocker eyedrops
Oramorph® SR (morphine)	Arthritis & Pain	Narcotics
Orasone® (prednisone)	Arthritis & Pain; Asthma, Emphysema, & Chronic Bronchitis	Corticosteroids
Oretic® (hydrochlorothiazide)	High Blood Pressure	Diuretics, thiazide
Orinase® (tolbutamide)	Diabetes	Sulfonylureas
Ortho-EST® (estropipate)	Osteoporosis; Urinary Problems	Estrogen
Ortho-Prefest® pill (estradiol/ norgestimate)	Osteoporosis; Urinary Problems	Estrogen
Orudis® (ketoprofen)	Arthritis & Pain	Nonsteroidal anti-inflammatory drugs (NSAIDs)
Oruvail® (ketoprofen)	Arthritis & Pain	Nonsteroidal anti-inflammatory drugs (NSAIDs)
Os-Cal 500® (calcium carbonate)	Osteoporosis	Calcium supplements
Oxazepam	Anxiety; Sleeping Difficulty	Benzodiazepines
Oxybutynin	Urinary Problems	Anticholinergic medications
Oxycodone	Arthritis & Pain	Narcotics
OxyContin® (oxycodone)	Arthritis & Pain	Narcotics
OxyFAST™ (oxycodone)	Arthritis & Pain	Narcotics
OxyIR® (oxycodone)	Arthritis & Pain	Narcotics
P.V. Carpine® (pilocarpine)	Glaucoma	Miotic medications
P_1E_1®, P_2E_1®, P_4E_1®, P_6E_1® (pilocarpine/epinephrine)	Glaucoma	Miotic medications; Epinephrine & *Propine*® (dipivefrin)
Pacerone® (amiodarone)	Irregular Heartbeat	Amiodarone
Pamelor® (nortriptyline)	Arthritis & Pain; Depression; Sleeping Difficulty; Urinary Problems	Tricyclic antidepressants
Pamine® (methscopolamine)	Irritable Bowel Syndrome	Antispasmodic medications
Panadol® (acetaminophen)	Arthritis & Pain	Acetaminophen
Parlodel® (bromocriptine)	Parkinson's Disease	*Parlodel*® (bromocriptine) & *Permax*® (pergolide)
Parnate® (tranylcypromine)	Depression	MAO inhibitors
Paxil® (paroxetine)	Depression	Selective serotonin reuptake inhibitors (SSRIs)

Name of Medication	Chapters	Medication Category
Paxipam® (halazepam)	Anxiety; Sleeping Difficulty	Benzodiazepines
Pentobarbital	Sleeping Difficulty	Barbiturates
Pepcid® (famotidine)	Heartburn, Ulcers, & Indigestion	H_2 blockers
Pepto-Bismol® (bismuth subsalicylate)	Heartburn, Ulcers, & Indigestion	*Pepto-Bismol®* (bismuth subsalicylate)
Pepto Diarrhea Control® (loperamide)	Irritable Bowel Syndrome	Loperamide
Percocet® (oxycodone/acetaminophen)	Arthritis & Pain	Narcotics; Acetaminophen
Percodan® (oxycodone/aspirin)	Arthritis & Pain	Narcotics; Aspirin & aspirin-like medications (salicylates)
Percolone® (oxycodone)	Arthritis & Pain	Narcotics
Perdiem® Fiber (psyllium)	Constipation	Laxatives, bulk-forming
Peri-Colace® (docusate sodium/casanthranol)	Constipation	Stool softeners; Laxatives, stimulant
Permax® (pergolide)	Parkinson's Disease	*Parlodel®* (bromocriptine) & *Permax®* (pergolide)
Perphenazine	Alzheimer's Disease	Neuroleptic medications
Persantine® (dipyridamole)	Stroke, Heart Attack, & Blood Clot Prevention	Dipyridamole (*Persantine®* & *Aggrenox®*)
Phenaphen® with Codeine (acetaminophen/codeine)	Arthritis & Pain	Acetaminophen; Narcotics
Phenobarbital	Sleeping Difficulty	Barbiturates
Phillips' Milk of Magnesia® (magnesium hydroxide)	Constipation; Heartburn, Ulcers, & Indigestion	Laxatives, saline; Antacids
Phospholine Iodide® (echothiophate iodide)	Glaucoma	Miotic medications
Pilocar® (pilocarpine)	Glaucoma	Miotic medications
Pilocarpine	Glaucoma	Miotic medications
Pilostat® (pilocarpine)	Glaucoma	Miotic medications
Pindolol	High Blood Pressure	Beta blockers
Piroxicam	Arthritis & Pain	Nonsteroidal anti-inflammatory drugs (NSAIDs)
Plavix® (clopidogrel)	Stroke, Heart Attack, & Blood Clot Prevention	*Plavix®* (clopidogrel) & *Ticlid®* (ticlopidine)
Plendil® (felodipine)	Coronary Artery Disease; High Blood Pressure	Calcium channel blockers
Polycarbophil	Constipation	Laxatives, bulk-forming
Posture® (tricalcium phosphate)	Osteoporosis	Calcium supplements
Prandin™ (repaglinide)	Diabetes	*Prandin™* (repaglinide)
Pravachol® (pravastatin)	High Cholesterol	Statins
Prazosin	High Blood Pressure; Urinary Problems	Alpha blockers
Precose® (acarbose)	Diabetes	*Precose®* (acarbose)

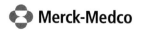

Name of Medication	Chapters	Medication Category
Prednisolone	Arthritis & Pain; Asthma, Emphysema, & Chronic Bronchitis	Corticosteroids
Prednisone	Arthritis & Pain; Asthma, Emphysema, & Chronic Bronchitis	Corticosteroids
Prelone® (prednisolone)	Arthritis & Pain; Asthma, Emphysema, & Chronic Bronchitis	Corticosteroids
Premarin® (conjugated estrogens)	Osteoporosis; Urinary Problems	Estrogen
Premphase® (conjugated estrogens/ medroxyprogesterone)	Osteoporosis; Urinary Problems	Estrogen
Prempro™ (conjugated estrogens/ medroxyprogesterone)	Osteoporosis; Urinary Problems	Estrogen
PREVACID® (lansoprazole)	Heartburn, Ulcers, & Indigestion	Proton pump inhibitors
Prevalite® (cholestyramine)	High Cholesterol	Bile acid binders
Prilosec® (omeprazole)	Heartburn, Ulcers, & Indigestion	Proton pump inhibitors
Primatene® Mist (epinephrine)	Asthma, Emphysema, & Chronic Bronchitis	Beta-adrenergic bronchodilators
Prinivil® (lisinopril)	Congestive Heart Failure; High Blood Pressure	ACE inhibitors
Prinzide® (hydrochlorothiazide/ lisinopril)	High Blood Pressure	Diuretics, thiazide; ACE inhibitors
Pro-Banthine® (propantheline)	Irritable Bowel Syndrome; Urinary Problems	Antispasmodic medications; Anticholinergic medications
Procainamide	Irregular Heartbeat	Procainamide
Procanbid® (procainamide)	Irregular Heartbeat	Procainamide
Procardia® (nifedipine)	Coronary Artery Disease; High Blood Pressure	Calcium channel blockers
Prolixin® (fluphenazine)	Alzheimer's Disease	Neuroleptic medications
Pronestyl® (procainamide)	Irregular Heartbeat	Procainamide
Propantheline	Irritable Bowel Syndrome; Urinary Problems	Antispasmodic medications; Anticholinergic medications
Propine® (dipivefrin)	Glaucoma	Epinephrine & Propine® (dipivefrin)
Propoxyphene	Arthritis & Pain	Narcotics
Propranolol	Congestive Heart Failure; Coronary Artery Disease; High Blood Pressure; Irregular Heartbeat	Beta blockers
Propulsid® (cisapride)	Heartburn, Ulcers, & Indigestion	Propulsid® (cisapride)
Propylthiouracil (PTU)	Thyroid Problems	Propylthiouracil (PTU) & Tapazole® (methimazole)
Proscar® (finasteride)	Urinary Problems	Proscar® (finasteride)
ProSom™ (estazolam)	Sleeping Difficulty	Benzodiazepines
Protonix® (pantoprazole)	Heartburn, Ulcers, & Indigestion	Proton pump inhibitors
Protriptyline	Depression	Tricyclic antidepressants

Name of Medication	Chapters	Medication Category
Proventil® (albuterol)	Asthma, Emphysema, & Chronic Bronchitis	Beta-adrenergic bronchodilators
Prozac® (fluoxetine)	Depression	Selective serotonin reuptake inhibitors (SSRIs)
Pseudoephedrine	Urinary Problems	*Sudafed*® (pseudoephedrine)
Psyllium	Constipation	Laxatives, bulk-forming
PTU	Thyroid Problems	Propylthiouracil (PTU) & *Tapazole*® (methimazole)
Pulmicort® (budesonide)	Asthma, Emphysema, & Chronic Bronchitis	Corticosteroids
Quarzan® (clidinium)	Irritable Bowel Syndrome	Antispasmodic medications
Questran® (cholestyramine)	High Cholesterol	Bile acid binders
Quinaglute Dura-Tabs® (quinidine gluconate)	Irregular Heartbeat	Quinidine
Quinidex® (quinidine sulfate)	Irregular Heartbeat	Quinidine
Quinidine	Irregular Heartbeat	Quinidine
Quinora® (quinidine sulfate)	Irregular Heartbeat	Quinidine
Ranitidine	Heartburn, Ulcers, & Indigestion	H$_2$ blockers
Reglan® (metoclopramide)	Heartburn, Ulcers, & Indigestion	*Reglan*® (metoclopramide)
Regular Insulin	Diabetes	Insulin
Relafen® (nabumetone)	Arthritis & Pain	Nonsteroidal anti-inflammatory drugs (NSAIDs)
Remeron® (mirtazapine)	Depression	*Remeron*® (mirtazapine)
Renese® (polythiazide)	High Blood Pressure	Diuretics, thiazide
Requip® (ropinirole)	Parkinson's Disease	*Mirapex*® (pramipexole) & *Requip*® (ropinirole)
Restoril® (temazepam)	Sleeping Difficulty	Benzodiazepines
Riopan® (magaldrate)	Heartburn, Ulcers, & Indigestion	Antacids
Riopan Plus® (magaldrate/simethicone)	Heartburn, Ulcers, & Indigestion	Antacids
Risperdal® (risperidone)	Alzheimer's Disease	Neuroleptic medications
Ritalin® (methylphenidate)	Depression	*Ritalin*® (methylphenidate)
Rolaids® (calcium carbonate)	Heartburn, Ulcers, & Indigestion; Osteoporosis	Antacids; Calcium supplements
Roxanol® (morphine)	Arthritis & Pain	Narcotics
Roxicet™ (oxycodone/ acetaminophen)	Arthritis & Pain	Narcotics; Acetaminophen
Rythmol® (propafenone)	Irregular Heartbeat	*Rythmol*® (propafenone)
Salflex® (salsalate)	Arthritis & Pain	Aspirin & aspirin-like medications (salicylates)
Salsalate	Arthritis & Pain	Aspirin & aspirin-like medications (salicylates)
Seconal® (secobarbital)	Sleeping Difficulty	Barbiturates

Name of Medication	Chapters	Medication Category
Sectral® (acebutolol)	High Blood Pressure	Beta blockers
Selegiline	Parkinson's Disease	Selegiline
Senna	Constipation	Laxatives, stimulant
Senokot® (senna)	Constipation	Laxatives, stimulant
Senokot-S® (senna/docusate)	Constipation	Laxatives, stimulant; Stool softeners
Serax® (oxazepam)	Anxiety; Sleeping Difficulty	Benzodiazepines
Serentil® (mesoridazine)	Alzheimer's Disease	Neuroleptic medications
Serevent® (salmeterol)	Asthma, Emphysema, & Chronic Bronchitis	Beta-adrenergic bronchodilators
Seroquel® (quetiapine)	Alzheimer's Disease	Neuroleptic medications
Serzone® (nefazodone)	Depression	*Desyrel®* (trazodone) & *Serzone®* (nefazodone)
Simaal™ (aluminum hydroxide/ magnesium hydroxide/simethicone)	Heartburn, Ulcers, & Indigestion	Antacids
Simply Sleep® (diphenhydramine)	Sleeping Difficulty	Antihistamines
Sinemet® (carbidopa/levodopa)	Parkinson's Disease	Levodopa
Sinequan® (doxepin)	Arthritis & Pain; Depression; Sleeping Difficulty; Urinary Problems	Tricyclic antidepressants
Singulair® (montelukast)	Asthma, Emphysema, & Chronic Bronchitis	Leukotriene modifiers
Sleep-eze 3® (diphenhydramine)	Sleeping Difficulty	Antihistamines
Slo-bid™ (theophylline)	Asthma, Emphysema, & Chronic Bronchitis	Theophylline
Slo-Niacin® (niacin)	High Cholesterol	Niacin
Slo-Phyllin® (theophylline)	Asthma, Emphysema, & Chronic Bronchitis	Theophylline
Sodium bicarbonate	Heartburn, Ulcers, & Indigestion	Antacids
Sodium diphosphate & sodium phosphate	Constipation	Enemas
Sodium phosphate	Constipation	Laxatives, saline
Sominex® (diphenhydramine)	Sleeping Difficulty	Antihistamines
Sonata® (zaleplon)	Sleeping Difficulty	*Sonata®* (zaleplon)
Sorbitrate Chewable® (isosorbide dinitrate)	Coronary Artery Disease	Nitrates
Sorbitrate® (isosorbide dinitrate)	Congestive Heart Failure; Coronary Artery Disease	Nitrates
Spironolactone	Congestive Heart Failure; High Blood Pressure	Diuretics, potassium-sparing
Spironolactone & hydrochlorothiazide	High Blood Pressure	Diuretics, potassium-sparing; Diuretics, thiazide
Stadol® (butorphanol)	Arthritis & Pain	Narcotics
Stelazine® (trifluoperazine)	Alzheimer's Disease	Neuroleptic medications

Name of Medication	Chapters	Medication Category
Sucralfate	Heartburn, Ulcers, & Indigestion	*Carafate*® (sucralfate)
Sudafed® (pseudoephedrine)	Urinary Problems	*Sudafed*® (pseudoephedrine)
Sular® (nisoldipine)	Coronary Artery Disease; High Blood Pressure	Calcium channel blockers
Sulindac	Arthritis & Pain	Nonsteroidal anti-inflammatory drugs (NSAIDs)
Sumycin® (tetracycline)	Heartburn, Ulcers, & Indigestion	Tetracycline
Surfak® (docusate calcium)	Constipation	Stool softeners
Surmontil® (trimipramine)	Arthritis & Pain; Depression; Sleeping Difficulty; Urinary Problems	Tricyclic antidepressants
Symmetrel® (amantadine)	Parkinson's Disease	*Symmetrel*® (amantadine)
Synthroid® (levothyroxine)	Thyroid Problems	Thyroid medications
Tagamet® (cimetidine)	Heartburn, Ulcers, & Indigestion	H_2 blockers
Talacen® (pentazocine/ acetaminophen)	Arthritis & Pain	Narcotics; Acetaminophen
Talwin® (pentazocine)	Arthritis & Pain	Narcotics
Tambocor® (flecainide)	Irregular Heartbeat	*Tambocor*® (flecainide)
Tapazole® (methimazole)	Thyroid problems	Propylthiouracil (PTU) & *Tapazole*® (methimazole)
Tarka® (trandolapril/verapamil)	High Blood Pressure	ACE inhibitors; Calcium channel blockers
Tasmar® (tolcapone)	Parkinson's Disease	*Tasmar*® (tolcapone)
Teczem® (diltiazem/enalapril)	High Blood Pressure	Calcium channel blockers; ACE inhibitors
Tegretol® (carbamazepine)	Arthritis & Pain	*Tegretol*® (carbamazepine) & *Trileptal*® (oxcarbazepine)
Temazepam	Sleeping Difficulty	Benzodiazepines
Tempo® (calcium carbonate/ aluminum hydroxide/ magnesium hydroxide)	Heartburn, Ulcers, & Indigestion	Antacids
Tenoretic® (chlorthalidone/atenolol)	High Blood Pressure	Diuretics, thiazide; Beta blockers
Tenormin® (atenolol)	Congestive Heart Failure; Coronary Artery Disease; High Blood Pressure; Irregular Heartbeat	Beta blockers
Terbutaline	Asthma, Emphysema, & Chronic Bronchitis	Beta-adrenergic bronchodilators
Tetracycline	Heartburn, Ulcers, & Indigestion	Tetracycline
Teveten® (eprosartan)	High Blood Pressure	A-II blockers
Theo-24® (theophylline)	Asthma, Emphysema, & Chronic Bronchitis	Theophylline
Theobid® (theophylline)	Asthma, Emphysema, & Chronic Bronchitis	Theophylline

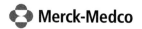

Name of Medication	Chapters	Medication Category
Theo-Dur® (theophylline)	Asthma, Emphysema, & Chronic Bronchitis	Theophylline
Theolair™ (theophylline)	Asthma, Emphysema, & Chronic Bronchitis	Theophylline
Theophylline	Asthma, Emphysema, & Chronic Bronchitis	Theophylline
Theo-X® (theophylline)	Asthma, Emphysema, & Chronic Bronchitis	Theophylline
Therevac® Plus (docusate sodium/ glycerin/benzocaine)	Constipation	Enemas
Therevac®-SB (docusate sodium/glycerin)	Constipation	Enemas
Thioridazine	Alzheimer's Disease	Neuroleptic medications
Thiothixene	Alzheimer's Disease	Neuroleptic medications
Thorazine® (chlorpromazine)	Alzheimer's Disease	Neuroleptic medications
Thyrolar® (liotrix)	Thyroid Problems	Thyroid medications
Tiamate® (diltiazem)	Coronary Artery Disease; High Blood Pressure; Irregular Heartbeat	Calcium channel blockers
Tiazac® (diltiazem)	Coronary Artery Disease; High Blood Pressure; Irregular Heartbeat	Calcium channel blockers
Ticlid® (ticlopidine)	Stroke, Heart Attack, & Blood Clot Prevention	*Plavix®* (clopidogrel) & *Ticlid®* (ticlopidine)
Ticlopidine	Stroke, Heart Attack, & Blood Clot Prevention	*Plavix®* (clopidogrel) & *Ticlid®* (ticlopidine)
Tilade® (nedocromil)	Asthma, Emphysema, & Chronic Bronchitis	*Intal®* (cromolyn) & *Tilade®* (nedocromil)
Timolide® (hydrochlorothiazide/ timolol)	High Blood Pressure	Diuretics, thiazide; Beta blockers
Timolol eyedrops	Glaucoma	Beta blocker eyedrops
Timolol tablets	Congestive Heart Failure; Coronary Artery Disease; High Blood Pressure; Irregular Heartbeat	Beta blockers
Timoptic® (timolol)	Glaucoma	Beta blocker eyedrops
Titralac® (calcium carbonate)	Heartburn, Ulcers, & Indigestion	Antacids
Titralac® Plus (calcium carbonate/ simethicone)	Heartburn, Ulcers, & Indigestion	Antacids
Tofranil® (imipramine)	Arthritis & Pain; Depression; Sleeping Difficulty; Urinary Problems	Tricyclic antidepressants
Tolazamide	Diabetes	Sulfonylureas
Tolbutamide	Diabetes	Sulfonylureas
Tolectin® (tolmetin)	Arthritis & Pain	Nonsteroidal anti-inflammatory drugs (NSAIDs)

Name of Medication	Chapters	Medication Category
Tolinase® (tolazamide)	Diabetes	Sulfonylureas
Tolmetin	Arthritis & Pain	Nonsteroidal anti-inflammatory drugs (NSAIDs)
Tonocard® (tocainide)	Irregular Heartbeat	*Tonocard*® (tocainide)
Toprol® (metoprolol)	Congestive Heart Failure; Coronary Artery Disease; High Blood Pressure; Irregular Heartbeat	Beta blockers
Toradol® (ketorolac)	Arthritis & Pain	Nonsteroidal anti-inflammatory drugs (NSAIDs)
Tornalate® (bitolterol)	Asthma, Emphysema, & Chronic Bronchitis	Beta-adrenergic bronchodilators
T-Phyl® (theophylline)	Asthma, Emphysema, & Chronic Bronchitis	Theophylline
Trandate® (labetalol)	Congestive Heart Failure; Coronary Artery Disease; High Blood Pressure	Beta blockers
Transderm-Nitro® (nitroglycerin)	Congestive Heart Failure; Coronary Artery Disease	Nitrates
Tranxene® (clorazepate)	Anxiety; Sleeping Difficulty	Benzodiazepines
Trazodone	Depression; Sleeping Difficulty	*Desyrel*® (trazodone) & *Serzone*® (nefazodone)
Triamcinolone	Arthritis & Pain; Asthma, Emphysema, & Chronic Bronchitis	Corticosteroids
Triamterene & hydrochlorothiazide	High Blood Pressure	Diuretics, potassium-sparing; Diuretics, thiazide
Triazolam	Sleeping Difficulty	Benzodiazepines
Trichlormethiazide	High Blood Pressure	Diuretics, thiazide
Tricor® (fenofibrate)	High Cholesterol	Fibrates
Trifluoperazine	Alzheimer's Disease	Neuroleptic medications
Trihexyphenidyl	Parkinson's Disease	Anticholinergic medications
Trilafon® (perphénazine)	Alzheimer's Disease	Neuroleptic medications
Trileptal® (oxcarbazepine)	Arthritis & Pain	*Tegretol*® (carbamazepine) & *Trileptal*® (oxcarbazepine)
Trilisate® (choline magnesium trisalicylate)	Arthritis & Pain	Aspirin & aspirin-like medications (salicylates)
Trusopt® (dorzolamide)	Glaucoma	Carbonic anhydrase inhibitors
Tums® (calcium carbonate)	Heartburn, Ulcers, & Indigestion; Osteoporosis	Antacids; Calcium supplements
TYLENOL® (acetaminophen)	Arthritis & Pain	Acetaminophen
TYLENOL® *with Codeine* (acetaminophen/codeine)	Arthritis & Pain	Acetaminophen; Narcotics
TYLENOL® PM (diphenhydramine/acetaminophen)	Arthritis & Pain; Sleeping Difficulty	Antihistamines; Acetaminophen
Tylox® (oxycodone/acetaminophen)	Arthritis & Pain	Narcotics; Acetaminophen

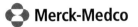

Name of Medication	Chapters	Medication Category
Ultra-Lente insulin	Diabetes	Insulin
Ultram® (tramadol)	Arthritis & Pain	*Ultram®* (tramadol)
Uni-Dur® (theophylline)	Asthma, Emphysema, & Chronic Bronchitis	Theophylline
Unifiber® (cellulose)	Constipation	Laxatives, bulk-forming
Uniphyl® (theophylline)	Asthma, Emphysema, & Chronic Bronchitis	Theophylline
Uniretic® (moexipril/ hydrochlorothiazide)	High Blood Pressure	ACE Inhibitors; Diuretics, thiazide
Unisom® (doxylamine)	Sleeping Difficulty	Antihistamines
Univasc® (moexipril)	Congestive Heart Failure; High Blood Pressure	ACE inhibitors
Urispas® (flavoxate)	Urinary Problems	Anticholinergic medications
Vagifem® (estradiol)	Urinary Problems	Estrogen
Valium® (diazepam)	Anxiety; Sleeping Difficulty	Benzodiazepines
Vanceril® (beclomethasone)	Asthma, Emphysema, & Chronic Bronchitis	Corticosteroids
Vascor® (bepridil)	Coronary Artery Disease; High Blood Pressure	Calcium channel blockers
Vaseretic® (hydrochlorothiazide/ enalapril)	High Blood Pressure	Diuretics, thiazide, ACE inhibitors
Vasotec® (enalapril)	Congestive Heart Failure; High Blood Pressure	ACE inhibitors
Ventolin® (albuterol)	Asthma, Emphysema, & Chronic Bronchitis	Beta-adrenergic bronchodilators
Verapamil	Coronary Artery Disease; High Blood Pressure; Irregular Heartbeat	Calcium channel blockers
Verelan® (verapamil)	Coronary Artery Disease; High Blood Pressure; Irregular Heartbeat	Calcium channel blockers
Viactiv® (calcium carbonate/ Vitamins D & K)	Osteoporosis	Calcium supplements; Vitamin D
Vicodin® (hydrocodone/ acetaminophen)	Arthritis & Pain	Narcotics; Acetaminophen
Vicoprofen® (hydrocodone/ ibuprofen)	Arthritis & Pain	Narcotics; Nonsteroidal anti-inflammatory drugs (NSAIDs)
Vioxx® (rofecoxib)	Arthritis & Pain	Cox-2 inhibitors
Visken® (pindolol)	High Blood Pressure	Beta blockers
Vistaril® (hydroxyzine)	Anxiety	Antihistamines
Vivactil® (protriptyline)	Depression	Tricyclic antidepressants
Vivelle® (estradiol)	Osteoporosis; Urinary Problems	Estrogen
Voltaren® (diclofenac)	Arthritis & Pain	Nonsteroidal anti-inflammatory drugs (NSAIDs)

Name of Medication	Chapters	Medication Category
Warfarin	Stroke, Heart Attack, & Blood Clot Prevention	*Coumadin*® (warfarin)
Wellbutrin® (bupropion)	Depression	*Wellbutrin*® (bupropion)
Wygesic® (propoxyphene/ acetaminophen)	Arthritis & Pain	Narcotics; Acetaminophen
Xalatan® (latanoprost)	Glaucoma	*Xalatan*® (latanoprost)
Xanax® (alprazolam)	Anxiety; Sleeping Difficulty	Benzodiazepines
Xopenex™ (levalbuterol)	Asthma, Emphysema, & Chronic Bronchitis	Beta-adrenergic bronchodilators
Zantac® (ranitidine)	Heartburn, Ulcers, & Indigestion	H_2 blockers
Zaroxolyn® (metolazone)	Congestive Heart Failure; High Blood Pressure	Diuretics, thiazide
Zebeta® (bisoprolol)	Congestive Heart Failure; Coronary Artery Disease; High Blood Pressure; Irregular Heartbeat	Beta blockers
Zestoretic® (hydrochlorothiazide/ lisinopril)	High Blood Pressure	Diuretics, thiazides; ACE inhibitors
Zestril® (lisinopril)	Congestive Heart Failure; High Blood Pressure	ACE inhibitors
Ziac® (hydrochlorothiazide/ bisoprolol)	High Blood Pressure	Diuretics, thiazide; Beta blockers
Zocor® (simvastatin)	High Cholesterol	Statins
Zoloft® (sertraline)	Depression	Selective serotonin reuptake inhibitors (SSRIs)
ZORprin® (aspirin)	Arthritis & Pain; Stroke, Heart Attack, & Blood Clot Prevention	Aspirin & aspirin-like medications (salicylates)
Zostrix® (capsaicin)	Arthritis & Pain	Capsaicin
Zydone® (hydrocodone/ acetaminophen)	Arthritis & Pain	Narcotics; Acetaminophen
Zyflo® (zileuton)	Asthma, Emphysema, & Chronic Bronchitis	Leukotriene modifiers
Zyprexa® (olanzapine)	Alzheimer's Disease	Neuroleptic medications

Manufacturer Listing

Complete names of manufacturers appear at the end of this list.

Name of Medication	Manufacturer
Accolate®	AstraZeneca
Accupril®	Pfizer
Accuretic™	Pfizer
Aceon®	Solvay
Achromycin®	American Home Products
AcipHex®	Eisai/Janssen
Actigall®	Novartis
Actonel®	Procter & Gamble
Actos®	Takeda/Eli Lilly
Acuprin 81®	Integrity
Adalat®	Bayer
Adsorbocarpine™	Alcon
Advil®	American Home Products
AeroBid®	Forest
Aggrenox®	Boehringer Ingelheim
Agoral®	Pfizer
Akineton®	Knoll
Alamag®	Goldline
Aldactazide®	Pharmacia
Aldactone®	Pharmacia
Aldoclor®	Merck
Aldomet®	Merck
Aldoril®	Merck
Aleve®	Procter & Gamble
Alka-Mints®	Bayer
Alkets®	Pharmacia

Name of Medication	Manufacturer
Allegra®	Aventis
Alora®	Procter & Gamble
Alphagan®	Allergan
Altace®	Monarch
AlternaGEL®	Johnson & Johnson/Merck
Alupent®	Boehringer Ingelheim
Alurate®	Roche
Amaryl®	Aventis
Ambien®	Pharmacia
Amen®	Carnrick
Amerge®	GlaxoWellcome
Amitone®	Menley and James
Amoxil®	SmithKline Beecham
Amphojel®	American Home Products
Anacin®	American Home Products
Anacin3®	American Home Products
Anafranil®	Novartis
Anaprox®	Roche
Anaspaz®	B. F. Ascher
Ansaid®	Pharmacia
Antabuse®	American Home Products
Anturane®	Novartis
Apresazide®	Novartis
Apresoline®	Novartis
Aquachloral®	PolyMedica
Aquatensen®	Wallace
Aricept®	Eisai/Pfizer
Aristocort®	Fujisawa
Armour® *Thyroid*	Forest
Artane®	American Home Products
Arthritis Pain Formula™	American Home Products
Arthrotec®	Pharmacia
Ascriptin®	Aventis
Asendin®	American Home Products
Aspirin Free Excedrin®	Bristol-Myers Squibb

Name of Medication	Manufacturer
AsthmaNefrin®	Numark
Atacand®	AstraZeneca
Atamet®	Elan
Atapryl™	Elan
Atarax®	Pfizer
Ativan®	American Home Products
Atromid-S®	American Home Products
Atrovent®	Boehringer Ingelheim
Augmentin®	SmithKline Beecham
Avalide®	Bristol-Myers Squibb
Avandia®	SmithKline Beecham
Avapro®	Bristol-Myers Squibb
Axid®	Eli Lilly
Azmacort®	Aventis
Azopt®	Alcon
Azulfidine®	Pharmacia
Bactrim®	Roche
Basaljel®	American Home Products
Baycol®	Bayer
Beclovent®	GlaxoWellcome
Bell/ans™	C.S. Dent
Benadryl®	Pfizer
Benemid®	Merck
Bentyl®	Aventis
Betagan®	Allergan
Betapace®	Berlex
Betaseron®	Berlex
Betoptic®	Alcon
Biaxin®	Abbott
Blocadren®	Merck
Brethaire®	Novartis
Brethine®	Novartis
Bricanyl®	Aventis
Bromo-Seltzer®	Pfizer
Bufferin®	Bristol-Myers Squibb

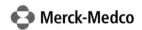

Name of Medication	Manufacturer
Bumex®	Roche
BuSpar®	Bristol-Myers Squibb
Butisol®	Wallace
Cafergot®	Novartis
Calan®	Pharmacia
Calcet Plus®	Mission
Calcimar®	Aventis
Caltrate®	American Home Products
Cantil®	Aventis
Capoten®	Bristol-Myers Squibb
Capozide®	Bristol-Myers Squibb
Capsin®	Fleming
Carafate®	Aventis
Carbatrol®	Shire
Carbex®	Endo
Carboptic®	Optopics
Cardene®	Roche
Cardioquin®	Purdue Frederick
Cardizem®	Aventis
Cardura®	Pfizer
Cartrol®	Abbott
Cataflam®	Novartis
Catapres®	Boehringer Ingelheim
Ceftin®	GlaxoWellcome
Cefzil®	Bristol-Myers Squibb
Celebrex®	Pfizer
Celestone®	Schering-Plough
Celexa™	Forest
Cenestin®	Elan
Cephulac®	Aventis
Cerebyx®	Pfizer
Chloromycetin®	Pfizer
Chooz®	Schering-Plough
Chronulac®	Aventis
Cipro®	Bayer

Name of Medication	Manufacturer
Citracal®	Mission
Citrocarbonate®	Shire
Citrucel®	SmithKline Beecham
Claritin®	Schering-Plough
Climara®	Berlex
Clinoril®	Merck
Clorpres®	Bertek
Clozaril®	Novartis
Cogentin®	Merck
Cognex®	Pfizer
Colace®	Mead Johnson
Colestid®	Pharmacia
CombiPatch®	Aventis
Combipres®	Boehringer Ingelheim
Combivent®	Boehringer Ingelheim
Compazine®	SmithKline Beecham
Comtan®	Novartis
Cordarone®	American Home Products
Coreg®	SmithKline Beecham
Corgard®	Bristol-Myers Squibb
Correctol®	Schering-Plough
Cortef®	Pharmacia
Cortone®	Merck
Corzide®	Bristol-Myers Squibb
Cosopt®	Merck
Cotazym®	Organon
Coumadin®	DuPont
Covera®	Pharmacia
Cozaar®	Merck
Creon®	Solvay
Crixivan®	Merck
Cycrin®	ESI Lederle
Cystospaz®	PolyMedica
Cytadren®	Novartis
Cytomel®	SmithKline Beecham

Name of Medication	Manufacturer
Cytotec®	Pharmacia
D.H.E.-45®	Novartis
Dalmane®	Roche
Danocrine®	Sanofi
Dantrium®	Procter & Gamble
Daranide®	Merck
Darvocet-N®	Eli Lilly
Darvon®	Eli Lilly
Darvon® Compound	Eli Lilly
Daypro®	Pharmacia
Decadron®	Merck
Declomycin®	American Home Products
Delta-Cortef®	Pharmacia
Demadex®	Roche
Demerol®	Sanofi
Depakene®	Abbott
Depakote®	Abbott
Deponit®	Schwarz
Desyrel®	Mead Johnson
Detrol®	Pharmacia
DiaBeta®	Aventis
Diabinese®	Pfizer
Diamox®	American Home Products
Diar-aid®	Thompson
Dicarbosil®	BIRA
Didronel®	Procter & Gamble
Diflucan®	Pfizer
Di-Gel®	Schering-Plough
Dilacor®	Watson
Dilantin®	Pfizer
Dilatrate®	Schwarz
Dilaudid®	Knoll
Diltia®	Andrx
Diocto-K®	Watson
Diovan HCT®	Novartis

Name of Medication	Manufacturer
Diovan®	Novartis
Disalcid®	3M
Ditropan®	Alza
Diucardin®	American Home Products
Diurese™	American Urologicals
Diuril®	Merck
Doan's® Pills	Novartis
Dolobid®	Merck
Donnatal®	American Home Products
Donnazyme®	American Home Products
Dopar®	Procter & Gamble
Doral®	Wallace
Doxidan®	Pharmacia
Dulcolax®	Novartis
Duphalac®	Solvay
Duragesic®	Janssen
Dyazide®	SmithKline Beecham
Dymelor®	Eli Lilly
Dynabac®	Sanofi
Dynacin®	Medicis
DynaCirc®	Novartis
Dyrenium®	SmithKline Beecham
E.E.S. 400®	Abbott
Ecotrin®	SmithKline Beecham
Edecrin®	Merck
Effexor®	American Home Products
Elavil®	AstraZeneca
ELDEPRYL®	Somerset
Eltroxin™	Shire
Empirin®	GlaxoWellcome
E-Mycin®	Knoll
Enduron®	Abbott
Epifrin®	Allergan
E-Pilo®	Novartis
EpiPen®	Dey

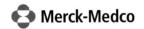

Name of Medication	Manufacturer
Equanil®	American Home Products
Equilet®	Mission
Ergamisol®	Janssen
Ergomar®	Lotus
Eryc®	Pfizer
Ery-Tab®	Abbott
Erythrocin®	Abbott
Esidrix®	Novartis
Eskalith®	SmithKline Beecham
Estrace®	Bristol-Myers Squibb
Estraderm®	Novartis
Estratab®	Solvay
Estratest®	Solvay
Estring®	Pharmacia
Ethmozine®	Shire
Etrafon®	Schering-Plough
Evista®	Eli Lilly
Excedrin P.M.®	Bristol-Myers Squibb
Excedrin® Migraine	Bristol-Myers Squibb
Exelon®	Novartis
Ex-Lax®	Novartis
Exna®	American Home Products
Extra Strength Excedrin®	Bristol-Myers Squibb
Felbatol®	Wallace
Feldene®	Pfizer
FemPatch®	Pfizer
Fiberall®	Novartis
FiberCon®	American Home Products
Fioricet®	Novartis
Fioricet® with Codeine	Novartis
Fiorinal®	Novartis
Fiorinal® with Codeine	Novartis
Flagyl®	Pharmacia
Fleet®	C.B. Fleet
Fleet® Bisacodyl	C.B. Fleet
Fleet® Phospho-soda	C.B. Fleet

Name of Medication	Manufacturer
Flexeril®	Merck
Flomax®	Boehringer Ingelheim
Flovent®	GlaxoWellcome
Floxin®	Ortho-McNeil
Flumadine®	Forest
Fosamax®	Merck
Furoxone®	Procter & Gamble
Gaviscon®	SmithKline Beecham
Gelusil®	Pfizer
Genapap™	Goldline
Glaucon®	Alcon
Glucophage®	Bristol-Myers Squibb
Glucotrol®	Pfizer
Glynase®	Pharmacia
Glyset®	Pharmacia
Grisactin®	American Home Products
Gris-PEG®	Allergan
Halcion®	Pharmacia
Haldol®	Ortho-McNeil
Halfprin®	Kramer
Halotestin®	Pharmacia
Hexadrol®	Organon
Hismanal®	Janssen
Humalog®	Eli Lilly
Humorsol®	Merck
Hycodan®	Endo
Hydrocet®	Carnrick
Hydrocortone®	Merck
HydroDIURIL®	Merck
Hydromox®	American Home Products
Hygroton®	Aventis
Hytrin®	Abbott
Hyzaar®	Merck
Imdur®	Schering-Plough
Imitrex®	GlaxoWellcome
Imodium®	McNeil

Name of Medication	Manufacturer
Inderal®	American Home Products
Inderide®	American Home Products
Indocin®	Merck
Intal®	Aventis
Intron® *A*	Schering-Plough
Iopidine®	Alcon
Ismelin®	Novartis
ISMO®	American Home Products
Isoptin®	Knoll
Isopto® *Carbachol*	Alcon
Isopto® *Carpine*	Alcon
Isordil®	American Home Products
Isuprel®	Sanofi
KADIAN®	Fielding
Kaopectate® *II*	Pharmacia
K-Dur®	Schering-Plough
Keflex®	Eli Lilly
Kemadrin®	GlaxoWellcome
Kerlone®	Pharmacia
Klonopin®	Roche
Klor-Con®	Upsher-Smith
Konsyl®	Konsyl
K-Tab®	Abbott
Kudrox®	Schwarz
Lanoxicaps®	GlaxoWellcome
Lanoxin®	GlaxoWellcome
Larodopa®	Roche
Lasix®	Aventis
Lescol®	Novartis
Levaquin®	Ortho-McNeil
Levatol®	Schwarz
Levbid®	Schwarz
Levo-Dromoran®	ICN
Levo-T®	American Home Products
Levothroid®	Forest

Name of Medication	Manufacturer
Levoxyl®	King
Levsin®	Schwarz
Levsinex®	Schwarz
Lexxel®	Merck
Librax®	Roche
Libritabs®	Roche
Librium®	ICN
Limbitrol®	ICN
Lipitor®	Pfizer
Lithobid®	Solvay
Lithonate®	Solvay
Lithotabs®	Solvay
LoCHOLEST®	Pfizer
Lodine®	American Home Products
Lodosyn®	Merck
Lomotil®	Pharmacia
Loniten®	Pharmacia
Lopid®	Pfizer
Lopressor®	Novartis
Lopressor HCT®	Novartis
Lorcet®	Forest
Lortab®	UCB
Lotensin®	Novartis
Lotensin HCT®	Novartis
Lotrel®	Novartis
Lovenox®	Aventis
Loxitane®	Watson
Lozol®	Aventis
Ludiomil®	Novartis
Luminal®	Sanofi
Luvox®	Solvay
Maalox®	Novartis
Magan®	Pharmacia
Magnalox®	Schein
Mallamint®	Shire

Name of Medication	Manufacturer
Maltsupex®	Wallace
Marblen™	Fleming
Marplan®	Oxford
Mavik®	Knoll
Maxair®	3M
Maxalt®	Merck
Maxzide®	Bertek
Mebaral®	Sanofi
Medihaler-Iso®	3M
Medrol®	Pharmacia
Mellaril®	Novartis
Menest®	Monarch
Meridia®	Knoll
Mesantoin®	Novartis
Mestinon®	ICN
Metamucil®	Procter & Gamble
Metandren®	Novartis
Metaprel®	Novartis
Methylin®	Mallinckrodt
Meticorten®	Schering-Plough
Mevacor®	Merck
Mexitil®	Boehringer Ingelheim
Miacalcin®	Novartis
Micardis®	Boehringer Ingelheim
MicroK®	American Home Products
Micronase®	Pharmacia
Microzide®	Watson
Midamor®	Merck
Migranal®	Novartis
Miltown™	Wallace
Minipress®	Pfizer
Minitran®	3M
Minizide®	Pfizer
Minocin®	American Home Products
Mintezol®	Merck

Name of Medication	Manufacturer
Mirapex®	Pharmacia
Mitrolan®	American Home Products
Moban®	Endo
Mobic®	Boehringer Ingelheim/Abbott
Mobidin®	B. F. Ascher
Moduretic®	Merck
Monoket®	Schwarz
Monopril®	Bristol-Myers Squibb
Motrin®	Pharmacia
MS Contin®	Purdue Frederick
MSIR®	Purdue Frederick
Mycobutin®	Pharmacia
Mylanta®	Johnson & Johnson/Merck
Nalfon®	Eli Lilly
Naprelan®	Carnrick
Naprosyn®	Roche
Naqua®	Schering-Plough
Nardil®	Pfizer
Nature's Remedy®	SmithKline Beecham
Naturetin®	Princeton
Navane®	Pfizer
Nembutal®	Abbott
Neo-Calglucon®	Novartis
Neoloid®	Doak
Neoral®	Novartis
Neptazane®	Bausch and Lomb
Neurontin®	Pfizer
Neutrexin®	U.S. Bioscience
Niaspan®	KOS
Nitrek®	Bertek
Nitro-Bid®	Aventis
Nitrodisc®	Shire
Nitro-Dur®	Schering-Plough
Nitrogard®	Forest
Nitroglyn®	Doak

Name of Medication	Manufacturer
Nitrol®	Savage
Nitrolingual®	Aventis
Nitrong®	Aventis
NitroQuick®	Ethex
Nitrostat®	Pfizer
Nitro-Time®	Time-Cap
Nizoral®	Janssen
Nolvadex®	AstraZeneca
Norco™	Watson
Normodyne®	Schering-Plough
Norpace®	Pharmacia
Norpramin®	Aventis
Norvasc®	Pfizer
Norvir®	Abbott
Novolin Prefilled™	Novo Nordisk
NovoPen® 3	Novo Nordisk
Nydrazid®	Apothecon
Nytol®	Block
Ocupress®	Otsuka America
Ocusert®	Alza
Ogen®	Pharmacia
OptiPranolol®	Bausch and Lomb
Oramorph® SR	Roxane
Orap®	Gate
Orasone®	Solvay
Oretic®	Abbott
Orinase®	Pharmacia
Ortho-EST®	Women First
Ortho-Prefest®	Ortho-McNeil
Orudis®	American Home Products
Oruvail®	American Home Products
Os-Cal 500®	SmithKline Beecham
OxyContin®	Purdue Frederick
OxyFAST™	Purdue Frederick
OxyIR®	Purdue Frederick

Name of Medication	Manufacturer
P.V. Carpine®	Allergan
P_1E_1®, P_2E_1®, P_4E_1®, P_6E_1®	Alcon
Pacerone®	Upsher-Smith
Pamelor®	Novartis
Pamine®	Doak
Panadol®	SmithKline Beecham
Pancrease®	Ortho-McNeil
Parlodel®	Novartis
Parnate®	SmithKline Beecham
Paxil®	SmithKline Beecham
Paxipam®	Schering-Plough
PCE®	Abbott
Peganone®	Abbott
Pen-Vee® K	American Home Products
Pepcid®	Merck
Pepto-Bismol®	Procter & Gamble
Pepto Diarrhea Control®	Procter & Gamble
Percocet®	Endo
Percodan®	Endo
Percolone®	Endo
Perdiem® Fiber	Novartis
Peri-Colace®	Mead Johnson
Permax®	Elan
Persantine®	Boehringer Ingelheim
Phenaphen® with Codeine	American Home Products
Phenergan®	American Home Products
Phillips' Milk of Magnesia®	Bayer
Phospholine Iodide®	American Home Products
Pilocar®	Novartis
Pilostat®	Bausch and Lomb
Plaquenil®	Sanofi
Plavix®	Bristol-Myers Squibb
Plendil®	AstraZeneca
Posture®	American Home Products
Prandin™	Novo Nordisk

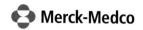
Name of Medication	Manufacturer
Pravachol®	Bristol-Myers Squibb
Precose®	Bayer
Prelone®	Muro
Premarin®	American Home Products
Premphase®	American Home Products
Prempro™	American Home Products
PREVACID®	Tap
Prevalite®	Upsher-Smith
Prilosec®	AstraZeneca
Primatene® Mist	American Home Products
Principen®	Apothecon
Prinivil®	Merck
Prinzide®	Merck
Pro-Banthine®	SCS
Procanbid®	Monarch
Procardia®	Pfizer
Prolixin®	Apothecon
Pronestyl®	Princeton
Propecia®	Merck
Propine®	Allergan
Propulsid®	Janssen
Proscar®	Merck
ProSom™	Abbott
Prostigmin®	ICN
Protonix®	American Home Products
Proventil®	Schering-Plough
Provera®	Pharmacia
Prozac®	Eli Lilly
Pulmicort®	AstraZeneca
Quarzan®	Roche
Questran®	Bristol-Myers Squibb
Quinaglute Dura-Tabs®	Berlex
Quinidex®	American Home Products
Quinora®	Schering-Plough
Reglan®	American Home Products

Name of Medication	Manufacturer
Relafen®	SmithKline Beecham
Remeron®	Organon
Renese®	Pfizer
Requip®	SmithKline Beecham
Rescriptor®	Pharmacia
Restoril®	Novartis
Retrovir®	GlaxoWellcome
Rheumatrex®	American Home Products
Rifadin®	Aventis
Rimactane®	Novartis
Riopan®	American Home Products
Riopan Plus®	American Home Products
Risperdal®	Janssen
Ritalin®	Novartis
Rogaine®	Pharmacia
Rolaids®	Pfizer
Roxanol®	Roxane
Roxicet™	Roxane
Rythmol®	Knoll
Salflex®	Carnrick
Sandimmune®	Novartis
Sansert®	Novartis
Seconal®	Eli Lilly
Sectral®	AstraZeneca
Seldane®	Aventis
Senokot®	Purdue Frederick
Senokot-S®	Purdue Frederick
Septra®	GlaxoWellcome
Serax®	American Home Products
Serentil®	Boehringer Ingelheim
Serevent®	GlaxoWellcome
Seroquel®	AstraZeneca
Serzone®	Bristol-Myers Squibb
Simaal™	Schein
Simply Sleep®	Johnson & Johnson

Name of Medication	Manufacturer
Sinemet®	DuPont
Sinequan®	Pfizer
Singulair®	Merck
Sleep-eze 3®	American Home Products
Slo-bid™	Aventis
Slo-Niacin®	Upsher-Smith
Slo-Phyllin®	Aventis
Slow-K®	Novartis
Soma®	Wallace
Sominex®	SmithKline Beecham
Sonata®	American Home Products
Sorbitrate®	AstraZeneca
Sorbitrate Chewable®	AstraZeneca
Spectrobid®	Pfizer
Sporanox®	Ortho Biotech/Janssen
Stadol®	Bristol-Myers Squibb
Stelazine®	SmithKline Beecham
Sudafed®	GlaxoWellcome
Sular®	AstraZeneca
Sumycin®	Apothecon
Surfak®	Pharmacia
Surmontil®	American Home Products
Sustiva®	DuPont
Symmetrel®	Endo
Synthroid®	Knoll
Tagamet®	SmithKline Beecham
Talacen®	Sanofi
Talwin®	Sanofi
Tambocor®	3M
Tapazole®	Eli Lilly
Tarka®	Knoll
Tasmar®	Roche
Tavist®	Novartis
Teczem®	Aventis
Tegretol®	Novartis

Name of Medication	Manufacturer
Tempo®	Thompson
Tenoretic®	AstraZeneca
Tenormin®	AstraZeneca
Testred®	ICN
Teveten®	SmithKline Beecham
Theo-24®	UCB
Theobid®	UCB
Theo-Dur®	Schering-Plough
Theolair™	3M
Theo-X®	Carnrick
Therevac® Plus	King
Therevac®-SB	King
Thorazine®	SmithKline Beecham
Thyrolar®	Forest
Tiamate®	Aventis
Tiazac®	Forest
Ticlid®	Roche
Tilade®	Aventis
Timolide®	Merck
Timoptic®	Merck
Titralac®	3M
Tofranil®	Novartis
Tolectin®	Ortho-McNeil
Tolinase®	Pharmacia
Tonocard®	AstraZeneca
Topamax®	Ortho-McNeil
Toprol®	AstraZeneca
Toradol®	Roche
Tornalate®	Elan
T-Phyl®	Purdue Frederick
Trandate®	Faro
Transderm-Nitro®	Novartis
Tranxene®	Abbott
Tricor®	Abbott
Trilafon®	Schering-Plough

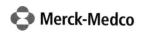

Name of Medication	Manufacturer
Trileptal®	Novartis
Trilisate®	Purdue Frederick
Trimox®	Apothecon
Trimpex®	Roche
Trusopt®	Merck
Tums®	SmithKline Beecham
TYLENOL®	McNeil
TYLENOL® with Codeine	Ortho-McNeil
TYLENOL® PM	Ortho-McNeil
Tylox®	Ortho-McNeil
Ultram®	Ortho-McNeil
Ultrase®	Scandipharm
Uni-Dur®	Schering-Plough
Unifiber®	Bertek
Uniphyl®	Purdue Frederick
Uniretic®	Schwarz
Unisom®	Pfizer
Univasc®	Schwarz
Urispas®	SmithKline Beecham
Urocit-K®	Mission
Urso®	Axcan
Vagifem®	Novo Nordisk
Valium®	Roche
Vanceril®	Schering-Plough
Vascor®	Ortho-McNeil
Vaseretic®	Merck
Vasotec®	Merck
Veetids®	Apothecon
Ventolin®	GlaxoWellcome
Verelan®	Schwarz
Viactiv®	Mead Johnson
Viagra®	Pfizer
Vibramycin®	Pfizer
Vicodin®	Knoll
Vicoprofen®	Knoll

Name of Medication	Manufacturer
Viokase®	Axcan
Vioxx®	Merck
Visken®	Novartis
Vistaril®	Pfizer
Vivactil®	Merck
Vivelle®	Novartis
Voltaren®	Novartis
Wellbutrin®	GlaxoWellcome
Wigraine®	Organon
Wygesic®	American Home Products
Xalatan®	Pharmacia
Xanax®	Pharmacia
Xopenex™	Sepracor
Zagam®	Bertek
Zantac®	GlaxoWellcome
Zaroxolyn®	Celltech Medeva
Zebeta®	American Home Products
Zestoretic®	AstraZeneca
Zestril®	AstraZeneca
Ziac	American Home Products
Zithromax®	Pfizer
Zocor®	Merck
Zoloft®	Pfizer
Zomig®	AstraZeneca
ZORprin®	Knoll
Zostrix®	GenDerm
Zovirax®	GlaxoWellcome
Zyban®	GlaxoWellcome
Zydone®	Endo
Zyflo®	Abbott
Zyloprim®	GlaxoWellcome
Zymase®	Organon
Zyprexa®	Eli Lilly
Zyrtec®	Pfizer

Following are the complete names of each manufacturer listed on previous pages:

Abbott Laboratories	Fujisawa Healthcare, Inc.
Alcon	Gate Pharmaceuticals
Allergan, Inc.	GenDerm Corporation
Alza Pharmaceuticals	GlaxoWellcome
American Home Products	Goldline Laboratories, Inc.
Andrx Pharmaceuticals, Inc.	Humco Holding Group, Inc.
Apothecon	ICN Pharmaceuticals
AstraZeneca	Integrity Pharmaceutical
Aventis Pharma	Janssen Pharmaceutica, Inc.
Axcan Pharma	Johnson & Johnson
B. F. Ascher	King Pharmaceuticals
Bausch and Lomb	Knoll Pharmaceutical Company
Bayer Corporation	Konsyl Pharmaceuticals
Berlex Laboratories	KOS Pharmaceuticals, Inc.
Bertek Pharmaceuticals, Inc.	Kramer
BIRA Corporation	Lotus
Block Drug Company, Inc.	Mallinckrodt, Inc.
Boehringer Ingelheim Pharmaceuticals, Inc.	McNeil Consumer Healthcare
Bristol-Myers Squibb Co.	Mead Johnson Company
C.B. Fleet Company, Inc.	Medicis, The Dermatology Company
Carnrick Laboratories	Menley and James Laboratories, Inc.
Celltech Medeva	Merck & Co., Inc.
Dey	Mission Pharmacal
Doak Dermatologics	Monarch Pharmaceuticals
DuPont Pharmaceuticals	Muro Pharmaceutical, Inc.
Eisai Inc.	Novartis Pharmaceuticals
Elan Pharmaceuticals	Novo Nordisk Pharmaceuticals, Inc.
Eli Lilly and Company	Numark
Endo Pharmaceuticals, Inc.	Optopics
ESI Lederle	Organon, Inc.
Ethex Corporation	Ortho Biotech, Inc.
Faro Pharmaceuticals	Ortho-McNeil Pharmaceutical
Fleming and Company	Otsuka America Pharma, Inc.
Forest Pharmaceuticals, Inc.	Oxford Pharmaceutical Services, Inc.

Pfizer Inc.

Pharmacia Corporation

PolyMedica Pharmaceuticals (U.S.A.), Inc.

Princeton Pharmaceutical Products

Procter & Gamble Pharmaceuticals, Inc.

Roche Pharmaceuticals

Roxane Laboratories, Inc.

Sanofi Pharmaceuticals

Savage Laboratories

Scandipharm, Inc.

Schein Pharmaceutical, Inc.

Schering-Plough

Schwarz Pharma

SCS Pharmaceuticals

Sepracor, Inc.

Shire Pharmaceuticals

SmithKline Beecham Pharmaceuticals

Solvay Pharmaceuticals, Inc.

Somerset Pharmaceuticals

Takeda Pharmaceuticals America, Inc.

Tap Pharmaceuticals, Inc.

The Fielding Pharmaceutical Company, Inc.

The Purdue Frederick Company

Thompson Medical

3M Pharmaceuticals

Time-Cap Laboratories, Inc.

UCB Pharma, Inc.

Upsher-Smith Laboratories

U.S. Bioscience, Inc.

Wallace Laboratories

Watson Pharmaceuticals, Inc.

Women First Healthcare, Inc.

Glossary of Medical Terms Used in This Book

A

Absorption: Uptake of a medication, food, or other substance from the digestive tract into the bloodstream.

Acid: A substance produced in the lining of the stomach that helps in breaking down (digesting) food.

Acute: Description of a condition or illness that starts suddenly and usually lasts for only a short time.

Addiction: A strong need or craving for a medication or substance (narcotics; alcoholic beverages such as beer, wine, whiskey, and others; nicotine; and others) to the point that not taking it may be difficult or cause physical or mental symptoms.

Addison's disease: A disease in which the adrenal glands do not produce enough hormones. Addison's disease may cause extreme weakness, weight loss, low blood pressure, stomach problems, and brownish skin color.

Aerosol medication: A medication that is sprayed as a fine mist.

Allergic reaction: A bad reaction to a medication, food, or substance that in most people causes no problems. Symptoms of an allergic reaction include rash (skin redness, bumps, itching, or irritation), swelling of the face and throat, or trouble breathing.

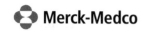

Alpha blockers: Medications that help relax blood vessels so blood can flow through arteries more easily. Alpha blockers may be used to help reduce the symptoms caused by an enlarged prostate or to treat high blood pressure. They include *Cardura®* (doxazosin), *Flomax®* (tamsulosin), *Hytrin®* (terazosin), and *Minipress®* (prazosin).

Amnesia: A problem with long-term memory.

Amputation: Surgical removal of an external body part, such as a toe, foot, or leg.

Analgesics: Medications used to help relieve pain. Analgesics include:

- **Acetaminophen:** *Anacin®*, *Genapap™*, *Panadol®*, *Panex®*, *Tylenol®*

- **Aspirin:** *Arthritis Pain Formula™*, *Ascriptin®*, *Bufferin®*, *Ecotrin®*, *Empirin®*, *Halfprin®*, *ZORprin®*, and others

- **Aspirin-like medications:** *Disalcid®* (salsalate), magnesium salicylate (*Doan's®*, *Magan®*, *Mobidin®*, and others), *Dolobid®* (diflunisal), *Trilisate®* (choline magnesium trisalicylate), and others

- **Medications that contain aspirin:** *Darvon®* Compound (propoxyphene/aspirin), *Percodan®* (oxycodone/aspirin), *Talwin®* Compound (pentazocine/aspirin), and others

- **Narcotic pain relievers:** *Darvon®* (propoxyphene), *Demerol®* (meperidine), *Dilaudid®* (hydromorphone), *Duragesic®* (fentanyl) *Hycodan®* (hydrocodone), morphine (*Kadian®*, *MS Contin®*, *Oramorph®*, and others) *Levo-Dromoran®* (levorphanol), *OxyContin®* (oxycodone), *Stadol®* (butorphanol), *Talwin®* (pentazocine), codeine, and others

- **Others:** *Ultram®* (tramadol), and others

Anaphylaxis: A life-threatening allergic reaction that causes a drop in blood pressure and is characterized by rash, swelling, difficulty breathing, fainting, and itching.

Anemia: The condition of not having enough red blood cells. Anemia can be caused by a decrease in red blood cell production, an increase in red blood cell destruction, or blood loss. Symptoms of anemia include fatigue (tiredness).

Anesthesia: A medication usually given to a person during surgery or a medical procedure to produce loss of sensation or pain. Anesthesia can be given with or without loss of consciousness.

Angina, angina pectoris: Chest pain caused by the heart not getting enough oxygen. See Coronary Artery Disease and Cardiac Chest Pain (Angina) chapter on page 193.

Angioedema: Swelling of the face, lips, tongue, arms, and legs.

Angioplasty: A medical procedure in which clogged arteries (blood vessels) are opened with a tiny balloon at the end of a flexible tube.

Angiotensin-converting enzyme (ACE) inhibitors: Medications that help to relax and open blood vessels. They are used to help treat high blood pressure, congestive heart failure, and other medical conditions. They include:
- *Accupril*® (quinapril)
- *Aceon*® (perindopril)
- *Altace*® (ramipril)
- *Capoten*® (captopril)
- Lisinopril (*Prinivil*®, *Zestril*®)
- *Lotensin*® (benazepril)
- *Mavik*® (trandolapril)
- *Monopril*® (fosinopril)
- *Univasc*® (moexipril)
- *Vasotec*® (enalapril)

Angiotensin II (A-II) blockers: Medications that help to relax the blood vessels by blocking angiotensin II, a substance in the body that causes the blood vessels to tighten (constrict). A-II blockers are used to help treat high blood pressure and other medical conditions. They include:
- *Atacand*® (candesartan)
- *Avapro*® (irbesartan)
- *Cozaar*® (losartan)

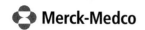

- *Diovan®* (valsartan)
- *Micardis®* (telmisartan)
- *Teveten®* (eprosartan)

Anorexia: Loss of appetite and/or an unwillingness to eat or a dislike for food.

Anorexia nervosa: An eating disorder in which a person eats almost nothing because of an extreme fear of becoming overweight. Also see Bulimia.

Antacids: Medications that help relieve stomach pain by neutralizing stomach acid so the stomach juices are less irritating to the stomach and esophagus (the tube that connects the mouth to the stomach). Antacids are used to help relieve the symptoms of heartburn, ulcers, indigestion, and other medical conditions. Antacids contain aluminum, calcium, magnesium, or sodium bicarbonate. They include:

- **Antacids, aluminum-containing:** *Alamag*™, *AlternaGEL®*, *Amphojel®*, *Basaljel®*, *Di-Gel®*, *Gaviscon®*, *Maalox®*, *Riopan®*, and others

- **Antacids, calcium-containing:** *Alka-Mints®*, *Alkets®*, *Amitone®*, *Chooz®*, *Dicarbosil®*, *Equilet®*, *Mallamint*™, *Rolaids®*, *Titralac® Plus*, *Titralac®*, *Tums®*, and others

- **Antacids, magnesium-containing:** *Alamag*™, *Alkets®*, *Di-Gel®*, *Gelusil®*, *Kudrox®*, *Maalox®*, *Magnalox*™, *Phillips® Milk of Magnesia*, *Mylanta®*, *Riopan®*, *Riopan Plus®*, *Rolaids®*, *Simaal*™, and others

- **Antacids, sodium bicarbonate-containing:** *Bell/ans*™, *Bromo-Seltzer®*, *Citrocarbonate®*, *Gaviscon®*, and others

Antibiotics: Medications that help destroy bacteria or prevent bacteria from growing. Antibiotics include:
- Amoxicillin (*Amoxil®*, *Trimox®*, and others)
- *Augmentin®* (amoxicillin/clavulanate)
- *Bactrim®* (cotrimoxazole)
- *Biaxin®* (clarithromycin)
- *Ceftin®* (cefuroxime)
- *Cefzil®* (cefprozil)
- *Cipro®* (ciprofloxacin)

- *Declomycin*® (demeclocycline)
- *Dynabac*® (dirithromycin)
- Erythromycin (*E-Mycin*®, *Eryc*®, *Ery-Tab*®, *Erythrocin*®, *PCE*®, and others)
- *Flagyl*® (metronidazole)
- *Furoxone*® (furazolidone)
- *Keflex*® (cephalexin)
- *Levaquin*® (levofloxacin)
- *Microsulfon*® (sulfadiazine)
- Minocycline (*Dynacin*®, *Minocin*®)
- *Mycobutin*® (rifabutin)
- *Neo-Tabs*™ (neomycin)
- *Nydrazid*® (isoniazid)
- Penicillin (*Pen-Vee*® K, *Veetids*®, and others)
- *Principen*® (ampicillin)
- *Rifadin*® (rifampin)
- *Septra*® (sulfamethoxazole/trimethoprim)
- *Spectrobid*® (bacampicillin)
- *Sumycin*® (tetracycline)
- *Trimpex*® (trimethoprim)
- *Vibramycin*® (doxycycline)
- *Zagam*® (sparfloxacin)
- *Zithromax*® (azithromycin)
- Others

Anticholinergic medications: Medications that help prevent transmission of acetylcholine (a chemical in the brain that transmits messages to the muscles and that nerve cells use to communicate and store memories). These medications are often used to help treat Parkinson's disease, irritable bowel syndrome, urge incontinence, and other medical conditions. These medications include:
- *Akineton*® (biperiden)
- *Artane*® (trihexyphenidyl)
- *Bentyl*® (dicyclomine)
- *Cantil*® (mepenzolate)
- *Cogentin*® (benztropine)
- *Detrol*® (tolterodine)
- *Ditropan*® (oxybutynin)
- *Donnatal*® (phenobarbital)

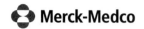

- Hyoscyamine (*Anaspaz®*, *Cystospaz®*, *Levsin®*, *Levsinex®*)
- *Kemadrin®* (procyclidine)
- *Librax®* (chlordiazepoxide/clidinium)
- *Lomotil®* (diphenoxylate/atropine)
- *Pamine®* (methscopolamine)
- *Pro-Banthine®* (propantheline)
- *Quarzan®* (clidinium)
- *Robinul®* (glycopyrrolate)
- *Urispas®* (flavoxate)
- Others

Anticoagulant: "Blood thinner" medication, which helps stop new blood clots from forming and existing clots from getting bigger, but does not actually "thin" the blood. Anticoagulants include *Coumadin®* (warfarin), heparin, and *Lovenox®* (enoxaparin).

Antidepressants: Medications that help prevent or relieve depression. Antidepressants include:

- **Monoamine oxidase (MAO) inhibitors:** *Marplan®* (isocarboxazid), *Nardil®* (phenelzine), *Parnate®* (tranylcypromine), and others.

- **Selective serotonin reuptake inhibitors (SSRIs):** *Celexa™* (citalopram), *Luvox®* (fluvoxamine), *Paxil®* (paroxetine), *Prozac®* (fluoxetine), *Zoloft®* (sertraline)

- **Tricyclic antidepressants:** *Anafranil®* (clomipramine), *Asendin®* (amoxapine), *Elavil®* (amitriptyline), *Norpramin®* (desipramine), *Pamelor®* (nortriptyline), *Sinequan®* (doxepin), *Surmontil®* (trimipramine), *Tofranil®* (imipramine), *Vivactil®* (protriptyline)

- **Others:** *Desyrel®* (trazodone), *Effexor®* (venlafaxine), *Ludiomil®* (maprotiline), *Remeron®* (mirtazapine), *Serzone®* (nefazodone), *Wellbutrin®* (bupropion), and others

Antihistamines: Medications that help block the effects of histamine, a natural substance that can make the nose stuffy and the eyes watery. Antihistamines are used to help relieve the symptoms of colds and allergies. Some antihistamines cause drowsiness and can be used to help relieve symptoms of anxiety or insomnia (trouble falling asleep or staying asleep). Antihistamines include:

- **Nonsedating antihistamines (do not cause drowsiness):** *Allegra*® (fexofenadine), *Claritin*® (loratadine), *Hismanal*® (astemizole), *Seldane*® (terfenadine), *Zyrtec*® (cetirizine), and others

- **Sedating antihistamines (cause drowsiness):** *Atarax*® (hydroxyzine), diphenhydramine (*Benadryl*®, *Nytol*®, *Sleep-Eze 3*®, *Sominex*®), *Excedrin P.M.*® (acetaminophen/diphenhydramine), *Tavist*® (clemastine), *Tylenol PM*® (diphenhydramine/acetaminophen), *Unisom*® (doxylamine), *Vistaril*® (hydroxyzine), and others

Anti-inflammatory: A medication that helps reduce the symptoms of inflammation, such as pain, swelling, and redness.

Antiplatelet medications: Medications that make blood platelets less likely to stick together and form blood clots or scabs. Antiplatelet medications include *Aggrenox*® (dipyridamole/aspirin), *Persantine*® (dipyridamole), *Plavix*® (clopidogrel), *Ticlid*® (ticlopidine), and others.

Antispasmodic medications: Medications that help prevent smooth muscle spasms or contractions. They are used to help relieve symptoms of irritable bowel syndrome and other medical conditions. Antispasmodics include:
- *Bentyl*® (dicyclomine)
- Hyoscyamine (*Anaspaz*®, *Cystospaz*®, *Levbid*®, *Levsin*®, *Levsinex*®)
- *Librax*® (clidinium/chlordiazepoxide)
- *Lomotil*® (diphenoxylate/atropine)
- *Pamine*® (methscopolamine)
- *Pro-Banthine*® (propantheline)
- *Quarzan*® (clidinium)
- *Robinul*® (glycopyrrolate)
- Others

Anxiety: A feeling of nervousness, fear, tension, or stress. See Anxiety (Nervousness) chapter on page 13.

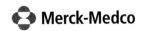

Anxiety medications: Medications that help relieve the symptoms of anxiety or nervousness. Anxiety medications include *BuSpar®* (buspirone), *Effexor®* (venlafaxine), meprobamate (*Equanil®*, *Miltown®*), and others.

Arrhythmia: Irregular (fast, slow, or abnormal) heartbeat. See Irregular or Abnormal Heartbeat chapter on page 451.

Artery: A blood vessel that carries blood from the heart to other parts of the body.

Arthritis: A medical condition usually caused by wear and tear on the joints or by inflammation (swelling, pain, and redness) from an overactive immune system. See Arthritis and Pain chapter on page 37.

Aspirin and aspirin-like medications (salicylates): Aspirin is a medication that helps relieve pain, fever, and inflammation. Aspirin, medications that contain aspirin, and aspirin-like medications (salicylates) include:

- **Aspirin:** *Arthritis Pain Formula™*, *Ascriptin®*, *Bayer®* Aspirin Maximum Strength, *Bayer®* Enteric-Coated, *Bufferin®*, *Ecotrin®*, *Empirin®*, *Halfprin®*, *ZORprin®*, and others

- **Aspirin-like medications:** *Disalcid®* (salsalate), *Dolobid®*, (diflunisal), magnesium salicylate (*Doan's®*, *Halprin®* 81, *Magan®*, *Mobidin®*), *Trilisate®* (choline magnesium trisalicylate), and others

- **Medications that contain aspirin:** *Aggrenox®* (dipyridamole/aspirin), *Darvon®* Compound-65 (propoxyphene/aspirin), *Percodan®* (oxycodone/aspirin), *Talwin®* Compound (pentazocine/aspirin), and others

Atherosclerosis: Hardening of the arteries from an accumulation of cholesterol and other material on the inside of the arteries (arterial plaques) that causes heart disease. See High Cholesterol chapter on page 431 and Coronary Artery Disease chapter on page 193.

Autoimmune disease: A group of medical conditions in which the body's immune system attacks itself. Examples of autoimmune diseases include rheumatoid arthritis and lupus.

B

Bacteria: Tiny, single-celled microorganisms commonly known as germs. Some bacteria cause infections or other medical problems.

Barbiturate: A highly addictive type of medication that helps cause sleep and has a calming effect (sedation). Barbiturates include:
- *Alurate*® (aprobarbital)
- *Amytal*® (amobarbital)
- *Butisol*® (butabarbital)
- *Luminal*® (phenobarbital)
- *Mebaral*® (mephobarbital)
- *Nembutal*® (pentobarbital)
- *Seconal*® (secobarbital)
- Others

Benign: Noncancerous.

Benign prostatic hypertrophy or hyperplasia (BPH): An enlarged prostate. See Urinary Problems chapter on page 663.

Benzodiazepines: Medications that help relax muscles and cause a calming effect (sedation). Benzodiazepines are sometimes used to help relieve symptoms of anxiety (nervousness), insomnia (trouble falling or staying asleep), muscle spasms, and other medical conditions. They include:
- *Ativan*® (lorazepam)
- Chlordiazepoxide (*Libritabs*®, *Librium*®)
- *Dalmane*® (flurazepam)
- *Doral*® (quazepam)
- *Halcion*® (triazolam)
- *Klonopin*® (clonazepam)
- *Librax*® (chlordiazepoxide/clidinium)
- *Paxipam*® (halazepam)
- *ProSom*™ (estazolam)
- *Restoril*® (temazepam)
- *Serax*® (oxazepam)
- *Tranxene*® (clorazepate)
- *Valium*® (diazepam)
- *Xanax*® (alprazolam)

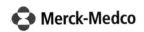

Beta-adrenergic bronchodilators: Medications that help to relax constricted (narrowed) breathing passages that cause shortness of breath in people with asthma and COPD, including chronic bronchitis and emphysema. This helps to open the breathing passages and allow air to pass in and out of the lungs more freely. Beta-adrenergic bronchodilators include:

- Albuterol (*Proventil®*, *Ventolin®*)
- *Combivent®* (ipratropium/albuterol)
- Epinephrine (*AsthmaNefrin®*, *Bronkaid Mist®*, *Primatene® Mist*)
- Isoproterenol (*Isuprel®*, *Medihaler-Iso®*)
- *Maxair®* (pirbuterol)
- Metaproterenol (*Alupent®*, *Metaprel®*)
- *Serevent®* (salmeterol)
- Terbutaline (*Brethaire®*, *Brethine®*, *Bricanyl®*)
- *Tornalate®* (bitolterol)
- *Xopenex™* (levalbuterol)
- Others

Beta blockers: Medications that help slow the heartbeat, prevent heart rhythm problems, decrease the heart's need for oxygen, and lower blood pressure. Beta blocker eyedrops can also be used to help treat glaucoma. Beta blockers include:

- *Betagan®* (levobunolol)
- *Betapace®* (sotalol)
- Betaxolol (*Betoptic®*, *Kerlone®*)
- *Blocadren®* (timolol)
- Carteolol (*Cartrol®*, *Ocupress®*)
- *Coreg®* (carvedilol)
- *Corgard®* (nadolol)
- *Cosopt®* (dorzolamide/timolol)
- *Inderal®* (propranolol)
- *Inderide®* (propranolol/hydrochlorothiazide)
- *Levatol®* (penbutolol)
- *Lopressor®* (metoprolol)
- *Normodyne®* (labetalol)
- *OptiPranolol®* (metipranolol)
- *Sectral®* (acebutolol)
- *Tenormin®* (atenolol)
- *Timoptic®* (timolol maleate)

- *Toprol®* (metoprolol)
- *Trandate®* (labetalol)
- *Visken®* (pindolol)
- *Zebeta®* (bisoprolol)
- *Ziac®* (hydrochlorothiazide/bisoprolol)
- Others

Bile acid binders: Medications that help to lower low-density lipoproteins (LDL or "bad" cholesterol) levels by binding cholesterol and helping prevent its reabsorption into the body. Bile acid binders include cholestyramine (*LoCHOLEST®*, *Prevalite®*, *Questran®*), *Colestid®* (colestipol), and others.

Bisphosphonates: Medications that help prevent bones from breaking down and becoming weaker. Bisphosphonates are used to help prevent and treat osteoporosis. These medications include *Actonel®* (risedronate), *Didronel®* (etidronate), and *Fosamax®* (alendronate).

Bladder: The body organ that stores urine.

Blood clot: A coagulated mass of blood. Blood clotting keeps a person from bleeding to death from small cuts, but a blood clot can also cause a stroke or a heart attack.

Blood pressure: The measurement of the pressure against the walls of the blood vessels by blood pumped by the heart throughout the body. See High Blood Pressure chapter on page 373.

Blood sugar: Sugar (glucose) in the blood.

Blood thinner: An inaccurate term for anticoagulant medication, which helps stop new blood clots from forming and existing clots from getting bigger, but does not actually "thin" the blood. See Anticoagulant.

Blood vessel: A living tube, such as a vein or an artery, that carries blood from one part of the body to another.

Bone density: Thickness and strength of bones. People with osteoporosis have low bone density.

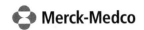

BPH (benign prostatic hypertrophy or hyperplasia): An enlarged prostate. See Urinary Problems chapter on page 663.

Bronchitis: Inflammation of one or more of the large air passages in the lungs (bronchi).

Bronchodilators: Medications that help relax the muscles around the airways of the lungs.

Buffer: A chemical that helps to control acid levels in the stomach. It is sometimes added to medications such as aspirin to help prevent stomach upset.

Bulimia: An eating disorder in which a person eats a great deal at a time (binges), then causes himself or herself to vomit, preventing the food from being fully digested, typically in an effort to lose weight. Also see Anorexia nervosa.

Bulk-forming laxatives: Medications that help cause the urge to have a bowel movement. Bulk-forming laxatives include:
- *Citrucel®* (methylcellulose)
- *Maltsupex®* (malt soup extract)
- Polycarbophil (*Fiberall®, FiberCon®, Mitrolan®*)
- Psyllium (*Konsyl®, Metamucil®, Perdiem® Fiber*)
- *Unifiber®* (cellulose)
- Others

Bursitis: Inflammation of a bursa, which is normally a small tissue space (sac) that is filled with fluid to make movement easier, such as in the knee or the elbow.

C

Calcium: A mineral in the body that strengthens teeth and bones. It is also essential for cell function, muscle contractions, transmission of nerve impulses, and blood clotting.

Calcium channel blockers: Calcium channel blockers help relax blood vessels, so that more blood and oxygen flow to the heart, and the heart does not have to work so hard to pump blood through the blood vessels. They are used to help treat high blood pressure, coronary artery disease, cardiac chest pain (angina), heart rhythm problems, and other medical conditions. They include:
- *Cardene*® (nicardipine)
- Diltiazem (*Cardizem*®, *Dilacor*®, *Diltia*®, *Tiamate*®, *Tiazac*®)
- *DynaCirc*® (isradipine)
- *Norvasc*® (amlodipine)
- Nifedipine (*Adalat*®, *Procardia*®)
- *Plendil*® (felodipine)
- *Sular*® (nisoldipine)
- *Vascor*® (bepridil)
- Verapamil (*Calan*®, *Covera*®, *Isoptin*®, *Verelan*®)

Calcium supplements: Medications that help increase the amount of calcium in the body. These include:
- *Calcet Plus*® (calcium carbonate)
- *Caltrate*® (calcium/vitamin D)
- *Citracal*® (calcium citrate)
- *Neo-Calglucon*® (calcium gluconate)
- *Os-Cal 500*® (calcium carbonate)
- *Posture*® (calcium phosphate)
- *Viactiv*® (calcium carbonate/vitamins D & K)
- Others

***Candida*:** A fungus that resembles yeast. Infections caused by *Candida* may include thrush, athlete's foot, and vaginitis.

Carbohydrate: A substance contained mainly in sugary and starchy foods (such as cereal, bread, pasta, grains, fruit, and vegetables) that is a main source of energy for the body.

Carbonic anhydrase inhibitors: Medications used to help treat glaucoma by helping to reduce the pressure in the eye caused from fluid buildup. These medications include:
- *Azopt*® (brinzolamide)
- *Cosopt*® (dorzolamide/timolol)

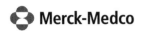

- *Daranide*® (dichlorphenamide)
- *Diamox*® (acetazolamide)
- *Neptazane*® (methazolamide)
- *Trusopt*® (dorzolamide)
- Others

Cardiac: Relating to the heart.

Cataract: A cloudy film (opacity) over part of the eye that makes it difficult or, over time, impossible to see.

CHF (Congestive Heart Failure): A medical condition that occurs when the heart cannot pump enough blood to meet the body's needs. See Congestive Heart Failure chapter on page 135.

Cholesterol: A fatty substance in the body found in the blood. See High Cholesterol chapter on page 431.

Cholinesterase inhibitors: Medications that help keep the amount of acetylcholine (a chemical in the brain that transmits messages to the muscles and that nerve cells use to communicate and store memories) at higher levels than it would be without these medications. They may temporarily help to improve memory or to keep it from getting worse. These medications include *Aricept*® (donepezil), *Cognex*® (tacrine), and *Exelon*® (rivastigmine).

Chronic: Long-lasting (the opposite of "acute").

Chronic obstructive pulmonary disease (COPD): A medical condition that also may be called emphysema or chronic bronchitis, which usually occurs as a result of damage to the lungs from long-standing exposure to inhaled irritants, the most common of which is cigarette smoke. See Asthma, Emphysema and Chronic Bronchitis chapter on page 97.

Circulation: The movement of blood through the vessels of the body caused by the pumping action of the heart.

Cirrhosis: A type of advanced liver disease, often caused by infections or drinking too many alcoholic beverages (such as beer, wine, whiskey, and others) over many years.

Closed-angle glaucoma (also called acute glaucoma or narrow-angle glaucoma): An uncommon type of glaucoma in which fluid buildup occurs quickly, causing a serious increase in eye pressure. See Glaucoma chapter on page 291.

Colonoscopy: A procedure used to look inside the colon using a long, flexible, fiberoptic tube (an instrument that transmits lights and images so structures inside the body can be viewed).

Coma: A state of unconsciousness from which a person cannot be awakened.

Combination medication: More than one medication in one pill or one eyedrop.

Congestive heart failure (CHF): A medical condition that occurs when the heart cannot pump enough blood to meet the body's needs. See Congestive Heart Failure chapter on page 135.

Conjunctivitis: A common eye problem in which the membrane that lines the inside of the eyelid or the exposed surface of the eyeball becomes inflamed (red, swollen, and/or painful).

Constipation: Having bowel movements less often than usual, difficulty having a bowel movement, or both. See Constipation chapter on page 169.

Constriction: Narrowing, such as the pupil of the eye.

Contract: To tighten or get smaller through a squeezing motion called a contraction (the opposite of "expand").

Contraction: A squeezing motion, such as in a muscle.

Controller medications: Medications that help prevent or control asthma so that asthma attacks do not occur. Controller medications are slow-acting and are usually used daily to help prevent an asthma attack from occurring.

COPD (chronic obstructive pulmonary disease): A medical condition that also may be called emphysema or chronic bronchitis, which usually occurs as a result of damage to the lungs from long-standing exposure to inhaled irritants,

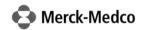
the most common of which is cigarette smoke. See Asthma, Emphysema and Chronic Bronchitis chapter on page 97.

Corneal abrasion: A scratch in the cornea, a part of the eye.

Coronary artery disease: A medical condition in which the arteries that bring blood to the heart muscle become clogged, and too little blood can flow to the heart muscle. See Coronary Artery Disease and Cardiac Chest Pain (Angina) chapter on page 193.

Corticosteroids (steroids): Anti-inflammatory medications that are used to help treat arthritis, asthma, and other medical conditions. These medications include:
- *AeroBid*® (flunisolide)
- Beclomethasone (*Beclovent*®, *Vanceril*®)
- Budesonide (*Pulmicort*®, *Pulmicort Inhaler*®)
- *Celestone*® (betamethasone)
- *Cortone*® (cortisone)
- Dexamethasone (*Decadron*®, *Hexadrol*®)
- *Flovent*® (fluticasone)
- Hydrocortisone (*Cortef*®, *Delta-Cortef*®, *Hydrocortone*®)
- *Medrol*® (methylprednisolone)
- Prednisone (*Deltasone*®, *Meticorten*®, *Orasone*®, *Prelone*®)
- Triamcinolone (*Aristocort*®, *Azmacort*®)
- Others

COX-2 inhibitor: Short for cyclooxygenase inhibitor, a COX-2 inhibitor is a type of nonsteroidal anti-inflammatory drug (NSAID). They are used to help relieve pain of arthritis and other conditions. These medications include *Celebrex*® (celecoxib) and *Vioxx*® (rofecoxib).

Crohn's disease: A chronic inflammatory disease of the digestive system usually affecting the intestines. It is also called regional enteritis, granulomatous, ileitis, and ileocolitis.

D

Decongestant: A type of medication that relieves congestion by constricting swollen blood vessels in mucous membranes in the nose.

Deficiency: Not enough of something that is needed by the body.

Dehydration: The loss of too much water from the body.

Delusion: A false belief that a person incorrectly believes to be true.

Dementia: A gradual decline in mental ability often caused by a brain disease, such as Alzheimer's disease.

Dependence: The need to take a medication to experience its effects or to keep from having the uncomfortable feelings that result when it is not taken.

Depression: A medical condition that can affect the whole body, the way you think, and the way you feel. See Depression chapter on page 219.

Dextrose: Another name for sugar or glucose.

Diabetes: A medical condition in which people have high blood sugar (glucose) levels (hyperglycemia). See Diabetes chapter on page 259.

Diabetes medications: Medications used to control the level of sugar (glucose) in the body. These include:
- *Actos*® (pioglitazone)
- *Amaryl*® (glimepiride)
- *Avandia*® (rosiglitazone)
- *Diabinese*® (chlorpropamide)
- *Dymelor*® (acetohexamide)
- *Glucophage*® (metformin)
- *Glucotrol*® (glipizide)
- Glyburide (*DiaBeta*®, *Glynase*®, *Micronase*®)
- *Glyset*® (miglitol)
- Insulin (*Humalog*®, *Humulin*®, Lente, Regular, *Novolin*®, *Novo-Nordisk*®, NPH, Ultra-lente, and others)
- *Orinase*® (tolbutamide)

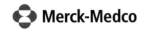

- *Prandin*™ (repaglinide)
- *Precose*® (acarbose)
- *Rezulin*® (troglitazone)
- *Tolinase*® (tolazamide)
- Others

Diaphragm: The large, dome-shaped muscle that separates the abdomen and chest and contracts and relaxes to make breathing possible.

Diarrhea: An increase in the volume, wateriness, or frequency of bowel movements.

Diastolic pressure: The measurement of blood pressure, in millimeters of mercury (mm Hg), between heartbeats, when the heart is at rest. This is the bottom (second) number in a blood pressure reading. Also see systolic pressure.

Diet: The types of food a person usually eats and drinks every day—not necessarily related to a weight-loss program.

Dilate: Widen, expand, enlarge.

Diuretics: Medications sometimes referred to as "water pills." They help the body remove excess water and salt and often cause people to urinate more than usual. Diuretics include:
- *Aldactazide*® (spironolactone/hydrochlorothiazide)
- *Aldactone*® (spironolactone)
- *Bumex*® (bumetanide)
- *Demadex*® (torsemide)
- *Diucardin*® (hydroflumethiazide)
- *Diuril*® (chlorothiazide)
- *Dyazide*® (triamterene/hydrochlorothiazide)
- *Dyrenium*® (triamterene)
- *Edecrin*® (ethacrynic acid)
- *Exna*® (benzthiazide)
- *HydroDIURIL*® (hydrochlorothiazide)
- *Hydromox*® (quinethazone)
- *Hygroton*® (chlorthalidone)
- *Lasix*® (furosemide)
- *Lozol*® (indapamide)

- *Maxzide*® (triamterene/hydrochlorothiazide)
- Methyclothiazide (*Aquatensen*®, *Enduron*®)
- *Midamor*® (amiloride)
- *Moduretic*® (amiloride/hydrochlorothiazide)
- *Naturetin*® (bendroflumethiazide)
- *Renese*® (polythiazide)
- Trichlormethiazide (*Naqua*®, *Diurese*™)
- *Zaroxolyn*® (metolazone)
- Others

Drowsiness: The feeling of being tired or about to drift off to sleep.

Dyspepsia: Indigestion. See Heartburn, Ulcers, and Indigestion chapter on page 323.

E

Edema: Swelling or puffiness of the feet, ankles, or lower legs.

Ejaculation: The act by a male of discharging semen during orgasm.

Electrolytes: Chemicals that help regulate the balance of fluids in the body and other cell functions.

Elixir: A liquid usually containing alcohol that is used in some liquid medications.

Embolism: Sudden blockage of a blood vessel caused by a clot or other material.

Emphysema: A medical condition that also may be called chronic obstructive pulmonary disease (COPD), which usually occurs as a result of damage to the lungs from long-standing exposure to inhaled irritants, the most common of which is cigarette smoke. See Asthma, Emphysema and Chronic Bronchitis chapter on page 97.

Endometrial cancer: Cancer of the lining of the uterus (the pear-shaped organ at the top of the vagina).

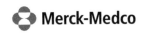

Endometriosis: A painful condition in which fragments of the lining of the uterus are found in other pelvic organs.

Endometrium: The lining of the uterus. The uterus is the pear-shaped organ at the top of the vagina.

Enema: A fluid that is inserted into the rectum through a syringe with a dull tip. By increasing the amount of fluid in the rectum and lower large intestine, enemas stretch the walls of the intestine, creating the urge to have a bowel movement. An enema may contain water alone or water combined with mineral oil, a stimulant medication, or a stool softener. Enemas include:
- *Fleet®* (sodium phosphate)
- *Fleet® Bisacodyl* (bisacodyl)
- *Therevac® Plus* (docusate sodium/glycerin/benzocaine)
- *Therevac®*-SB (docusate sodium/glycerin)
- Others

Enlarged prostate: A condition, also known as benign prostatic hypertrophy or hyperplasia (BPH), in which the prostate (the gland that lies between the bladder and the rectum in males) gets larger. See Urinary Problems chapter on page 663.

Enteric coating: Protective coatings on some medication tablets and capsules that help to prevent stomach upset or help prevent the medication from breaking down in the acid of the stomach.

Epilepsy: A disorder of the nervous system in which there is a tendency to have recurring seizures.

Erectile dysfunction: Trouble getting or keeping an erection; also called impotence.

Erythromycin: An antibiotic that helps to treat many bacterial and mycoplasmal infections. This type of medication includes: *EES®*, *ERYC®*, *E-Mycin®*, *Ery-Tab®*, *Erythrocin®*, *Ilosone®*, *PCE®*, and others.

Esophagus: The tube that connects the mouth to the stomach; the swallowing tube.

Estrogen: A hormone produced primarily by the ovaries that is responsible for many of the characteristics that distinguish women from men. Men's bodies also produce estrogen but in a much smaller amount. Estrogens include:
- *CombiPatch*™ (estradiol/norethindrone)
- Conjugated estrogens (*Cenestin®, Premarin®*)
- Conjugated estrogens/medroxyprogesterone (*Premphase®, Prempro*™)
- Esterified estrogens (*Estratab®, Menest®*)
- Estradiol (*Alora®, Climara®, E₂III*™, *Estrace®, Estraderm®, Estring®, FemPatch®, Ortho-Prefest®, Vagifem®, Vivelle®*)
- Estropipate (*Ogen®, Ortho-Est®*)
- Others

F

Fatal: Causing death.

Fatigue: Tiredness or sluggishness.

Fiber: An indigestible part of some fruits, vegetables, and whole grains that helps maintain healthy functioning of the bowels and helps prevent constipation.

Fibrates: Also called fibric acid derivatives, these medications help lower triglyceride levels and low-density lipoproteins (LDL or "bad " cholesterol). They may also raise HDL ("good" cholesterol). Fibrates include *Atromid-S®* (clofibrate), *Lopid®* (gemfibrozil), and *Tricor®* (fenofibrate).

Fibroid: A noncancerous growth of tissue that commonly occurs in the uterus. The uterus is the pear-shaped organ at the top of the vagina.

Fissures: Small tears around the opening of the rectum.

Flu: See Influenza.

Flushing: Reddening of the face.

Fracture: The breaking, cracking, or opening of a bone.

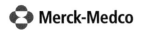

G

Gastroesophageal reflux disease (GERD): A condition, also known as heartburn, in which small amounts of food and acid from the stomach come up into the swallowing tube (esophagus). See Heartburn, Ulcers, and Indigestion chapter on page 323.

Gastrointestinal: Having to do with the part of the digestive system that includes the mouth, esophagus, stomach, and intestines.

Gastroparesis: Slow digestion.

Gel: The combination of a solid and a liquid to create a substance with a texture like that of jelly or glue.

Genetics: A branch of biology that deals with the heredity and variation of organisms.

GERD (Gastroesophageal reflux disease): A condition, also known as heartburn, in which small amounts of food and acid from the stomach come up into the swallowing tube (esophagus). See Heartburn, Ulcers, and Indigestion chapter on page 323.

Glaucoma: An eye disease in which fluid builds up inside the eye, and this fluid buildup puts pressure on the eye that can damage the optic nerve. See Glaucoma chapter on page 291.

Glucose: A type of sugar that is the main energy source for the body. Glucose most often comes from a type of food called carbohydrates (sugars, fruits, vegetables, breads, and pasta).

Glucose meter: A device used to measures a person's blood sugar (glucose).

Gout: A very painful type of arthritis caused by uric acid deposits in and around the joints.

Grave's disease: A medical condition associated with an overactive thyroid. See Thyroid Problems chapter on page 653.

H

H$_2$ Blockers: Medications that help reduce acid production in the stomach. They are used to help relieve symptoms of heartburn, ulcers, indigestion, and other medical conditions. These medications include *Axid*® (nizatidine), *Pepcid*® (famotidine), *Tagamet*® (cimetidine), and *Zantac*® (ranitidine).

Hallucinations: Seeing or hearing things that are not there.

HDL (high-density lipoprotein): A type of cholesterol that carries fatty deposits to the liver for elimination from the body. HDL is sometimes called "good" or "healthy" cholesterol because if fatty deposits are not removed and build up, they can cause heart disease or stroke.

Heartburn: A condition, also known as gastroesophageal reflux disease (GERD), in which small amounts of food and acid from the stomach come up into the swallowing tube (esophagus). See Heartburn, Ulcers, and Indigestion chapter on page 323.

Heart failure: A medical condition that occurs when the heart cannot pump enough blood to meet the body's needs. See Congestive Heart Failure chapter on page 135.

Heart rhythm medications: Medications that help prevent or control abnormal heart rhythms or irregular heartbeat (palpitations). They may also be called antiarrhythmic medications. Heart rhythm medications include:
- Amiodarone (*Cordarone*®, *Pacerone*®)
- *Betapace*® (sotalol)
- Digoxin (*Lanoxin*®, *Lanoxicaps*®)
- Diltiazem (*Cardizem*®, *Dilacor*®, *Tiazac*®)
- *Mexitil*® (mexiletine)
- *Norpace*® (disopyramide)
- Procainamide (*Procanbid*®, *Pronestyl*®)
- Quinidine (*Cardioquin*®, *Quinaglute*®, *Quinidex*®, *Quinora*®)
- *Rythmol*® (propafenone)
- *Tambocor*® (flecainide)
- *Tonocard*® (tocainide)
- Verapamil (*Calan*®, *Covera*®, *Isoptin*®, *Verelan*®)
- Others

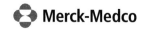

Heat stroke: A life-threatening condition resulting from extreme overexposure to heat, which disrupts the body's system of regulating temperature.

Hemorrhage: Severe bleeding that may occur either inside or outside of the body.

Hemorrhoid: A bulging vein at either the opening of the anus or just inside it.

High blood pressure (hypertension): Having a systolic pressure above 140 mm Hg, a diastolic pressure above 90 mm Hg, or both. See High Blood Pressure chapter on page 373.

High-density lipoprotein (HDL): A type of cholesterol that carries fatty deposits to the liver for elimination from the body. HDL is sometimes called "good" or "healthy" cholesterol because if fatty deposits are not removed and build up, they can cause heart disease or stroke.

Histamine: A natural substance that can increase the blood flow to the skin or increase stomach acid. Histamine is often responsible for the symptoms of allergic reactions, such as watery eyes and runny nose.

Hives: An itchy, inflamed (red, swollen, or painful) rash that often results from an allergic reaction.

Hormone: A chemical produced by a gland or tissue that is released into the bloodstream and controls such body functions as growth, sexual development, and other organ functions.

Hot flash, hot flush: A sudden warm or hot feeling with sweating and reddening of the face and neck. Many women have hot flashes while they are entering menopause.

Hydrogenated fat: A type of fat that can increase cholesterol and cause coronary artery disease and is found in such foods as palm and coconut oils.

Hypercalcemia: Too much calcium in the blood.

Hypercholesterolemia: High level of cholesterol in the blood. See High Cholesterol chapter on page 431.

Hyperglycemia (high blood sugar): Too much sugar (glucose) in the blood. See Diabetes chapter on page 259.

Hyperkalemia: Too much potassium in the blood.

Hypertension (high blood pressure): Having a systolic pressure above 140 mm Hg, a diastolic pressure above 90 mm Hg, or both. See High Blood Pressure chapter on page 373.

Hyperthyroidism: A condition in which a person's thyroid is overactive and produces too much thyroid hormone. See Thyroid Problems chapter on page 653.

Hypocalcemia: Low level of calcium in the blood.

Hypoglycemia (low blood sugar): Low level of sugar (glucose) in the blood.

Hypokalemia: Low level of potassium in the blood.

Hypotension: Abnormally low blood pressure that causes symptoms such as dizziness and fainting.

Hypothyroidism: A condition in which a person's thyroid is underactive and does not produce enough thyroid hormone. See Thyroid Problems chapter on page 653.

Hysterectomy: An operation in which the uterus (the pear-shaped organ at the top of the vagina) is removed.

I

IBS (irritable bowel syndrome): A condition, sometimes called spastic colon, that affects the intestines and in which the digestive system is often sensitive to stress, diet, and medications. See Irritable Bowel Syndrome chapter on page 509.

Immune system: The cells, substances, and structures in the body that protect against infection and illness.

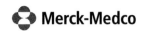

Incontinence, functional: A type of urinary incontinence in which there is nothing wrong with the bladder itself, but a physical problem (such as an inconvenient or unsuitable living situation) makes it hard for the person to get to a bathroom in time to urinate. See Urinary Problems chapter on page 663.

Incontinence, overflow: A type of urinary incontinence in which urine may leak out because the bladder cannot squeeze hard enough to empty very well, so it is left full almost all of the time. See Urinary Problems chapter on page 663.

Incontinence, stress: A type of urinary incontinence in which small amounts of urine leak out when a person exercises, coughs, laughs, or sneezes, because of pressure on the muscles that keep urine in the bladder. See Urinary Problems chapter on page 663.

Incontinence, urge: A type of urinary incontinence in which a person feels a sudden need to urinate because the bladder squeezes inward (contracts) more often than it should without giving the usual warning that it is time to urinate. See Urinary Problems chapter on page 663.

Incontinence, urinary: Loss of bladder control. See Urinary Problems chapter on page 663.

Indigestion (dyspepsia): A condition in which there is pain, discomfort, nausea, uncomfortable fullness, or bloating in the stomach soon after eating. See Heartburn, Ulcers, and Indigestion chapter on page 323.

Infection: Disease-carrying microorganisms that enter the body, multiply, and damage cells or release toxins (poisonous substances).

Inflammation: Pain, redness, and swelling in one or more parts of the body. When inflammation occurs, the part of the body affected is said to be inflamed.

Inflammatory bowel disease: Inflammation of the intestines, including ulcerative colitis and Crohn's disease.

Influenza (flu): A viral infection that causes a fever, runny nose, cough, headache, a feeling of illness (malaise), and inflammation of the lining of the nose and airways. See influenza section on page xxi.

Inhalant: A medication, such as that used for asthma, that is breathed directly into the lungs.

Inhaler: A device for breathing a medication into the lungs (inhaling), such as for asthma.

Injection: A way to receive a dose of medication through a needle; a "shot."

Insomnia: Difficulty in falling asleep or staying asleep. See Sleeping Difficulty (Insomnia) chapter on page 583.

Insulin: A hormone produced by the pancreas that helps regulate the level of glucose (blood sugar) in the body.

Interaction: A process in which two or more things act on each other, creating a situation that would not exist if either one were not there. A drug interaction (sometimes called a drug-drug interaction) is the effect on a person of taking two or more particular medications. A food-drug interaction is the effect of eating a particular type of food while taking a certain kind of medication.

Intolerance: Inability to endure something, such as having side effects from a medication that make it too difficult to continue taking the medication comfortably.

Intravenous (IV): Inside of or into a vein.

Involuntary: Happening without choice.

Irritable bowel syndrome (IBS): A condition, sometimes called spastic colon, that affects the intestines and in which the digestive system is often sensitive to stress, diet, and medications. See Irritable Bowel Syndrome chapter on page 509.

Isolated systolic hypertension: A type of high blood pressure with a high systolic (top number) and a normal diastolic (low number). Having isolated systolic hypertension is just as serious as having both numbers high. See High Blood Pressure chapter on page 373.

IU (international unit): A quantity of a biologic (such as a vitamin) that produces a particular effect agreed upon as an international standard.

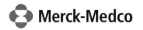

J

Jaundice: A symptom of liver problems that causes the skin, the whites of the eyes, or both to look yellowish.

L

Lactic acidosis: An abnormal buildup of acid in the body characterized by a strong odor to the breath, drowsiness, muscle aches and spasms, nausea, slow heartbeat, stomach pain, tiredness or sluggishness, trouble breathing, or shortness of breath. Advanced lactic acidosis can be serious, possibly even fatal.

Laxative: A medication that helps to relieve constipation.

LDL (low-density lipoprotein): A type of cholesterol that is deposited in the arteries, causing a buildup of fat there. Because these fatty deposits can be harmful to health, LDL is sometimes called "bad" or "lousy" cholesterol, although having some LDL in the blood is necessary.

Libido: Sex drive or interest in sex.

Lipoproteins: Substances containing lipids and proteins, making up most fats in the body.

Lithium: A medication used to treat manic episodes of manic-depressive disorders. Some brands of this medication include *Eskalith®*, *Lithobid®*, *Lithonate®*, *Lithotabs®*, and others.

Low-density lipoprotein (LDL): A type of cholesterol that is deposited in the arteries, causing a buildup of fat there. Because these fatty deposits can be harmful to health, LDL is sometimes called "bad" or "lousy" cholesterol, although having some LDL in the blood is necessary.

Lupus (lupus erythematosus): A disorder of the immune system that causes inflammation of connective tissue.

M

Magnesium: A mineral that is essential for many body functions, including nerve impulse transmission, formation of bones and teeth, and muscle contraction.

Manic depression (manic depressive disorder): A mental condition characterized by extreme mood swings, including either mania, depression, or a continuing shift between the two extremes.

MAO (monoamine oxidase inhibitors): A group of antidepressant medications that increase the level of specific substances in the central nervous system to help relieve depression. These medications include *Marplan*® (isocarboxazid), *Nardil*® (phenelzine), *Parnate*® (tranylcypromine), and others.

Medical history: A medical history should include all diseases and medical conditions that a person has had, as well as medications taken and responses to them. Additionally, medical conditions of close blood relatives are important for a healthcare professional to know because many conditions can run in the family.

Melanoma: A life-threatening form of skin cancer.

Microorganism: Any tiny, single-celled organism (such as a bacterium, virus, or fungus).

Migraine: A severe headache, usually accompanied by vision problems and/or nausea and vomiting.

Milligram: A unit of weight in the metric system that is used to describe dosage strengths of medications. Abbreviated as mg.

Miotic: Short for "miotic medication." A medication that temporarily causes the pupil of the eye to shrink (become smaller). Miotics include:
- *E-Pilo*® (pilocarpine/epinephrine)
- *Humorsol*® (demecarium)
- *Isopto*® *Carbachol* (carbachol)
- Pilocarpine (*Adsorbocarpine*™, *Isopto*® *Carpine*, *Ocusert*®, *P.V. Carpine*®, *Pilocar*®, *Pilostat*®)

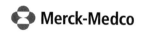

- $P_1E_1^®$, $P_2E_1^®$, $P_4E_1^®$, $P_6E_1^®$ (pilocarpine/epinephrine)
- *Phospholine Iodide*® (echothiophate)
- Others

Monoamine oxidase (MAO) inhibitors: A group of antidepressant medications that increase the level of specific substances in the central nervous system to help relieve depression. These medications include *Marplan*® (isocarboxazid), *Nardil*® (phenelzine), *Parnate*® (tranylcypromine), and others.

Monounsaturated fat: A type of fat that is thought to be beneficial in the prevention of coronary artery disease, found in such foods as olive oil and peanut oil.

Mucus: The sticky secretions in the mucous membranes, such as in the nose.

Multivitamin: A single pill that contains many different vitamins and, usually, minerals.

Muscle relaxants: Medications used to treat muscle spasms. These medications include *Dantrium*® (dantrolene), *Flexeril*® (cyclobenzaprine), *Soma*® (carisoprodol), and others.

Myasthenia gravis: A medical condition in which the muscles (mainly those in the face, eyes, throat, and limbs) become weak and tire quickly; caused by the body's immune system attacking the receptors in the muscles that pick up nerve impulses.

Mydriatic: A medication that causes the pupil of the eye to dilate (become wider or larger). It reduces the pressure in the eye caused from fluid buildup by increasing the flow of fluid out of the eye and decreasing the amount of fluid produced in the eye. These medications include:
- Epinephrine (*Epifrin*®, *Glaucon*®, and others)
- Epinephrine/pilocarpine (*E-Pilo*®, $P_1E_1^®$, $P_2E_1^®$, $P_4E_1^®$, $P_6E_1^®$)
- *Propine*® (dipivefrin)
- Others

Myocardial infarction (MI): Heart attack. See Stroke, Heart Attack, and Blood Clot Prevention chapter on page 623 and Coronary Artery Disease and Cardiac Chest Pain (Angina) chapter on page 193.

N

Narcotic: A medication made from opium or any medication that has similar effects. Narcotics help relieve moderate to severe pain. Narcotics include:
- Acetaminophen/codeine (*Phenaphen®* with Codeine, *Tylenol with Codeine®*)
- Codeine
- *Demerol®* (meperidine)
- *Dilaudid®* (hydromorphone)
- *Duragesic®* (fentanyl)
- *Hycodan®* (hydrocodone)
- Hydrocodone (*Lorcet®*, *Lortab®*, *Vicodin®*)
- Morphine (*Duramorph®*, *Kadian™*, *MS Contin®*, *MSIR®*, *Oramorph®*, *Roxanol®*)
- Oxycodone (*Endocodone®*, *OxyContin®*, *OxyFAST®*, *OxyIR®*, *Percocet®*, *Percodan®*, *Percolone®*, *Roxicet™*, *Roxicodone®*, *Roxiprin®*, *Tylox®*)
- Pentazocine (*Talacen®*, *Talwin®*)
- Propoxyphene (*Darvocet-N®*, *Darvon®*, *Wygesic®*)
- *Stadol®* (butorphanol)
- Others

Nasal congestion: Stuffy nose.

Nebulizer: A small machine for breathing medication into the lungs (inhaling) for asthma and other lung diseases. The medication starts as a liquid and is turned into a spray mist inside the nebulizer.

Neuroleptic medications: Medications that can be used for behavior problems in Alzheimer's disease and other dementias. These medications may also be used for mental conditions like schizophrenia and may be called tranquilizers. Neuroleptic medications include:
- *Clozaril®* (clozapine)
- *Haldol®* (haloperidol)
- *Loxitane®* (loxapine)
- *Mellaril®* (thioridazine)
- *Moban®* (molindone)
- *Navane®* (thiothixene)
- *Orap®* (pimozide)
- *Prolixin®* (fluphenazine)

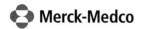
- *Risperdal*® (risperidone)
- *Serentil*® (mesoridazine)
- *Seroquel*® (quetiapine)
- *Stelazine*® (trifluoperazine)
- *Thorazine*® (chlorpromazine)
- *Trilafon*® (perphenazine)
- *Zyprexa*® (olanzapine)
- Others

Neuropathy: Disease or damage to the nerves.

Niacin: A vitamin important in many chemical processes in the body; also known as vitamin B_3.

Night vision: The capacity to see things in faint light, as at night.

Nitrates: Medications that help relieve chest pain from angina and symptoms of heart failure. Nitrates open (dilate) blood vessels and increase the supply of oxygen to the heart. Nitrates include:
- Nitroglycerin (*Deponit*®, *Minitran*®, *Nitro-Bid*®, *Nitrodisc*®, *Nitro-Dur*®, *Nitrogard*®, *Nitroglyn*®, *Nitrol*®, *Nitrolingual*®, *Nitrong*®, *NitroQuick*®, *Nitrostat*®, *Transderm-Nitro*®)
- Isosorbide dinitrate (*Dilatrate*®, *Isordil*®, *Sorbitrate*®)
- Isosorbide mononitrate (*Imdur*®, *ISMO*®, *Monoket*®)
- Others

Nitroglycerin: See Nitrates.

Nonsteroidal anti-inflammatory drugs (NSAIDs): Medications that help relieve pain and reduce inflammation and fever. NSAIDs include:
- *Ansaid*® (flurbiprofen)
- *Arthrotec*® (diclofenac/misoprostol)
- *Celebrex*® (celecoxib)
- *Clinoril*® (sulindac)
- *Daypro*® (oxaprozin),
- Diclofenac (*Cataflam*®, *Voltaren*®)
- *Dolobid*® (diflunisal)
- *Feldene*® (piroxicam)

- Ibuprofen (*Advil®*, *Motrin®*)
- *Indocin®* (indomethacin)
- Ketoprofen (*Orudis®*, *Oruvail®*)
- *Lodine®* (etodolac)
- *Nalfon®* (fenoprofen)
- *Naprosyn®* (naproxen)
- Naproxen (*Aleve®*, *Anaprox®*)
- *Ponstel®* (mefenamic acid)
- *Relafen®* (nabumetone)
- *Tolectin®* (tolmetin)
- *Toradol®* (ketorolac)
- *Vioxx®* (rofecoxib)
- Others

NSAIDs: See Nonsteroidal anti-inflammatory drugs.

Nutrient: Any substance that the body can use to maintain its health.

O

Obsessive-compulsive disorder (OCD): A mental illness in which a person frequently or constantly worries about one or more specific things (obsession) or does one thing repeatedly (compulsion), such as washing his or her hands over and over again.

OCD: See Obsessive-compulsive disorder.

Ointment: A thick, greasy form of medication to be spread on the skin that usually comes in a tube or jar.

Open-angle glaucoma (also called chronic or wide-angle glaucoma): This most common form of glaucoma usually has no symptoms but usually responds well to medication, especially if diagnosed and treated early. See Glaucoma chapter on page 291.

Optic nerves: Important nerves that send images from the eye to the brain.

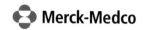

Osteoarthritis: Arthritis caused by wear and tear on the joints, it is the most common type of arthritis in people over 65. See Arthritis and Pain chapter on page 37.

Osteoporosis: A medical condition in which bones become thin, weak, and brittle, so they break more easily. See Osteoporosis chapter on page 521.

Overactive bladder: A condition in which the bladder squeezes inward (contracts) more often than it should, which can cause urinary incontinence.

Over-the-counter (OTC) medication: A medication that can be bought without a prescription.

Oxygen: A gas that is colorless, odorless, and tasteless, essential to almost all forms of life.

P

Pacemaker: A small electronic device that is surgically implanted to stimulate the heart muscle to provide a normal heartbeat.

Paget's disease: A disorder in which bone does not form properly, causing bone weakening, thickening, and deformity.

Pain receptors: Nerves in the brain that receive pain signals from other nerves throughout the body.

Palpitations: An unusual or unpleasant sensation, usually in the chest from an irregular or forceful heartbeat. Palpitations may be caused by heart rhythm problems (arrhythmias) where the heart beats too slowly, too rapidly, or irregularly.

Pancreas: A large gland between the spleen and intestine that produces insulin and some of the enzymes that are needed to digest food.

Panic attack/disorder: An emotional disorder characterized by sudden attacks of anxiety (nervousness), fear, or panic.

Parkinson's disease: An illness that affects the part of the brain that controls body movement. See Parkinson's Disease chapter on page 547.

Penicillins: A type of antibiotic that kills bacteria and is used to treat various infections. Penicillins include:
- Amoxicillin (*Amoxil®*, *Trimox®*, and others)
- *Augmentin®* (amoxicillin/clavulanate)
- Penicillin (*Pen-Vee®* K, *Veetids®*, and others)
- *Principen®* (ampicillin)
- *Spectrobid®* (bacampicillin)
- Others

Peptic ulcer disease (PUD): Also known as ulcers; irritations in the lining of the stomach or small intestine that are formed when this lining is damaged. See Heartburn, Ulcers, and Indigestion chapter on page 323.

Peripheral vascular disease (PVD): The narrowing of blood vessels in the legs or arms, causing pain and possibly tissue death (gangrene) as a result of a reduced flow of blood to areas supplied by the narrowed vessels.

Personal medical identification bracelet or necklace: A bracelet or necklace containing medical information about the person who is wearing it. This information may be that the person has a particular allergy or chronic condition (such as epilepsy) or takes a certain medication (such as for seizures). In an emergency, if the person cannot speak, the bracelet or necklace gives important information to medical professionals who are trying to help.

Phlebitis: Redness, pain, and swelling caused by a clot that forms in the veins and blocks the normal flow of blood.

Phlegm: Abnormal quantity of thick mucus secreted from the nasal or lung passages.

Phobia: An abnormal fear of something, such as bridges, dogs, spiders, or heights.

Plaque: A deposit of something that is different from its surroundings, such as fatty deposits in the arteries, hardened areas on muscle or soft tissue, or a film on the teeth where bacteria can grow.

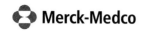

Platelets: Tiny cell-like particles in the bloodstream that help the blood to clot.

Pneumonia: Inflammation of the lungs due to a bacterial or viral infection, which causes fever, shortness of breath, and the coughing up of phlegm. See Advice about the Flu and Pneumonia on page xxi.

Polyp: An abnormal overgrowth of tissue in the body, such as in the nose (nasal polyp) or intestines (intestinal polyp).

Postherpetic neuralgia: Also called shingles; an infection or reactivation of the chickenpox virus. It causes inflammation of the nerves and is often very painful.

Potassium: A mineral that plays an important role in the body, helping to maintain water balance, normal heart rhythm, conduction of nerve impulses, and muscle contraction.

Potassium supplements: Pills and liquids that contain potassium used to help prevent or correct a low potassium level in the body. These include *Kaochlor*®, *Kay Ciel*®, *K-Dur*®, *K-Lyte*®, *K-Tab*®, *Klor-Con*®, *Klorvess*®, *Klotrix*®, *Micro-K*®, *Slow K*®, *Ten-K*®, and others.

Potassium-sparing diuretics: Medications used to help lower high blood pressure. These diuretics (water pills) increase the amount of urine that the body makes without causing the body to lose potassium. These medications include:
- *Aldactazide*® (spironolactone/hydrochlorothiazide)
- *Aldactone*® (spironolactone)
- *Dyrenium*® (triamterene)
- *Midamor*® (amiloride)
- *Moduretic*® (amiloride/hydrochlorothiazide)
- Triamterene/hydrochlorothiazide (*Dyazide*®, *Maxzide*®)
- Others

PPIs: See Proton pump inhibitors.

Priapism: A lasting, painful erection. Priapism is a medical condition that requires treatment by a healthcare professional.

Progestin/Progesterone: A female sex hormone that is taken with estrogen to help reduce the risk of endometrial cancer in women who have not had a hysterectomy.

Propellant: Gas kept under pressure that drives the medication out of an inhaler when pressed.

Proteins: Large molecules made up of amino acids that play many major roles in the body, including forming the basis of body structures such as skin and hair, and important chemicals such as enzymes and hormones.

Proton pump inhibitors (PPIs): Medications that help prevent the stomach from making acid. Proton pump inhibitors are usually prescribed for heartburn and peptic ulcer disease. These medications include *Aciphex*® (rabeprazole), *Prevacid*® (lansoprazole), *Prilosec*® (omeprazole), and *Protonix*® (pantoprazole).

Prostate, prostate gland: A small gland in men that lies between the bladder and rectum and is involved in male sexual function.

Pulmonary embolism: A blood clot in the arteries that supply blood to the lungs.

Q

Quick-relief medications: Quick-relief medications help reduce or relieve shortness of breath and wheezing during an asthma attack. Quick-relief medications are fast-acting and are usually used as needed when asthma symptoms start.

Quinidine: A medication that is used to treat atrial fibrillation and flutter and other heart rhythm problems. This medication works by changing the electrical impulses in the heart to help control abnormal heart rhythms. Quinidines include *Cardioquin*®, *Quinaglute*®, *Quinalan*®, *Quinidex*®, *Quinora*®, and others.

Quinolone: A type of antibiotic that kills bacteria and is used to treat various infections. These medications include:
- *Avalox*® (moxifloxacin)
- *Cipro*® (ciprofloxacin)
- *Floxin*® (ofloxacin)
- *Levaquin*® (levofloxacin)
- *Maxaquin*® (lomefloxacin)
- *Noroxin*® (norfloxacin)
- *Zagam*® (sparfloxacin)
- Others

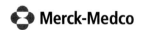
R

Rash: Skin redness, bumps, itching, or irritation.

Raynaud's disease: A condition in which there is poor blood flow to the hands.

Rectum: The end of the large intestine, ending at the anus.

Restless leg syndrome: A disorder that occurs just before falling asleep, causing vaguely uncomfortable sensations in the legs, along with spontaneous, uncontrollable leg movements.

Retinal detachment: Separation of the retina of the eye from its underlying support.

Reye's syndrome: A serious, even fatal illness in children that may occur if aspirin is given to children with flu-like symptoms. Do not give aspirin or any medication containing aspirin to children before checking with a doctor or other healthcare professional.

Rheumatoid arthritis: A type of arthritis that is caused by inflammation. See Arthritis and Pain chapter on page 37.

Rhinitis: Inflammation of the lining of the nose, which can cause sneezing, runny nose, congestion, and pain; when caused by substances in the air, it is called allergic rhinitis or hay fever.

Room temperature: The usual range of temperatures indoors (59° F to 86°).

S

Salicylates: Aspirin and aspirin-like compounds; pain-relieving medications in the aspirin family. They include:

- **Aspirin:** *Arthritis Pain Formula*™, *Ascriptin*®, *Bufferin*®, *Ecotrin*®, *Empirin*®, *Halfprin*®, *ZORprin*®, and others

- **Aspirin-like medications:** *Disalcid®* (salsalate), *Dolobid®*, (diflunisal), magnesium salicylate (*Doan's®*, *Magan®*, *Mobidin®*), *Trilisate®* (choline magnesium trisalicylate), and others

- **Medications that contain aspirin:** *Aggrenox®* (dipyridamole/aspirin), *Darvon® Compound-65* (propoxyphene/aspirin), *Percodan®* (oxycodone/aspirin), *Talwin® Compound* (pentazocine/aspirin), and others

Salicylism: A condition caused by a reaction to salicylates. The symptoms of salicylism include dizziness, diarrhea, confusion, headache, sweating, and fast, troubled breathing (hyperventilation).

Saturated fats: The type of fat in the diet most likely to raise blood cholesterol levels that cause plaque to form in the lining of arteries

Schizophrenia: A mental illness that causes delusions and hallucinations.

Sedative: A medication that has a calming effect. It helps to reduce anxiety (nervousness). Barbiturates, benzodiazepines, meprobamate, neuroleptic medications, and sleep medications may be used as a sedative.

Seizure: An abnormal or uncontrollable stimulation in the brain that can cause convulsions (sudden, involuntary contractions of a group of muscles), thought disturbances, or other minor physical changes.

Seizure medications: Medications used to treat or prevent seizures. Also known as "anticonvulsants." These include:
- *Cerebyx®* (fosphenytoin)
- *Depakene®* (valproic acid)
- *Depakote®* (divalproex sodium)
- *Dilantin®* (phenytoin)
- *Felbatol®* (felbamate)
- *Mesantoin®* (mephenytoin)
- *Neurontin®* (gabapentin)
- *Peganone®* (ethotoin)
- *Tegretol®* (carbamazepine)
- *Topamax®* (topiramate)
- *Trileptal®* (oxcarbazepine)
- Others

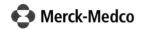

Selective serotonin reuptake inhibitors (SSRIs): A group of antidepressant medications that work by helping to restore the balance of chemical signals in the brain. These medications include:
- *Celexa*™ (citalopram)
- *Luvox*® (fluvoxamine)
- *Paxil*® (paroxetine)
- *Prozac*® (fluoxetine)
- *Zoloft*® (sertraline)

Serotonin: A chemical that transmits nerve impulses that cause blood vessels to constrict (narrow). Serotonin levels in the brain also affect mood.

Shingles: An infection or reactivation of the chickenpox virus. It causes inflammation of the nerves and is often very painful. Shingles is also called postherpetic neuralgia.

Side effect: Any unwanted effect that results from the use of a medication. Sometimes called an adverse effect.

Social phobia: More than normal anxiety (nervousness) in common social situations that causes a person to either avoid social situations or endure them with great distress.

Sodium: A mineral that plays a role in the body's water balance, heart rhythm, nerve impulses, and muscle contraction; present in table salt (sodium chloride).

Spacer: A small device that attaches to an inhaler to make it easier to use and help prevent some of the side effects.

Spasm: Sudden, involuntary contraction of a muscle or group of muscles.

SSRIs (selective serotonin reuptake inhibitors): A group of antidepressant medications that work by helping to restore the balance of chemical signals in the brain. These medications include:
- *Celexa*™ (citalopram)
- *Luvox*® (fluvoxamine)
- *Paxil*® (paroxetine)
- *Prozac*® (fluoxetine)
- *Zoloft*® (sertraline)

Statins: Medications used to lower cholesterol levels. Some statins can also help lower triglyceride levels and help raise HDL ("good") cholesterol levels. These medications include:
- *Baycol*® (cerivastatin)
- *Lescol*® (fluvastatin)
- *Lipitor*® (atorvastatin)
- *Mevacor*® (lovastatin)
- *Pravachol*® (pravastatin)
- *Zocor*® (simvastatin)

Sternum: The breastbone.

Stimulant laxatives: Medications that help to create the urge to have a bowel movement. These include:
- *Agoral*® (mineral oil/phenolphthalein)
- Bisacodyl (*Correctol*®, *Dulcolax*®, *Fleet*®)
- Docusate/casanthranol (*Doxidan*®, *Peri-Colace*®)
- *Nature's Remedy*® (cascara sagrada/aloe)
- *Neoloid*® (castor oil)
- Senna (*Ex-Lax*®, *Senokot*®)
- *Senokot-S*® (senna/docusate sodium)
- Others

Stool: Bowel movement.

Stool softener: A medication that helps to soften bowel movements inside the intestines so that they can pass more easily and with less pain. Stool softeners include *Colace*® (docusate sodium), *Diocto-K*® (docusate potassium), *Surfak*® (docusate calcium), and others.

Stricture: An abnormal narrowing of a bodily passage or that narrowed part.

Stroke: What happens when a blood clot blocks one of the blood vessels going to the brain, causing tissue damage due to lack of oxygen. See Stroke, Heart Attack, and Blood Clot Prevention chapter on page 623.

Sublingual: Under the tongue.

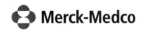

Sulfonylureas: Medications that increase the release of insulin and are used in the treatment of diabetes. These medications include:
- *Amaryl®* (glimepiride)
- *Diabinese®* (chlorpropamide)
- *Dymelor®* (acetohexamide)
- *Glucotrol®* (glipizide)
- Glyburide (*DiaBeta®*, *Glynase®*, *Micronase®*)
- *Orinase®* (tolbutamide)
- *Tolinase®* (tolazamide)
- Others

Sunblock or sunscreen: An ointment, cream, or lotion containing chemicals that help protect the skin exposed to sunlight from harmful rays to prevent skin cancer, aging of the skin, and sunburn.

Supplement: Something added to what a person eats to provide more of the ingredient that the body needs, such as vitamins or minerals.

Suppository: A medication that is inserted in the rectum.

Suppressant: A medication that is used to help reduce in intensity rather than stop entirely (as in appetite).

Sustained- or controlled-release dosage forms: Medications that are specially formulated to release their ingredients slowly, usually over 12 hours or more.

Synthetic: Something produced artificially by a chemical process (not from a natural source).

Systolic pressure: The measurement of blood pressure, in millimeters of mercury (mm Hg), during the part of the heartbeat when blood is being squeezed out of the heart. The top (first) number in a blood pressure reading. Also see Diastolic pressure.

T

Tetracycline: A type of antibiotic that prevents bacteria from growing that is used to treat various infections. These medications include *Declomycin®* (demeclocycline), minocycline (*Dynacin®*, *Minocin®*), tetracycline (*Achromycin®*, *Sumycin®*), *Vibramycin®* (doxycycline), and others.

Theophylline: A medication that helps to open the breathing passages and helps the diaphragm (muscle under the lungs) bring air into the lungs. Theophylline is used to help prevent symptoms of asthma and COPD from occurring. Theophylline comes in different brand names such as *Slo-bid™*, *Slo-Phyllin®*, *Theo-24®*, *Theobid®*, *Theo-Dur®*, *Theolair™*, *T-Phyl®*, *Uni-Dur®*, *Uniphyl®*, and others.

Thrombus: A blood clot that forms in the heart or a blood vessel (vein or artery).

Thrush: A yeast infection of the mouth that is often caused by *Candida* (yeast). It may look like a white rash and cause soreness.

Thyroid: A small gland located in the front of the neck that produces natural chemicals (hormones) that control energy-producing functions in the body and releases them into the bloodstream.

Thyroid medications: Medications used to increase the amount of thyroid hormone in the body when the body's thyroid gland is not making enough thyroid hormone (hypothyroidism). These medications include *Armour®* *Thyroid* (thyroid hormone), *Cytomel®* (liothyronine), levothyroxine (*Eltroxin™*, *Levo-T®*, *Levothroid®*, *Levoxine®*, *Levoxyl®*, *Synthroid®*), *Thyrolar®* (liotrix), and others.

Tic: A jerking motion or uncontrollable, repetitive movement of the face, neck, and/or arms.

Tinnitus: Ringing in the ears; a possible side effect of some medications.

Toxic: Poisonous.

Toxicity: The effect of a poison or toxin.

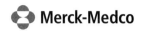

Tranquilizer: A medication used to reduce nervousness (anxiety) or tension.

Transdermal: Through the skin.

Travelers' diarrhea: Diarrhea that occurs when traveling in a foreign country, caused by contaminated food or water.

Tremor: An involuntary trembling or shaking motion.

Tricyclic antidepressants: Medications used to treat depression and other conditions such as pain. These medications include:
- *Anafranil*® (clomipramine)
- *Asendin*® (amoxapine)
- *Elavil*® (amitriptyline)
- *Norpramin*® (desipramine)
- *Pamelor*® (nortriptyline)
- *Sinequan*® (doxepin)
- *Surmontil*® (trimipramine)
- *Tofranil*® (imipramine)
- *Vivactil*® (protriptyline)
- Others

Trigeminal neuralgia: A disorder of a cranial nerve that causes attacks of pain in the lips, cheeks, gums, or chin on one side of the face.

Triglyceride: A type of fat in the blood.

Triptans: Medications that constrict vessels in the brain to help treat migraine headaches. These include *Amerge*® (naratriptan), *Imitrex*® (sumatriptan), *Maxalt*® (rizatriptan), and *Zomig*® (zolmitriptan).

Tuberculosis: An infectious bacterial disease transmitted through the air that mainly affects the lungs.

Type 1 diabetes: The type of diabetes in which the pancreas does not make enough insulin. See Diabetes chapter on page 259.

Type 2 diabetes: The type of diabetes in which the body is resistant to the insulin the pancreas makes. See Diabetes chapter on page 259.

Tyramine: Natural substance in food and beverages that can stimulate the nervous system and must be avoided while taking MAO inhibitors.

U

Ulcer: Also known as peptic ulcer disease (PUD); irritation in the lining of the stomach or small intestine that is formed when this lining is damaged. See Heartburn, Ulcers, and Indigestion chapter on page 323.

Ulcerative colitis: A chronic inflammatory disease of the digestive system usually affecting the large intestine (colon).

Urethra: The tiny tube that carries urine from the bladder to the outside of the body.

Urinary incontinence: Loss of bladder control. See Incontinence, and Urinary Problems chapter on page 663.

Urinary retention: The lack of ability to empty the bladder, so that urine is retained (held) there.

V

Vaccination: Administering a vaccine to prevent a disease.

Vaccine: A solution containing a killed or altered form of a virus to help make a person resistant to the disease it causes.

Vaginal ring: A device that contains medication that can be placed into the vagina. The device delivers medication slowly over time for a few months.

Vasodilator: A medication that relaxes the walls of blood vessels so that they open more widely, allowing blood to flow through them more freely.

Vein: A blood vessel that carries blood to the heart from various parts of the body.

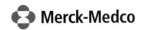

Venous: Having to do with a vein.

Venous thrombosis: A clot in the vein of a leg that may form after surgery or after long periods of bed rest or inactivity.

Verapamil: A calcium channel blocker that may be used to treat heart rhythm problems, high blood pressure, cardiac chest pain (angina pectoris), and other conditions. Brand names of verapamil include *Calan*®, *Covera HS*®, *Isoptin*®, *Verelan*®, and others.

Vial: A small glass or plastic container. Vials are often used to store prescription pills or liquids.

W

Water pills: See Diuretics.

Weight-bearing exercise: Exercise that puts stress on bones, such as walking, weightlifting, gardening, and others. Weight-bearing exercise helps build up bone density and prevent the bones from becoming brittle.

Withdrawal symptoms: Problems that develop as a direct result of stopping a particular medication abruptly.

Y

Yeast infection: An infection caused by an overgrowth of *Candida*. It can cause mouth infections, diaper rash, vaginitis, and other infections.

Understanding Prescriptions

Understanding the Information That is on Your Prescription Label

This is a sample of a prescription label. While the same information appears on all prescription labels, the look of the label may change from pharmacy to pharmacy.

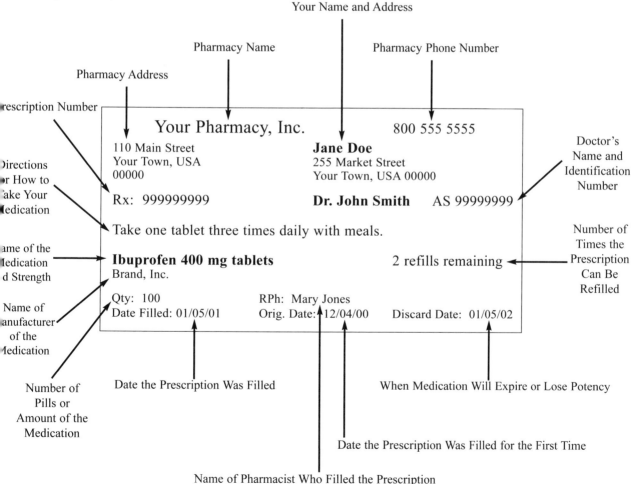

Your Name and Address

Pharmacy Name

Pharmacy Phone Number

Pharmacy Address

Prescription Number

Directions or How to Take Your Medication

Name of the Medication and Strength

Name of Manufacturer of the Medication

Your Pharmacy, Inc.   800 555 5555

110 Main Street
Your Town, USA
00000

Jane Doe
255 Market Street
Your Town, USA 00000

Rx: 999999999   **Dr. John Smith   AS 99999999**

Take one tablet three times daily with meals.

Ibuprofen 400 mg tablets   2 refills remaining
Brand, Inc.

Qty: 100   RPh: Mary Jones
Date Filled: 01/05/01   Orig. Date: 12/04/00   Discard Date: 01/05/02

Doctor's Name and Identification Number

Number of Times the Prescription Can Be Refilled

Number of Pills or Amount of the Medication

Date the Prescription Was Filled

When Medication Will Expire or Lose Potency

Date the Prescription Was Filled for the First Time

Name of Pharmacist Who Filled the Prescription

793

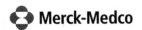

Auxiliary Labels

Labels similar to the examples that appear below may also be placed on your prescription bottle. They provide additional important information on how to take your medication safely and effectively. Be sure to read all labels carefully and follow all directions as stated.

 MAY CAUSE **DROWSINESS**. **ALCOHOL** MAY INTENSIFY THIS EFFECT. **USE CARE** WHEN OPERATING A CAR OR DANGEROUS MACHINERY.

 YOU SHOULD **AVOID** PROLONGED OR EXCESSIVE EXPOSURE TO DIRECT AND/OR ARTIFICIAL **SUNLIGHT** WHILE TAKING THIS MEDICATION

 IT IS VERY **IMPORTANT** THAT YOU TAKE OR USE THIS **EXACTLY AS DIRECTED**. DO NOT SKIP DOSES OR DISCONTINUE UNLESS DIRECTED BY YOUR DOCTOR

(Labels appear about 2 times actual size.)

KEEP IN REFRIGERATOR
DO NOT FREEZE

OBTAIN MEDICAL ADVICE
BEFORE TAKING NONPRESCRIPTION
DRUGS. SOME MAY AFFECT THE
ACTION OF THIS MEDICATION.

FOR EXTERNAL USE
ONLY

Resources for Help and Information

This is a list of organizations in the United States that provide assistance for people with various health problems. Most of these are national organizations, but many have local chapters. Most are not-for-profit organizations that offer information or support rather than actual healthcare or legal services. Telephone numbers and Internet Web sites are included when available. However, such information changes frequently. Additional information is available through healthcare professionals, local libraries, telephone listings, and the Internet.

Aging

American Association of Retired People
601 E Street NW
Washington, DC 20049
800-424-3410; 202-434-2277
www.aarp.org

American Geriatrics Society Foundation for Health in Aging (FHA)
The Empire State Building
350 Fifth Avenue, Suite 801
New York, NY 10118
212-755-6810
www.healthinaging.org

National Association of Area Agencies on Aging
1112 16th Street NW
Washington, DC 20036
202-296-8130
www.n4a.org

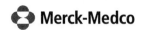

National Council on the Aging
409 Third Street SW, Suite 200
Washington, DC 20024
202-479-1200
www.ncoa.org

National Institute on Aging
Public Information Office
Room 5C27
31 Center Drive, MSC 2292
Bethesda, MD 20892-2292
800-222-2225; 301-496-1752
www.nih.gov/nia

Older Women's League
666 11th Street NW, Suite 700
Washington, DC 20001
202-783-6686
www.owl-national.org

Alcohol

Alcoholics Anonymous
PO Box 459
Grand Central Station
New York, NY 10163
212-870-3400
www.alcoholicsanonymous.org

National Council on Alcoholism & Drug Dependence
12 West 21st Street
New York, NY 10010
800-NCA-CALL; 212-206-6770
www.ncadd.org

Alzheimer's Disease

Alzheimer's Association
919 N Michigan Avenue, Suite 1100
Chicago, IL 60611-1676
800-272-3900
www.alz.org

Alzheimer's Disease Education & Referral Center
PO Box 8250
Silver Spring, MD 20907-8250
800-438-4380; 301-495-3311
www.alzheimers.org

Amputation
(see also Disability and Rehabilitation)

National Amputation Foundation
38-40 Church Street
Malverne, NY 11565
516-887-3600

Arthritis

Arthritis Foundation
1330 W Peachtree Street
Atlanta, GA 30309
800-283-7800; 404-872-7100
www.arthritis.org

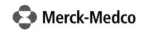

National Institute of Arthritis & Musculoskeletal & Skin Diseases
National Institutes of Health
Building 31, Room 4C-05
31 Center Drive, MSC 2350
Bethesda, MD 20892-2350
301-496-8190
www.nih-gov/niams

Blindness and Vision Problems

American Association of the Deaf & Blind
814 Thayer Avenue, Suite 302
Silver Spring, MD 20910
301-588-6565 (TTY)

American Foundation for the Blind
11 Penn Plaza, Suite 300
New York, NY 10001
800-232-5463; 212-502-7600
www.afb.org

**Association for the Education & Rehabilitation
of the Blind & Visually Impaired**
4600 Duke Street, Suite 430
PO Box 22397
Alexandria, VA 22304
703-823-9690
www.aerbvi.org

Glaucoma Research Foundation
200 Pine Street, Suite 200
San Francisco, CA 94104
800-826-6696; 415-986-3162
www.glaucoma.org

National Association for Visually Handicapped
22 West 21st Street, 6th Floor
New York, NY 10010
212-889-3141
www.navh.org

Breathing and Lung Problems

American Lung Association
1740 Broadway
New York, NY 10019
800-586-4872; 312-315-8700
www.lungusa.org

Cancer

American Cancer Society
1599 Clifton Road NE
Atlanta, GA 30329-4251
800-ACS-2345; 404-320-3333
www.cancer.org

National Coalition for Cancer Survivorship
1010 Wayne Avenue, Suite 505
Silver Spring, MD 20910
877-622-7937
www.cansearch.org

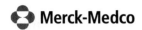

Death and Dying

Choice in Dying
475 Riverside Drive
Room 1852
New York, NY 10115
212-870-2003
National Office:
1035 30th Street NW
Washington, DC 20007
202-338-9790
www.choices.org

National Hospice Organization
1901 N Moore Street, Suite 901
Arlington, VA 22209
800-658-8898; 703-243-5900
www.nho.org

Diabetes

American Diabetes Association
1660 Duke Street
Alexandria, VA 22314
800-232-3472; 703-549-1500
www.diabetes.org

Disability and Rehabilitation

Disabled American Veterans
National Headquarters:
3725 Alexandria Pike
Cold Spring, KY 41076
606-441-7300
www.dav.org

National Rehabilitation Information Center
1010 Wayne Avenue, Suite 800
Silver Spring, MD 20910
800-346-2742
www.naric.com

General Medicine

American Medical Association
515 North State Street
Chicago, IL 60610
312-464-5000
www.ama-assn.org

Centers for Disease Control and Prevention
1600 Clifton Road NE
Atlanta, GA 30333
404-639-3311
www.cdc.gov

National Council on Patient Information & Education
4915 St. Elmo Avenue, Suite 505
Bethesda, MD 20814-6053
301-656-8565
www.talkaboutrx.org

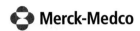

National Institutes of Health
9000 Rockville Pike
Bethesda, MD 20892
301-496-4000
www.nih.gov/science/campus

US Department of Health and Human Services
200 Independence Avenue SW
Washington, DC 20201
202-619-0257
www.os.dhhs.gov

US Food and Drug Administration
Office of Consumer Affairs
Inquiry Information Line
888-463-6332
www.fda.gov

Heart Problems

American Heart Association
7272 Greenville Avenue
Dallas, TX 75231
214-373-6300
www.americanheart.org

Inflammatory Bowel Problems

Crohn's & Colitis Foundation of America
386 Park Avenue South
New York, NY 10016
800-932-2423
212-685-3440
www.ccfa.org

Kidney Problems

American Association of Kidney Patients
100 S Ashley Drive, Suite 280
Tampa, FL 33602
800-749-2257
www.aakp.org

Liver Problems

American Liver Foundation
75 Maiden Lane, Suite 603
New York, NY 10038-4810
800-223-0179; 973-256-2550
www.liverfoundation.org

Mental Health

National Mental Health Association
1021 Prince Street
Alexandria, VA 22314-2971
800-969-NMHA; 703-684-7722
www.nmha.org

Osteoporosis

National Osteoporosis Foundation
1232 22nd Street NW
Washington, DC 20037
202-223-2226
www.nof.org

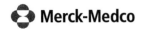

Pain Relief

American Chronic Pain Association
PO Box 850
Rocklin, CA 95677
916-632-0922
www.theacpa.org

Parkinson's Disease

American Parkinson Disease Association
1250 Hylan Boulevard
Staten Island, NY 10305
800-223-2732; 718-981-8001
www.apdaparkinson.com

Prostate Problems

The Prostatitis Foundation
1063 30th Street, Box 8
Smithshire, IL 61478
888-891-4200
www.prostate.org

Sleep Problems

National Sleep Foundation
1522 K Street NW, Suite 500
Washington, DC 20005
202-347-3471
www.sleepfoundation.org

Stroke and Nerve Damage

National Institute of Neurological Disorders and Stroke
Office of Communications and Public Liaison
PO Box 5801
Bethesda, MD 20824
800-352-9424; 301-496-5751
www.ninds.nih.gov

National Stroke Association
9707 East Easter Lane
Englewood, CO 80112
800-STROKES (787-6537)
www.stroke.org

Thyroid Problems

Thyroid Foundation of America
Ruth Sleeper Hall, RSL350
40 Parkman Street
Boston, MA 02114
617-726-8500
www.tsh.org

Urinary Problems

National Association for Continence
PO Box 8310
Spartanburg, SC 29305
800-BLADDER; 864-579-7900
www.nafc.org

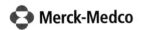

Women's Health

National Women's Health Network
514 10th Street NW, Suite 400
Washington, DC 20004
202-347-1140
www.womenshealthnetwork.org

Personal Medication Record

Name _____   Primary Care Doctor's Name _____   Doctor's Telephone _____

I am allergic to: _____

Name of medication (prescription and/or nonprescription)	Dose	When are you taking this medication?				Taken with food/ liquid?	List any problems you have with this medication	Date of next refill
		A.M.	Noon	P.M.	Bedtime			

Please fill out this table so you can take it with you the next time you visit your doctor, pharmacist, nurse, or other healthcare professional.

Merck-Medco
Live life well™

809

Index

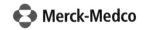

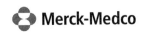

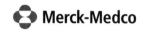

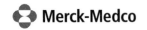

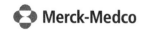

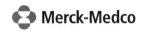

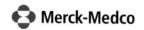

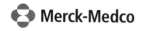

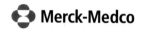

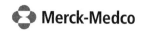

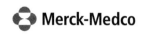